HOSPITAL FOR SPECIAL SURGERY ORTHOPAEDICS MANUAL

HOSPITAL FOR SPECIAL SURGERY ORTHOPAEDICS MANUAL

EDITORS

Thomas P. Sculco, MD
*Surgeon-in-Chief and Korein-Wilson Professor
   of Orthopedic Surgery
Hospital for Special Surgery
Chairman of the Department of Orthopedic Surgery
Professor of Orthopedic Surgery
Weill Cornell Medical College
New York, New York*

Moe R. Lim, MD
*Assistant Professor of Orthopaedics
University of North Carolina–Chapel Hill
Chapel Hill, North Carolina*

Andrew D. Pearle, MD
*Associate Professor of Orthopaedic Surgery
Weill Cornell Medical College
Associate Attending Orthopaedic Surgeon
Shoulder and Sports medicine Service
Hospital for Special Surgery
New York, New York*

Anil S. Ranawat, MD
*Assistant Professor of Orthopaedic Surgery
Weill Cornell Medical College
Assistant Attending Orthopaedic Surgeon
New York–Presbyterian Hospital
Assistant Attending Orthopaedic Surgeon
Hospital for Special Surgery
New York, New York*

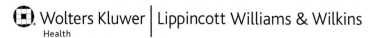

. Wolters Kluwer | Lippincott Williams & Wilkins
Health

Philadelphia • Baltimore • New York • London
Buenos Aires • Hong Kong • Sydney • Tokyo

Executive Editor: Brian Brown
Product Manager: Dave Murphy
Manufacturing Manager: Beth Welsh
Design Manager: Doug Smock
Compositor: Aptara, Inc.

Printed in China

Library of Congress Cataloging-in-Publication Data

Hospital for Special Surgery orthopaedic manual / editors, Thomas P. Sculco ... [et al.].
 p. ; cm.
 Orthopaedic manual
 Includes bibliographical references and index.
 ISBN 978-0-7817-6467-4 (pbk.)
 1. Orthopedics–Handbooks, manuals, etc. 2. Orthopedic surgery–Handbooks, manuals, etc.
3. Musculoskeletal system–Diseases–Handbooks, manuals, etc. I. Sculco, Thomas P. II. Hospital
for Special Surgery. III. Title: Orthopaedic manual.
 [DNLM: 1. Orthopedic Procedures–Handbooks. 2. Musculoskeletal Diseases–diagnosis–
Handbooks. 3. Musculoskeletal Diseases–surgery–Handbooks. 4. Musculoskeletal System–
anatomy & histology–Handbooks. WE 39]
 RD701.H69 2013
 616.7–dc22

                                                                                    2011006402

Care has been taken to confirm the accuracy of the information presented and to describe generally
accepted practices. However, the authors, editors, and publisher are not responsible for errors or
omissions or for any consequences from application of the information in this book and make no
warranty, expressed or implied, with respect to the currency, completeness, or accuracy of the
contents of the publication. Application of the information in a particular situation remains the
professional responsibility of the practitioner.

The authors, editors, and publisher have exerted every effort to ensure that drug selection and
dosage set forth in this text are in accordance with current recommendations and practice at
the time of publication. However, in view of ongoing research, changes in government regulations,
and the constant flow of information relating to drug therapy and drug reactions, the reader is urged
to check the package insert for each drug for any change in indications and dosage and for added
warnings and precautions. This is particularly important when the recommended agent is a new or
infrequently employed drug.

Some drugs and medical devices presented in the publication have Food and Drug
Administration (FDA) clearance for limited use in restricted research settings. It is the responsibility of the health care provider to ascertain the FDA status of each drug or device planned for use
in their clinical practice.

To purchase additional copies of this book, call our customer service department at (800) 638-3030
or fax orders to (301) 223-2320. International customers should call (301) 223-2300.

*Visit Lippincott Williams & Wilkins on the Internet: at LWW.com. Lippincott Williams
& Wilkins customer service representatives are available from 8:30 am to 6 pm, EST.*

                                    10 9 8 7 6 5 4 3 2 1

CCS0813

To my wife, Sora, and my sons, Alex, Andy, Henry, and Holden.

ML

I would like to thank my many mentors who have guided me during my surgical training and career at the Hospital for Special Surgery. I would like to acknowledge my co-editors, Drs. Moe Lim and Andy Pearle, who were my senior residents and great role models of what an "HSS resident" was supposed to be. I also have to thank two senior mentors, my present surgeon-in-chief, Dr. Thomas Sculco, who has been supportive of me since I was a medical student, and of course my father, Dr. C.S. Ranawat , who has been the single greatest driving force in my life and career. His advice and example have truly defined the word, mentor. And, of course, I have to thank my wife, Dana, and my two children, Cooper and Viviana, who have shown me unwavering love and support. I love you guys, and this book is for you.

AR

As residents at Hospital for Special Surgery, we were surrounded by some of the greatest minds in orthopedics. Over a century of ever-expanding orthopedic wisdom was passed on through the residency program. While we could never capture the intricacies of this wisdom in a book, this publication represents a "Cliff-Notes" version of the teachings at the Hospital for Special Surgery.

I would like to thank the many clinicians and residents who contributed to this book. Without their expertise, it would not have been possible to bring this project together. I would also like to thank our mentors at the Hospital for Special Surgery who continue to pass on their knowledge and expertise.

Finally, I would like to thank my wife Katherine and my kids Allison, Alex, and Charlie who inspire me every day.

AP

CONTENTS

Contributors   ix

Introduction   xi

CHAPTER 1   Arthroplasty   1
MORTEZA MEFTAH, ANNA N. MILLER, ANNE H. JOHNSON, EDWIN P. SU, ANIL S. RANAWAT

CHAPTER 2   Sports   66
JOSHUA S. DINES, ANDREW D. PEARLE, CHRISTOPHER C. DODSON

CHAPTER 3   Pediatrics   111
PETER D. FABRICANT, KRISTIN K. WARNER, DANIEL W. GREEN

CHAPTER 4   Trauma   185
MILTON LITTLE, MICHAEL J. GARDNER, DEAN G. LORICH

CHAPTER 5   General/Basic Science   422
MATTHEW E. CUNNINGHAM, JOSEPH M. LANE

CHAPTER 6   Tumors   448
MOE R. LIM, JOHN H. HEALEY

CHAPTER 7   Hand   509
SCOTT J. ELLIS, AARON DALUISKI, MARK C. DRAKOS, ALISON F. KITAY

CHAPTER 8   Foot and Ankle   551
TONY S. WANICH, MATTHEW H. GRIFFITH, JOHN G. KENNEDY, PADHRAIG F. O'LOUGHLIN

CHAPTER 9   Spine   591
CHRISTOPHER R. GOOD, WAKENDA K. TYLER, RUSSEL C. HUANG

Index   657

CONTRIBUTORS

MATTHEW E. CUNNINGHAM, MD, PHD
Director, John Cobb Scoliosis Fellowship
Assistant Professor, Orthopaedic Surgery
Weill-Cornell Medical College, Cornell University
Assistant Attending Orthopaedic Surgeon
Hospital for Special Surgery
Assistant Scientist, Research Division
Hospital for Special Surgery
New York, New York

AARON DALUISKI, MD
Assistant Attending Orthopaedic Surgeon
Hospital for Special Surgery
Assistant Professor of Orthopaedic Surgery
Weill Cornell Medical College
Chief of Hand Service
New York–Presbyterian Hospital
New York, New York

JOSHUA S. DINES, MD
Assistant Professor of Orthopedic Surgery
Weill Cornell Medical College
Sports Medicine and Shoulder Service
Hospital for Special Surgery
New York, New York

CHRISTOPHER C. DODSON, MD
Assistant Professor of Orthopaedic Surgery
Jefferson Medical College
Orthopaedic Surgery
Rothman Institute
Philadelphia, Pennsylvania
New York, New York

MARK C. DRAKOS, MD
Assistant Attending Orthopedic Surgeon
Hospital for Special Surgery
New York, New York

SCOTT J. ELLIS, MD
Assistant Professor of Orthopaedic Surgery
Weill Cornell Medical College
Assistant Attending Orthopaedic Surgeon
Hospital for Special Surgery
New York, New York

PETER D. FABRICANT, MD, MPH
Resident in Orthopaedic Surgery
Hospital for Special Surgery
New York, New York

MICHAEL J. GARDNER, MD
Assistant Professor
Department of Orthopaedic Surgery
Washington University School of Medicine
St. Louis, Missouri

CHRISTOPHER R. GOOD, MD
Department of Orthopaedic Surgery, Spine Section
Reston Hospital Center
Reston, Virginia

DANIEL W. GREEN, MD, MS, FAAP, FACS
Director, Pediatric Orthopaedic Surgery
Hospital for Special Surgery
Associate Attending Orthopedic Surgeon
Hospital for Special Surgery
Associate Professor of Orthopaedic Surgery
Weill Cornell Medical College
New York, New York

MATTHEW H. GRIFFITH, MD
Attending Orthopaedic Surgeon
Department of Orthopaedic Surgery
Reston Hospital Center
Reston, Virginia

JOHN H. HEALEY, MD
Chief of Orthopaedic Surgery
Memorial Sloan-Kettering Cancer Center
Attending Surgeon
Hospital for Special Surgery
Professor of Orthopaedic Surgery
Weill Cornell Medical College
New York, New York

RUSSEL C. HUANG, MD
Director of Spine Surgery Clinic
Hospital for Special Surgery
Assistant Attending Orthopaedic Surgeon
Hospital for Special Surgery
Assistant Professor of Orthopaedic Surgery
Weill Cornell Medical College
Assistant Attending Orthopaedic Surgeon
New York–Presbyterian Hospital
New York, New York

ANNE H. JOHNSON, MD
Foot and Ankle Orthopaedic Surgeon
Instructor in Orthopaedic Surgery
Harvard Medical School
Boston, Massachusetts

JOHN G. KENNEDY, MD
Assistant Attending Orthopaedic Surgeon
Hospital for Special Surgery
Assistant Professor of Orthopaedic Surgery
Weill Cornell Medical College
New York, New York

ALISON F. KITAY, MD
Department of Hand and Upper Extremity Surgery
Hospital for Special Surgery
New York, New York

JOSEPH M. LANE, MD
Chief Metabolic Bone Disease Service
Orthopaedic Attending Trauma Service
Hospital for Special Surgery
New York, New York

MOE R. LIM, MD
Assistant Professor of Orthopaedics
University of North Carolina–Chapel Hill
Chapel Hill, North Carolina

MILTON LITTLE, MD
Resident in Orthopaedic Surgery
Hospital for Special Surgery
New York, New York

DEAN G. LORICH, MD
Associate Director of Orthopaedic Trauma Service
Hospital for Special Surgery
Associate Professor of Orthopaedic Surgery
Weill Cornell Medical College
New York, New York

MORTEZA MEFTAH, MD
Ranawat Orthopaedic Center
Hospital for Special Surgery
New York, New York

ANNA N. MILLER, MD
Assistant Professor
Department of Orthopaedic Surgery
Wake Forest University Baptist Medical Center
Winston Salem, North Carolina

PADHRAIG F. O'LOUGHLIN, MD
Orthopaedic Research Fellow
Orthopaedic Surgery
Hospital for Special Surgery
Orthopaedic Resident
Trauma and Orthopaedic Surgery
Hospital for Special Surgery
Mater Misericordiae University Hospital
New York, New York

ANDREW D. PEARLE, MD
Associate Professor of Orthopaedic Surgery
Weill Cornell Medical College
Associate Attending Orthopaedic Surgeon
Shoulder and Sports medicine Service
Hospital for Special Surgery
New York, New York

ANIL S. RANAWAT, MD
Assistant Professor of Orthopaedic Surgery
Weill Cornell Medical College
Assistant Attending Orthopaedic Surgeon
New York–Presbyterian Hospital
Assistant Attending Orthopaedic Surgeon
Hospital for Special Surgery
New York, New York

EDWIN P. SU, MD
Associate Attending Orthopaedic Surgeon
Hospital for Special Surgery
Associate Professor of Orthopedic Surgery
Weill Cornell Medical College
New York, New York

WAKENDA K. TYLER, MD MPH
Assistant Professor Orthopaedic Surgery
Division of Musculoskeletal Oncology
University of Rochester Medical Center
Rochester, New York

TONY S. WANICH, MD
Assistant Professor
Department of Surgery
Albert Einstein College of Medicine
Attending Physician
Department of Orthopaedic Surgery
Montefiore Medical Center
Bronx, New York

KRISTIN K. WARNER, MD
Carolina Orthopaedics and Sports Medicine
New Bern, North Carolina

INTRODUCTION

The study of orthopaedic surgery has become more challenging, with a need to master an ever-increasing fund of knowledge. In the age of the Internet search engines, we now rely on instant information that covers a wide breadth of topics. In this book, we have compiled nine chapters of accurate, relevant, and, most important, high-yield orthopaedic facts, organized by the subspecialties. These facts have been gathered from textbooks, journal articles, and lectures from our training program at the Hospital for Special Surgery. As residents, we were surrounded by some of the greatest minds in orthopedics. We have tried to compile over a century of ever-expanding orthopedic wisdom into a quick reference user-friendly format that can be applicable on either paper or a handheld device. While we could never capture the intricacies of this wisdom in a book, this publication represents a "Cliff Notes" version of the teachings at the Hospital for Special Surgery.

We hope that the orthopaedic trainee or clinician will use this resource for rapid access to clinically relevant and reliable information. We would like to thank the many clinicians and residents who contributed to this book. Without their expertise and dedication, it would not have been possible to bring this project to fruition. Finally, we would like to acknowledge our many teachers and mentors at the Hospital for Special Surgery, especially our co-editor and surgeon-in-chief, Dr. Thomas Sculco. We are greatly indebted to them for their knowledge, dedication, and inspiring ethic to advance orthopaedic care and knowledge.

Moe Lim
Anil Ranawat
Andy Pearle
Thomas Sculco

HOSPITAL FOR SPECIAL SURGERY ORTHOPAEDICS MANUAL

CHAPTER 1

Arthroplasty

Morteza Meftah, Anna N. Miller, Anne H. Johnson, Edwin P. Su, Anil S. Ranawat

Background
  Inflammatory Arthritis
  Osteoarthritis (OA)
Hip Section
  Anatomy
  Approaches
  Avascular Necrosis (Osteonecrosis)
  Developmental Dysplasia of the Hip
  Nonsurgical Management For Hip Arthritis
  Nonarthroplasty Options For Hip Arthritis
  Total Hip Arthroplasty
  Total Hip Arthroplasty Templating
  Implant Type—Acetabulum
  Implant Type—Femur
  Bearing Surfaces
Knee Section
  Biomechanics, Anatomy, and Approaches
  Avascular Necrosis and Osteonecrosis
  Nonsurgical Management
  Nonarthroplasty Options
  Total Knee Arthroplasty
  Total Knee Operative Technique
  Partial Knee Replacement
  Computer-Assisted Surgery
  Implant Types—Femur
  Implant Types—Tibia
  Bearing Surfaces
Complications
  Infection
  Venous Thromboembolic Disease
  Soft Tissue Complications
  Heterotopic Ossification
  Wear and Loosening in THA
  Hip Dislocation
  Periprosthetic Femoral Fractures
  Patellar Problems
  Wear and Loosening in TKA
  Periprosthetic Knee Fractures

Revision
  Revision Total Hip Replacement
  Revision Total Knee Arthroplasty

Background

INFLAMMATORY ARTHRITIS

Rheumatoid Arthritis (RA)

Presentation
- Symmetric polyarthritis (especially hand/foot) with joint swelling
- Morning stiffness for >1 hour
- Joint deformity
- Subcutaneous nodules
- Rheumatoid factor (RF) positive in 80%
- Elevated erythrocyte sedimentation rate (ESR), C-reactive protein (CRP)
- Creates disability and shortens life expectancy

Pathology
- Autoimmune disorder through cytokine (interleukin [IL]-1, IL-8) and tumor necrosis factor (TNF) release (initiates innate immune response, activates and differentiates macrophages, increases vascular permeability)
- Chronic inflammatory disease with synovial hyperplasia, angiogenesis, mononuclear cell infiltration, pannus formation, cartilage erosion, and, ultimately, joint destruction
- 0.5%–1% of population
- Three times more prevalent in women than men
- Increases with age
- Considered autoimmune disease but humoral and cellular response to autoantigens rheumatoid factor (RF) not specific to disease
- Role of T cells and major histocompatibility complex-II or viral hypothesis as pathogenesis

- Anticyclic citrullinated peptide antibody specific for RA

Imaging
- Plain film:
    - Juxta-articular erosions, bone loss
    - Concentric joint erosion
    - Joint deformity, but no osteophytes
    - Periarticular bone erosion
    - Protrusio acetabuli in advanced disease

Treatment
Medical Management
- Nonsteroidal anti-inflammatory drugs (NSAIDs)
- Glucocorticoids
- Sulfasalazine, gold
- Plaquenil
- Disease-modifying antirheumatic drugs: methotrexate, hydroxychloroquine (administer low-dose folic acid with methotrexate to prevent toxicity)
- TNF-α inhibitors (etanercept—fusion protein of Fc receptor that is soluble binder of TNF and given SQ; infliximab—monoclonal antibody given IV)
- IL-1 receptor antagonist (Humira, anakinra)
- Pyrimidine synthesis inhibitor (leflunomide)
- Advanced disease requires combination therapy

Surgical Management
- Synovectomy
- Soft tissue realignment
- Arthrodesis
- Arthroplasty

Other Inflammatory Diseases
Systemic Lupus Erythematosus
- Second most common inflammatory disease
- More prevalent in women and African Americans
- Symptoms include rash, fever, and polyarthralgia
- Similar radiographic findings to RA

Juvenile Rheumatoid Arthritis
- Occurs in first two decades of life
- Symptoms include rash, fever, morning stiffness, and joint pain
- Risk factor for protrusion acetabuli
- Treatment includes high-dose salicylates, physiotherapy, synovectomy, arthrodesis, and arthroplasty

Crystal Disease
- Gout
    - Monosodium urate crystals, negatively birefringent
    - Flares due to chemotherapy, tyrosine, trauma, surgery
    - Treatment: indomethacin, colchicine, allopurinol, débridement, arthroplasty

- Chondrocalcinosis
    - Chondrosis, pseudogout, hypothyroidism, hemochromatosis
    - Mediated by neutrophils
    - Calcification of cartilage, weakly positive birefringent crystals
- Calcium hydroxyapatite deposition
    - Calcium salt crystals in joint
    - Most common in knee and shoulder

Bibliography
Conn DL. Resolved: low-dose prednisone is indicated as a standard treatment in patients with rheumatoid arthritis. Arthritis Rheum 2001; 45(5):462–467.
Ilowite NT. Current treatment of juvenile rheumatoid arthritis. Pediatrics 2002; 109(1):109–115.
Jenkins JK, et al. The pathogenesis of rheumatoid arthritis: a guide to therapy. Am J Med Sci 2002; 323(4):171–180.
Reimold AM. New indications for treatment of chronic inflammation by TNF-alpha blockade. Am J Med Sci 2003; 325(2): 75–92.

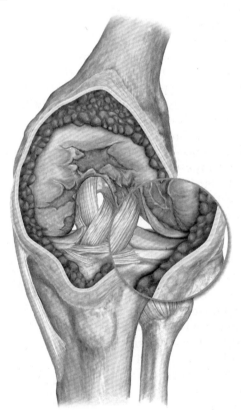

Joints affected by rheumatoid arthritis—left knee. (Asset provided by Anatomical Chart Co.)

OSTEOARTHRITIS (OA)

General
- Affects 40 million people in United States
- Leading cause of physical disability—twice as prevalent in women as men
- Noninflammatory degenerative joint disease

- Risk factors: age, gender, genetic predisposition, mechanical stresses, joint trauma, obesity
- Classification (American College of Rheumatology): "heterogenous group of conditions that lead to joint symptoms and signs which are associated with defective integrity of articular cartilage, in addition to related changes in the underlying bone and the joint margins"

Types
Clinical/Laboratory—knee pain and 5 of 9 factors:
- Age >50 yr
- Morning stiffness
- Crepitus
- Bone, joint line tender to palpation (TTP)
- Bony enlargement (osteophytes)
- No warmth
- ESR <40
- RF <1:40
- Synovial fluid consistent with OA

Diagnosis:
Clinical/Radiographic: knee pain and 1 of 3 factors:
- Age >50 yr
- Morning stiffness
- Crepitus

Clinical Only: knee pain and 3 of 6 factors:
- Age >50 yr
- Morning stiffness
- Crepitus
- Bone TTP
- Bony enlargement
- No palpable warmth

Posttraumatic Osteoarthritis/Meniscectomy
- Fairbanks changes of postmeniscectomy include condylar squaring, ridging, and narrowing; sclerosis is also included

Imaging
- Plain film:
  - Narrowing joint line (articular degeneration)
  - Subchondral sclerosis
  - Squaring of condyles
  - Osteophyte formation
  - Subchondral cysts

Pathophysiology
Articular Cartilage (Wet Weight) Contents
- Sparse chondrocytes (5%)
- Type II collagen (gives tensile strength and 90%–95% of total collagen in cartilage [V/VI 10%–20%])

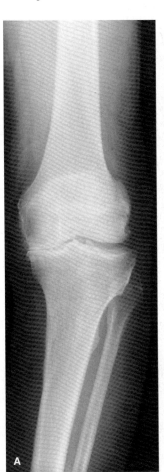
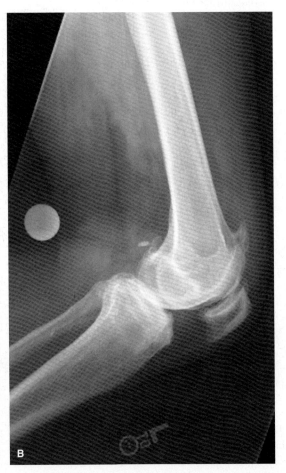

Preoperative weight-bearing radiographs demonstrate osteoarthritis wit varus deformity, antero-posterior (**A**) and lateral (**B**) views

- Proteoglycans (10%–15%)
- Other proteins
- Water (65%–80%) not distributed homogeneously, responsible for nutrition and lubrication
- Water concentration increases in OA; leads to decrease in Young's modulus, increased permeability, and decreased strength

Stage 1
- Disruption of cartilage matrix
- Increased water content

Stage 2
- Chondrocyte response
- Increased matrix synthesis

Stage 3
- Decline in chondrocyte response
- Loss of cartilage
- Poorly understood

Bibliography
Buckwalter JA. Articular cartilage injuries. Clin Orthop 2002; (402):21–37.

Buckwalter JA, et al. Articular cartilage and osteoarthritis. Instr Course Lect 2005; 54:465–480.

Fairbank TJ. Knee joint changes after meniscectomy. J Bone Joint Surg B 1948; 30(4):664–670.

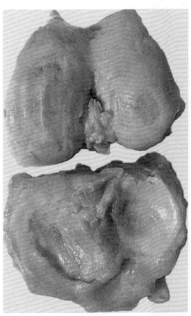

Arthrosis

Stage four arthrosis. (From Moore KL, Dalley AF II. Clinical Oriented Anatomy, 4th ed. Baltimore: Lippincott Williams & Wilkins; 1999.)

Lippiello L, et al. Collagen synthesis in normal and osteoarthritic human cartilage. J Clin Invest 1977; 59(4): 593–600.

Mankin HJ. The response of articular cartilage to mechanical injury. J Bone Joint Surg Am 1982; 64(3):460–466.

Martin JA, Buckwalter JA. Aging, articular cartilage chondrocyte senescence and osteoarthritis. Biogerontology 2002; 3(5):257–264.

Hip Section

ANATOMY

Surface
Anterior
- Anterior superior iliac spine (sartorius insertion)
- Anterior inferior iliac spine (rectus femoris insertion)

Posterolateral
- Greater trochanter (GT)
- Posterior superior iliac spine

Muscle/Tendon
- 24 muscles cross the hip joint

Flexors
- Iliacus
- Psoas
- Iliocapsularis
- Pectineus
- Rectus femoris
- Sartorius

Extensors
- Gluteus maximus
- Semimembranosus
- Semitendinosus
- Biceps femoris

Abductors
- Gluteus medius
- Gluteus minimus
- Tensor fascia lata
- Iliotibial band

Adductors
- Adductor brevis
- Adductor longus
- Gracilis
- Adductor magnus (anterior)

External Rotators
- Piriformis
- Quadratus femoris
- Inferior gemellus
- Superior gemellus

– Obturator internus
– Obturator externus

Five Insertions into Greater Trochanter
– Gluteus minimus
– Gluteus medius
– Piriformis
– Obturator internus (with gemellus)
– Obturator externus

Neurovascular
– Ten neurovascular structures that enter posteriorly:
  – Above piriformis
    – Superior gluteal artery, gluteal nerve (gluteus medius, gluteus minimus, tensor fascia lata)
  – Below piriformis (*POP'S IQ*)
    – *P*udendal artery and nerve
    – Nerve to *o*bturator internus (superior gemellus)
    – *P*osterior femoral cutaneous nerve
    – *S*ciatic nerve
    – *I*nferior gluteal artery and nerve (gluteus maximus)
    – Nerve to *q*uadratus femoris (inferior gemellus)

Superficial Lateral Femoral Cutaneous Nerve
– Most commonly injured during surgery
– Passes either through or underneath lateral aspect of inguinal ligament, and finally travels on to innervate lateral thigh

Obturator Nerve
– Injured by aggressive retractor behind transverse acetabular ligament
– From L2 to L4 of lumbar plexus
– Comes out of pelvis in obturator foramen
– Anterior superficial branch hits adductor longus, brevis, and gracilis, with sensory to distal medial thigh
– Posterior deep branch hits obturator externus, adductor magnus, and pectineus, with sensory to hip joint

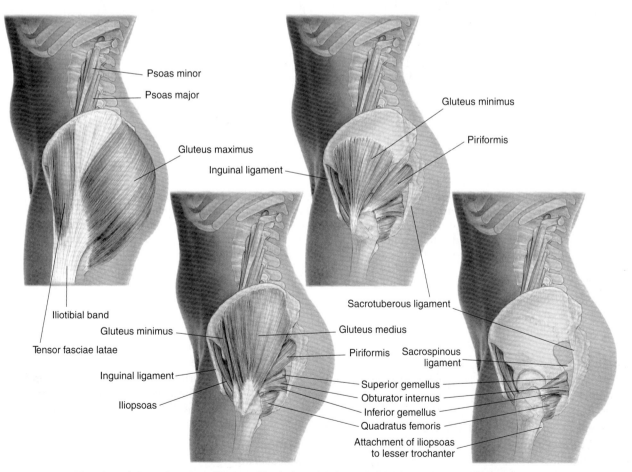

Muscles of the pelvis, lateral view. (From Clay JH, Pounds DM. Basic Clinical Massage Therapy: Integrating Anatomy and Treatment. Baltimore: Lippincott Williams & Wilkins; 2003.)

Cross-section of Hip Joint Area

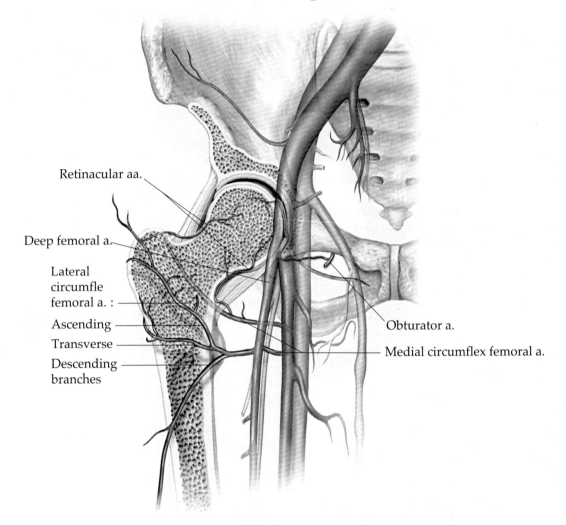

Retinacular aa.

Deep femoral a.

Lateral circumfle femoral a. :

Ascending

Transverse

Descending branches

Obturator a.

Medial circumflex femoral a.

Anatomy and injuries of the hip. Blood supply, cross section of hip joint area. Blood supply to the head of femur: blood flow to the head of the femur is supplied by arteries passing through the capsule and ligament. When a fracture or dislocation tears the capsule and ligament, the head of the femur loses its blood supply and deteriorates (avascular necrosis [AVN]). (Asset provided by Anatomical Chart Co.)

Sciatic Nerve
- Travels without arterial counterpart
- Exits out greater sciatic foramen with posterior femoral cutaneous nerve

Vascular
- Extensions from internal and external iliac arteries supply most of hip
- Internal iliac supplies:
  - Superior/inferior gluteal arteries
  - Obturator artery
- External iliac:
  - Divides into profunda (deep) and superficial artery
  - Femoral artery → profunda → medial and lateral circumflex arteries—supply hip

- Medial femoral circumflex
  - Runs between iliopsoas and pectineus, lies on upper border of adductor longus, and then winds around interval between quadratus femoris and adductor magnus
  - Three branches: ascending, deep, trochanteric
  - Ascending is primary blood supply to femoral head
  - Distal section of the Profunda artery is posterior to adductor longus

Bone
Acetabulum
- Consists of three bones: pelvis, ileum, pubis
- Y-shaped triradiate cartilage
- Fuse by 16 yr

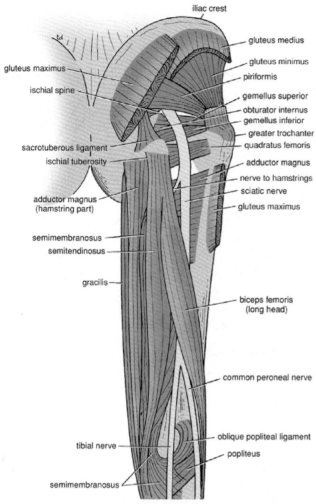

Structures in the posterior aspect of the right thigh. (From Snell RS. Clinical Anatomy by Regions, 8th ed. Philadelphia: Lippincott Williams & Wilkins; 2008.)

Femur
- Two growth centers: femoral epiphysis, trochanteric apophysis
- Ossify by 16–18 yr
- Neck shaft angle 125 degrees
- Anteversion 15 degrees

APPROACHES

- Anterior—Smith Peterson
- Anterolateral—Watson Jones
- Lateral—Hardinge
- Posterior—Southern or Moore or Kocher-Langenbeck
- Medial—Ludloff

Anterior
- Position: supine with sandbag under buttocks
- Incision: anterior one-half iliac crest to anterior superior iliac spine (ASIS), then curve inferiorly 8–10 cm toward lateral
- Superficial plane: between sartorius (femoral n.) and tensor fascia lata (superior gluteal n.)
- Deep plane: between rectus femoris (femoral n.) and gluteus medius (superior gluteal n.)
- Detach two rectus heads off anterior inferior iliac spine (AIIS) and superior lip of acetabulum
- Anterior joint capsule lies below
- Beware: lateral femoral cutaneous n. over sartorius, 2.5 cm inferior to ASIS; femoral n. medial to rectus femoris

Anterolateral
- Position: supine with buttocks over table edge
- Incision: 15 cm vertical, centered over GT
- Superficial plane: between posterior tensor fascia lata and anterior edge of gluteus medius (both superior gluteal n.)
- Retract gluteus laterally and tensor fascia lata anterior-medially, revealing fat over anterior joint capsule
- Deep plane: detach abductors via trochanteric osteotomy or tag and remove gluteus medius from GT
- Reflect head of rectus from anterior joint caps
- Beware: femoral n. compression via strong medial retraction of anterior structures, femoral artery and vein can be damaged by acetabular retractors

Lateral
- Higher heterotopic ossification, fewer dislocations (0.3%), 10% limp at 2 yr
- Position: spine with buttocks over table edge
- Incision: 8 cm caudal to GT at anterior femoral border to GT, and then curve posteriorly, ending at level of ASIS
- Incise tensor fascia lata and reflect anteriorly, reflect gluteus maximus posteriorly
- Incise anterior gluteus medially, leaving cuff off GT, and continue gluteus medius fibers proximally in line with its fibers
- Resect gluteus minimus with joint capsule off anterior GT to expose joint
- Danger: femoral n., artery, and vein with anterior retractors

Posterior
- Increased rate of posterior dislocation, less abductor lurch if SER and capsule are repaired.
- Position: true lateral
- Incision: start 6–8 cm superior-posterior to GT, curve in line with gluteal fibers to GT and then inferiorly down femoral shaft 5–7 cm
- Superficial plane: through fascia and split gluteus maximus fibers
- Deep plane: tag and cut short external rotators and piriformis, then capsule, to expose the joint

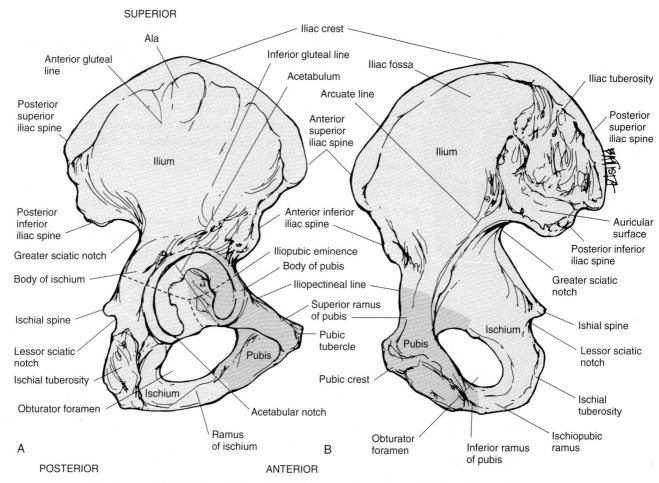

Hip bone (right). **A:** Lateral view. **B:** Medial view. (From Oatis CA. Kinesiology: The Mechanics and Pathomechanics of Human Movement. Baltimore: Lippincott Williams & Wilkins; 2003.)

- Beware: sciatic n. usually posterior to external rotator insertion, inferior gluteal artery branches to gluteus maximus when splitting muscle

Medial

- For developmental dysplasia of the hip (DDH), biopsy of femoral neck, psoas release, and obturator neurectomy
- Position: supine with hip externally rotated, abducted, and flexed
- Superficial plane: between gracilis and adductor longus (obturator n.)
- Deep plane: between adductor brevis (obturator n.) and adductor magnus (obturator and sciatic n.) below to expose lesser trochanter (LT) and psoas insertion
- Beware: anterior division of obturator n. lies between adductor longus and brevis; post division of obturator n. lies on adductor magnus, under adductor brevis

Surgical Dislocation

- Trochanteric osteotomy that preserves the gluteus medius, minimus and vastus lateralis
- Safe anterior dislocation of the hip joint

Bibliography

Gibson A. Posterior exposure of the hip joint. J Bone Joint Surg Br 1950; 32:183–186.

Hardinge K. The direct lateral approach to the hip. J Bone Joint Surg 1982; 64B:17.

Hoppenfeld S, deBoer P. Surgical Exposures in Orthopaedics. Philadelphia: Lippincott Williams & Wilkins; 2003.

Ludloff K. The open reduction of the congenital hip dislocation by an anterior incision. Am J Orthop Surg 1913; 10: 438–454.

Smith-Petersen MN. Approach to and exposure of the hip joint for moldarthroplasty. J Bone Joint Surg Am 1949; 31: 40–46.

Watson-Jones R. Fractures of the neck of the femur. Br J Surg 1935; 23:787.

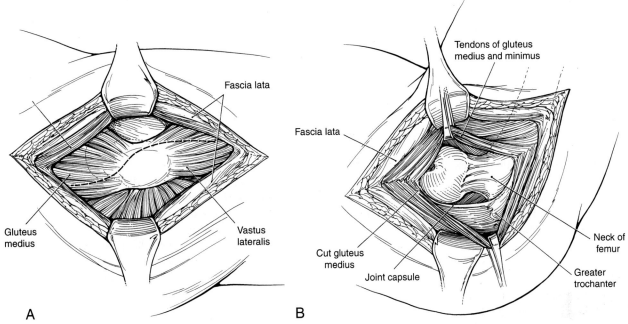

A

B

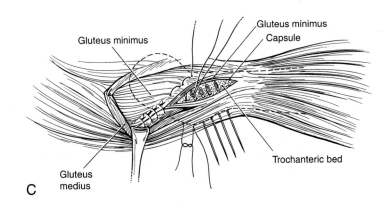

C

A: Lateral approach: Dissection of the gluteus medius is done along the anterior two-thirds, leaving the posterior tendon attached to the greater trochanter. A cuff of the vastus lateralis is dissected to create a continuous musculotendinous sleeve. **B:** The anterior hip joint capsule is exposed and released. The femoral head can be dislocated with extension, external rotation, and adduction of the femur. **C:** The abductor tendon sleeve is reattached to the greater trochanter. (From Craig EV, et al. Clinical Orthopedics. Philadelphia: Lippincott Williams & Wilkins; 1999.)

AVASCULAR NECROSIS (OSTEONECROSIS)

Presentation

Pain
- Groin, knee, buttock
- Represents 10% of total hip arthroplasty (THA)
- 20,000 patients annually

Age
- Mean age 35–40 yr

Risk Factors
- External compression
- Venous, arterial emboli, thrombosis
- Alcoholism, steroids
- Sickle cell, dysbarism, Gaucher disease, systemic lupus erythematous (SLE)

Imaging

Plain Film
- Changes usually occur after 3 mo
- Anterolateral head most commonly affected
- Collapse of articular surface at 6–12 mo
- Gradual increase in pain due to increased intraosseous pressure
- Obtain magnetic resonance image (MRI) of other hip

MRI
- On T1: peripheral band of low signal intensity surrounding central variable signal intensity marrow
- On T2: inner border of peripheral band has high signal intensity in 80% ("serpentine double line" sign)
- Differential diagnosis by MRI—transient osteoporosis: atypically, may have bone edema pattern with diffuse area of low signal intensity on T1 and high signal intensity on T2 without double line. Cannot

distinguish this from transient osteoporosis on MRI initially—avascular necrosis (AVN) will lead to typical appearance, whereas transient osteoporosis resolves in 4–10 months

Modified Ficat Classification System of Osteonecrosis
- I—No x-ray (XR) signs, positive MRI
- IIA—Sclerotic or porotic changes
- IIB—Subchondral lucency (crescent sign)
- III—Head collapse, normal joint space
- IV—Degenerative joint disease (DJD) of acetabulum

Steinberg Classification System
Note: There are A, B, and C subclasses within each stage.
- I—Normal XR, abnormal bone scan
- II—Sclerosis/cyst formation
- III—Crescent sign present indicating subchondral collapse
- IV—Femoral head flattening
- V—Joint space narrowing
- VI—Advanced degenerative changes

Ozhono (1992) Location Classification
- A—Medial, best prognosis
- B—Central, intermediate prognosis
- C—Lateral, worst prognosis

Kerboull Size Classification
- Add angle from center of head to necrotic area on orthogonal views (250 degrees has worse prognosis)

Treatment Options
- Core decompression
- Restricted weight bearing (Mont et al., 1996)
- Vascularized fibular graft (Urbaniak et al., 1995)
  - 80% success precollapse
  - 70% success postcollapse
- Osteotomy
- Hemiarthroplasty
- Femoral head surface replacement
- THA

Core Decompression
Indication
- Treatment of early osteonecrosis (Ficat stage I or early stage II)

Results
- Immediate pain relief
- Only effective precollapse
- Pathogenesis did not affect success
- Continued steroid use leads to worse prognosis
- Prognosis better if sclerotic medial to weight-bearing dome and if smaller lesion

Technique
- Enter femur on inferior edge of GT to avoid major stress riser

Studies
- Ficat (1985):
  - 133 hips, 9.5-yr follow-up on decompressions
  - 90% clinical success (I—94%, II—82%), based on pain, ROM, and XR
  - 79% XR success (I—87%, II—67%)
- Mont et al. (1996):
  - 42 studies from 1963 to 1993
  - Assessed XR, clinical, need for THA
  - 1,206 core decompression versus 819 nonsurgically treated patients
  - 23% success for nonsurgical group, 34-mo follow-up (I—35%, II—31%, III—13%)
  - 64% success for decompression, 30-mo follow-up (I—84%, II—65%, III—47%)

Caveats
- Weight bearing must be protected for 2–3 mo to decrease risk of postoperative fracture
- Has been combined with cancellous or fibular (vascularized or nonvascularized) graft, but did not show significant difference in results

Bibliography
Ficat P, Arlet J. [Dysplasias, osteoarthritis and osteonecrosis of the hip]. Sem Hop 1974; 50(8):567–579.
Merledaubigne R. Idiopathic necrosis of the femoral head in adults. Ann R Coll Surg Engl 1964; 34:143–160.
Steinberg ME. Osteonecrosis of the hip: summary and conclusions. Semin Arthroplasty 1991; 2(3):241–249.

References
Ficat RP. Idiopathic bone necrosis of the femoral head: early diagnosis and treatment. J Bone Joint Surg Br 1985; 67(1): 3–9.
Mont MA, et al. Core decompression versus nonoperative management for osteonecrosis of the hip. Clin Orthop 1996; (324):169–178.
Ohzono K, et al. The fate of nontraumatic avascular necrosis of the femoral head. A radiologic classification to formulate prognosis. Clin Orthop Relat Res 1992; (277):73–78.
Urbaniak JR, et al. Treatment of osteonecrosis of the femoral head with free vascularized fibular grafting: a long-term follow-up study of one hundred and three hips. J Bone Joint Surg Am 1995; 77(5):681–694.

DEVELOPMENTAL DYSPLASIA OF THE HIP

Presentation/Epidemiology
- Deficient lateral coverage of femoral head
  - Loss of continuity with Shenton's line: head is displaced superiorly, anteriorly, or superolaterally from medial wall of acetabulum

- Anterior center-edge angle of <25 degrees indicates dysplasia

Childhood Diagnosis
- 1–1.5/1,000 live births
- Encompasses spectrum from subluxation to dislocation
- Physical exam:
  - Positive Ortolani or Barlow test
  - Limited abduction
  - Asymmetric gluteal folds
  - Limb length discrepancy
- Risk factors:
  - Breech position
  - Female
  - Family history
  - Torticollis

Sequelae
- Increased contact stress
- Degenerative disease with time
- Up to 50% of patients with acetabular dysplasia had surgery before age 60 yr

Imaging
Studies
- Anteroposterior (AP)/Judet pelvis/hips
- AP/lateral affected femur
- Computed tomography (CT) for assessing Crowe grade III

Crowe/Ranawat Classification
- I: <50% subluxation
- II: 50%–75% subluxation
- III: 75%–100% subluxation
  - Loss of superior acetabular roof
  - Thin medial rim
  - Anterior and posterior columns intact
- IV: Complete dislocation
  - True acetabulum deficient but recognizable

Treatment
- Options to bring femur down include:
  - Soft tissue release
  - Swan-neck femoral custom implant
  - Trochanteric slide osteotomy (up to 3 cm)
  - Subtrochanteric osteotomy

Considerations
- Lengthening >2.5 cm risks sciatic nerve palsy
- Must ream more posteriorly to avoid damage to lateral rim
- Severe contractures may require tenotomies
- Femoral head deformity exists, but head–neck junction is usually reproducible with use of modular stems

- Porous ingrowth for acetabular component with more anteversion shows better results
- Bone graft for deficient acetabulum
- Femur can be in severe anteversion; if >40 degrees, consider derotational osteotomy

Results
- Radiographic evidence of failure (33%–40%)
- High percentage of revision (6%–15%)

Bibliography
Cabanela ME. Total hip arthroplasty for developmental dysplasia of the hip. Orthopedics 2001; 24(9):865–866.

Crowe JF, et al. Total hip replacement in congenital dislocation and dysplasia of the hip. J Bone Joint Surg Am 1979; 61(1):15–23.

DiFazio F, et al. Long-term results of total hip arthroplasty with a cemented custom-designed swan-neck femoral component for congenital dislocation or severe dysplasia: a follow-up note. J Bone Joint Surg Am 2002; 84(2):204–207.

Harris WH. Etiology of osteoarthritis of the hip. Clin Orthop 1986; (213):20–33.

Ito H, et al. Intermediate-term results after hybrid total hip arthroplasty for the treatment of dysplastic hips. J Bone Joint Surg Am 2003; 85(9):1725–1732.

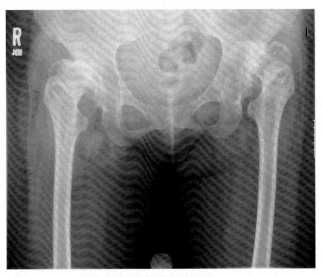

Radiograph of bilateral congenital dislocation of the hip showing that the femoral heads are not within the shallow acetabular fossae.

NONSURGICAL MANAGEMENT FOR HIP ARTHRITIS

Physical Therapy
- Aerobic exercise:
  - Increase stamina
  - Decrease pain
  - Weight loss
- Assistive devices:
  - Cane/crutch in opposite hand to decrease weight through hip
  - Provides balance

Pharmacologic Therapy
- Tylenol
  - Analgesic
  - Liver toxicity
- NSAIDs
  - Cyclooxygenase-1 (COX-1) (ibuprofen, indomethacin, naproxen)
    - Gastrointestinal symptoms
- Cyclooxygenase-2 (COX-2) (Celebrex, Vioxx, Bextra, Mobic)
  - Decreased gastrointestinal toxicity
  - Increased cardiac toxicity
  - Complications increase with age
- Hyaluronan
  - Mixed study results
- Intra-articular steroid injections
  - Require ultrasound or fluoroscopy
  - Good results
  - Possible increased risk of infection after arthroplasty
- Glucosamine/chondroitin
  - Glucosamine: stimulates production of glycosaminoglycans and hyaluronic acid
  - Chondroitin: inhibits enzymes that break down articular cartilage
  - Study funded by National Institutes of Health showed improvement in moderate and moderately severe OA in knee
  - Beware of brand quality, no U.S. Food and Drug Administration regulation

Bibliography

Barnhill JG, et al. Chondroitin product selection for the glucosamine/chondroitin arthritis intervention trial. J Am Pharm Assoc 2006; 46(1):14–24.

Blount WP. Don't throw away the cane. J Bone Joint Surg Am 1956; 38(3):695–708.

Clegg DO, et al. Glucosamine, chondroitin sulfate, and the two in combination for painful knee osteoarthritis. N Engl J Med 2006; 354(8):795–808.

Fries JF, Bruce B. Rates of serious gastrointestinal events from low dose use of acetylsalicylic acid, acetaminophen, and ibuprofen in patients with osteoarthritis and rheumatoid arthritis. J Rheumatol 2003; 30(10):2226–2233.

NONARTHROPLASTY OPTIONS FOR HIP ARTHRITIS

Arthrodesis

Indications
- Advanced, debilitating, unilateral OA—patient too young for THA
- High-demand patient (strenuous laborer)

Contraindications
- Inflammatory arthritis
- AVN (unless no risk of contralateral disease—rule out with MRI)

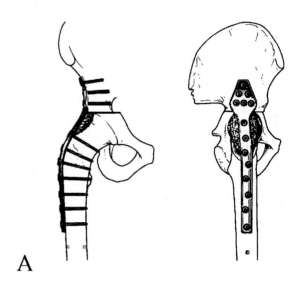

A

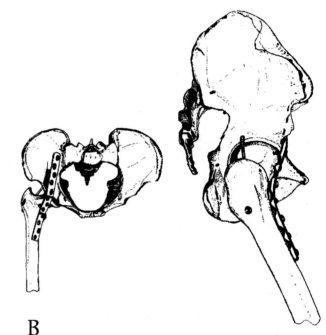

B

A: The Cobra plate technique for hip arthrodesis is performed through a lateral approach. (Reprinted with permission from Lechti R. Hip Arthrodesis and Associated Problems. New York: Springer-Verlag; 1978.) **B:** Anterior plating technique for hip arthrodesis. (Reprinted with permission from Matta JM, et al. Hip fusion through an anterior approach with the use of a ventral plate. Clin Orthop 1997; 337:129–139.)

- Ipsilateral knee disease or laxity
- Low back pain or spine disease
- Contralateral hip OA

Technique
- Arthrodesis position
  - 30 degrees flexion

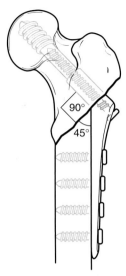

A valgus osteotomy. (From Bucholz RW, Heckman JD. Rockwood & Green's Fractures in Adults, 5th ed. Lippincott Williams & Wilkins; 2001.)

- 5 degrees adduction to 5 degrees abduction (foot close to midline)
- No rotation
- Put knee in center of mechanical axis
- Check AP pelvis before final fixation
- Cobra plate
  - Position: lateral
  - Approach: lateral, trochanteric osteotomy, anterior arthrotomy
  - Plate contoured to ilium, femoral neck, and lateral femoral shaft
  - Disadvantages: injures abductors
- Anterior
  - Position: supine

- Approach: iliofemoral with femoral exposure, anterior arthrotomy
- Limited-contact dynamic compression plate to iliac fossa, anterior acetabular margin, and femoral neck and shaft
- ±7-mm cannulated screws from femoral neck and head to post column of acetabulum

Results
- 10%–25% nonunion rate
- Patients usually satisfied
- Long-term degenerative changes in other joints: lumbar spine (55%–100%), ipsilateral and contralateral knee (45%–65%), contralateral hip (25%–60%)

Osteotomy
- Usually done in young patients to temporize problem before age/activity level appropriate for THA

Indications
- Coxa valga
- AVN: most commonly leads to collapse of anterior/superior femoral head (must have some joint space—Ficat stage III or less)
- Femoral neck nonunion: change of biomechanics to help bone healing
- Slipped capital femoral epiphysis
- Acetabular dysplasia (acetabular ostomies)

Intertrochanteric versus Periacetabular Osteotomy
Intertrochanteric Osteotomy
- Goal: alter biomechanics of hip joint to relieve pain and improve function

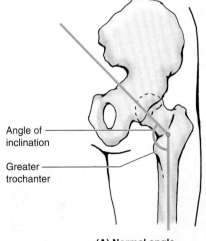

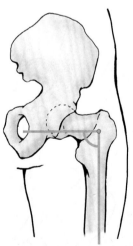

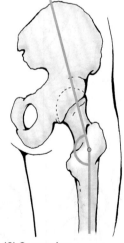

(A) Normal angle of inclination

(B) Coxa vara (abnormally decreased angle of inclination)

(C) Coxa valga (abnormally increased angle of inclination)

Coxa vara and coxa valga. (From Moore KL, Dalley AF II. Clinical Oriented Anatomy, 4th ed. Baltimore: Lippincott Williams & Wilkins; 1999.)

Types of intertrochanteric osteotomies. (Reprinted with permission from Schatzker J, ed. The Intertrochanteric Osteotomy. New York: Springer-Verlag; 1984.)

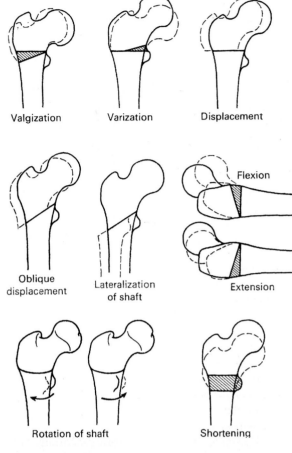

Valgization   Varization   Displacement

Oblique displacement   Lateralization of shaft   Flexion / Extension

Rotation of shaft   Shortening

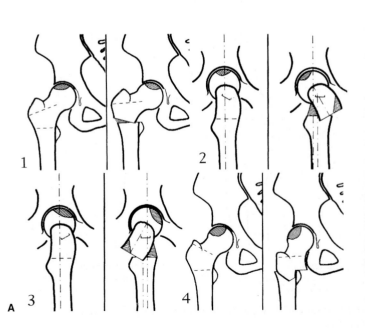

A

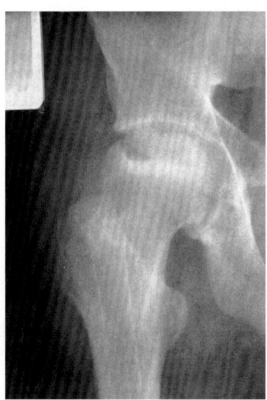

B

Osteotomy and Arthrodesis of the Hip

Procedure	Indications	Technique	Anatomy	Pitfalls
Intertrochanteric osteotomy	• Coxa valga • Avascular necrosis • Femoral neck nonunion • SCFE • Femoral head lesion	• Preoperative planning • Lateral approach • Osteotomy above the lesser trochanter • Blade plate fixation	• Medial femoral circumflex vessels • Perforating vessels	• Poor planning • Malpositioned chisel • Femoral neck perforation • Insufficient bone bridge • Insufficient correction
Periacetabular osteotomy	• Acetabular dysplasia	• Smith-Petersen or ilioinguinal approach • Open capsule for labral tears • Cut through the ilium, ischium, and pubis • Screw fixation	• Femoral nerve • Lateral femoral cutaneous nerve • Femoral vessels • Obturator neurovascular bundle • Sciatic nerve • Superior gluteal vessels	• Nerve injury • Vascular injury and bleeding • Joint violation • Blind ischial cut • Poor acetabular mobilization • Insufficient correction
Greater trochanteric advancement	• Relative overgrowth of the trochanter • Impingement on the ilium • Abductor muscle weakness	• Lateral approach • Mobilize the trochanter • Screw fixation	• Medial femoral circumflex vessels	• Blood supply to femoral head • Insufficient mobilization of trochanter • Inadequate fixation
Hip arthrodesis	• Severe hip arthritis • Unilateral hip pathology	• Lateral or anterior approach • Spare the greater trochanter and abductors • Confirm the hip position • Plate fixation with supplemental screws	• Femoral nerve • Lateral femoral cutaneous nerve • Superior gluteal neurovascular bundle • Inadequate fixation	• Poor hip position • Neurovascular injury • Bleeding • Blood supply to femoral head injured

From Craig EV, et al. Clinical Orthopedics. Philadelphia: Lippincott Williams & Wilkins; 1999.

– Mechanism (can change angulation/displacement/rotation/length):
  1) Replace damaged head segment with area still retaining articular cartilage (e.g., flexion osteotomy for AVN and slipped capital femoral epiphysis)
  2) Improve acetabular coverage of femoral head
  3) Move osteonecrotic area away from acetabular pressure
  4) Correct deformity
  5) Improve ROM
– Technique—preoperative planning very important:
  1) Straight lateral approach
  2) Intraoperative fluoroscopy
  3) 90-degree osteotomy blade plate for varus osteotomy
  4) 110/120/130-degree blade plate for valgus osteotomy (e.g., femoral neck nonunion)
  5) Steinman pins placed above/below osteotomy before cuts made to rotate fragments and measure

  6) Chisel into head at angle measured for blade plate
  7) Osteotomy at superior border of LT
  8) At least 2 cm of bone between chisel path and osteotomy site
  9) Medialization of varus osteotomies and lateralization of valgus osteotomies correct mechanical axis of leg
  10) In rotational osteotomies, incise capsule to allow greater rotation of femoral head

Periacetabular Osteotomy
– Goal: increase acetabular coverage in acetabular insufficiency
– Mechanism:
  1) Stabilize femoral head in acetabulum
  2) Increase contact between femoral head and acetabulum
  3) Move labrum to more peripheral location to prevent further labral deterioration

– Technique—preoperative planning very important:
  1) Ilioinguinal or iliofemoral approach
  2) Several types of osteotomies described, but most are more applicable to pediatric patients because most of hemipelvis must be mobilized
  3) Ganz:
     a. First cut: lateral surface of ischium below acetabulum (blind cut)
     b. Second cut through superior pubic ramus medial to iliopectineal eminence
     c. Third cut through ilium above AIIS
     d. Fourth cut 120 degrees to iliac cut and extended down posterior column
  4) Meticulous closure important to prevent herniation in ilioinguinal approach

Arthroscopy
Advantages
– Ability to thoroughly inspect hip joint
– Removal of offending tissues/foreign bodies
– Minimally invasive compared to arthrotomy

Indications
– Ideally with minimal arthritis
  1) Treatment of FAI (Femoroacetabilar Impingement) with or without labral tears
  2) Labral tears secondary to other disorders such as dysplasia, instability, etc.
– Patients with reproducible symptoms and physical findings, functionally limited status after failed trial of conservative management and chondral flaps

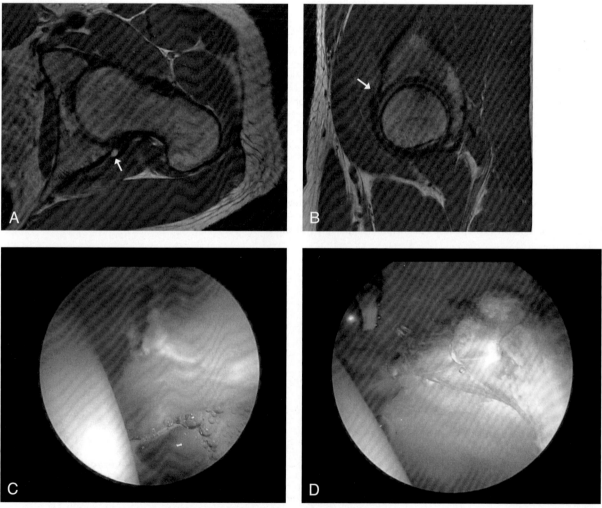

High-resolution coronal plane **(A)** and sagittal plane **(B)** magnetic resonance imaging (MRI) views showing a tear of the anterosuperior acetabula labrum and cyst formation (*arrow*). Intraoperative arthroscopic views of the labral tear before **(C)** and after **(D)** resection. (From Craig EV, et al. Clinical Orthopedics. Philadelphia: Lippincott Williams & Wilkins; 1999.)

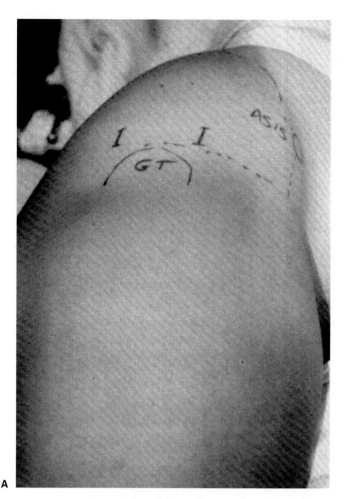

A: Arthroscopic portals for hip arthroscopy. **B:** Relevant anatomy in relation to arthroscopic portal location. (From Craig EV, et al. Clinical Orthopedics. Philadelphia: Lippincott Williams & Wilkins; 1999.)

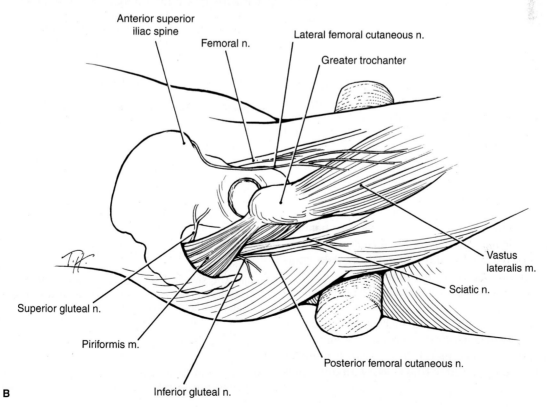

1) Removal of loose bodies (diagnosed on radiographs or by history: mechanical symptoms)
2) Treatment of septic joint (joint decompression, removal of necrotic debris, and copious lavage)
3) Synovial disorders including Synovial chondromatosis
4) Osteochondritis desiccans

Operative Technique
– Accurate portal placement essential for optimal visualization
  1) Distraction necessary to visualize intra-articular structures
     a. General anesthesia and skeletal muscle relaxation
     b. Puncture joint capsule to release negative intra-articular pressure
     c. Force should be longitudinal and lateral (in line with femoral neck)
  2) Positioning: supine or lateral, depending on surgeon's comfort with ports
  3) Instrumentation
     a. Extra-long arthroscopic instrumentation
     b. Fluoroscopy
     c. 30- and 70-degree arthroscopes necessary

Portals
1) Anterior (anterolateral): at intersection of perpendicular lines drawn laterally from superior aspect of symphysis pubis and inferiorly from ASIS
   a. Insert spinal needle from this point medially and superiorly at 45 degrees
   b. Visualize anterior femoral neck, anterior aspect of joint, superior retinacular fold, ligamentum teres (anterior labrum and acetabulum with 70-degree arthroscope only)
   c. Dangers: portal close to lateral femoral cutaneous nerve; if scope inferior to neck, lateral femoral cutaneous artery at risk; femoral neurovascular bundle is 3–4 cm medial to insertion site (find femoral pulse and avoid)
2) Anterior paratrochanteric: 2 cm anterior and 1 cm proximal to anterosuperior corner of GT
   a. Insert trocar at intertrochanteric line
   b. Visualize femoral head, anterior neck, anterior intrinsic capsular folds, synovial tissues beneath zona orbicularis, and anterior labrum
   c. Dangers: trochar too anterior and deep, risks injuring femoral neurovascular bundle
3) Proximal trochanteric: 2 cm proximal to superior tip of GT
   a. Insert trocar medially and slightly superiorly, directly toward superior dome of acetabulum
   b. Visualize fovea, femoral head, and acetabular labrum (mostly used to triangulate with other portals)

   c. Dangers: like anterior paratrochanteric portal if aimed too anteriorly
4) Posterior paratrochanteric: 2–3 cm posterior to tip of GT at level of anterior paratrochanteric portal
   a. Insert trocar with femur in neutral/slight internal rotation
   b. Visualize posterior femoral head, posterior labrum, posterior capsule, ligament of Weitbrecht, and inferior edge of ischiofemoral ligament
   c. Dangers: sciatic nerve close if hip in external rotation
5) Posterior: use only with small incision and dissection down to capsule
   a. Visualize posterior joint
   b. Danger: injury to sciatic nerve and superior gluteal vessels
– Theoretic risk of accelerating AVN if hip scope done in these patients due to high pressure in joint capsule

Bibliography

Amstutz HC, Le Duff MJ, Campbell PA, et al. Clinical and Radiographic Results of Metal-on-Metal Hip Resurfacing with a Minimum Ten-Year Follow-up. J Bone Joint Surg Am 2010; 92:2663–2671.

Ball S, Le Duff MJ, Amstutz HC. Early results of conversion of a failed femoral component in hip resurfacing arthroplasty. J Bone Joint Surg Am 2007; 89:735–41.

Byrd JWT, et al. Hip arthroscopy: an anatomic study of portal placement and relationship to the extra-articular structures. Arthroscopy 1995; 11(4):418–423.

Callaghan JJ, et al. Hip arthrodesis: a long-term follow-up. J Bone Joint Surg Am 1985; 67(9):1328–1335.

De Haan R, Campbell PA, Su EP, De Smet KA. Revision of metal-on-metal resurfacing arthroplasty of the hip: the influence of malpositioning of the components. J Bone Joint Surg Br 2008; 90:1158–63.

De Haan R, Pattyn C, Gill HS, et al. Correlation between inclination of the acetabular component and metal ion levels in metal-on metal hip resurfacing replacement. J Bone Joint Surg Br 2008; 90:1291–7.

Dvorak M, et al. Arthroscopic anatomy of the hip. Arthroscopy 1990; 6(4):264–273.

Ganz R, et al. A new periacetabular osteotomy for the treatment of hip dysplasias: technique and preliminary results. Clin Orthop 1988; 232:26–36.

Graves S. Annual Report. Australian Orthopaedic Association. National joint replacement registry. Adelaide: Australian Orthopaedic Association; 2009.

Millis MB, et al. Osteotomies about the hip for the prevention and treatment of osteoarthrosis. Instr Course Lect 1996; 45:209–226.

Mont MA, Seyler TM, Ulrich SD, et al. Effect of changing indications and techniques on total hip resurfacing. Clin Orthop Relat Res 2007; 465:63–70.

Müller ME. Intertrochanteric osteotomy: indication, preoperative planning, technique. In: Schatzker J, ed. The Intertrochanteric Osteotomy. Berlin: Springer-Verlag; 1984: 25–66.

Pollard, et al. Treatment of the young active patient with osteoarthritis of the hip: a five- to seven-year comparison of hybrid total hip arthroplasty and metal-on-metal resurfacing. J Bone Joint Surg Br 2006; 88(5):592–600.

Poss R. The roles of osteotomy in the treatment of osteoarthritis of the hip. J Bone Joint Surg Am 1984; 66:144–151.

Stover MD, et al. Hip arthrodesis: a procedure for the new millennium? Clin Orthop 2004; (418):126–133.

Villar RN. Arthroscopic debridement of the hip: a minimally invasive approach to osteoarthritis. J Bone Joint Surg Br 1991; 73(suppl 1):170–171.

TOTAL HIP ARTHROPLASTY

TOTAL HIP ARTHROPLASTY TEMPLATING

Acetabulum

Cup Size
- Teardrop is inferior edge of acetabulum
- Medial edge of cup should be 5 mm lateral to teardrop
- Ilioischial Köhler line should never be violated by cup
- Approximate subchondral bone

Cup Placement
- Cup should be 35 to 40 degrees abducted
- Balance bony coverage of cup versus abduction

- May have up to one-third of cup uncovered
- Should correspond to intraoperative coverage
- Draw in cup and mark center of rotation
- Based on the magnification of the x-ray, the templating may be over or undersized.

Protrusio Templating
- Point A is 5 mm lateral to intersection of Köhler (ilioischial) line and Shenton line
- Draw parallel lines at top of ilium and bottoms of ischium
- Draw horizontal line at one-fifth of distance
- Vertical line from A that intersects one-fifth line is point B
- Make horizontal line BC that is same length as AB to make triangle

Femur

Stem Size
- Template to zero neck/head so intraoperatively higher or lower option available

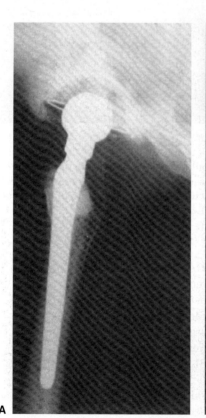
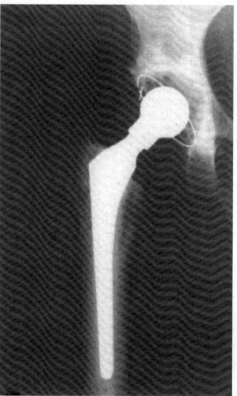

A   B

Lateral **(A)** and anteroposterior **(B)** views showing the 10-yr follow-up of a total hip replacement (THR) that was inserted with cement using second-generation techniques. (From Craig EV, et al. Clinical Orthopedics. Philadelphia: Lippincott Williams & Wilkins; 1999.)

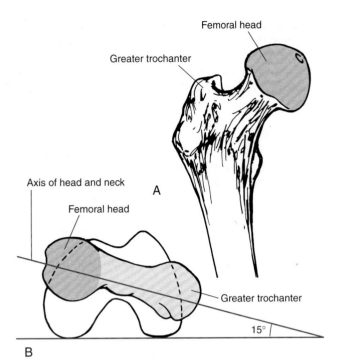

Orientation of the femoral head. **A:** An anterior view of the femur reveals that it faces medially and superiorly. **B:** A superior view of the femur reveals that it faces anteriorly. (From Oatis CA. Kinesiology—The Mechanics and Pathomechanics of Human Movement. Baltimore: Lippincott Williams & Wilkins; 2004.)

– Adjust height of implant in canal so distance from cup center of rotation to stem center of rotation corresponds to LLD

Neck Cut
– Be conservative—it is always easy to take more bone if necessary

Lesser Trochanter to Center of Head
– Measure LTC or rotation of stem
– Use inter-teardrop line as reference
– Measure to LT to check LLD
– Measure to acetabular centers of head and femoral centers of head to make sure leg lengths will be equal
– Fit cup and draw new proposed center of head using template cup
– If no LLD, go directly horizontal from new center
– For cementing femoral stems, template femur to fit with 1- to 2-mm cement mantle in shaft and zero head/neck along line of new acetabular center (with LLD adjusted)
– Femoral offset measured by tip of trochanter to center of rotation
– Pick extended offset if femoral center of head is lateral to acetabular center of head
– Mark off level off neck cut based on LT

Bibliography

Della Valle AG, et al. Preoperative planning for primary total hip arthroplasty. J Am Acad Orthop Surg 2005; 13(7):455–462.
Ranawat CS, Zahn MG. Role of bone grafting in correction of protrusio acetabuli by total hip arthroplasty. J Arthroplasty 1986; 1(2):131–137.

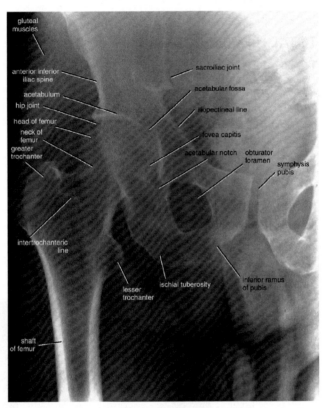

Anteroposterior radiograph of the hip joint. Note that the inferior margin of the neck of the femur should form a continuous curve with the upper margin of the obturator foramen (Shenton line). (From Snell RS. Clinical Anatomy by Regions, 8th ed. Philadelphia: Lippincott Williams & Wilkins; 2008.)

THA—Brief Operative Note
Preop Diagnosis:
Postop Diagnosis:
Procedure:
Surgeon/Assistants:
Anesthesia:
EBL:
IVF:
Drains:
Specimen:
Implants:
Complications:
Disposition:
Posterior approach

Resurfacing Arthroplasty

Procedure
– Replacement of both femoral and acetabular sides of joint without violating femoral canal

History
– Surface replacement first developed in 1970s by Amstutz, Wagner, and Freeman (concurrently) to preserve bone stock in younger patients. However, at the time, materials consisted of large-diameter cobalt chromium ball and thin polyethylene socket. Fixation was cemented on both femoral and acetabular sides, so this led to removal of large amount of acetabular bone. In addition, large metal ball on thin polyethylene socket led to tremendous amount of osteolysis, leading to high failure rate by 5 yr. Although concept was sound, materials of time were limiting factor.
– In 1990s, metal-on-metal technology became more reproducible, with better manufacturing tolerances, higher sphericity, and tighter clearances. Current generation of hip resurfacing implants, developed by Derek McMinn, has been in use in United Kingdom since 1997. Harlan Amstutz also developed metal-on-metal resurfacing device around this time. Both devices are designed for press-fit insertion of socket and cemented femoral fixation. Current devices also now employ short metaphyseal stem, which helps guide alignment of implant. U.S. Food and Drug Adminis-

tration first approved hip resurfacing implant in June 2006.

Advantage
– Better activity and quality-of-life scores, lower risk of dislocation

Problems
– Maintaining viability of bone under resurfaced femoral head
– Loosening of socket with substantial acetabular bone loss
– Femoral neck fracture
– Metal ion generation with current resurfacing implants (cobalt and chromium)
– Metal sensitivity (skin test is not reliable, blood test is more accurate)
– ALVAL (aseptic lymphocyte-dominated vascular associated lesion) or ARMD (adverse reactions to metal debris)
– Technique dependent (use of navigation)
– Design dependent (Recall of Depuy resurfacing cups in 2010)

Results
– Long-term studies are not yet available, but 5-yr results suggest slightly higher short-term failure rate from mechanisms such as femoral neck fracture and femoral loosening

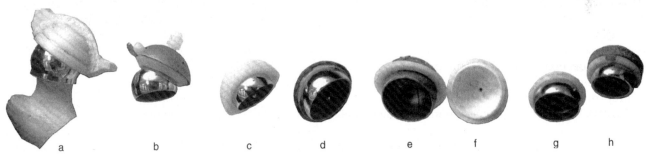

a   b   c   d   e   f   g   h

Resurfacing arthroplasty—replacement of both the femoral and acetabular sides of the joint without violating the femoral canal—was investigated in the 1970s. Problems with maintaining the viability of the bone under the resurfaced femoral head, eventual loosening of the socket with substantial acetabular bone loss due to the large size of the component, and femoral neck fractures were all problematic in most series. Note that methacrylate fixation was popular on both sides of the articulation until porous ingrowth became available. **A:** 1971 Italian design of Paltrinieri-Tretani. **B:** M.A.R. Freeman design from 1979. Note the use of flanged polyethylene pegs instead of cement for fixation of the cup. **C, D:** The Indiana Conservative Cup designed in Indianapolis by Eicher in the late 1960s and early 1970s, and redesigned by William Capello, his student, in the late 1970s. Note metal backing of acetabular liner. **E, F:** The original Wagner design with metal head and metal-backed polyethylene socket with low-profile metal backing. Harlan Amstutz of the University of California, Los Angeles, continued to modify his THARIES resurfacing arthroplasty from the cemented all-polyethylene cup **(G)** of the late 1970s through the porus ingrowth of the early 1990s, as seen in the fixation surface of the cup **(H).** (From Callaghan JJ, et al. The Adult Hip. Philadelphia: Lippincott Williams & Wilkins; 1998.)

Indications
- Younger patients—patients who may outlast their primary hip arthroplasty
- Patients who require high ROM (martial artists, dancers)
- Patients who want to participate in impact sports
- Patients with proximal femoral deformity or retained hardware that would preclude stemmed total hip replacement (THR)

Contraindications
- Absolute:
  - Patients on dialysis (because of metal ion buildup)
  - Patients with anatomical abnormalities that would not support resurfacing
- Relative:
  - Femoral head cysts
  - Osteoporosis
  - Person with inflammatory arthritis, in whom a stemmed THR may last entire life
  - Women who plan to have children (because of metal ions)
  - Major leg length discrepancy (LLD) that is from femur (because resurfacing should not be used to lengthen leg)
  - Severe acetabular dysplasia (if screws necessary, then dysplasia cup must be obtained)

THA—Operative Technique for Posterior Approach
Procedure
- Combined spinal epidural anesthesia
- Lateral decubitus position—axillary roll, pad bony prominences
- Prep, drape limb
- Tip of GT, anterior and posterior borders of femur palpated
- 8-cm curved incision starting proximally posterior to the tip of GT, along posterior border of GT, in line with femoral shaft
- Incise through skin and fat, down to fascia lata
- Fascia lata incised in middle of GT, but small hole created first; if no muscle herniates, then in good position
- When gluteus maximus seen, curve posteriorly over fascia and then split muscle bluntly
- Dissect with fingers under fascia to free up from underlying bursa
- Two moist lap pads and Charnley retractor placed to retract fascia
- Internally rotate hip, placing tension on short external rotators (SERs)
- Excise trochanteric bursa

- Place thin bent Hohmann retractor under Gluteus medius and minumus, place Aufranc retractor proximal to quadratus
- Take SER off close to insertion using Bovie
- Detach tendon of gluteus maximus, complete or partial.
- Make trapezoidal-shaped capsulotomy
- Tag capsule and SER in one or two layers with Ethibond suture
- Take proximal quadratus femoris down with Bovie to expose LT
- Dislocate hip with flexion, adduction, and internal rotation
- Measure center head to LT distance and mark neck cut
- Make neck cut with reciprocating or oscillating saw
- Remove femoral head
- Turn attention to acetabulum
- Airplane table toward surgeon
- Place C-retractor over anterior lip, Steinman pin superiorly, wide bent Hohmann posteriorly, and Aufranc inferiorly
- Anterior capsule and reflected head of rectus may be released for more exposure
- Excise labrum with long-handled knife
- Remove soft tissue of pulvinar with curette and rongeur
- Begin sequential reaming of acetabulum with small reamer
- First ream medially until cancellous bone reached, then position reamer in 45-degree abduction and 15-degree anteversion until good bony coverage reached
- Impact trial component and check position and fit, check with angled guide
- Impact final component
- Remove any overlying osteophytes with osteotome
- Place lap pad in acetabulum and prepare femur
- Place jaw retractors under anterior femoral neck, Aufranc retractor below LT, and thin bent Hohmann on abductors—excise remaining soft tissue from trochanteric fossa
- Use gouge to remove remainder of lateral femoral neck
- Place canal finder into femoral canal carefully
- Ream canal sequentially with straight reamers, taking care to ream laterally
- Broach sequentially, again taking care to lateralize and maintain 15- to 20-degree anteversion
- Place trial stem
- Ream calcar to create flush stem–calcar interface
- Place trail neck and head on trial stem
- Measure lesser trochanter to center of head (LTC) distance and compare native LTC
- Reduce hip and check ROM: check if stable to push/pull, adduction, in extension with external rotation,

flexion to beyond 90 degrees, and internal rotation to 75–80 degrees at 90 degrees of flexion
- Co-planar test: Combined anteversion of 30–45 degrees.
- Dislocate and remove trial components

If cementing:
- Impact cement restrictor down canal
- Irrigate canal and pack with gauze to keep dry
- Cement pressurized into canal and insert final component with careful attention to anteversion and lateralization
- Remove excess cement
- Hold stem until cement is hard
- Impact final head onto stem
- Inspect acetabulum for loose bodies

If cementless:
- After placement of the final components, irrigate then reduce hip
- Check ROM again
- Place two drill holes in GT, and place shuttle sutures
- Shuttle tag sutures for SER and capsule through drill holes and tie sutures down
- Place one/two drain(s) (optional)
- Copiously irrigate wound with pulse irrigator repair gluteus maximus tendon
- Close fascia lata, deep subcutaneous tissue, superficial subcutaneous tissue, and skin in separate layers
- Place sterile dressing and Ace wrap around hips place abduction pillow
- Check XR in recovery room after transfer

Bibliography

Pellicci PM, et al. Posterior approach to total hip replacement using enhanced posterior soft tissue repair. Clin Orthop 1988; (355):224–228.

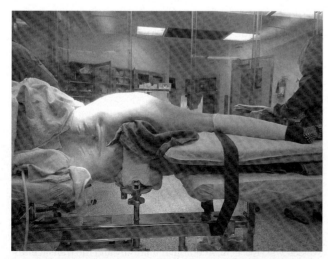

Use of a lateral position to hold the patient in a lateral decubitus position.

IMPLANT TYPE—ACETABULUM

Noncemented

Indications
- Biological potential for bone ingrowth over more than 60% of implant surface
- Any patient indicated for THA

Contraindications
- Severe bone loss/osteopenia
- Radiation necrosis
- Primary/metastatic periacetabular tumor
- Severe metabolic bone disease (no bony ingrowth)

Bony Ingrowth
- Implant must be biocompatible
- Titanium better than cobalt-chromium in some studies
- 100–400 μm is ideal pore size
- Intimate contact with host bone
- Micromotion >50–100 μm causes failure of ingrowth
- Mechanical fixation devices of various shapes showed high rates of failure
- Now use chromium-cobalt alloy, pure titanium, or titanium-based alloy
- Porous coated: sintered beads, fiber metal, plasma-sprayed titanium particles

Technique
- Ream to 1–2 mm less than final size for press fit, depending on manufacturer
- Screws only for implants with significant motion, inadequate anterior/posterior column bone, or >25% lateral cup exposure
- Goal is biological ingrowth/fixation (screws only for initial stability)

Cup Positioning
- 35–45 degrees of abduction (inclination)
- 15–30 degrees of anteversion

Screw Positioning
- Use four-quadrant system (Wasielewski et al., 1990)
- Anterior *not* safe (external iliac vein superiorly, obturator vein inferiorly)
- Posterosuperior: use screws up to 35 mm in length
- Posteroinferior: use screws up to 25 mm in length

Outcomes
- Nonporous, threaded: 4%–30% revision at ~4 yr
  - Early failure: only 9% surface area contact (aseptic loosening)

– Porous/grit, threaded: 1%–5% revision at 8–10 yr
– Hydroxy-apatite coated (smooth, press fit): 11%–14% revision at 5–8 yr
  – Early failure: poor initial fixation
– Overall: better 10-yr results compared with cemented cups

Complications
– Osteolysis for cemented or noncemented
– Acetabular fracture (more problematic with noncemented press fit)
– Polyethylene wear
– Failure of locking mechanism with modular implants
– Osteopenia in ilium (stress shielding from rim fit of cup)

Cemented

Indications (rare)
– Osteoarthritis with adequate bone stock
– Elderly patient
– Radiation Necrosis
– Extensive Bone Destruction due to tumor

Contraindications
– Inflammatory arthropathies
– Developmental dysplasia of the hip
– Protrusio acetabuli
– Extensive cyst formation/weak bone
– Significant cardiopulmonary disease (risk of embolization secondary to cement pressurization)

Technique
– Implants have increased surface area of polyethylene contact to increase resistance to torsional loads
– Thicker polyethylene decreases stress on adjacent subchondral bone and in polyethylene itself
– 2- to 4-mm circumferential cement mantle
– Increase surface area by making burr holes in which to pack cement
– Finger-pack holes, then maintain pressure on component until cement fully polymerized

Radiographic Evidence of Loosening
– Obvious migration of socket
– Progressive radiolucency of >2 mm throughout interface
– Radiographic evidence for loosening more common than clinical loosening

Outcomes
– Overall, up to 17% revision rate at 18 yr
– Up to 43% revision rate for metal-backed cemented cups, possibly due to accelerated wear of polyethylene on metal

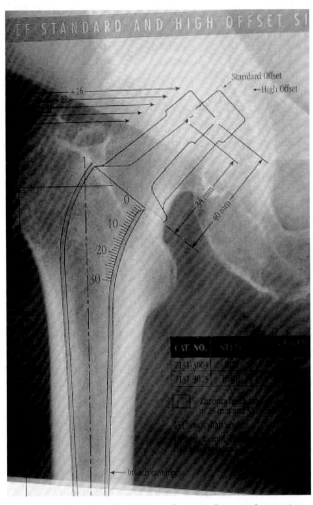

Cemented stem template. Use of a template to determine the optimal femoral stem size. (From Koval KJ, Zuckerman JD. Atlas of Orthopaedic Surgery: A Multimedia Reference. Philadelphia: Lippincott Williams & Wilkins; 2004.)

– 100% failure rate of cemented cups in patients with juvenile RA and ankylosing spondylitis, 25% in Legg-Calve-Perthes, >10% in RA and acetabular dysplasia

Bibliography

Illgen R II, Rubash HE. The optimal fixation of the cementless acetabular component in primary total hip arthroplasty. J Am Acad Orthop Surg 2002; 10(1):43–56.

Wright JM, et al. Bone density adjacent to press-fit acetabular components: a prospective analysis with quantitative computed tomography. J Bone Joint Surg Am 2001; 83(4):529–536.

References

Wasielewski RC, et al. Acetabular anatomy and the transacetabular fixation of screws in total hip arthroplasty. J Bone Joint Surg Am 1990; 72(4):501–508.

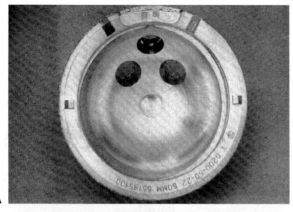

A

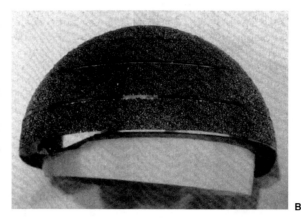

B

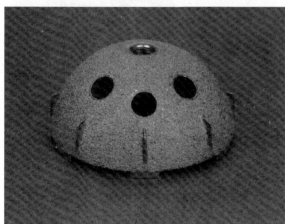

C

A: The Trilogy acetabular component is a modular hemispherical cup with a porous coating. It is available with screw holes, limited screw holes (cluster), or no screw holes. (Reprinted with permission from Zimmer, Inc., Warsaw, IN.) **B:** The Implex acetabular component is a nonmodular, elliptical cup with a porus coating. It does not have screw holes. (Reprinted with permission from Implex Corporation, Allendale, NJ.) **C:** The Mallory-Head acetabular component is a spherical cup with a porous coating. It has fins that augment fixation. (Reprinted with permission from Biomet, Inc., Warsaw, IN. From Craig EV, et al. Clinical Orthopedics. Philadelphia: Lippincott Williams & Wilkins; 1999.)

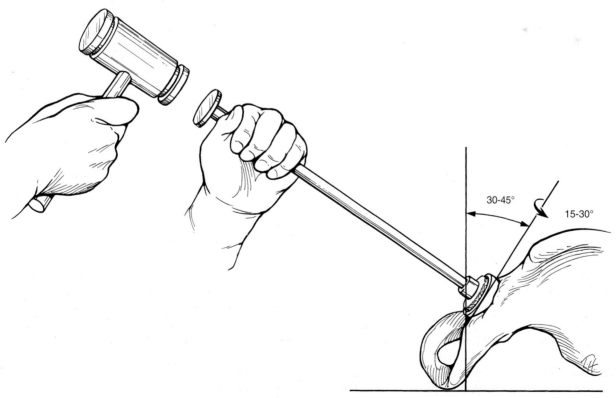

30-45°   15-30°

The ideal acetabular component is impacted in 30 to 45 degrees of abduction from the horizontal plane with 15 to 30 degrees of anteversion. (From Craig EV, et al. Clinical Orthopedics. Philadelphia: Lippincott Williams & Wilkins; 1999.)

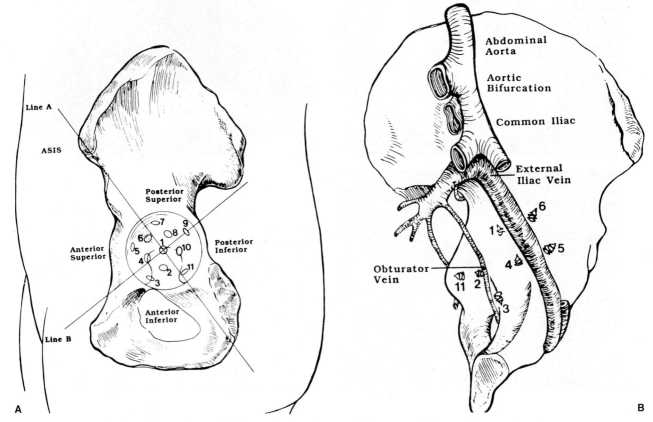

A: The quadrant system for determining safe screw placement. The anterior quadrants should be avoided. **B:** Note the proximity of the anterior acetabular screws to vital intrapelvic neurovascular structures. *1–11,* screw positions; ASIS, anterior-superior iliac spine. (Reprinted with permission from Wasielewski RC, et al. Acetabular anatomy and the transacetabular fixation of screws in total hip arthroplasty. J Bone Joint Surg Am 1990; 72:501–508.)

IMPLANT TYPE—FEMUR

Surface Finish

Matte/Rough Surfaces
- Cement is stronger in compression than tension
- Use cement as grout: transmit load to prosthesis–cement interface via tension, shear, and compression
- Cement–prosthesis interface motion: generates large amounts of abrasion, high failure rates
- Grit blasted gives ongrowth
- Porous coated gives ingrowth

Smooth Surfaces
- Use cement as glue and have weak bone–cement adhesion
- Transmit load at interface via compression, which results in higher cement stresses but less cement abrasion with interface motion
- Micromotion at stem–cement interface protects bone–cement interface

Noncemented

Biology
- Hip sees two to eight times body weight at 1 million cycles/yr
- Porous-coated metallic = bone ingrowth
- Grit-blasted metallic = bone ongrowth
- Porous-coated optimal pore size 50–350 μm, porosity 40%–50%
- Micromotion >150 μm leads to fibrous tissue ingrowth and pain
- Avoid micromotion with press fit and rigid fixation
- Gap between prosthesis and bone <50 μm
- Hydroxyapatite added to surface for osteoinduction
- Fully porous = complete porous coated, bone ingrowth occurs in diaphysis, with stress shielding at proximal femur
- Proximal porous = metaphyseal or upper metadiaphyseal region porous coated, results in less stress shielding, proximal bone ingrowth

Indications
- Now is standard of care in US, especially in young, active patients.
- Young, active individuals
- Good bone stock

Contraindications
- Absence of adequate bone stock

Technique
- Technique became more feasible with advent of modular systems for better cortical contact
- Cortical contact better for strength than cancellous contact
- Ream canal to diameter less than stem size

Outcomes
- Axial micromotion is minimal, rotational micromotion is harmful
- Straight or curved stem types
- Straight can be proximally or extensively coated
- Curved are all proximally coated for metaphyseal "fit and fill"
- Extensive coated stems are for diaphyseal fit and fill
- Collar does not improve rotational stability
- Distal fixers say proximal fixation is less predictable because of variable patient anatomy
- Proximal fixers say stress shielding is problem with distal fixation
- The newer stems are proximal fixation designs
- Clinically similar results are seen between proximally and extensively coated stems
- When seating implant, resistance is only with last 1–2 cm in proximally coated versus resistance throughout for extensively coated stems
- No clear difference between titanium and CoCr for uncemented stems
- Cannot see bony ingrowth on XR
- Stress shielding increases with extensively coated porosity, increased component radius, and stem stiffness

Cemented
Indications
- Less complication rate than cementless
- Older population

Contraindications
- Static cement fixation: microfracture with high activity can cause loosening

Fixation
- Only by interdigitation to bone
- Lower viscosity gets higher interdigitation in vitro but worse in vivo and clinically due to bleeding
- Pores decrease fatigue strength

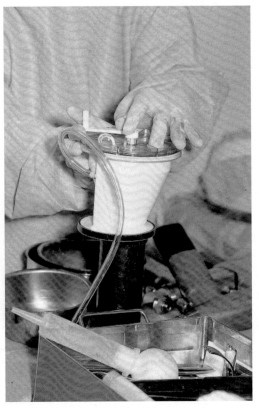

Vacuum mixing the cement. (From Koval KJ, Zuckerman JD. Atlas of Orthopaedic Surgery: A Multimedia Reference. Philadelphia: Lippincott Williams & Wilkins; 2004.)

- Highest intramedullary pressure during stem insertion, depends most on rate of insertion and stem geometry
- Early failure of rough cement stems seen

Technique
- First-generation cement technique
    - Finger packing
    - 20% failure at 5 yr, 40% at 10 yr
- Second-generation cement technique (1975)
    - Cement gun
    - Cement restrictor (ideal 2 cm from stem tip)
    - Canal brush and dry
    - Stem collar
- Third-generation cement technique (1982)
    - Porosity reduction of cement using vacuum
    - Pressurization
    - Precoated or preheated stem
    - Stem centralizer
- Forth-generation cement technique
    - Distal plug
    - Pulsatile lavage
    - Vaccum mixing
    - Cement gun
    - Distal centralizer
    - Proximal rubber seal to pressurize cement

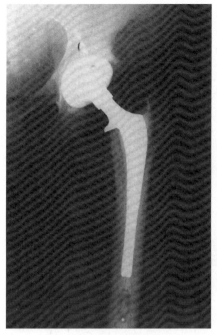
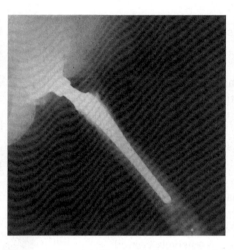
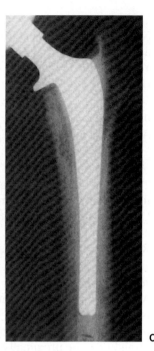

A,B
C

Anteroposterior **(A)** and lateral **(B)** views showing the central placement of the femoral stem with a good cement mantle. **C:** Close-up of the femoral cement mantle showing a complete whiteout, which indicates good pressurization technique. (From Craig EV, et al. Clinical Orthopedics. Philadelphia: Lippincott Williams & Wilkins; 1999.)

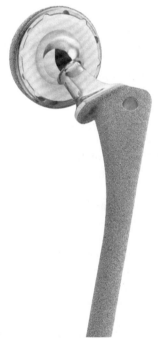
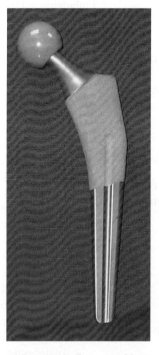
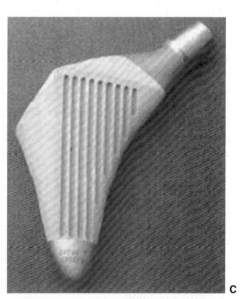

A,B
C

An example of a noncemented extensively coated long stem (**A:** AML stem, DePuy, Inc., Warsaw, IN From Callaghan JJ, et al. The Adult Hip Volume 2, Philadelphia: Lippincott Williams & Wilkins; 2007), a regular sized stem with proximal porous coating (**B:** Accolade stem, Stryker, Mahwah, NJ) and a short stem (**C:** Ultra Short Stem, DePuy, Inc., Warsaw, IN From Santori FS, et al. Avascular Necrosis of the Femoral Head: Current Trends, Milan: Springer-Verlag Italia; 2004).

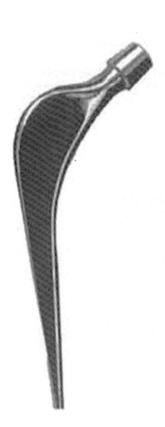
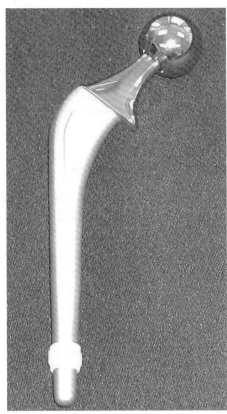

An example of a polished collarless cemented stem (**A:** Exeter stem, Stryker, Mahwah, NJ From Callaghan JJ, et al. The Adult Hip. Philadelphia: Lippincott Williams & Wilkins, 1998) and a cemented stem with collar (**B:** Accolade C stem, Stryker, Mahwah, NJ)

Operative Technique
- Cobalt-chrome (CoCr) is metal of choice for cemented stem
- Mantle should be >2 mm
- Avoid mantle defects
- Center stem within mantle (may use centralizer)
- Distal plugging 2–3 cm distal to component tip; this maintains adequate cement pressurization and equalizes distance
- No reaming
- Pressurized lavage to decrease embolism and prevent intrusion
- Varus orientation can lead to aseptic loosening

BEARING SURFACES

Combinations
Traditional
- "Hard on soft" cobalt or titanium on polyethylene cup
- Titanium should be avoided due to increased third-body debris
- Wear related to roughness of surface

Polyethylene
Biomechanics
- Ultra-high-molecular-weight polyethylene (UHMWPE)
- Avoid calcium stearate; it decreases strength of UHMWPE

- Sterilization via irradiation favors cross-linking, which improves resistance to wear, but in presence of oxygen promotes oxidation, which is detrimental
- Cross-linking also reduces Young's modulus, yield strength, and fracture toughness
- Oxidation causes molecular chain scission, leading to accelerated wear and failure
- Sterilization via gas plasma and ethylene oxide has no effect on cross-linking
- Use of HCLPE is now the standard of care
- New Antioxidant HIGHLY CROSSLINKED polyethylene, Vitamin E enhanced

Alternate Bearing Surfaces
Ceramic on Highly Crosslinked Polyethylene (HCLPE)
- Aluminum oxide first used—brittle
- Zirconium oxide introduced later
- Tribologic properties: more lubrication, less friction, less wear
- Inert due to highly oxidized states and does not release ions
- Several studies have shown better survivorship and lower wear of ceramic, especially with modern highly cross linked poly
- Newer ceramic composites are more scratch resistance and lower fracture
- Ceramic head fracture associated with:
- Vertical cup—high stress at rim
- Small ceramic head—high focal contact stress

- Skirted head—impingement
- Must have exact Morse taper to avoid hoop stresses

Ceramic on Ceramic

- First generation—poorly designed tapered locks led to component malpositioning and fracture
- Rigidity and low energy absorption of ceramic leads to load transfer to periacetabular bone, leading to implant migration in osteoporotics
- To reduce rigidity, "sandwiches" with metal shell, polyethylene middle, and ceramic articulating surfaces have been used

Metal on Metal

- Tribologic properties, but concerns of ion release and cancer exist
- High blood levels of metal found in blood, but clinical significance is unknown
- Possible hypersensitivity reactions may be seen, leading to premature osteolysis
- ALVAL (aseptic lymphocytic vasculitis-associated lesions) is a Type IV Hypersensitivity reaction from metal on metal bearing.

References

Pandit H, Glyn-Jones S, McLardy-Smith P, et al. Pseudotumours associated with metal-on-metal hip resurfacings. J Bone Joint Surg Br 2008; 90-B:847–51.

Willert HG, Buchhorn GH, Fayyazi A, et al. Metal-on-metal bearings and hypersensitivity in patients with artificial hip joints: a clinical and histomorphological study. J Bone Joint Surg Am 2005; 87-A:28–36.

Knee Section

BIOMECHANICS, ANATOMY, AND APPROACHES

Biomechanics

- Normal femoral-tibial angle of anatomical axis is 5–7 degrees of valgus; mechanical axis should pass through center of medial tibial spine
- Approximately 3 degrees of varus at joint line and 10 degrees of posterior slope of proximal tibia
- Normal weight bearing is 60% in medial compartment, 40% in lateral

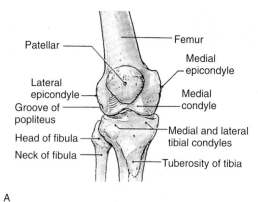

A

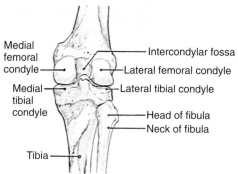

B

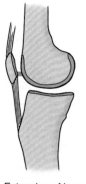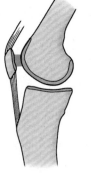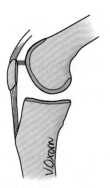

C

Bones of the right knee joint. **A:** Anterior view. **B:** Posterior view. **C:** Patella. Posterior view. Position of the patella during knee movements. (From Moore KL, Agur A. Essential Clinical Anatomy, 2nd ed. Philadelphia: Lippincott Williams & Wilkins; 2002.)

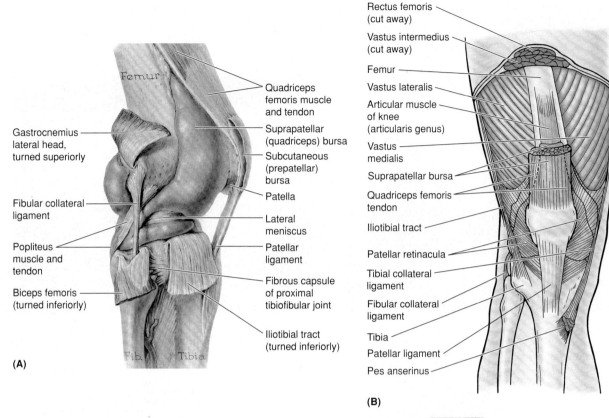

(A)

Femur

Quadriceps femoris muscle and tendon

Gastrocnemius lateral head, turned superiorly

Suprapatellar (quadriceps) bursa

Subcutaneous (prepatellar) bursa

Patella

Fibular collateral ligament

Lateral meniscus

Popliteus muscle and tendon

Patellar ligament

Biceps femoris (turned inferiorly)

Fibrous capsule of proximal tibiofibular joint

Iliotibial tract (turned inferiorly)

Fib.   Tibia

(B)

Rectus femoris (cut away)

Vastus intermedius (cut away)

Femur

Vastus lateralis

Articular muscle of knee (articularis genus)

Vastus medialis

Suprapatellar bursa

Quadriceps femoris tendon

Iliotibial tract

Patellar retinacula

Tibial collateral ligament

Fibular collateral ligament

Tibia

Patellar ligament

Pes anserinus

Right knee joint in extension. **A:** Lateral view. Latex was injected into the joint cavity to demonstrate the extensive synovial capsule. Observe the extent of the synovial capsule deep to the quadriceps, forming the suprapatellar bursa. **B:** Anterior view, demonstrating the bursae around the knee. **C:** Lateral view of the bones of the right knee region showing the attachment sites of muscles and ligaments. (From Moore KL, Dalley AF II. Clinical Oriented Anatomy, 4th ed. Baltimore: Lippincott Williams & Wilkins; 1999.)

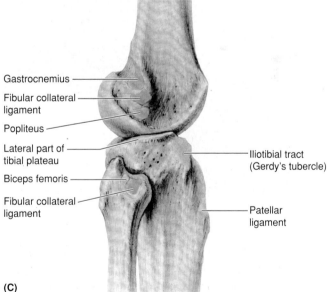

Gastrocnemius

Fibular collateral ligament

Popliteus

Lateral part of tibial plateau

Biceps femoris

Fibular collateral ligament

Iliotibial tract (Gerdy's tubercle)

Patellar ligament

(C)

Anatomy

- Three compartments: medial, lateral, and patello-femoral, more than simple hinge or ginglymus
- Also proximal tibiofibular joint—plane or gliding joint supported by anterior/posterior ligaments of head of fibula
- Patella: largest sesamoid—enhances quad function as fulcrum (after patellectomy drops 30%–60%), protects knee, lubricates/nutritional source to knee. Medial and lateral facets separate by vertical ridge; lateral is broader and deeper. Patella usually fully ossifies between second and sixth years of life; if it does not, patients may have a "bipartite patella" (usually super-olateral corner, be sure to distinguish from a fracture)
- Tibia: concave/oval/thicker posteriorly; medial condyle supports larger medial femoral condyle

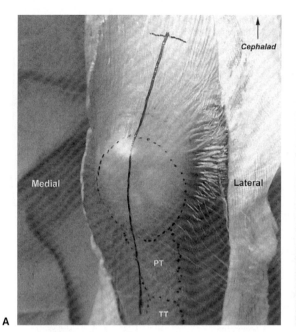

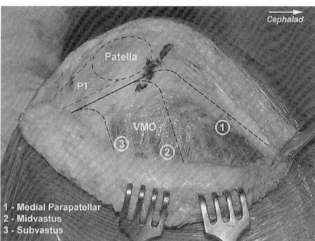

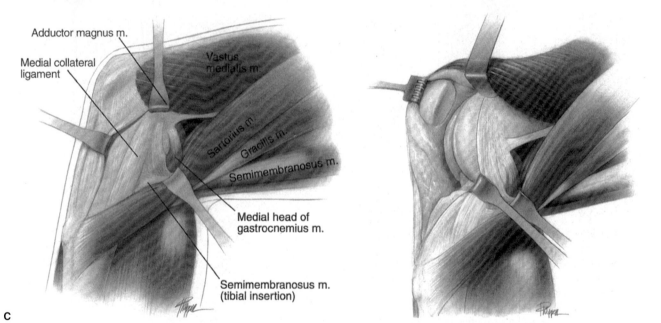

C

A: Authors' preferred skin incision. The skin and fat are incised with the knee in flexed position. **B:** Medial perspective of the flexed knee after dissection of the superficial tissues. **C:** The subvastus approach. (A, B: From photo library of the Department of Orthopaedics [Adult Reconstruction], London Health Sciences Centre, London, Ontario, Canada, with permission; C: From Insall N, Scott WN, eds. Surgery of the Knee, 3rd ed. Philadelphia: WB Saunders; 2000, with permission.)

(MFC); convex/circular lateral condyle. Medial meniscus is "C" shaped and fixed; lateral is "O" shaped and mobile. Tibial tubercle—oblong anterior elevation for patella ligament; Gerdy tubercle is iliotibial band (ITB) insertion laterally

– Femur: MFC is larger, prominent medial epicondyle supports adductor tubercle, lateral femoral condyle (LFC) is raised and longer. *Note:* Anatomical TKA designs take LFC in consideration but more expensive versus universal components

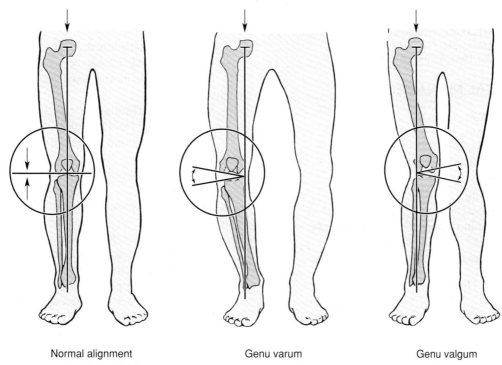

Normal alignment   Genu varum   Genu valgum

Knee deformities: normal alignment, genu varum, genu valgum. (From Moore KL, Dalley AF II. Clinical Oriented Anatomy, 4th ed. Baltimore: Lippincott Williams & Wilkins; 1999.)

- Articular cartilage (see Osteoarthritis section)
- Collateral, cruciate ligaments, patellofemoral ligaments, meniscotibial ligaments, plicas, and anatomy of posterolateral corner (see Sports section)

Medial Parapatellar Arthrotomy
- Gold standard, best exposure, lateral parapatellar arthrotomy can be done for valgus knee

Subvastus Approach
- Integrity of quad tendon and vastus medialis oblique (VMO) not violated, but at expense of limited visualization of lateral compartment

Midvastus Snip Approach
- Integrity of quad tendon not violated, but "snip" VMO muscle belly medially for better exposure than the subvastus
- Other approaches and the anatomical layers of knee are in the Sports section

AVASCULAR NECROSIS AND OSTEONECROSIS

- Primary AVN (spontaneous, may or may not be due to trauma) versus secondary (due to systemic diseases, such as SLE, sickle cell, steroid use)

- In knee, most common in MFC (LFC more common if secondary AVN)
- Sudden acute pain, effusion, like meniscus tear, nontraumatic
- Patient usually >70 yo, often female
- Bone scan better for diagnosis earlier in disease
- Natural history
  - Insall (1983): >70% heal in 9 mo
- Differential diagnosis: transient osteoporosis (insufficiency fracture)
  - Diffuse bone scan uptake
  - Partial weight bearing, calcitonin, heals in 6 mo
- Surgical options
  - Drill, microfracture
  - Autograft/allograft plugs
  - Osteotomy—if deformity present
  - Unicompartmental knee arthroplasty
  - Total knee arthroplasty—if joint collapsed already

Insufficiency Fracture
- Most common in LFC, also called transient osteoporosis
- Sudden acute pain, atraumatic (similar to AVN in middle-aged pts), but seen in younger patients
- MRI shows small chondral fracture, AVN much bigger, much more marrow edema on T2 compared with AVN
- Protected weight bearing, calcitonin and bisphosphonates, most get better conservatively

References

Aglietti P, et al. Idiopathic osteonecrosis of the knee. Aetiology, prognosis and treatment.

J Bone Joint Surg Br 1983; 65(5):588–597.

NONSURGICAL MANAGEMENT

Physical Therapy

- Aerobic exercise:
  - Increase stamina
  - Decrease pain
  - Weight loss
- Unloader bracing
- Assistive devices:
  - Cane/crutch in opposite hand to decrease weight through knee
  - Provides balance

Pharmacologic Therapy

- Tylenol
  - Analgesic
  - Liver toxicity
- NSAIDs
  - Cyclooxygenase-1 (COX-1) (ibuprofen, indomethacin, naproxen)
  - Gastrointestinal symptoms
- Cyclooxygenase-2 (COX-2) (Celebrex, Vioxx, Bextra, Mobic)
  - Decreased gastrointestinal toxicity
  - Increased cardiac toxicity
  - Complications increase with age
- Hyaluronan
  - Mixed study results
- Intra-articular steroid injections
  - Require ultrasound or fluoroscopy
  - Good results
  - Possible increased risk of infection after arthroplasty
- Intra-articular viscosupplementation (Synvisc, hyaluronic acids)
  - Modulation does not alter course of DJD, conflicting data regarding viscosupplementation, depends on purity, dose, methods, etc.
- Unloader bracing/physical therapy (PT), NSAIDs, COX-2, steroid injections, viscosupplementation (Synvisc, hyaluronic acids)
- Recent studies show that intra-articular Lidocaine or Marcaine have toxic effect on cartilage.
- Modulation does not alter course of DJD, conflicting data regarding viscosupplementation, depends on purity, dose, methods, etc.

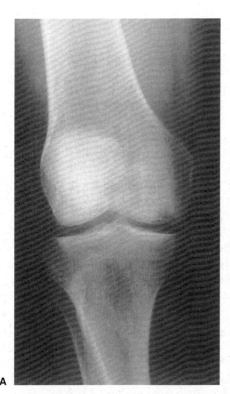 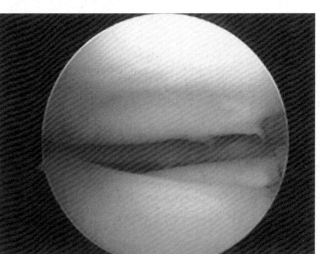

A   **B**

Avascular necrosis of the medial femoral condyle within 4 mo of a simple posterior horn medial meniscotomy in a 48-yo male. **A:** Routine weight-bearing anteroposterior radiograph demonstrating foci of avascular necroses. **B:** Arthroscopic evaluation in the same patient demonstrating softening over area of collapsed subchondral bone. (From Callaghan JJ, et al. The Adult Knee. Philadelphia: Lippincott Williams & Wilkins; 2003.)

NONARTHROPLASTY OPTIONS

Osteotomies
- Only if the underlying issue is alignment
- Realign mechanical axis
- Ideal pt: isolated compartment arthritis, deformity <10 degrees, ligamentous balance, young/active
- Contraindications: inflammatory arthritis, tri-comp disease, flexion arc <90 degrees, marked tibiofe-

moral subluxation or meniscectomy in contralateral comp
- Relative contraindications: age >60; patellofemoral (PF) arthritis, collateral insufficiency, lateral tibial subluxation, or varus deformity >10 degrees; cruciate ligament insufficiency (may do if stable insufficiency)
- Varus deformity—lateral closing high tibial osteotomy (HTO)
- 12- to 15-degree deformity, use dome osteotomy

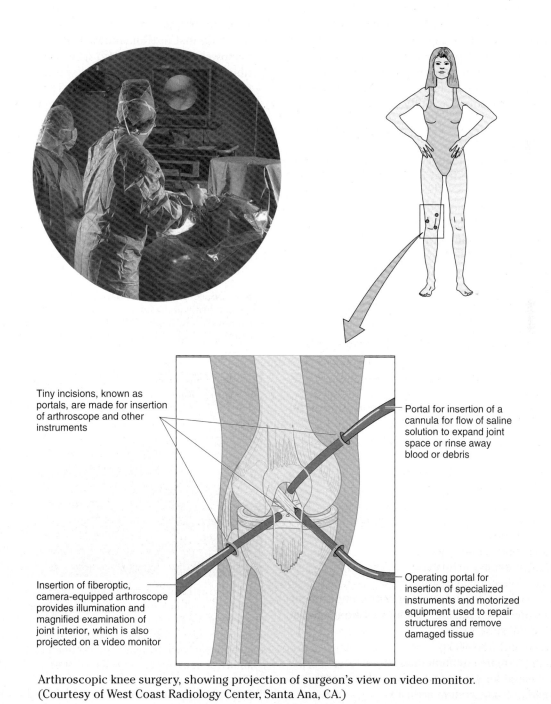

Tiny incisions, known as portals, are made for insertion of arthroscope and other instruments

Portal for insertion of a cannula for flow of saline solution to expand joint space or rinse away blood or debris

Insertion of fiberoptic, camera-equipped arthroscope provides illumination and magnified examination of joint interior, which is also projected on a video monitor

Operating portal for insertion of specialized instruments and motorized equipment used to repair structures and remove damaged tissue

Arthroscopic knee surgery, showing projection of surgeon's view on video monitor. (Courtesy of West Coast Radiology Center, Santa Ana, CA.)

– Newer techniques include medial opening wedge (Puddu plate)
– Benefits of opening wedge is less shortening of leg and bone preservation
– Want to aim for valgus alignment at end of case (relative overcorrection)
– HTO not as well tolerated by women because of cosmetic deformity of having "knock-knees"
– Valgus deformity—medial closing wedge HTO (12–15 degrees)
– Distal femur osteotomy (usually do osteotomy on femoral side because of joint line obliquity)
– Open reduction and internal fixation (ORIF) versus external fine wire fixation; higher rates of nerve palsy, nonunion, and infections with frames, but most data with less modern frame constructs; with more modern techniques, these numbers are improving, and external fixation gives surgeon ability to gradually correct deformity

Arthroscopy for DJD
– Highly controversial, recent article in VA population showed no difference from placebo (Moseley et al., 2002)
– Useful for carefully selected patients with acute mechanical symptoms—meniscal or loose body, normal alignment, minimal radiographic changes, and short duration of symptoms
– Poor outcome indicator: malalignment, loading symptoms, severe radiographic changes, previous surgeries or chronic symptoms

Synovectomy
– Either arthroscopic or open for inflammatory arthritides
– Long-term follow-up (up to 23 yr) reveals satisfactory results in 60%
– Scope—better results early on, but more similar results to open surgery

Unicondylar
– Relies on more normal kinematics
– No angular deformity like HTO
– Requirements/indications:
  – Correctable valgus or varus deformity
  – At least 90 degrees flexion
  – Flexion contraction <10 degrees
  – Noninflammatory arthritis
  – No patellofemoral symptoms
  – Stress XRs showing normal opposite compartment
  – Intact anterior cruciate ligament without medial and lateral subluxation
  – Body weight <80–90 kg
– Medial much more common than lateral
– Best indicated for young and active patients with isolated medial compartment arthritis

– Survivorship is 87% to 98% at 10 yr, but recent study by Engh had failure rate up to 18% at 10 yr (Eikmann et al., 2006)
– Failure by poly wear and progressive DJD in other compartments
– Conversion to TKA is difficult and results are worse due to bone deficiencies in medial compartment, also will need PS for conversion, results are better
– Advantages—in middle-aged patients: better success rate than HTO, fewer complications, better cosmetic limb alignment than valgus; in elderly patients: faster recovery, less medical morbidity, shorter hospitalization, and cheaper implants
– Role of mini-Uni (Romanowski & Repicci, 2002); Romanowski and Repicci also champion for pure poly tibial component for medial side versus modular components for lateral tibial plateau. They state isolated medial and lateral disease are different pathological processes. Former is extension gap disease, while the latter is flexion gap disease (due to hypoplastic LFC)
– Problems: technically demanding and strict indications

References

Eickmann TH, et al. Survival of medial unicondylar arthroplasties placed by one surgeon 1984-1998. Clin Orthop Relat Res 2006; 452:143–149.

Laskin RS, van Steijn M. Total knee replacement for patients with patellofemoral arthritis. Clin Orthop Relat Res 1999; (367):89–95.

Moseley JB, et al. A controlled trial of arthroscopic surgery for osteoarthritis of the knee. N Engl J Med 2002; 347(2):81–88.

Romanowski MR, Repicci JA. Minimally invasive unicondylar arthroplasty: eight-year follow-up. J Knee Surg 2002; 15(1): 17–22.

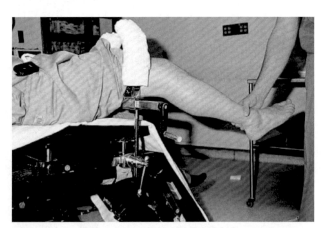

Diagnostic arthroscopy of the knee. The thigh can be placed in a leg holder for the arthroscopic procedure. **A:** The foot of the bed is dropped, and the leg can hang free or be manipulated. **B:** Valgus or varus stress can be applied to the knee by using the leg-holding device for countertraction. (From Koval KJ, Zuckerman JD. Atlas of Orthopaedic Surgery: A Multimedia Reference. Philadelphia: Lippincott Williams & Wilkins; 2004.)

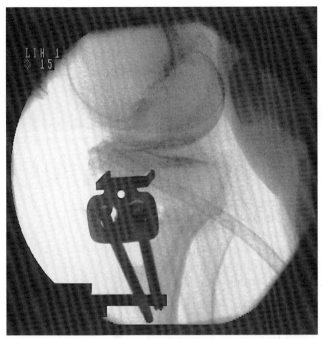

High tibial osteotomy. Postoperative lateral fluoroscopy of a completed high tibial osteotomy. (From Koval KJ, Zuckerman JD. Atlas of Orthopaedic Surgery: A Multimedia Reference. Philadelphia: Lippincott Williams & Wilkins; 2004.)

TOTAL KNEE ARTHROPLASTY
TOTAL KNEE OPERATIVE TECHNIQUE

Procedure (anterior referencing)
- Administration of combined spinal/epidural
- Prepped and draped
- Exsanguinated with Esmarch, tourniquet inflated to 250 mm Hg (Some surgeons use tourniquet only during cementation)
- Midline incision was taken down through skin medial to tibial tubercle
- Medial parapatellar arthrotomy, taking care to leave cuff of tissue on patella for closure and taking anterior horn of medial menisci
- Proximal medial tibia exposed using subperiosteal dissection and thin bent Hohmann, taking care to preserve sMCL
- Patella everted (or subluxed), knee flexed
- Fat pad excised, taking care to preserve patellar tendon
- Anterior collateral ligament (ACL) and PCL (off femur), anterior horn lateral menisci taken down with Bovie
- Patellofemoral ligaments taken
- Tibia externally rotated, subluxated anteriorly using the Hohmann

- Hohmann posterior and lateral
- External tibial cutting guide placed, tibial cut made referencing off most uninvolved side; take at least 10 mm—2 mm for metal, 8 mm for poly
- Take less bone if there is soft-tissue stretching
- Guide placed to make posterior slope and medially by ankle to make more valgus cut (assuming varus knee)
- Proximal tibia removed with Kocher and Bovie
- Alignment rod to middle of ankle mortis
- Femoral punch created starting point for insertion of femoral IM drill and cutting guide
- Jig set with 3- or 5-degree valgus (5 degrees for varus, 3 degrees for valgus)
- Confirm external rotation of femoral component
- Anterior rough cut (do not notch—saw from side)
- Distal cutting block placed, IM rod and anterior rough cut guide removed (headless pins), distal cut made (osteotome protects tibia)
- Femur measuring device to choose femoral component size
- Appropriately sized anteroposterior cutting guide
- Anterior and posterior cuts (can also do chamfers with this, but then cannot do gaps)
- Laminar spreaders placed into joint line
- Menisci removed, taking care to leave small cuff on medial side to preserve MCL
- Posterior osteophytes and soft tissue removed
- Flexion and extension gaps assessed with spacer block and found to be satisfactory
- Final chamfer cutting guide for chamfer cuts as well as box cut, taking care to lateralize femoral component
- Trial size—implant placed on femur
- Tibia anteriorly subluxed
- Size—tibial tray placed with anterior midpoint being at junction of middle and medial one-third of tubercle (Insall) and held with pins
- Tibial canal drilled, punched
- Size—tibial poly placed on tibial tray, knee was reduced
- If CCK, tray removed and CCK/trial poly assembly impacted in
- Found to extend and flex fully, stable in flexion and extension to valgus and varus stress, good tension on MCL and LCL, good passive flexion
- Patella everted
- Patellar cut made with cutting guide and oscillating saw
- Three drill holes, taking care to medialize and superiorize button (lateral with patella everted)
- Size—patellar trial button
- Excess bone trimmed
- Patellar tracking found to be satisfactory
- Trial components removed
- Vigorously irrigated, towel dried

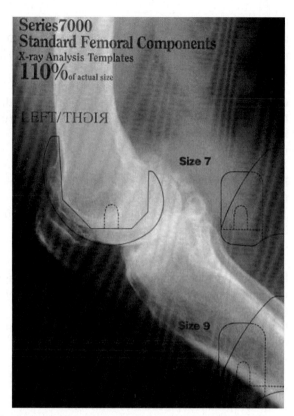

Total knee arthroplasty. Preoperative template in the lateral projection is used to estimate the implant's size. (From Koval KJ, Zuckerman JD. Atlas of Orthopaedic Surgery: A Multimedia Reference. Philadelphia: Lippincott Williams & Wilkins; 2004.)

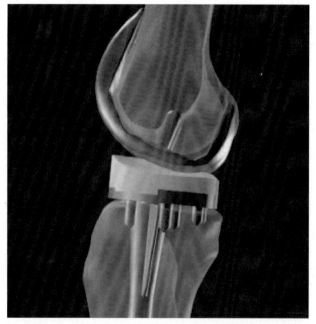

Total knee arthroplasty, lateral. Lateral view of a total knee arthroplasty. (LifeART image copyright © 2007 Lippincott Williams & Wilkins. All rights reserved.)

– Final components cemented into place, starting with patella, followed by femur, and then tibia (attached to poly for Wright)
– Excess cement removed
– Tibial poly impacted into place, knee reduced, held in full extension until the cement polymerized
– Tourniquet released
– Hemostasis
– Vigorously irrigated
– Two subfascial ConstaVac drains
– Fascia 0 Vicryl
– Deep SQ 0 Vicryl
– Superficial SQ 2-0 Vicryl
– Skin staples
– Sterile dressing
– Sponge, needle, instrument
– Tolerated procedure
– Transported to recovery room

Knee Balancing Techniques
Coronal Balancing
– Goal to restore mechanical, not anatomical, alignment
– Femoral cut perpendicular to mechanical axis, which means cut is 5–7 degrees valgus to anatomical axis, best used with IM device; be careful with bilateral with fat emboli
– If varus deformity is correctable on physical examination, then less medial release

Order of release in severe varus deformity
– Medial osteophytes
– Posterior cruciate ligament (PCL), especially is subluxed
– Deep medial collateral ligament (MCL) (intimate with capsule), with piecrusting
– Posteromedial capsule, if there is flexion contracture
– Attachment of semimembranosus
– Partial release of uperficial MCL (sMCL), which attaches near pes anserinus distally

Order of release in severe valgus deformity
– Lateral osteophytes
– Posterolateral capsule (can release with pie-crusting technique)
– ITB Z-type release or off Gerdy's if lateral tight in extension
– Popliteus tendon if lateral tight in flexion or subluxation
– Partial release of lateral collateral ligament (LCL)

- Considered constrained prosthesis if LCL or MCL requires extensive release (condylar constrained knee [CCK])

Component Rotational Positioning
- Femoral component rotation is vital for balancing flexion space and PF tracking
- Methods include transepicondylar axis, posterior condylar axis, and anterior-posterior line of femoral sulcus (Whiteside's line)
- Desire 3 degrees of external rotation of femur
- Posterior lateral femoral condyle deficient in valgus knee; thus, cannot use posterior condyles to judge external rotation of femoral component

Patellar Tracking
- Patellar instability can be from femur, tibia, or patella
- PF tracking is Q-angle management (angle of extensor mechanism from axis vs. patella ligament)
- Maintain normal Q angle (10–15 degrees) without compromising mechanical or ligament stability
- Must not increase Q angle
  - Externally rotate femoral component 3 degrees to posterior condylar axis because proximal tibia is normally 3 degrees varus (medial proximal tibial angle [MPTA], which is angle between mechanical axis of hip to ankle, vs. medial proximal joint line, which is 87 degrees). However, proximal tibia is cut at 90 degrees to tibial/mechanical axis. Thus, femoral put in neutral, it would be loose laterally. External rotation of femoral component compensates for 90-degree cut (i.e., creates rectangular flexion gap vs. internal rotated femoral cut, which will create trapezoidal flexion gap)
  - Epicondylar axis is slightly externally rotated in comparison to posterior condylar axis, so component should parallel epicondylar axis
  - Can also use posterior condyles or AP axis (line down trochlea) to determine external rotation of femur
  - Avoid internal rotation of tibial component
  - Center tibial poly over medial third of tubercle
  - Medialize smaller patellar button
  - Femoral component lateralized for better patellar tracking
- Summary: depends on all three cuts
- Femur: take care to lateralize femoral component with 3 degrees of external rotation
- Tibia: avoid excessive internal rotation, just medial to tubercle (most surgeons try to align it with medial one-third of tubercle, not medial to tubercle)
- Patella: medialize/superiorize patella (with it everted, lateralizes it), partial lateral facetectomy if needed

- Other: avoid excess valgus of femur with some varus of tibia—most common cause of maltracking; keep alignment neutral; also manipulate joint line
- When assessing tracking, no finger is required to hold the patella in the middle of the femoral trochlea groove if one finger can hold tracking, then inadequate PF tracking (rule of no thumb). Ideally, tourniquet down when assessing tracking, eliminate binding effect of tourniquet on quad

Sagittal Balance
- If preoperative flexion contraction significant, may need to take larger optional cut for distal femur and the posterior capsule should be released
- Measure flexion contraction with palm versus fist versus fist sideways under knee (5, 10, or 15 degree contracture, respectively)
- Knee has two radii of curvature—for patellofemoral articulation and for weight-bearing articulation
- Stability in extension and flexion is provided by different parts of collaterals (like metacarpal heads)
- If gap symmetric (same problem in flexion and extension), adjust tibia
- If gap asymmetric, adjust femur
- Better to place tibial component too posteriorly, allowing tibia to go anteriorly, giving quad better mechanical advantage; also avoid excessive interior rotation of tibia, but place just medial off tubercle

Symmetric Gaps
- Tight extension, tight flexion
- Cut more proximal tibia

Asymmetric Gaps
Note: Some of these corrective maneuvers are based on anterior referencing TKA systems only
- Problems with flexion, aka error in AP of distal femur, adjust femoral component size
- Good extension, loose flexion (cut too much posterior femur)
- Upsize femur
- Good extension, tight flexion
- Downsize femur
- Recess PCL
- Make sure enough tibial posterior slope
- Problems with extension, aka error in distal femur, adjust distal femur
- Extension loose, flexion good
- Augment distal femur
- Downsize femur, thicker poly
- Thicker poly, address tight flexion gap (PCL, posterior slope)

- Tight extension (flexion contraction), good flexion
- Release posterior capsule
- Take more distal femur

Measured Resection vs Gap Balancing

Measured Resection
- Femoral component is placed according to bony landmarks (femoral epicondyles, posterior femoral condyles, AP axis)
- Hard to identify these bony landmarks, may cause malrotation

Gap Balancing
- Symmetrical balancing the extension and flexion gaps
- Rectangular balanced gap with lamina spreaders
- Extension gap first, flexion gap second is our preferred technique
- Femoral component is placed parallel to the resected proximal tibia

Patellar Resurfacing
- Pros: to lessen anterior knee pain, obviate need for second surgery, control global destructive process of RA/OA
- Cons: longer surgery, maintaining bone stock, and avoiding complication (i.e., AVN, fracture) of resurfacing

Mini-TKA
- Pros: two types—small incision versus true mini with smaller instruments. Theoretically, less bleeding, dissection—primarily with violation of suprapatellar pouch—lead to less pain, easier PT (midvastus snip).
- Cons: limited prospective studies, "mini-TJA gives maxi-complications," what you gain with less exposure—poorer visualization

PARTIAL KNEE REPLACEMENT

- Short-term good to excellent results in 90%
- Improved kinematics, preserves both cruciates
- Quicker short term recovery compared to TKA
- Better quality and activity level than TKA since it is done in younger, more active patients with less bony deformity

Indication
- Young and active patient
- Isolated antero-medial compartment OA
- Intact ACL
- Correctable varus deformity
- Fixed Flexion Deformity less than 15°

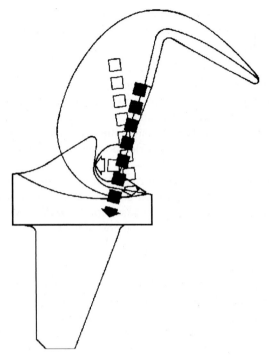

Posterior-stabilized knee implants replace the function of the posterior cruciate ligament with a mechanism by which a post on the tibial component impacts a cam on the femoral component as the joint flexes. The resultant force on the tibia (*solid arrow*) is composed of the joint contact force and the shear force of the cam on the post (*two open arrows*). (From Callaghan JJ, et al. The Adult Knee. Philadelphia: Lippincott Williams & Wilkins; 2003.)

Limitations
- Limited and precise indications
- Progression of lateral or PF compartment
- Failure Rate increases with longer follow-up, at 10–15 years between 15%–30%
- Component positioning and Cement technique are critical
- Patient specific instruments/implants or Haptic Robotic are used for precise positioning

Tibial Hemiarthroplasty
- McKeever, MacIntosh, and UniSpacer (high complication rate: 20% revision in first year)
- All slightly different, but are medial plateau inserts with no bone cuts or fixation. Mobile inserts, but high dislocation rates. UniSpacer theoretically improved because it is a more mobile, self-centering spacer that allows conformity with femoral condyle and tibial plateau in full extension and less patient loading
- Potential role in obese young pts (35–55 yr)—bone-preserving procedure

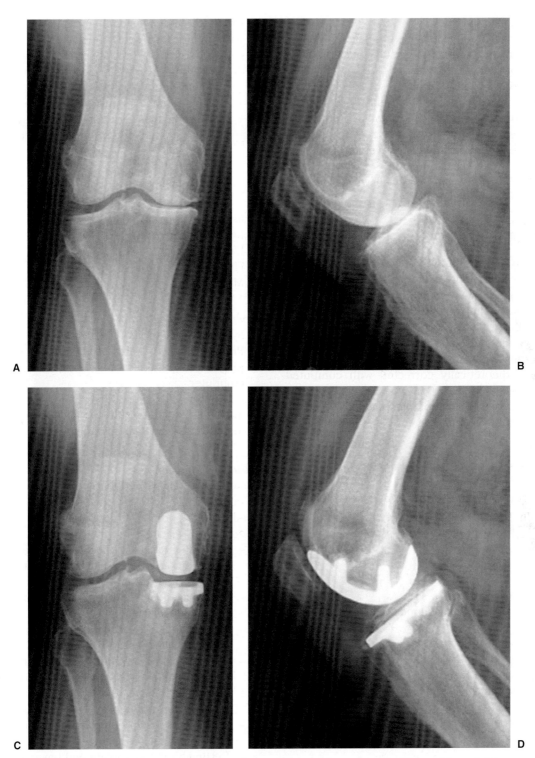

Medial unicompartmental replacement: Pre-operative antero-posterior **(A)** and lateral **(B)** views of stage III osteoarthritis with erosion of the medial femoral condyle and tibial plateau. Postoperative antero-posterior **(C)** and lateral **(D)** views showing satisfactory alignment of unicompartmental components. (From Weale AE, et al. Perceptions of outcomes after unicompartmental and total knee replacement. Clin Orthop 2001; 382:143–145, with permission.)

Patellofemoral Arthroplasty
- Laskin and van Steijn (1999) have article for TKA for isolated PF arthritis with good results, but isolated PF replacement is at early stages
- Other surgical options limited
- Indicated in severe and isolated PF disease, noninflammatory and no active chondrocalcinosis, minimal angular tibiofemoral deformity, intact cruciate ligaments
- Key is to preserve bone for later conversion, best done for dysplastics and posttraumatic
- Idiopathic PF tends not to do as well: will get progression in the other compartments

COMPUTER-ASSISTED SURGERY

- Anatomical alignment of TKA important for long-term implant survival, as previously discussed
- Computer-assisted navigation surgery can give excellent accuracy of implant placement
  - Within 0.5–1 mm and 1 degree of planned
  - Most common errors with TKA are poorly aligned tibial cuts and poorly aligned or rotated femoral cuts → theoretically corrected with computed-assisted surgery
  - German group OrthoPilot: most had 50% decrease in tibial cut malalignment

Pros
- Navigation system user friendly and increasingly popular
- No violation of femoral canal, so decreased bleeding and pulmonary problems
- Theoretically, can obtain an almost "perfect" implant placement

Cons
- Increased surgical time
- Computers can only make good results with good input data
  - Studies have shown that surgeons do not agree well on reference points
- Expensive startup costs
- Bulky instrumentation
- Computer has to be able to "see" pointers at all times; difficult with multiple people moving around operating room

Claims
- Patient-specific anatomy included in operative planning
- Preoperative and intraoperative planning can be visualized in three dimensions
  - Includes visualizing bone cuts and gaps before any actual sawing done

- Create three-dimensional model based on landmarks with pointer from computer system
  - Preoperative or intraoperative CT scanning to delineate bone versus bone surface points used to align navigational marker
  - Fixed reference points put into computer, compared to labeled structure in field (e.g., implant or instrument), and then triangulated in x, y, and z coordinates
  - All points digitally programmed into computer for three-dimensional guide to patient's anatomy

System Types
- Imageless
- CT based
- Fluoroscopy based
- MRI based

Operative Planning
- Systems allow surgeon to create operative plan
- Preprogrammed templates automatically create plan when patient's anatomical data entered into computer
- Computer will give actual values for varus/valgus alignment, degrees of flexion and extension, and flexion and extension gap distances

Intraoperative Planning
- Reference arrays attached to femoral and tibial bone
- Alignment points programmed at beginning of surgery
  - Computer requests specific points to be touched with pointer so that calculations about patient's anatomy can be made
  - In CT-based systems, patient's anatomy is already downloaded into computer
  - Physician can fine-tune any discrepancies at this point
  - Computer system then automatically plans implants based on preprogrammed algorithm
  - Surgeon again can adjust implants' size or orientation as appropriate
  - Surgery is then performed similar to non–computer-assisted technique
  - Cutting blocks are positioned based on navigation system
  - Computer can be used to recheck alignment after cuts have been made
  - Extension gap is balanced according to conventional technique
  - Computer can guide this balancing by showing exact alignment of gap

- Flexion gap is perfected using computer assistance
- Computer measures flexion gap, and then recommends femoral component orientation
- Studies of tourniquet time, continuous passive motion (CPM), and postoperative pain regimen show no statistically significant difference with or without computer navigation
- One study showed decreased drain output with navigation (possibly due to lack of femoral canal invasion)

Bibliography

Chin PL, et al. Randomized control trial comparing radiographic total knee arthroplasty implant placement using computer navigation versus conventional technique. J Arthroplasty 2005; 20(5):618–626.

Decking R, et al. Leg axis after computer-navigated total knee arthroplasty: a prospective randomized trial comparing computer-navigated and manual implantation. J Arthroplasty 2005; 20(3):282–288.

IMPLANT TYPES—FEMUR

Cemented
- Standard of care
- 89%–95% survivorship at 10–20 years

Technique
- Cement should be applied on both surfaces, bone and implant
- Apply continues pressure
- 2 to 4-mm circumferential cement mantle
- Increase surface area by drilling the hard chondral surface
- No cement over the box area since it is not under pressure

Radiographic Evidence of Loosening
- Obvious migration of the implant
- Progressive radiolucency of >2 mm throughout interface
- Radiographic evidence for loosening more common than clinical loosening

Noncemented
- Biological potential for bone ingrowth using beads or plasma spray
- Implant must be biocompatible
- Titanium better than cobalt-chromium in some studies
- 100–400 μm is ideal pore size

- Intimate contact with host bone
- Micromotion >50–100 μm causes failure of ingrowth

Contraindications
- Severe bone loss/osteopenia
- Radiation necrosis
- Primary/metastatic tumor
- Severe metabolic bone disease (no bony ingrowth)

IMPLANT TYPES—TIBIA

Cemented
- Standard of care
- 89%–95% survivorship at 10–20 years

Technique
- Cement should be applied on both surfaces, bone and implant
- Apply continues pressure
- 2- to 4-mm circumferential cement mantle
- Increase surface area by drilling the hard surface

Noncemented
- Results of noncemented tibia varies
- Screws commonly used for initial stability
- Goal is biological ingrowth/fixation

BEARING SURFACES

PCL Retaining versus Posterior Stabilized
Retaining
- Normal femoral rollback is produced by ACL and PCL where femoral–tibial contact point moves posteriorly with flexion, allowing femur to clear tibia to give more flexion
- Initial unconstrained TKA sacrificed both ACL and PCL; no rollback led to flex only to 95 degrees and femur dislocated anteriorly in flexion
- By saving PCL, rollback preserved and anterior dislocation in flexion prevented
- However, because no ACL, rollback was actually roll and slide, leading to increased wear; also, poly was flat to allow rollback, thus higher contact stresses because decreased surface contact area between femur and poly
- Recent PCL retainers changed to more congruent poly, but this decreased rollback and changed PCL to static stabilizer against anterior subluxation
- However, in vivo function of PCL different than in vitro analysis. PCL does not have truly normal rollback

function. Instability can occur with PCL-retaining design because of preoperative deterioration, intra-operative injury, or postoperative injury or attenuation

(Posterior Stabilized)
– Tibial post engages femoral cam to prevent anterior femoral displacement
– In addition, this engagement forces femur posteriorly with further flexion, leading to mechanical rollback
– If flexion gap is loose, femur can jump over tibial post in hyperflexion and dislocate
– Indicated in
  – Prior patellectomy
    – Weak extensor allows for easier femoral dislocation, even if PCL retained
  – Inflammatory arthritis (PCL can rupture)
    – PCL rupture or iatrogenic overrelease
– Several studies show similar results between PS and CR knees. In some studies, PS has better ROM

Rotating Platform
– Pros: developed to reduce poly wear and prosthetic loosening, and thus enhance survival of implant by reducing mechanical poly contact stress and fatigue wear by conforming surface design.
– Cons: knee must be properly balanced (more technically demanding to put in), cases of spinout, (with cruciate sacrificing designs like LCS, not with PS designs) and limited evidence that wear is less
– New high-flexion rotating platform design aim for >130 ROM

Tensioners
– Pros: soft tissue balancing is critical to TKA, controlled and calibrated tensioners more accurate than blocks and laminar spreaders, even possible to balance knee and calculate correct bone cuts prior to cuts
– Cons: dangerous with distorted anatomy like valgus knee, better to use bony landmarks that are more reliable

Alternate Bearings
– Pros: standard alloy is CoCrMo (cobalt-chrome-molybdenum), newer ones are zirconium and niobium, harder after oxidation to oxidized zirconium ceramic surface than traditional alloy and 50% less friction than UHMWPE
– Cons: fatigue strength is not issue; issue is poly, especially on the backside, not femorotibial component

Complications

INFECTION

Total Hip Arthroplasty
Epidemiology
– Incidence 1% in Medicare population, 0.06% in specialized centers

Presentation
– Pain
– Fever
– Elevated ESR, CRP, white blood cell (WBC) count
– CRP normalizes faster and more accurately identifies infection
– Recently, several molecular markers in joint fluid are used for diagnosis of infection: interleukin 6, interleukin 8, α(2)-macroglobulin, C-reactive protein, and vascular endothelial growth factor
– for all revision cases, infection should always be investigated.

Risk Factors
– Infection rate decreases as hospitals perform >100/yr
– Laminar airflow operating rooms, dedicated orthopaedic nursing decreases rates
– Postoperative wound drainage and hematoma increase risk

Radiographic Evaluation
– XR—progressive loosening, determined by comparing old XR to see femoral loosening (difficult to assess acetabular loosening) look for demarcation in AP and lateral (false profile) views
– Arthrogram—to evaluate acetabular loosening
– Bone scan—60% sensitive, 65% specific
– Gallium scan—67% sensitive, 75% specific
– Indium scan—86% sensitive, 87% specific; can distinguish between aseptic loosening, septic loosening, and secure implant in dogs; more accurate than gallium scan

Aspiration
– Gold standard to diagnose infection is aspiration, but false-negative rate is high
– Patient must be off antibiotics of 2–6 wk
– Finds causal bug in two-thirds infected THA
– Most commonly *Staphylococcus epidermidis* (late) and *Staphylococcus aureus* (early)
– Late infection often caused by dental work (*Peptostreptococcus*)
– Growth in broth requires less innoculum
  – Consider significant if patient had been on antibiotics
  – Broth will also grow anaerobes
  – Anaerobes will not grow on plating unless specifically requested to lab

Hip Aspiration Technique
- Anterior approach: palpate femoral artery in line between ASIS and pubic tubercle; go 2 cm lateral to pulse and enter (this is also 2 cm distal to inguinal ligament), aiming medially
- Lateral approach: palpate anterior and superior to the tip of GT; enter parallel to floor slightly cephalad, go along neck until joint entered

Histology
- Bacteria in tissue without presence of polys suggests contaminant

Classification
- I—Early, acute postop (<1 mo)
  - Cannot differentiate deep from superficial infection using any radiographic study
  - If fascia is intact in operating room (OR), consider infection superficial
  - If fascia violated, deep infection is present, and need to open, irrigate and débride entire wound and close over drains
- II—Acute, late hematogenous (<1 mo, other site)
  - Arthroscopic incision and drainage (I&D) if sensitive bacteria found
  - 6 wk of IV antibiotics, PO prophylaxis thereafter
  - After 5-yr follow-up, one-twelfth needed more surgery
- III—Chronic, late infection (>1 mo)
  - Remove implant, place antibiotic spacer, 6 wk IV antibiotics
  - 3.6 g tobramycin, 1 g vancomycin in spacer
  - Achieve 1:8 postpeak serum bactericidal titer against specific bug
  - 70% reimplanted with 6.5% recurrence rate, 40-mo follow-up

Treatment Options
- Aspiration, antibiotics
  - 15% success
  - Two-thirds short-term success (Europe)
  - Really only for patients unfit for surgery
- Open I&D
  - For early infection within 3 wk of initial surgery
  - With sensitive bacteria
  - 50% failure
- Direct implant exchange
  - 70% success with nonantibiotic cement
  - 85% success with antibiotic cement
  - Better success if bacteria present is without glycocalyx
  - One-half *S. epidermidis* and one-fourth *S. aureus* isolates make glycocalyx
  - Palacos cement gives higher and more sustained local antibiotic concentration, but Simplex cement is easier to inject

- Two stage revision
  - Standard of care
  - 92% success with antibiotic cement
  - Choose cement antibiotic that bacteria is sensitive to
  - Removal of infected components, through debridement, insertion of antibiotic coated articulating cement spacers
  - 6 weeks of intravenous antibiotics
  - 2 weeks of antibiotic holiday
  - re-implantation when aspiration is negative and inflammatory markers (ESR, CRP) are normal
  - Frozen section in OR should show less than 5 WBC per high-powered field (HPF)
- Resection arthroplasty
  - Contraindicated when extensive proximal femoral bone loss is present or bilateral THA present
- Arthrodesis
- Amputation

Prevention
- Infection decreases 50%–80% with preoperative antibiotics
- Prophylaxis for dental and other procedures with amoxicillin 2 g or clindamycin 600 mg 1 hr before (and 1 g amoxicillin 6 hr after procedure) for 2 yr after surgery

Bibliography

Charnley J, Eftekhar N. Postoperative infection in total prosthetic replacement arthroplasty of the hip-joint: with special reference to the bacterial content of the air of the operating room. Br J Surg 1969; 56(9):641–649.

Ghanem E, Parvizi J, Burnett RS, Sharkey PF, Keshavarzi N, Aggarwal A, Barrack RL. Cell count and differential of aspirated fluid in the diagnosis of infection at the site of total knee arthroplasty. J Bone Joint Surg Am 2008 Aug; 90(8):1637–1643.

Hyman JL, et al. The arthroscopic drainage, irrigation, and debridement of late, acute total hip arthroplasty infections: average 6-year follow-up. J Arthroplasty 1999; 14(8):903–910.

Jacovides CL, Parvizi J, Adeli B, Jung KA. Molecular Markers for Diagnosis of Periprosthetic Joint Infection. J Arthroplasty 2011 May 12.

Lieberman JR, et al. Treatment of the infected total hip arthroplasty with a two-stage reimplantation protocol. Clin Orthop 1994; (301):205–212.

McDonald DJ, et al. Two-stage reconstruction of a total hip arthroplasty because of infection. J Bone Joint Surg Am 1989; 71(6):828–834.

Parvizi J, Suh DH, Jafari SM, Mullan A, Purtill JJ. Aseptic loosening of total hip arthroplasty: infection always should be ruled out. Clin Orthop Relat Res 2011 May; 469(5):1401–1405.

Total Knee Arthroplasty
- 3%–4% complication rate in TKA
  - Biological—infection, loosening
  - Technical

- Components
  - Associated with specific diagnosis
- Infection incidence 1%–12%, 1.2% at Mayo
- Higher rate than hips
- Infection risk factors
  - RA, RA male
  - Psoriatic arthritis
  - Skin ulcers
  - Prior knee surgery
- Hinged cemented IM stem implants have very high infection rates
- Windsor (1990)—52 TKRs
  - 96% of infections have pain (most common presenting complaint)
  - 77% swelling
  - 27% drainage
  - 27% fevers
  - ESR >30 is 60% sensitive, 65% specific
  - Average ESR in infection is 63
  - Average WBC count is 8
  - ESR takes about 1 yr to normalize
- Peersman (2001)
  - 6,120 TKRs at HSS 1993 to 1999
  - 0.39% deep infection in primary
  - 0.97% deep infection in revisions
  - Risk factor—diabetes mellitus, smoking, prior open knee surgery, obesity, low K^+, nutrition, immunosuppression
  - Increased risk if surgery longer than 2.5 hr
  - No difference between 24- and 48-hr antibiotics
  - 20% of patients, no organism found; all had been given antibiotics at outside hospital
  - New pain without apparent cause assumed to be infection until proven otherwise
  - XRs, bone scans, gallium scans do not really help with diagnosis; combined technetium and indium

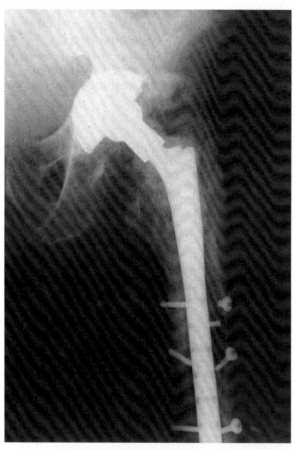

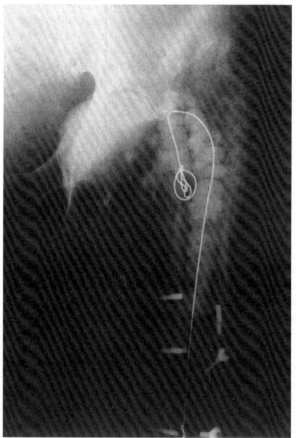

A: An 88-yo patient who presented with a failed and infected Kent prosthesis (Biomet, Warsaw, IN) and broken screws within the medullary canal of the femur. Significant periosteal reaction suggests pan-diaphyseal osteomyelitis. **B:** Because of the patient's age and degree of infection, he was treated with a definitive Girdlestone arthroplasty. Antibiotic-loaded cement was left within the joint cavity and medullary canal of the femur as an antibiotic depot, supplementing intravenous antibiotic therapy. (From Craig EV, et al. Clinical Orthopedics. Philadelphia: Lippincott Williams & Wilkins; 1999.)

Infected Total Hip Replacement and Treatments for Different Indications

Procedure	Indications	Technique	Pitfalls
Débridement and irrigation	• Acute early infection • Acute hematogenous infection	• Wide exposure • Avoid devascularization • Exchange modular components	• Components loose • Débridement too late • Inadequate débridement
Girdlestone arthroplasty	• Debilitated patient • Uncooperative patient • Recurrent infection	• Extensile exposure • Femoral osteotomy if necessary • Antibiotic beads • Special techniques for removing solidly fixed components	• Poor function • Worse function if deficient bone stock
One-stage exchange	• Infection with less virulent organism • No draining sinuses • Adequate bone stock for cemented femoral fixation	• Special techniques for removing solidly fixed components • Reconstruct with antibiotic-loaded cement	• Lower infection control rate • Cannot use cementless femoral fixation • Cannot use bone graft
Two-stage exchange	• Used for most patients • Avoid in unwell or uncooperative patients	• First operation similar to Girdlestone • May use an articulated spacer • Intravenous antibiotics for 6 weeks • Then reimplant	• Long treatment protocol • Expensive

(From Craig EV, et al. Clinical Orthopedics. Philadelphia: Lippincott Williams & Wilkins; 1999.)

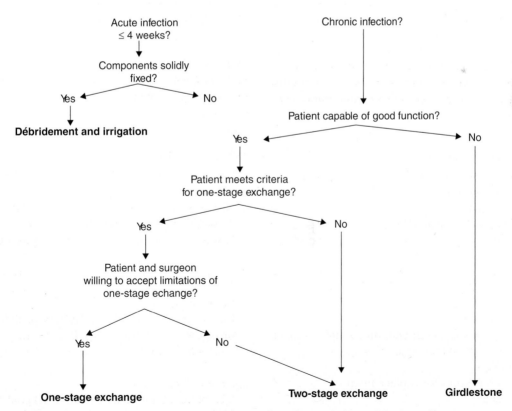

Treatment Algorithm for Infected THA. (From Craig EV, et al. Clinical Orthopedics. Philadelphia: Lippincott Williams & Wilkins; 1999.)

(WBC-labeled) increase sensitivity and specificity to 100% and 97%, respectively
- Aspiration is gold standard
  - 55% sensitivity, 96% specificity, 84% accuracy
  - 100% sensitivity and specificity if off antibiotics
- Worry if knee WBC count >25,000, (some studies as low as 2,000) 75% polys
- Glucose in synovial fluid usually equal to plasma but lower in infection; protein levels higher in infection
- Most common in TKR: *S. aureus*
- Intraoperative frozen section
  - 43% sensitivity, 97% specificity if 5 polys/HPF used as positive criteria

Treatment
- Depends on type:
  - Early postoperative or early hematogenous (2–4 wk): can retain components if early I&D and poly exchange, then postoperative IV antibiotics for 6 wk. If reinfection occurs, must remove implant, but prognosis is good. Usual cause is *S. aureus*. Rarely, one use just if acute pain <48 hr, with obvious hematogenous source and very sensitive bug such as pneumococcus or streptococcus and patient is unable to have surgery
  - Late chronic infection (>4 wk from surgery or hematogenous seeding): gold standard—two-stage explant with antibiotics spacer (vancomycin, tobramycin, gentamicin) and IV antibiotics for 6 wk and then replantation, two-stage arthrodesis with interval period of spacer/antibiotics (resistant cases), resection arthroplasty (components out and ± antibiotics spacer) and amputation. Often, cause is *S. epidermis*

Arthrodesis
- Fusion rate 50% in infection
- 90% fusion in surface replacement removal because more bone preserved
- Two-stage replant
  - 90% success with single IM rod
- Four methods: single IM rod, articulating rod, dual-frame half-pin external fixation, plates/screws
- Arthrodesis position is 10–15 degrees of flexion and 5–7 degrees of valgus

Indications for Fusion
- Extensor mechanism destroyed; functional result of revised TKA is worse than arthrodesis
- Resistant infection
- Inadequate bone stock for replacement
- Younger patient
- Medically compromised
- Bad wound, high risk of reinfection

Bibliography

Windsor RE, Insall JN, Urs WK, Miller DV, Brause BD. Two-stage reimplantation for the salvage of total knee arthroplasty complicated by infection. Further follow-up and refinement of indications. J Bone Joint Surg Am. 1990 Feb;72(2):272–8.

Peersman G, Laskin R, Davis J, Peterson M. Infection in total knee replacement: a retrospective review of 6489 total knee replacements. Clin Orthop Relat Res. 2001 Nov;(392):15–23.

VENOUS THROMBOEMBOLIC DISEASE

Embolism
Fat Embolism
- PMMA monomer (vasodilator and myocardial suppressant) levels during cementing not high enough to cause hypotension, hypoxia
- Air emboli are eliminated by retrograde filling of canal and rubber nozzle to pressurize
- Higher intramedullary pressure is associated with higher pulmonary shunts
- Higher intramedial pressures seen with cemented
- 28% intraoperative shunt in cemented versus none in uncemented stems
- Concluded fat/marrow emboli as cause

Pulmonary Embolism
- Prevalence in THR without prophylaxis 0.7%–30% and fatal in 0.1%–0.4%
- 90% originate in proximal vein (popliteal and higher)
- Venography is gold standard
- Other diagnostic tests: spiral CT, chest XR, electrocardiogram (ECG), D-dimer

Deep Vein Thrombosis (DVT)
Virchow Triad
- Vessel wall damage
- Venous stasis
- Blood coagulability

Epidemiology
- DVT is most common reason for readmission after THA and TKR
- 45%–57% of patients after THA without prophylaxis, 23%–36% have proximal DVT
- Historical mortality rates from pulmonary embolism (PE) after THA 2%–3%
- Meta-analysis showed rate of fatal PE without chemical prophylaxis is 0.1%; thus, prophylactic use questioned by Europe
- United States' use of prophylaxis based on smaller prospective studies shows fatal PE rate <0.1% with chemical prophylaxis

Coumadin Prophylaxis
- International normalized ratio (INR) goal 1.8–2.4
- DVT
  - 90% in calf, 10% in thigh

- Thigh DVTs are segmental, no communication with calf clots
- Total DVT rate 20%, proximal DVT rate 2%–5%
- Warfarin with epidural
  - Total DVT rate 9%
  - Proximal DVT rate 2%–3%, all clots were connected to distal clots (no primary proximal clots)

New Potent Anticoagulant Agents
- Lovenox (enoxaparin)
- Fondaparin
- Rivaroxaban: oral factor Xa inhibitor

Compression Boots
- No difference in total DVT rate
- Fewer distal clots, more proximal clots

Studies
Freedman et al. (2000)
52 randomized controlled trials (RCTs), venograms, 10,929 patients

	DVT	Proximal DVT	Sx PE
Placebo	48%	26%	1.5%
ASA	31%		1.3%
Coumadin	23%	6.3%	0.16%
LMWH	18%	7.7%	0.36%
Mini-Heparin	31%		
Boots	21%		0.26%

- Boots: lowest risk distal clot
- Proximal DVT rate—13% in boots, 8% in low-molecular-weight heparin (LMWH), 6% in Coumadin
- ASA alone had higher PE rates
- Minor wound bleeds: 9% in LMWH, 7.6% in mini-Heparin, 2.2% in placebo
- Conclusion—warfarin most effective, safest

Westrich et al. (1999)
- Protocol of ASA, hypotensive anesthesia, compression hose, early ambulation
- 2,592 primary THAs
- 2,037 with normal risk had venograms
- 555 with high risk received warfarin and no venograms
- 10.3% DVT in those with venogram
- Proximal DVT rate 4.3%
- Symptomatic PE 1% (diagnosis by ventilation/perfusion [V/Q])
- Overall 0.04% fatal PE

DiGiovanni et al. (2000)
- Same protocol as above plus intraoperative heparin
- Decreased overall DVT 7%, proximal DVT rate 2%

DVT in TKR
Literature
Boots (Intermittent Pneumatic Compression)
- Combined foot calf maybe better than foot alone, but no clinical support
- More effective than any chemical prophylaxis; some cite that any mechanical prophylaxis reduces DVT 25%–82%
- Two mechanisms: increases venous return and increases endothelial products in clotting cascade, which reduced thrombogenesis

ASA/Boots (Westrich & Sculco, 1996)
- 164 TKR with ASA alone or ASA with boots
- DVT rate 27% for combo versus 59% for ASA alone
- Proximal DVT rate 0% for combo versus 14% for ASA alone
- Boots prevent DVT, but unclear if they prevent PE

ASA/Boots versus Lovenox/Boots (Westrich et al., 2006)
- At postoperative day 3, DVT rates were 17.9 (A/B) versus 15.9 (L/B); rate at 4 wk, 5.5% versus 1.3%—not significantly different

TKA/Intraoperative Heparin (Westrich & Sculco, 1999)
- Intraoperative heparin makes no difference for TKRs

TKA Meta-Analysis (Westrich et al., 2000)
- 23 articles, 6,001 TKR patients
- Routine venogram, V/Q, angiogram

	DVT	ASx PE	Sx PE
ASA	53%	11.7%	1.3%
Coumadin	45%	8.2%	0.4%
LMWH	25%	—	0.5%
Boots	17%	6.3%	0%

- All historic data, not all using pumps and hypotensive anesthesia but isolated prophylaxis
- For anticoagulation, keep in mind that wound hematoma is much less well tolerated in TKR than THR
- Remove boot from side ipsilateral to DVT

Prophylaxis
- Based on risk stratification from HSS Memo Committee on DVT/PE Prophylaxis 7/1/03 (unpublished data)
- High risk: age >65 yr with comorbidity, prolonged immobility, stroke/paralysis, prior DVT, family history of venous thromboembolism (VTE), cancer, obesity (BMI >30), venous insufficiency, cardiac dysfunction, indwelling central line, nephritic syndrome, estrogen, smoking, thrombophilia/hypofibrinolysis, bilateral TKA

– Very high risk: antiphospholipid syndrome, protein C/S deficiency, anti-III deficiency or history of PE
– TKA (all boot and hypotensive epidurals): low risk: ASA or Coumadin or LMWH; high risk: Coumadin or LMWH; very high risk: LMWH ± inferior vena cava (IVC) filter

Complications
– Bleeding complications (wound hematomas, gastrointestinal bleeds):
  – 5% for INR 1.5–2.0
  – 1% for INR 1.3–1.5
– Bleeding complications two times higher with LMWH versus warfarin

Anatomy
– Lesser and greater saphenous veins—superficial
– Popliteal vein—deep at knee
– Anterior tibial vein—deep below knee
– Posterior tibial vein—deep below knee

Diagnosis
– Doppler after total joint replacement
  – Compared with venogram
  – 82% sensitive
  – 97% specific
  – Better diagnosis with proximal clots
– Clot above knee or popliteal fossa
  – Common femoral vein, superficial femoral vein, popliteal vein
  – Treatment = LMWH (1 mg/kg q12) and/or Coumadin (INR 2.0–2.5 for 3–6 mo)
– Clot below knee (calf clot)
  – Peroneal vein
  – Surgeon/medical attending specific
  – Most arthroplasty surgeons treat with LMWH and INR 2.0–2.5 for 3–6 mo, ± repeat Doppler; some may give SQH or 0.5 mg/kg LMWH
  – Most sports/medical attendings treat with LMWH 0.5–1.0 mg/kg and INR 2.0–2.5 for 3–6 mo, ± repeat Doppler
– No clot
  – INR 1.8–2.5 for 6 wk (this number changing, used to be 1.5–2.0 and some say 1.8–2.5, by new warfarin nomogram [Anderson et al., 2002])

Physiology
– Clotting pathway
  – Prothrombin time (PT) affected by extrinsic (PeT, involves tissue factor)
  – Partial thromboplastin time (PTT) affected by intrinsic (PiTT, involves only blood components)
  – These two pathways converge with activation of factor X, which activates thrombin (factor II), which converts fibrinogen to fibrin
  – Plasmin digests fibrin

– ASA
  – Irreversibly inhibits clotting for life span of platelet
– Warfarin (Coumadin)
– Vitamin K is cofactor in postribosomal synthesis of these clotting factors
– Warfarin blocks regeneration of vitamin K epoxide
– Half-lives
– Prot C: 8 hr
– Prot S: 30 hr
– II: 60 hr
– VII: 4–6 hr
– IX: 24 hr
– X: 48–72 hr
– Thus, warfarin affects VII, IX, X, and then II sequentially
– Effects occur within 24 hr
– Peak may be delayed 72–96 hr
– Duration of single dose is 2–5 days
– Peak concentration reached in 4 hr
– Patients >60 yr have higher INR response
– Asians have higher INR response
  – Chinese average 3.3 mg daily for INR 2–2.5
– Men >180 lb have highest risk of being subtherapeutic
– Maintenance dose of 4–5 mg usually achieves INR 2.0 in 4–5 days
– 1 mg PO vitamin K is effective to reduce INR 4.5–9.5 in nonbleeding patient to INR 2–3 within 24 hr
– Cimetidine and Bactrim slow warfarin breakdown via competing for P450
– phenobarbital, rifampin speed up warfarin breakdown by revving up P450
– LMWH (enoxaparin, Lovenox)
  – One-third less heparin-induced thrombocytopenia (HIT) versus heparin
  – Blocks Xa more than IIa
  – IIa needed for local hemostasis
  – Xa is essential in thrombosis
  – More bioavailable than heparin
  – Same bleeding rate as heparin
– Fondaparinux
  – Synthetic pentasaccharide that selectively inhibits activated factor X
  – DVT at day 11 after hip fracture ORIF was 8.3% in fondaparinux group and 19.1% in Lovenox group. No difference in bleeding (Eriksson et al., 2001)
  – DVT at day 11 was 12% after major knee surgery versus 28% with Lovenox (Bauer et al., 2001)
– Heparin
  – Binds to antithrombin III and increases its inhibition of IIa and Xa equally
  – Less effective than LMWH in prevention of proximal DVT after THR

Anterior view

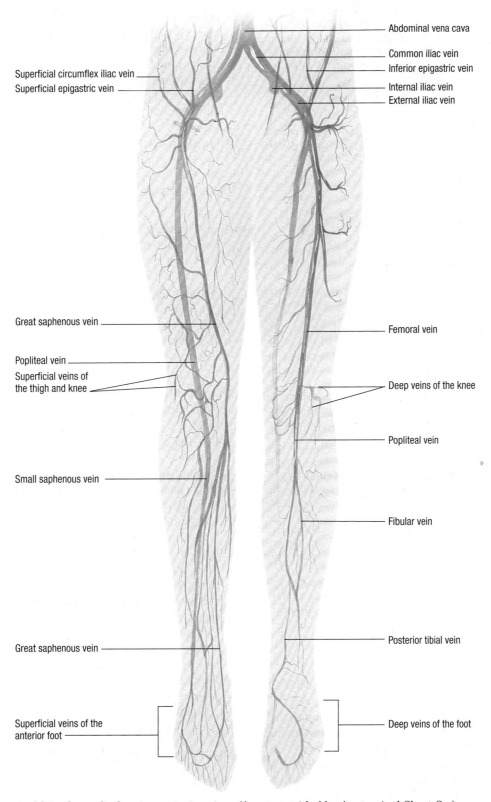

Superficial circumflex iliac vein
Superficial epigastric vein

Abdominal vena cava
Common iliac vein
Inferior epigastric vein
Internal iliac vein
External iliac vein

Great saphenous vein

Popliteal vein

Superficial veins of
the thigh and knee

Small saphenous vein

Great saphenous vein

Superficial veins of the
anterior foot

Femoral vein

Deep veins of the knee

Popliteal vein

Fibular vein

Posterior tibial vein

Deep veins of the foot

Major lower limb veins: anterior view. (Asset provided by Anatomical Chart Co.)

Bibliography

Eriksson BI, et al. Prevention of deep-vein thrombosis and pulmonary embolism after total hip replacement: comparison of low-molecular-weight heparin and unfractionated heparin. J Bone Joint Surg Am 1991; 73(4):484–493.

Ries MD, et al. Pulmonary function during and after total hip replacement: findings in patients who have insertion of a femoral component with and without cement. J Bone Joint Surg Am 1993; 75(4):581–587.

References

Anderson DR, et al. Comparison of a nomogram and physician-adjusted dosage of warfarin for prophylaxis against deep-vein thrombosis after arthroplasty. J Bone Joint Surg Am 2002; 84:1992–1997.

Bauer KA, et al. Steering Committee of the Pentasaccharide in Major Knee Surgery Study. Fondaparinux compared with enoxaparin for the prevention of venous thromboembolism after elective major knee surgery. N Engl J Med 2001; 345(18):1305–1310.

DiGiovanni CW, et al. The safety and efficacy of intraoperative heparin in total hip arthroplasty. Clin Orthop 2000; (379):178–185.

Eriksson BI, et al. Steering Committee of the Pentasaccharide in Hip-Fracture Surgery Study. Fondaparinux compared with enoxaparin for the prevention of venous thromboembolism after hip-fracture surgery. N Engl J Med 2001; 345(18):1298–1304.

Freedman KB, et al. A meta-analysis of thromboembolic prophylaxis following elective total hip arthroplasty. J Bone Joint Surg Am 2000; 82(7):929–938.

Westrich GH, Sculco TP. Prophylaxis against deep venous thrombosis after total knee arthroplasty. Pneumatic plantar compression and aspirin compared with aspirin alone. J Bone Joint Surg Am 1996; 78(6):826–834.

Westrich GH, et al. The incidence of venous thromboembolism after total hip arthroplasty: a specific hypotensive epidural anesthesia protocol. J Arthroplasty 1999; 14(4):456–463.

Westrich GH, et al. Meta-analysis of thromboembolic prophylaxis after total knee arthroplasty. J Bone Joint Surg Br 2000; 82(6):795–800.

Westrich GH, et al. Thromboembolic disease prophylaxis in total knee arthroplasty using intraoperative heparin and postoperative pneumatic foot compression. J Arthroplasty 1999; 14(6):651–656.

Westrich GH, et al. VenaFlow plus Lovenox vs VenaFlow plus aspirin for thromboembolic disease prophylaxis in total knee arthroplasty. J Arthroplasty 2006; 21(6 Suppl 2):139–143.

SOFT TISSUE COMPLICATIONS

Neurovascular

- Arterial complication very little from 0.2% to 0.3%, increasing with Minimal incision TKA
- Complications are usually occlusion/thrombus, partial or total arterial division, and arteriovenous malformation (AVM) or false aneurysm
- Thrombus most associated with atherosclerotic disease, requires emergent thrombectomy/bypass
- Preoperative evaluation of patients with peripheral vascular disease (PVD) is recommended with vascular studies, bypass if needed
- Role of tourniquet with these PVD patients and old bypass patients is controversial
- Peroneal palsy most common from 0.3% to 4.0%, associated with valgus knees, large flexion contracture, and prior knee surgery (HTO)
- Mechanisms are aggressive retraction/limb realignment (traction neurapraxia) or direct pressure (hematoma/tight bandage)
- Patients at high risk should have loose bandages, and knee should stay flexed until peroneal function returns
- Usually partial palsies return, sensory better than motor, while complete have more variable courses
- No role for primary neurolysis, but with residual deficit at 3 mo, it may be indicated

Wound Problems

- Beware of large, thin skin flaps, if lifting flaps keep all SQ with it
- Parallel incisions should have ratio 1:4 from distance between them versus length of incision
- Use longest and most lateral scar, avoid larger lateral flap
- May need plastics preoperatively and tissue expander
- Bisect transverse incisions at 90 degrees

Arthrofibrosis

- Most common cause of stiffness is poor preoperative ROM
- Can also be caused by flexion contracture in contralateral knee
- Walking needs 60 degrees flexion
- Stair climbing needs 90 degrees flexion
- Getting out of chair needs 100 degrees flexion
- Manipulation under anesthesia (MUA) may be effective in first 3 mo postop, after that time, increased risk of fracture
- Also arthroscopic versus open arthrolysis—better than MUA because can use to rule out infection
- Preoperative ROM is the strongest predictor of postoperative ROM usually
- Flexion contractures that are corrected at time of surgery and that return postoperatively are usually due to hamstring tightness due to quad inhibition
- Hamstring tightness resolves by 6 mo postoperatively
- Beware other causes: low-grade infection, reflex sympathetic dystrophy (RSD), overstuffed components

HETEROTOPIC OSSIFICATION

Requirements

- Pluripotential cells
- Transforming stimulus
- Suitable local environment

Risk Factors
- Hypertrophic arthritis
- Ankylosing spondylitis
- Diffuse idiopathic skeletal hyperostosis, aka Forestier disease
- Posttraumatic arthritis
- Male > female
- Cemented arthroplasty
- Direct lateral (aka Harding) approach
- Prior history of heterotopic ossification (HO), especially if seen on contralateral hip
- Prior hip fusion
- Extensive soft tissue dissection or bony resection

Incidence
- Approximately 13% (3%–50%), but only 2%–7% have significant limitations due to HO
- Significant reduction due to use of NSAIDs in post-op pain protocols

Symptoms
- Limited ROM
- Usually not painful
- No associated muscle weakness

Brooker Classification (Based on AP XR)
- I—bony islands in soft tissue
- II—>1 cm between opposing bone
- III —<1 cm between opposing bone
- IV—XR ankylosis
- Histologically similar to myositis ossificans (may even see areas of marrow)
- Once HO is evident on XR, no treatment is available to prevent further progression
- Maturity assessed by XR to determine time for excision
- If excised, *must* use prophylaxis to prevent recurrence

Treatment/Prophylaxis
- Older diphosphonates
- Inhibits matrix mineralization
- HO appears after medications stopped: no long-term prophylaxis seen
- Largely abandoned
- Postoperative radiation: 700 cGy within 72 hr (within 48 hr optimal)
  - Shield porous ingrowth parts of new THA/TKA (i.e., noncemented areas)
  - Reports of bone sarcoma with doses as low as 1,200 cGy
- Indomethacin 75 mg PO QD for 6 wk

Bibliography

Brooker AF, et al. Ectopic ossification following total hip replacement: incidence and a method of classification. J Bone Joint Surg Am 1973; 55(8):1629–1632.

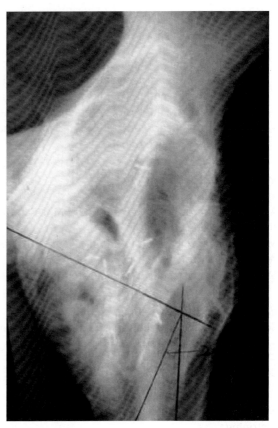

Anteroposterior hip demonstrating Brooker IV heterotopic bone formation. (From Chapman ME, et al. Chapman's Orthopaedic Surgery. Philadelphia: Lippincott Williams & Wilkins; 2001.)

Healy WL, et al. Single-dose irradiation for the prevention of heterotopic ossification after total hip arthroplasty: a comparison of doses of five hundred and fifty and seven hundred centigray. J Bone Joint Surg Am 1995; 77(4):590–595.
Hedley AK, et al. The prevention of heterotopic bone formation following total hip arthroplasty using 600 rad in a single dose. J Arthroplasty 1989; 4(4):319–325.
Purtill JJ, et al. Heterotopic ossification: incidence in cemented versus cementless total hip arthroplasty. J Arthroplasty 1996; 11(1):58–63.

WEAR AND LOOSENING IN THA

Polyethylene Wear

Biology
- Particles are phagocytized, macrophages release cytokines
- Cytokines promote local inflammation and periprosthetic bone resorption
- Particle release from components:
  - Adhesion: surface pressure pulls particles away from weaker material
  - Abrasion: mechanical process where particles are cut away from softer material

– Fatigue: local stresses exceed fatigue strength of material and release material
– Wear rates:
  – Function of number of cycles, not time
  – Higher wear rates are associated with increased activity level, male gender, younger age, larger (36 and 40 mm) head size has more volumetric wear rate
  – Measured by linear wear rates: >0.2 mm/yr have increased prevalence of osteolysis

Component Loosening
Osteolysis
– Activated macrophages activated by PMMA and particulate debris
– Macrophages release arachidonic acid and bone-resorbing factors
– Startup thigh pain indicates loose stem

Radiographic Signs of Loosening
– Seven Gruen zones surrounding femoral component
  – 1 is proximal lateral
  – 4 is distal
  – 7 is calcar

Modes of Loosening
– Pistoning
  – Stem in cement
  – Cement mantle in bone
– Media (mid)stem pivot
  – Proximal stem goes medially
  – Distal stem goes laterally
– Calcar pivots
  – Distal hang-up "windshield wiper" effect
– Cantilever bending
  – Loss of proximal support, good distal fixation
  – Leads to stem fracture

Reference
Lachiewicz PF, Heckman DS, Soileau ES, Mangla J, Martell JM. Femoral head size and wear of highly cross-linkedpolyethylene at 5 to 8 years. Clin Orthop 2009; 467:3290–3296.

HIP DISLOCATION

– 1.5% in bipolar hemiarthroplasty
– 2%–3% (0%–9%) dislocation in primary, lower rate of dislocation with anterior approach than posterior. Posterior soft-tissue repair, use of large femoral heads and proper combined anteversion significantly reduced the dislocation rate in posterior approach.
– 10% (up to 30%) dislocation in revision
– Of dislocators, 35%–40% need surgery, and despite it, 30% redislocate
– 1% of all THA need surgery for dislocation
– Elderly patients (>80 yr) who previously had surgery for femoral neck fracture, then converted to primary THA have highest number of dislocations (up to 80%)
– 80% of dislocations occur in first 3 mo
– Early dislocation caused by incomplete soft tissue healing is less likely to become recurrent

Natural History
– In one study, 35% stable after first dislocation, total 65% stable after second or third
– This justifies use of three strikes rule (i.e., patient can dislocate three times before a revision is considered)

Risk Factors for Dislocation
– Alcoholism
– Neuromuscular conditions
– Females > males
– Elderly patients
– Obese patients
– Highest risk in patients >80 yo with conversion from failed ORIF (80%)
– Posterolateral approach
– Smaller femoral head size
– Trochanteric nonunion
– Revision surgery
– Surgeon experience—rate levels off after first 30 THA, rate decreases 50% for every 10 THA done annually (Swedish study)

Stability
– Four factors influence stability:
  – Component design
  – Component position
  – Soft tissue tension
  – Soft tissue function
    – Many of these coexist

Component Design
– Head:neck ratio affects primary arc range (the amount of arc the ball can move before impingement). Avoid heads with skirts. Bigger heads get more volumetric wear
– Excursion is distance ball must travel from point of impingement to dislocation—it is equal to half of head diameter
– Elevated liners decrease primary arc but are proven to have fewer dislocations (2.2% vs. 3.9% for no liner) in one study with 5,000 THA
– Femoral offset restores tension of soft tissues
– Narrow neck taper increases head:neck ratio (increases stability)

Component Position
– Goal is to center prosthetic primary arc in center of patient's functional range

- Ideally 45-degree cup lateral abduction (35–45 degrees), 20-degree anteversion (15–30 degrees)
- Too vertical or too much or too little anteversion causes dislocation
- Optimal femoral anteversion is 15 degrees
- Avoid placing cup too medial or superior
- Very important to trial components at extremes intraoperatively

Soft Tissue Tension
- Abductors (especially gluteus medius and minimus) are key to hip stability
- Re-create anatomical head offset and neck length (based on preoperative templating)
- Must optimize abductor tension and avoid GT impingement

Soft Tissue Function
- Central problems (brain, brainstem, spinal cord): uncoordinated muscle firing, spasticity
- Peripheral problems (peripheral nerves, muscles): neuropathy, soft tissue trauma
- Think infection as possible dislocation due to fluid accumulation and failed healing of capsular tissues

- Osteophytes and cement that are not removed during surgery may cause impingement leading to dislocation

Relocation
- Dislocation diagnosed with excess pain on ROM, usually shortened/internally rotated in posterior dislocation
- Understand direction of dislocation
- Examine ROM under anesthesia after relocation (increased chance of needing revision if dislocates easily)
- Knee immobilizer for posterior dislocations to avoid hip and knee flexion during ADLs
- Abduction brace for 4–8 wk after reduction
- Two-thirds will only dislocate once

Options for Revision
- Study factors that caused dislocation (usually one of four overrides others)
- Increase head size to change primary arc range
- GT advancement to increase abductor tension
- Reposition components
- Constrained liner if soft tissue function is poor

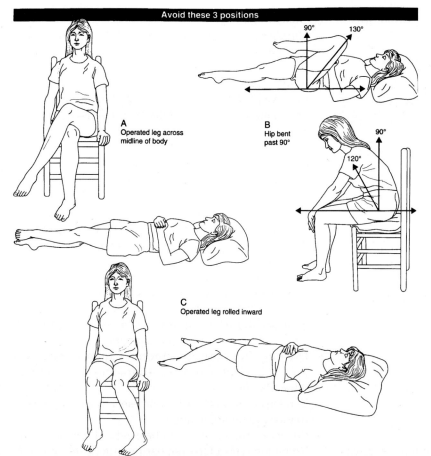

These hip precautions are taught to all total hip arthroplasty patients to prevent dislocation. (From Maher AB, et al., eds. Orthopaedic Nursing. Philadelphia: WB Saunders; 1994:552.)

- Conversion to hemiarthroplasty with large head
- Resection arthroplasty

Wound Closure (Mahoney & Pellicci, 2003; Pellicci et al., 1998)
- Meticulous posterior repair of capsule, external rotators, quadratus, and gluteus maximus tendon
- For Pellicci et al. (1998), dislocation rate was 4% in 395 with external rotator only repair and decreased to 0% in additional 395 with full repair (1-yr follow-up)
- For Poss (Pellicci et al., 1998), 6.2% dislocated in 160 patients with no posterior repair versus 0.8% in 124 hips after full repair (6-mo follow-up)

Bibliography

Ekelund A. Trochanteric osteotomy for recurrent dislocation of total hip arthroplasty. J Arthroplasty 1993; 8(6):629–632.

Fackler CD, Poss R. Dislocation in total hip arthroplasties. Clin Orthop 1980; (151):169–178.

Khatod M, et al. An analysis of the risk of hip dislocation with a contemporary total joint registry. Clin Orthop 2006; 447: 19–23.

References

Mahoney CR, Pellicci PM. Complications in primary total hip arthroplasty: avoidance and management of dislocations. Instr Course Lect 2003; 52:247–255.

Pellicci PM, et al. Posterior approach to total hip replacement using enhanced posterior soft tissue repair. Clin Orthop Relat Res 1998; (355):224–228.

PERIPROSTHETIC FEMORAL FRACTURES

Epidemiology
- Address fracture union and prosthetic stability
- Intraoperative fracture in 3.5% uncemented primaries, in 0.4% cemented
- Postoperative periprosthetic fracture incidence 0.1%
- Ingrowth tends to fracture within 6 mo
- Cemented tends to fracture after >5 yr

Classification
Vancouver Classification
- Classify by region, pattern, and prosthetic stability
  - A: fracture proximal to prosthesis (around greater or LT) stable versus unstable
  - B: fracture at or just below stem
    - B1: femoral component fixed
    - B2: femoral component loose
    - B3: severe bone loss
  - C: fracture well below stem tip

Treatment
Proximal Region
- Usually longitudinal splits
- Stable if split proximal to LT
- Unstable is complete two-part fracture that requires cerclage wiring, ± long stem
- Consider prophylactic cerclage wiring in osteopenia

Middle Region
- Between LT and implant tip
- 50% associated with prosthesis loosening
- High union rate regardless of treatment
- Distal stem may provide stability
- Noncomminuted more stable
- To prevent intraoperative fracture, leave old hardware in place until after hip dislocated and cut neck before dislocation
- If previously loose stem, revise to long stem
- If well fixed, treat the fracture

Distal Region
- 25%–40% nonunion if nonoperative treatment
- Low rates of implant loosening
- At tip or distal to tip
- Can be intraoperative with straight implant affecting anterior bow of femur
- Intraoperative stem perforation—need bone graft, long stem replacement
- Leave implant in place if not loose
- ORIF with cerclage and plate
- Nonprosthetic retrograde intramedullary nail if fracture distal enough

Combinations
- Mid/distal fracture associated with nonunion and loosening

Prosthetic Function
- Remove prostheses that have high failure rate regardless of stability (nonmodular titanium head)
- Remove poorly functioning prostheses

Results
- Treatment based on status of prosthesis and bone quality
- Timely revision prevents progression of fracture
- If adequate diaphyseal bone stock, long stem provides intramedullary fixation and can be inserted without cement
- Impaction grafting or cemented revision long stem may be needed if deficient diaphyseal bone
- In unreconstructable proximal femur, consider allograft/prosthesis composite in young and proximal femoral replacement in old patients
- Fracture in loose prosthesis requires long-stem porous implant that bypasses fracture by two times bone diameter
- Cerclage fixation alone is poor, use only as supplement to intramedullary fixation
- Cortical strut allograft can be used as biological plate
- Nonunion rates of treated periprosthetic femoral fracture is 3%

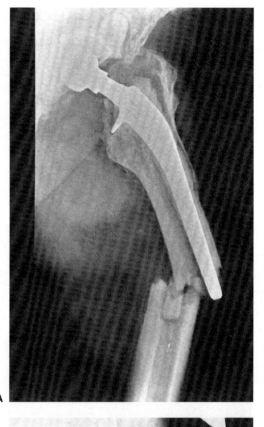

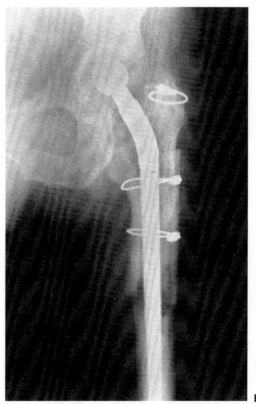

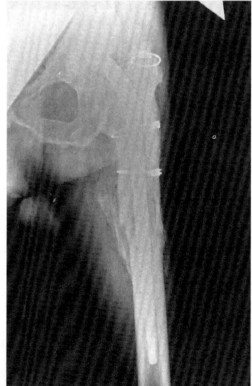

A: A periprosthetic fracture of the femur with extensive lateral cortical bone loss type IIIB and implant loosening. **B:** Immediate postoperative view showing the transfemoral approach with a distally fixed uncemented stem. **C:** After 2 yr, the osteotomy has healed, and the proximal bone stock has been reconstructed. (From Craig EV, et al. Clinical Orthopedics. Philadelphia: Lippincott Williams & Wilkins; 1999.)

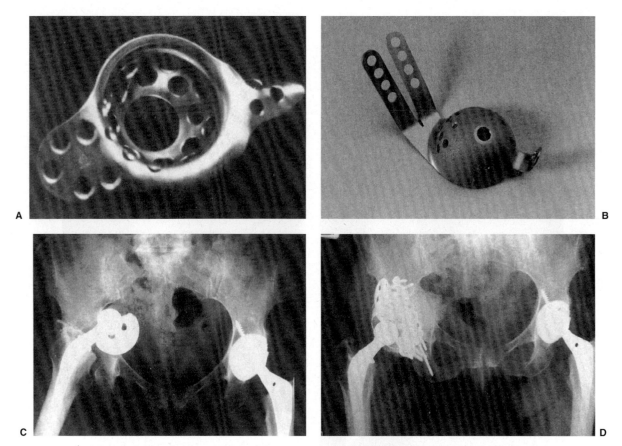

A: A Burch-Schneider ring is a type of antiprotrusio cage. **B:** The GAP (Osteonics, Allendale, NJ) cup has a teardrop hook and ilium plates to counteract protrusion. **C:** Pelvic discontinuity following intraoperative fracture and socket migration. **D:** Anteroposterior view 2 yr after reconstruction with a Burch-Schneider ring and morcelized bone graft. (From Craig EV, et al. Clinical Orthopedics. Philadelphia: Lippincott Williams & Wilkins; 1999.)

Bibliography

Brady OH, et al. The reliability and validity of the Vancouver classification of femoral fractures after hip replacement. J Arthroplasty 2000; 15(1):59–62.

Haddad FS, et al. Periprosthetic femoral fractures around well-fixed implants: use of cortical onlay allografts with or without a plate. J Bone Joint Surg Am 2002; 84(6):945–950.

PATELLAR PROBLEMS

– Most common cause of reoperation
– Incidence is 2%–10% of TKA
– Instability, fracture, loosening, surf erosion
– Malalignment > accelerated wear

Patellar Instability/Malalignment
– Tilting, subluxation, dislocation
– Varies 1%–20%
– Best goal is prevention: externally rotate femoral component, lateralize femoral component, medialize button, tibia centered at medial one-third of tubercle—not in internal rotation

– CT useful in workup
– Lateral release only works if components well aligned; if not, then femoral-tibial component revision is necessary

Patellar Clunk Syndrome (Soft Tissue Impingement)
– Seen in PCL-sacrificing TKA
– Fibrous lump on superior pole of patella gets caught in box of PCL sacrificed femoral component as knee extended from 60 to 30 degrees
– Common in IB-II TKAs because sudden edge from trochlea into box
– Scope or open débridement
– Incidence of asymptomatic crepitation: 10–15%
– Incidence of painful crepitation: 5%

Patellar Component Wear/Loosening
– Relatively uncommon <1%
– Factors associated with it are osteonecrosis of patella, patella fracture, subluxation, osteoporosis, malposition, improper patellar resection, improper cement

fixation, osteolysis, altered joint line, and metal-backed implants

Patella Baja
- Most common after HTO or tubercle transfer or fracture
- Impinges in flexion
- Avoid bone cuts that raise joint line, most common with PS knees
- Put smaller button superiorly
- Trim patellar and tibial poly at impingement points
- Risk factor for fracture
- Patellar fracture
  - Incidence 0.05%–1%
  - Technique dependent
  - Usually in small patella, females, one peg button
  - Requires screw fixation or cable

Other Complications
- Extensor mechanism rupture
  - Rare but devastating, 0.17%–2.3%
  - Etiology is mechanical, vascular, and surgical
  - Acute surgical repair has best results, may need semitendinosus or allograft for supplementation, acute from iatrogenic
  - Chronic will need extensor mechanism allograft, chronic from impingement on tibial insert, manipulation, or distal tubercle realignment procedure

WEAR AND LOOSENING IN TKA

Evaluation of Painful TKA
- History, physical examination (P/E), imaging studies, labs
- Differential diagnosis: surgical—prosthetic loosening/failure, component wear, component overhang, PF maltracking, instability, sepsis, osteolysis, arthrofibrosis, intra-articular soft tissue impingement, effusion/synovitis; nonsurgical—referred pain (back/hip), RSD, bursitis/tendonitis (pes, patella, popliteal), gout/calcium pyrophosphate dihydrate deposition disease (CPPD), neurovascular problems (neuropathy, radiculopathy, claudication, thrombophlebitis/DVT, fibromyalgia, psych, secondary gain)
- Imaging studies: x-rays, CT (component rotational position), radionucleotide studies: note bone scan is hot in uncemented knee up to 1 yr
- Well-fixed, aligned painful uninfected TKR without identified mechanical problem has only 40% success with revision

Poly Wear
- Multifactorial: surgical technique (component malalignment, instability), patient selection, and implant design (Old poly insert, less conforming implants)
- Presenting symptoms: pain, swelling, progressive osteolysis, change in component position (loosening), instability, clicking/grinding

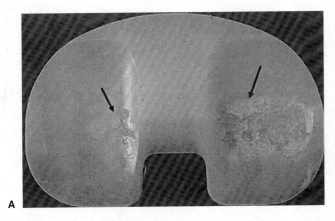

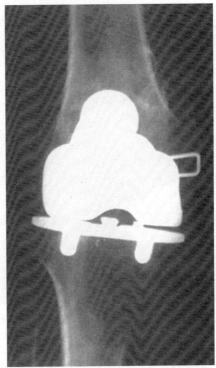

A: An example of delamination on the articular surface of a surgically retrieved polyethylene tibial insert. The delaminations (*arrows*) are well accepted and have a strong correlation with oxidation-induced embrittlement secondary to gamma sterilization. **B:** Anteroposterior radiograph of a patient with signs of failure due to polyethylene wear. (From Callaghan JJ, et al. The Adult Hip. Philadelphia: Lippincott Williams & Wilkins; 1998.)

- Poly wear patterns: post and backside wear
- Wear pattern seen on poly post in posterior stabilized knees from rotational impingement, tibial component loosening more common than femur or patella. Speculated "backside wear" is from excess motion between backside surface of poly insert and tibial component. This wear mechanism may result in loosening of the tibial component secondary to generation of poly wear debris and lysis
- Treatment: simple poly exchange unsuccessful, especially if procedure <5 yr from primary; revised TKA indicated if poly wear has associated osteolysis

Causes of Failure/Revision
- Instability
  - Ligaments
  - Malposition
  - Loosening
- Infection
- Massive wear
- Fracture
- Ankylosis
- Unexplained pain

PERIPROSTHETIC KNEE FRACTURES

Periprosthetic Fracture
- 0.3%–2%, most common in elderly females
- Other risk factors: RA, osteoporosis, chronic steroid use, and notching of anterior femoral cortex
- Goal of treatment: restore prefracture functional status (ROM of knee), well-aligned knee, well-fixed components, and healed fracture
- Must assess if components are loose and fracture is displaced!

Supracondylar Fracture
- Debatable whether anterior notch weakens bone, one study (Culp et al., 1987) shows 29.2% decrease in torsional strength of distal femur such as RA versus study (Ritter, 1988) with no correlation between notching and fracture
- Can be caused by excess force at MUA
- Many classifications systems—Neer, Digioia/Rubash, Chen, and Lewis/Rorabaeck—not widely used in older patients or not cleared for surgery

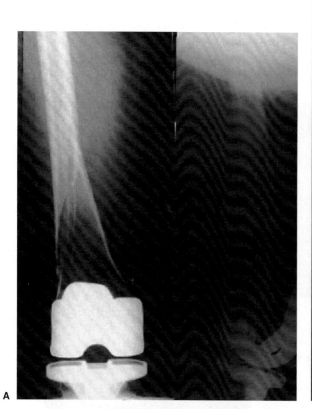
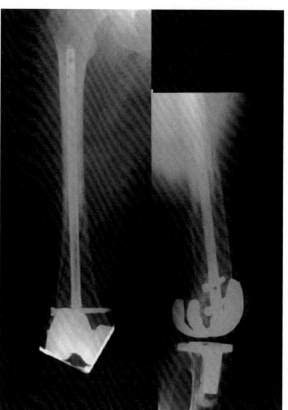

A: Periprosthetic distal femoral fracture 3 mo after a successful total knee arthroplasty. **B:** Closed reduction and static locked reamed full-length retrograde femoral intramedullary nail fixation. (From Bucholz RW, Heckman JD. Rockwood & Green's Fractures in Adults, 5th ed. Philadelphia: Lippincott Williams & Wilkins; 2001.)

- Treatment: long leg cast (LLC)/traction, buttress plates/fixed-angle device, less invasive stabilization system (LISS) plate, retrograde IM nail, anterograde IM nail, revised TKA with stems (Su et al., 2004)

Tibial Fracture
- Uncommon but fundamental principle is the same; if components are well fixed, then traditional fracture methods based on displacement (LLC vs. plate, etc.); if components are loose, then long-stem revision for distal fixation ± proximal tibia reconstruction

Patella Fracture
- Associated with patella cuts <10–15 mm, this cut substantially increases patella strain
- Also associated with osteonecrosis (sacrifice of lateral geniculate artery) or patella baja
- Treatment based on pattern (Goldberg classification)
- <2 mm displacement, nonoperative with cast in extension
- >2 mm displacement, surgical fixation, less reliable outcome; Windsor (1989) indicates all patella fractures be treated in LLC unless cement–prosthesis interface is disrupted, then best treated with patellectomy

References
Culp RW, et al. Supracondylar fracture of the femur following prosthetic knee arthroplasty. Clin Orthop Relat Res 1987; (222):212–222.
Ritter MA, et al. Anterior femoral notching and ipsilateral supracondylar femur fracture in total knee arthroplasty. J Arthroplasty 1988; 3(2):185–187.
Su ET, et al. Periprosthetic femoral fractures above total knee replacements. J Am Acad Orthop Surg 2004; 12(1): 12–20.
Windsor RE, et al. Patellar fractures in total knee arthroplasty. J Arthroplasty 1989; 4 Suppl:S63–S67.

Revision

REVISION TOTAL HIP REPLACEMENT

THA—Revision Cup
Epidemiology
- In cemented THA, the most common reason for failure is cup
- In uncemented THA, the most common reason for failure is stem
- Groin pain
- Loose cup is better tolerated than loose femur
- Indications include component loosening, polyethylene wear, and osteolysis

DeLee-Charnley Zones for Cup
- Vertical and horizontal lines drawn from center head
  - Zone 1—superolateral
  - Zone 2—superomedial
  - Zone 3—inferomedial
- Acetabulum loose if:
  - >2 mm lucency in all three zones
  - Progressive lucency in zones 1 and 2
  - Component position changes

Acetabular Deficiencies (Paprosky's classification)
- I—little migration and osteolysis
  - Uncemented hemisphere cup ± screws
- II—superior migration <2 cm
- IIa—superomedial migration, rim intact
  - Morcellized bone graft, large uncemented cup
- IIb—superolateral migration, segmental loss of superior rim
  - Oblong cup
  - Uncemented cup with modular augment
  - Small cup placed high hip center
- IIc—teardrop lysis, loss of medial wall
  - Jumbo noncement cup
- IIIa—>2 cm socket migration, ischial osteolysis, missing rim
  - Requires strut graft
- IIIb—Kohler line disrupted indicating profound medial loss, ± pelvic discontinuity
  - Needs antiprotrusio cage
  - Pelvic reconstruction plates to ORIF
  - Acetabular allograft

Acetabular Deficiencies (American Academy of Orthopaedic Surgeons Hip Committee)
- I—defect in column
- II—cavitary defect within rim of bone
  - Most common
- III—combined cavitary and segmental bone loss
- IV—pelvic discontinuity
- V—prior arthrodesis

Treatment
- First choice is porous hemisphere cup with superior screws
  - More than two-thirds of rim must remain
  - Needs good rim fit
  - Cavitary defect with intact rim filled with particulate graft
- Strut allograft with reconstruction cage
  - For rim and/or cavitary defect
  - All polyethylene cup cemented into cage
  - 50% failure if cemented or noncemented cup placed on strut graft without cage
- Use large, noncemented cup if anterior and posterior columns are intact
  - Fill defects with morselized bone

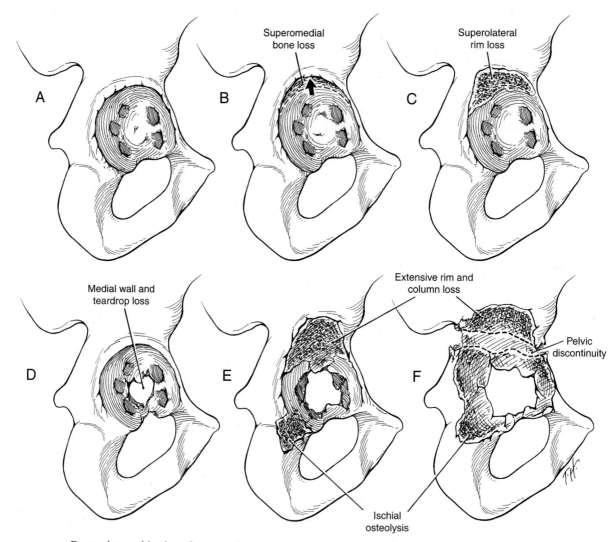

Paprosky et al.'s classification of acetabular bone loss in revision total hip replacement: **(A)** type 1, **(B)** type 2A, **(C)** type 2B, **(D)** type 2C, **(E)** type 3A, and **(F)** type 3B. (From Craig EV, et al. Clinical Orthopedics. Philadelphia: Lippincott Williams & Wilkins; 1999.)

- Bone stock lost if anterior and posterior columns widened to fit jumbo cup to provide superior coverage
- Indications for cage:
  - In severe disruption of acetabular bone stock, when cementless acetabular component cannot be stabilized in bed of structurally sound viable host bone, with or without strut graft
  - In pelvic discontinuity, to provide link between ischium and ilium
  - Cup should have at least 8 mm of thickness as it is cemented into cage

THA—Revision Stem
Epidemiology
- Hip sees two to eight times body weight at 1 million cycles/yr
- Startup thigh pain indicates loose stem

- Gruen zones 1–7
  - 1 is proximal lateral
  - 4 is distal
  - 7 is calcar

Modes of Loosening
- Pistoning
  - Stem in cement
  - Cement mantle in bone
- Media (mid)stem pivot
  - Proximal stem goes medially
  - Distal stem goes laterally
- Calcar pivots
  - Distal "windshield wiper" effect
- Cantilever bending
  - Loss of proximal support, good distal fixation
  - Leads to stem fracture

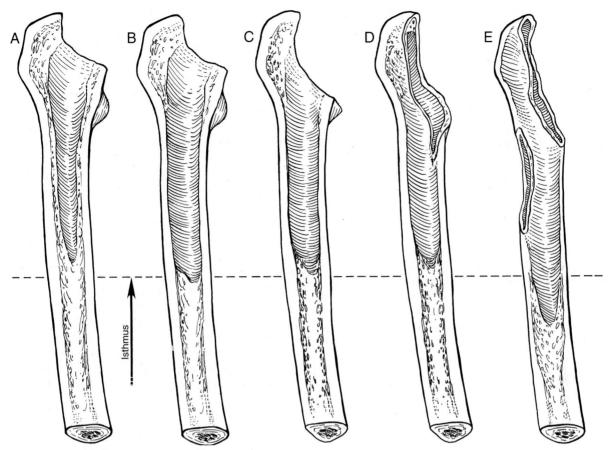

Mallory's classification of femoral bone loss in revision total hip replacement: **(A)** type I, **(B)** type II, **(C)** type IIIA, **(D)** type IIIB, and **(E)** type IIIC. (From Craig EV, et al. Clinical Orthopedics. Philadelphia: Lippincott Williams & Wilkins; 1999.)

Femoral Bone Defects (Mallory)
- I—intact cortex, cancellous remains
  - Cemented or noncemented will work
- II—no cancellous endosteum
  - Needs noncement stem
  - Can cement into distal cancellous bone but will not restore bone stock, and next revision will be harder
  - Possible Ling impaction graft
- IIIa—cortex gone to level of LT
  - Napkin ring allograft did poorly
  - May need calcar replacing stem
- IIIb—cortex gone to level of isthmus
  - If noncement, need extensive coat to fix implant in diaphyseal bone
  - If cement, need proximal femoral replacement or allograft
- IIIc—cortex gone to beyond isthmus
  - May need proximal femoral replacement or allograft
  - Cannot achieve distal fixation with extensively coated stem because canal now diverges

- May need to cement distal stem and reconstruct proximal with porous stem and bone grafting

Treatment
- Consider prophylactic cerclage wires
- First choice is uncemented, extensively coated long stem (2–3 cm below original stem), anatomical medullary locking stem
- If cortex is violated, long stem should pass hole by >2.5 shaft diameters
- Fill ectatic cavitary defects with particulate graft
- Reconstruct segmental defects with cortical strut, cables
- Ling impaction bone grafting
- Morsel fresh-frozen allograft packed tightly into ectatic canal
- Smooth tapered stem cemented into allograft
- Requires intact cortical tube

Caveats
- Intraoperative stability is a must
- Cemented stem leads to failure compared to uncemented because cement fixation requires cancellous

interstices, which is gone after old cement comes out

- No need to bypass old cement plug unless cortical bone is thinned and needs to be bypassed

Surgical Approaches

Transfemoral Approach

- First split GT in half in coronal plane
- Extend split into abductors
- Second osteotomy just anterior to linea aspera
- Distal cut at end of cement mantle
- Must keep vastus lateralis attached to lateral femur

Extended Trochanteric Osteotomy

- In standard trochanteric osteotomy, vastus origin is taken 1 cm distal to vastus ridge, then flat or chevron osteotomy, anterior and posterior capsule released, and entire GT is reflected proximally with abductors attached
- In extended trochanteric osteotomy, entire GT is elevated, but distal osteotomy is made farther down the shaft

Bibliography

Callaghan JJ, et al. Results of revision for mechanical failure after cemented total hip replacement, 1979 to 1982: a two to five-year follow-up. J Bone Joint Surg Am 1985; 67(7):1074–1085.

Engh CA Jr, et al. Extensively porous-coated femoral revision for severe femoral bone loss: minimum 10-year follow-up. J Arthroplasty 2002; 17(8):955–960.

Padgett DE, et al. Revision of the acetabular component without cement after total hip arthroplasty: three to six-year follow-up. J Bone Joint Surg Am 1993; 75(5):663–673.

Paprosky WG, et al. Acetabular defect classification and surgical reconstruction in revision arthroplasty: a 6-year follow-up evaluation. J Arthroplasty 1994; 9(1):33–44.

Pellicci PM, et al. Long-term results of revision total hip replacement: a follow-up report. J Bone Joint Surg Am 1985; 67(4):513–516.

REVISION TOTAL KNEE ARTHROPLASTY

Stages

- Exposure—extensile, may need to add V-Y quad plasty, tubercle osteotomy or quad snip
- Component removal—minimize further bone loss/ fracture, generally 4 mm of bone is removed for well-fixed implant; if significant osteolysis, then thorough synovectomy
- Soft tissue balancing—same principles, effectiveness of collateral ligament repair/advancement in revision situation, more likely to use constrained CCK. CCK does not make up for flexion-extension gaps. CCK for varus/valgus and anterior/posttranslation. Need flexion-extension gaps to be symmetric
- Bone resection/assessment of bone loss—as minimal as possible, balance a fresh smooth cancellous bed versus large defect. May need to resect more bone from femur notch if converting to PS
- Joint-line restoration—assuming one lost 4–8 mm of distal femur, will need augments to restore joint line. In addition, 2–4 mm of tibia can be lost; restore it by adding 2 mm to insert. Joint line should be 2 cm above fib head; look at patella for joint height re-creation
- PF joint—restore PF tracking as primary; landmarks can be eroded. Scarring can create patella infera—can elevate patella by using smaller implant more proximally/superiorly on native patella. Role of extensor mechanism allograft for severe cases

Other Issues

Stems

- IM stems are used when there is need for additional constraint or for enhanced rigidity when significant bone loss compromises normal fixation. Stems come in various lengths, widths, and configurations
- Usually "press-fit" stems with cemented metaphysis (Bostrom & Haas, 1996; 85% G/E at 3-yr follow-up, 85% 8-yr survival), although cemented stems are occasionally used
- Recent trend toward using longer stems with real press fit into bone, careful for fracture
- Stems >125 mm may need to be bowed for more length and more stability
- in infection cases, all cement should be removed
- in non-infection cases, in cement mantle is good, cement-in-cement technique can also be used

Constraint (Laxity)

- Mild laxity—PS
- More laxity—CCK
- Collateral insufficiency—hinged prosthesis/Finn/distal femur replacement or proximal tibia replacement

Bone Defects

- Classification systems designed to determine bone graft (BG) supplementation and type of prosthesis
- Types of supplementation are autogenous BG, morcellized or bulk allograft, cement, bone substitutes, and modular metal augmentation
- Tibial defects by percent and degree
- Contained (cortical rim intact)—particulate graft and/or cement
- Noncontained (no rim)—prosthetic augment (in defects up to 15 mm)
- Massive—structural allograft (defects >2 cm)
- Anderson Orthopaedic Research Institute
  - Type 1—intact bone, normal joint line, use primary style component

- Type 2—damaged bone, with loss of cancellous bone and incorrect joint line, need revision modular component with stems
  - Type 2A—one condyle
  - Type 2B—both condyles
- Type 3—large osteolytic legion, severe component migration, epicondyles are flared away; options include hinged or custom-designed implant, or repair of metaphysis with allograft and long stem
- Signs of poor revision (Bostrom & Haas, 1996)
  - Very small femur
  - Flexion gap composed of thick poly with patella baja and high joint line
- Haas and Bostrom (1996)
  - Establish femoral size using prior landmarks and posterior augments
  - Adjust flexion gap first
  - Then adjust extension gap by adding on distal femur
  - Some implants (Genesis II) already have distal augment built in
- Overall goals
  1) Re-establish tibial platform
  2) Reconstruct flexion gap
     - Femoral rotation, size, poly thickens
  3) Stabilize knee in position of extension

References

Bostrom MP, Haas SB. Revision total knee arthroplasty due to aseptic failure. Am J Knee Surg 1996; 9(2):91–98.

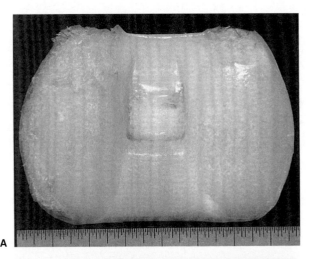

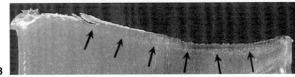

A: A retrieved posterior-stabilized tibial component showing severe wear damage. **B:** A thin cross section taken through the component shows the bearing surface of one of the plateaus (*top*). The *arrows* highlight a damaged subsurface band that contributes to the delamination; the region can be confirmed as highly degraded through density or infrared spectroscopy measurements. (From Callaghan JJ, et al. The Adult Knee. Philadelphia: Lippincott Williams & Wilkins; 2003.)

CHAPTER 2

Sports

Joshua S. Dines, Andrew D. Pearle, Christopher C. Dodson

Anatomy of Knee
ACL
PCL
MCL
LCL
Menisci
Patella
Anatomy of Medial Knee
Anatomy of Posterolateral
Knee
Knee Physical Exam
PF Joint
Varus, Valgus Instability
ACL
PCL
PLc
Menisci
Patella
Knee X-Ray
Meniscal Tears
Classification by Location
Type of Tear
Popliteal Cysts
Fairbanks Changes
Partial Meniscectomy
Meniscal Repair Techniques
Ideal Indications for Repair
Complications
Postrepair MRI
Knee MRI
Basics
Menisci
Grades
Cruciates
Meniscofemoral Ligaments
Collaterals
Cartilage
OCD (Osteochondritis Dessicans)
Classification

Chondromalacia
Outerbridge Classification for
Chondromalacia
Patellar Dislocation
Anatomy
Natural History
Patellar Tendonitis (Jumper's Knee)
Patellofemoral Pain
Patellar Subluxation
Merchant View
Nonoperative
Operative
Patellar Tilt
Rehab
**Anterior Cruciate Ligament
(ACL)**
Pathophysiology
Natural History
Grafts
Treatment
Rehab
ACL—Arthroscopic Procedure Transtibial
Technique
ACL—Pediatric
Posterior Cruciate Ligament
MRI
Primary Repair
Reconstruction
Indications
Posterolateral Corner
Anatomy
Physical Examination
Imaging
Treatment
Chondral Defects
Acute Cartilage Injury
Options
Treatment Based On

High Tibial Osteotomy (HTO)
Medial Opening Technique
Lateral Closing Technique
Hip Pain in Athlete
Differential Diagnosis
Differential Diagnosis by
Physical Exam
Hip Snapping
Anatomy of Shoulder
Anatomy of Shoulder—Nerves
Shoulder Physical Exam
Block to ER (Active = Passive) Differential
Diagnosis
Wright
Roos Test
Glenohumeral Translation
Sulcus Sign
Generalized Laxity
Impingement Sign
Shoulder X-ray Studies
True AP
Axillary Lateral
West Point
Stryker Notch
Garth
Zanca
Hobbs
Serendipity
Supraspinatus Outlet
30-Degree Caudal Tilt View
Bicipital Groove View
Shoulder MRI
Systematic Approach
RTC Tear
Labrum
Biceps Tendon
Acromioclavicular (AC)
Joint Injury
Anatomy
Classification
Imaging
Treatment
Arthroscopic Acromioplasty
Indications
Contraindications
Results
Categories of Failures
Adhesive Capsulitis
Classification
Differential Diagnosis
Evaluation
Clinical Stages
Treatment
Rotator Cuff Disease
Pathophysiology

Imaging
Treatment
Subscapularis Tear
Isolated Tear
Irreparable Tear
Scapular Winging
Medial
Lateral
Internal Impingement
MR Findings
Shoulder Dislocation
Recurrence
Shoulder Dislocation:
Complications
Shoulder Instability—Anterior
Static Restraints
Biomechanics
Pathologic Lesions
Shoulder Instability—Multidirectional (MD)
Pathophysiology
History and Physical Examination
Treatment
Shoulder Instability—Posterior
Pathophysiology
Imaging
Treatment
Chronic Locked Posterior
Dislocation
Anterior Instability—Arthroscopic
Repairs
Transglenoid Suture
Cannulated Suretac
Anterior Instability—Open Repairs
Helfet-Bristow Procedure
Magnuson-Stack
Nicola
Putti-Platt
Bone Blocks
Open Bankart
Capsular Shift
Shoulder Arthroscopy—Operative
Pearls
SLAP (Superior Labral Tears Anterior
to Posterior)
Bankart
SAD/RTC repair
Capsular Shift
SLAP Lesions
Classification
Differential Diagnosis
Treatment
Suprascapular Neuropathy
Thoracic Outlet Syndrome
Wright
Roos Test

Throwing Phases
Wind-up
Early Cocking
Late Cocking
Acceleration
Follow-through
Total Shoulder Arthroplasty
Contraindications
Technique
Rehabilitation
Results
Total Shoulder Arthroplasty:
Operative Pearls
Total Shoulder Arthroplasty Indications
Distal Biceps Rupture
Anatomy
Natural History
Operative Techniques
Results
Elbow Arthroscopy
Lateral Portals
Medial Portals
Posterior
Elbow MCL Injury
Anatomy
Pathophysiology
Medial Pain
Anterior Pain
Lateral Pain
Physical Examination
X-ray Studies
Arthroscopic Test
Remedy—Rehabilitation
Remedy—Repair
Remedy—Reconstruction
Concussions
Runner—Leg Pain Differential Diagnosis
Medial Tibial Stress Syndrome
Exertional Compartment Syndrome
Stress Fractures
Popliteal Artery Entrapment Syndrome

Anatomy of Knee

ACL

- 33 mm long, 11 mm diameter
- Anteromedial tight in flexion, isometric
- Posterolateral tight in extension, nonisometric
- (First part of name is origin on femur and second part is insertion on tibia)
- 90% type I, 10% type III collagen
- Blood supply from midgeniculate
- Secondary stabilizer to valgus stress after MCL is shot

PCL

- 38 mm long, 13 mm diameter
- Three components
  - Anterolateral tight in flexion and stronger
  - Posteromedial tight in extension
  - Meniscofemoral ligaments
- Higher tensile strength than ACL
- Both ACL and PCL help with screw home mechanism—ER of tibia with terminal extension
- Middle geniculate artery also
- PAL: PCL anterolateral
- MCL strongest, lateral collateral ligament (LCL) weakest

MCL

- Superficial MCL (sMCL) from medial femoral epicondyle to proximal tibial periosteum, deep to pes anserinus
- Deep MCL (dMCL) is capsular thickening that blends with sMCL on tibia
- Two times stiffness and tensile strength as ACL

LCL

- On lateral femoral epicondyle post and superior to popliteus and inserts on lateral fibular head
- Because behind axis of rotation, tightest in extension

MENISCI

- Mainly type I collagen
- Lateral open "O", attaches near ACL
- Medial "C", separated attachments
- Lateral plateau convex
- Medial plateau concave, thicker A to P
- Lateral moves A to P 12 mm
- Medial moves A to P 6 mm
- Menisci attached peripherally to tibia via coronary ligaments except at popliteal hiatus of lateral meniscus
- Post horn medial meniscus becomes primary anterior stabilizer in ACL-deficient knee
- Medial and lateral connected anteriorly by transverse ligament
- Meniscofemoral ligaments of Humphrey and Wrisberg to lateral meniscus
- Circumferential fibers lead to hoop tension
- Medial—50% of joint contact
- Lateral—75% of joint contact
- Medial two times thicker posteriorly
- Blood supply
- Center of rotation moves posteriorly with flexion

PATELLA

- Sees forces of three to five times body weight (BW)
- Thickest cartilage in body

- Seven facets, lateral is biggest
- Contact area moves proximally as knee is flexed
- Bipartite usually superior-lateral corner
  - Do lateral release if painful due to pull of vena lateralis

ANATOMY OF MEDIAL KNEE

Layer I
- Deep crural fascia
- Invests sartorius
- Posteriorly invests two heads of gastrocnemius and popliteal nerve structures
- Anteriorly fuses with layer II
- Saphenous nerve post to sartorius
- Tendons of gracilis and semitendinosus between layer I and layer II

Layer II
- Defined by parallel fibers of superficial MCL
- Anterior to sMCL is split in layer II
- Anterior to split is the connection of the quad mechanism to tibia
- Posterior fibers of sMCL become more oblique above and below joint
- Posteriorly merges with layer III and tendon sheath of semimembranosus to form posteromedial corner
- Semimembranosus tendon sheath sends fibers over medial condyle and across back of knee to lateral condyles to form oblique popliteal ligament
- Semimembranosus tendon anteriorly attaches to bone deep to sMCL (II) and distally to capsule (III)

Layer III
- True knee capsule with attachment at margins of articular surfaces
- Anteriorly it envelops fat pad
- Beneath the sMCL is the deep MCL
- Posteriorly II and III fuse to form posteromedial corner
- Three layers are distinct only over where fascia is directly over sMCL and dMCL

Reference
Warren LF, Marshall JL. The supporting structures and layers on the medial side of the knee: an anatomical analysis. J Bone Joint Surg Am 1979; 61(1):56–62.

ANATOMY OF POSTEROLATERAL KNEE

Layer I
- Iliotibial tract and anterior expansion
- Prepatellar bursa anteriorly
- Superfemoral biceps and post expansion
- Peroneal nerve on deep side of layer I posterior to biceps tendon

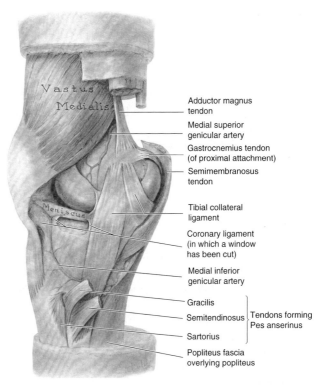

Medial view

Dissection of the right knee joint, medial view. (From Moore KL, Dalley AF II. Clinical Oriented Anatomy, 4th ed. Philadelphia: Lippincott Williams & Wilkins; 1999.)

Labels on image:
- Adductor magnus tendon
- Medial superior genicular artery
- Gastrocnemius tendon (of proximal attachment)
- Semimembranosus tendon
- Tibial collateral ligament
- Coronary ligament (in which a window has been cut)
- Medial inferior genicular artery
- Gracilis
- Semitendinosus — Tendons forming Pes anserinus
- Sartorius
- Popliteus fascia overlying popliteus

Layer II
- Very anteriorly, sticks to layer I
- Quad retinaculum anteriorly
- Posteriorly incomplete with two patellofemoral ligaments and patellomeniscal ligament

Layer III
- Lateral part of joint capsule
- Divided into superficial and deep lamina
- Superficial lamina
  - Invests LCL
  - Ends at fabellofibular ligament
  - Inferior lateral genicular vessels are between the two lamina
- Deep lamina
  - Coronary ligament
  - Popliteal hiatus
  - Ends at arcuate ligament (popliteofibular ligament)

Three anatomic variations
1. Arcuate ligament alone (13%)
   - No fabella
2. Fabellofibular ligament alone (20%)
   - Visible fabella on x-ray view
3. Both arcuate and fabellofibular (67%)
   - Cartilage fabella not seen on x-ray view
   - Palpable on physical exam

Posterolateral Corner

- LCL
  - Lateral femoral epicondyle to lateral edge of fib head (medial to biceps)
- Popliteus muscle
  - From posterior tibia, runs obliquely and inserts deep, anterior, and distal to LCL in lateral femoral epicondyle
- Popliteofibular ligament
  - From fibular head posterior and medial to biceps insertion and joins popliteus tendon just proximal to its muscle-tendon junction
- Arcuate/fabellofibular ligament
  - Arcuate is condensation of fascia over popliteus muscle
  - Arcuate runs with fabellofibular ligament from posterior apex of fibular styloid to lateral head of gastrocnemius, joined by oblique ligament of Winslow
- Capsule
  - anterior—supported by quad retinaculum
  - mid—meniscofemoral and meniscotibular ligaments
  - post—supported by arcuate ligament
- Biceps femoris
  - Short head from femur
  - Long head from ischium
  - Both insert into fibular head most posteriorly and most laterally
  - Wide attachments at iliotibial band (ITB), Gerdy, LCL
  - Externally rotates tibia
- ITB —
  - Joins intermuscular septum at its insertion into supracondylar tubercle of femur
  - Distally inserts into patella, patellar tendon, and Gerdy
  - In flexion, it externally rotates and posterially pulls tibia

Reference

Seebacher JR, et al. The structure of the posterolateral aspect of the knee. J Bone Joint Surg Am 1982; 64(4):536–541.

Knee Physical Exam

PF JOINT

- Crepitation elicited by resisted knee extension with one hand on knee
- Patellar tendonitis felt by palpating undersurface of distal patella while patella is depressed proximally

VARUS, VALGUS INSTABILITY

- Done at 0 degrees and 30 degrees with one hand on joint line

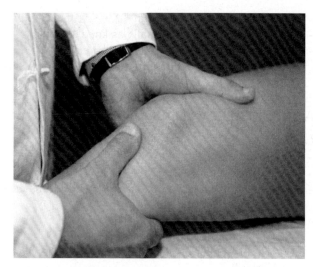

The Lachman test for anterior cruciate ligament insufficiency. (From Bucholz RW, Heckman JD. Rockwood & Green's Fractures in Adults, 5th ed. Philadelphia: Lippincott, Williams & Wilkins; 2001.)

- Opening only at 30 degrees flexion indicates isolated collateral injury
- Opening at 0 degrees and 30 degrees indicates additional injuries
- >10 degrees varus laxity at full extension suggests PCL tear with LCL

ACL

*- Lachman
  - Done at 30 degrees
  - Put pillow behind thigh if big patient
  - Most sensitive acutely
  - Measure translation and endpoint
  - If translation with firm endpoint, it may be the PCL that is torn
  - Graded I (0–5 mm), II (5–10 mm), or III (>10 mm); A firm, B soft
- *Pivot shift (Bach et al., 1988)
  - Anterior tibial subluxation at extension reduces with flexion to ~30 degrees
  - Hip abduction flexion 30 degrees, foot externally rotated, valgus stress, fingers only on tibia gently
  - Foot IR increases specificity
  - Hip abduction and ER increases pivot because ITB
  - No axial load needed
  - Grade 1+ for minimal slide to 3+ for subluxation with sensation of locking

Reference

Bach BR Jr, et al. The pivot shift phenomenon: results and description of a modified clinical test for anterior cruciate ligament insufficiency. Am J Sports Med 1988; 16(6):571–576.

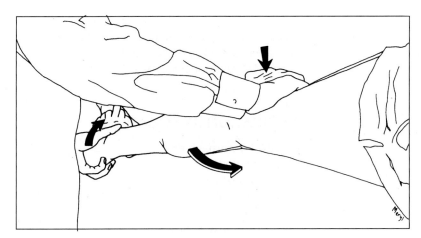

Lateral pivot shift test. Valgus force is applied to knee, fibula is pushed anteriorly, the leg is internally rotated, and the knee is then flexed. (Medi Clip image copyright © 2003 Lippincott Williams & Wilkins. All rights reserved.)

PCL

- *Posterior drawer
  - Sit on foot
  - Most sensitive for PCL
  - Grade I, II, or III
  - If drawer decreases in IR of foot, ligaments of Humphry/Wrisberg or posterolateral corner (PLc) may be OK
- Posterior sag sign
- *Quad active drawer test
  - Ask patient to move foot down table as you sit on it
  - Tibia moves anteriorly with quad contraction at ~70 degrees flexion

PLC

- *Prone passive ER test
  - Medial foot border versus femur
  - Increase by 10 degrees compared with contralateral is positive
  - Palpate tibial condyles to rule out anteromedial instability mimicking PLRI
  - Increased ER at 30 degrees that lessens at 90 degrees is isolated PLc injury
  - Increased ER at 30 degrees and 90 degrees is both PCL and PLc injured
- *Varus/valgus stress test
  - Increased varus at 30 degrees is LCL and possible additional PLc injury
  - Slightly increased varus at full extension is LCL with additional PLc injury
  - Significant increase in varus at full extension is combined PLc and PCL, and possibly ACL too
  - Increased valgus is MCL injury, which is seen commonly with PCL
- External rotation recurvatum test
  - Tibia externally rotates, varus, and recurvatum as hallux lifted off bed
  - Thought to indicate isolated PLc but if significant, ACL and maybe PCL also injured
- Posterolateral drawer test
  - Foot externally rotated for drawer
  - Not specific
- Reverse pivot shift
  - Reduction felt when flexed, externally rotated knee is extended with valgus stress
  - Positive in 35% of normal knees due to laxity, thus significant only when different from opposite side

MENISCI

- Squat test: duck walk causes pain
- McMurray test
  - IR/ER done at near maximum flexion
  - Valgus/varus stress and tibial rotation while extending knee from fully flexed position causes clicking and pain in joint line
- Apley compression test

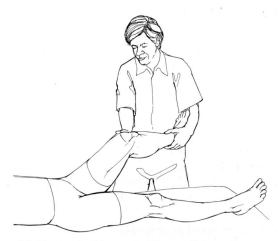

McMurray test to assess the medial meniscus.

- Steinmann test
  - Brisk tibial rotation in flexed knee
- Forced hyperextension test—posterior pain

PATELLA

- Q angle—ASIS, patella, tibial tubercle
- J sign—patella deviates laterally in terminal extension
- Apprehension
- Passive patellar tilt in extended knee
- Track patella in ER and IR; ER increases Q-angle
- Medial and lateral glide in 30-degree flexion

Knee X-Ray

- Standard anteroposterior
- 45 degrees posteroanterior weight-bearing view—joint space
- Lateral with 30 degrees flexion
- On lateral, anterior facet of lateral femoral condyle bigger to accommodate bigger lateral patellar facet. Lateral femoral condyle has two bumps versus one bump for medial
- On lateral, medial femoral condyle protrudes distally and posteriorly and appears bigger because of magnification and because it is slightly bigger
- Segond fracture—avulsion off lateral tibial plateau compared with ACL rupture
- Pellegrini-Stieda lesion—MCL calcium density
- Lateral femoral condylar notch sign
  - Sulcus terminalis deeper in chronically ACL-deficient knee
- Blumensaat line intersects bottom on patella with knee 30 degrees flexed
- Insall-Salvati ratio
- Merchant view—45 degrees flexed, to assess subluxation
- Laurin view—20 degrees flexed, to assess tilt

MENISCAL TEARS

- Accounts for 50% of knee injuries requiring surgery
- Medial three times more common than lateral in stable knee
- Posterior horn medial most common
- Anterior horn lateral least common
- Lateral tears along with ACL tears
- Traumatic
  - More peripheral
- Degenerative
  - More complex tear, posterior horn medial meniscus (PHMM)
- Location
  - Red-red (most peripheral)
  - Red-white

- White-white
- Fibers mostly longitudinal to allow compression with some radial fibers to hold it together
- Surface with random mesh for shear

CLASSIFICATION BY LOCATION

- A—posterior horn, medial
- B—body, medial
- C—anterior horn, medial
- D—anterior horn, lateral
- E—body, lateral
- F—posterior horn, lateral
- 0—capsule
- 1—red/red
- 2—red/white
- 3—white/white

TYPE OF TEAR

- Vertical versus horizontal
- Longitudinal versus radial
- Fixed ones are vertical longitudinal

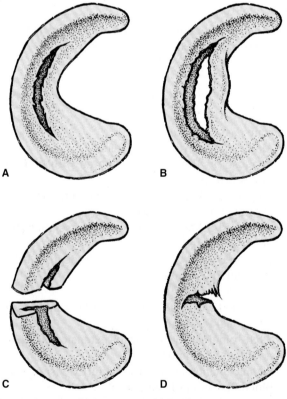

Meniscal tears: **(A)** longitudinal, **(B)** bucket-handle, **(C)** horizontal, **(D)** parrot beak. (Figure © Neil O. Hardy, Westport, CT.)

POPLITEAL CYSTS

- Between medial gastrocnemius and semimembranosus
- Along with degenerative meniscal tears in adults but not in children
- Cysts can be from very small tears not even seen by MR

FAIRBANKS CHANGES

- After total meniscectomy
- Condyle squaring
- Ridging off condyle
- Joint space narrowing

PARTIAL MENISCECTOMY

- OA risk proportional to amount removed
- Lateral meniscectomy predisposes to OA more than medial

MENISCAL REPAIR TECHNIQUES

- Healing by fibrochondrocyte
  1. Open
     - For extreme periphery
  2. Arthroscopic inside out
     - Most popular
     - Laterally, stay anterior to biceps tendon to avoid peroneal nerve
     - Medially, stay anterior to sartorius and retract deep to layer I to protect saphenous nerve
     - Better suture orientation for posterior horn
     - Need special equipment, higher rate of chondral iatrogenic injury
  3. Arthroscopic outside in
     - Better for anterior horn, allografts
     - Avoid neurovascular injury without large incision
     - Posterior horn difficult
  4. Arthroscopic all inside—FasT-Fix
     - Lower neurovascular complications
     - Shorter operation time

IDEAL INDICATIONS FOR REPAIR

- Young, no OA, no deformity
- 1–2 cm acute longitudinal tear that is unstable (moves >3 mm by probe)
- Peripheral (<3 mm from periphery)
- Repaired with ACL reconstruction because meniscus repair fails in ACL-deficient knee
- Better results with repair of lateral meniscus
- Poor prognosis if remnant has abnormal intrasubstance signal
- After repair, high signal persists for up to 2 yr indicating healing tissue. However, fluid signal indicates a failed repair or retear

COMPLICATIONS

- Saphenous nerve injury most common (9% in medial repairs)

POSTREPAIR MRI

- Increased signal (usual grade 3 or 4) is OK
- Fluid signal, however, is indicative of retear or failure of repair. Thus, look at meniscus in windows with bright fluid marker
- When meniscus repairs fail, they fail inferiorly

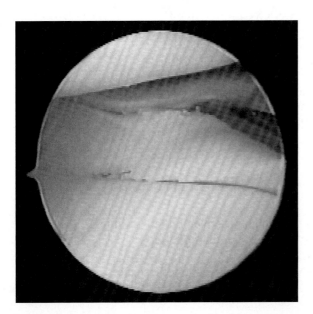

Diagnostic arthroscopy of the knee. Visualization of the posterior horn of the lateral meniscus, demonstrating a tear. The probe is placed in the superior surface of the tear. (From Koval KJ, Zuckerman JD. Atlas of Orthopaedic Surgery: A Multimedial Reference. Philadelphia: Lippincott Williams & Wilkins; 2004.)

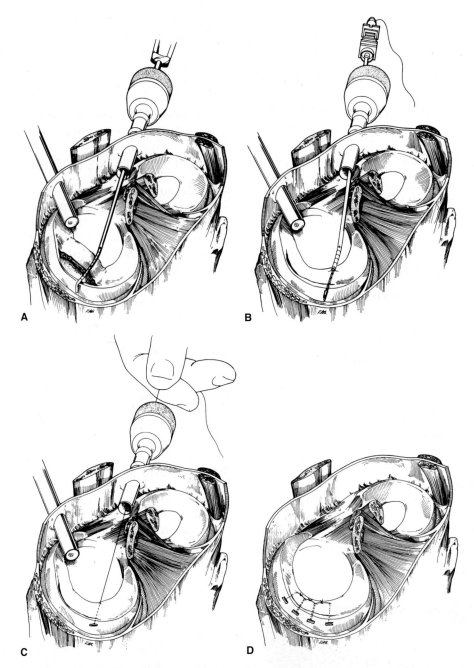

All-inside technique with the T-fix. **A:** The meniscal rim is probed and the width of the meniscus measured. **B:** The T-fix with the suture engages the meniscal tear and the peripheral rim. **C:** The T-fix and suture engaged. **D:** Multiple sutures are placed and tied within the joint. (Courtesy of Smith & Nephew)

Reference

Rodeo SA, et al. Histological analysis of human meniscal allografts. A preliminary report. J Bone Joint Surg Am 2000; 82-A(8):1071–1082.

Knee MRI

– Systematic approach
  – ACL, PCL
  – Popliteus
  – Menisci
  – MCL, LCL
  – Cartilage
– Very high negative predictive value
– Fat suppressed for overview
– Sagittal T1 or proton density for meniscus
– Sagittal T2 spin echo for cruciates
  – Knee externally rotated 10 degrees to see cruciates

- T2 coronals for collaterals and meniscocapsular separations
- Axial T2 to see patellofemoral cartilage and medial plica
- Fast spin echo for cartilage

BASICS

- T1–fluid dark, fat bright, TR <1,000
- T2–fluid bright, muscle dark, fat intermediate, TR >1,000
- T2 ~"fat suppression"

MENISCI

- Lateral more "O", medial "C"
- Lateral plateau convex
- Medial plateau concave
- Meniscus low signal on T1 and T2
- Any signal within meniscus on T1 is abnormal except in children (vascularity)
- If signal does not disrupt surface, then intrasubstance myxoid degeneration
- Most common pattern is oblique tear extending to inferior surface of posterior medial meniscus
- Posterior horn of medial meniscus two times bigger than anterior horn. If not, think displaced tear. Lateral meniscus similar size anterior and posterior
- Sagittals for horn tears
- Coronals for body tears
- Axials for radial tears
- Coronals for tibial attachments
- Sagittals for popliteal fasciculi. Lateral meniscus hypermobile if torn, but amount of mobility cannot be assessed by MR; must scope.
- Cysts associated with horizontal tears
- Pseudotear seen on lateral meniscus upper margin of anterior horn from insertion of transverse ligament and popliteal hiatus. Transverse ligament can be followed across fat pad into anterior horn of medial meniscus. Also, can be differentiated from real tear by estimating size of whole meniscus. In pseudotear, the whole meniscus would be too big
- Meniscocapsular separation with line of fluid high signal distinguished from normal meniscosynovial recesses, which are nubbins from above and below without connecting

GRADES

- I—fuzzy intrasubstance signal
- II—linear signal, not to joint
- III—linear, goes into joint
- IV—irregular, abnormal shape, followed up
- All radial tears are vertical

- Not all vertical tears are radial
- Bucket handle is vertical
- Posterior horn lateral meniscus tears have low specificity on MRI
- Bucket-handle tear
  - Meniscus is 10–12 mm in width
  - Sagittal cuts are 4-5 mm
  - Thus, bowtie in two contiguous sagittal images. If only one bowtie seen, displaced bucket-handle or parrot beak tear
  - Double PCL sign for displaced bucket handle seen on sagittal
- Discoid meniscus
  - Seen laterally in 3%
  - Coronal shows meniscus extending into notch
  - Sagittals with more than two bowties

CRUCIATES

- T2 needed because edema obscures ligament on T1 images
- Normal uniform low signals
- Normal PCL is curved but if torn, diffuse intermediate signal seen throughout
- Anterior lateral condyle and posterior lateral plateau contused in 90% of torn ACLs
- LCL only seen on one coronal image due to knee subluxation
- PCL buckles in torn ACL

MENISCOFEMORAL LIGAMENTS

- Low-signal round structures
- Medial femoral condyle to posterior horn of lateral meniscus
- Anterior to PCL: Humphry
- Posterior to PCL: Wrisberg (medial femoral condyle to posterior lateral meniscus)
- Insertions look like pseudotears

COLLATERALS

- Meniscocapsular separation seen near MCL on T2 with joint fluid between capsule/MCL and meniscus
- LCL complex from anterior to posterior is ITB, then LCL, then biceps tendon

CARTILAGE

- Fibrocartilage is higher signal than hyaline because higher free water content

OCD (Osteochondritis Dessicans)

- Classically at lateral aspect of medial femoral condyle

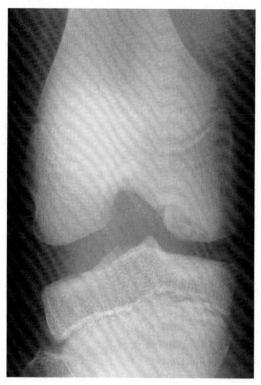

Osteochondritis dissecans. The tunnel view clearly shows a defect of the subchondral bone. (From Fleisher GR, et al. Atlas of Pediatric Emergency Medicine. Philadelphia: Lippincott Williams & Wilkins; 2004.)

- Tends to be more central when in lateral femoral condyle (LFC)
- Children with open physis do well regardless of remedy (boys <14 yo, girls <12 yo do well)
- Wilson sign—pain with IR and extension of knee, relieved by ER
- Notch or flexed weight-bearing view

CLASSIFICATION

- I—in situ
- II—early separation
- III—incomplete detached
- IV—completely detached
- In situ lesion
  - Retrograde drilling
  - ± bone grafting
- Early separation
  - Secured with K-wire, screws
- Incompletely detached
  - Remove fibrous tissue
  - Chondroplasty
  - Reduce and fix flap
- Completely detached
  - Remove loose body

- Abrasion chondroplasty
- Possible osteochondral allograft if big

Chondromalacia

OUTERBRIDGE CLASSIFICATION FOR CHONDROMALACIA

- I - softening
- II - fissures, clefts
- III - crabmeat, deep fissures, partial thick flap
- IV - exposed subchondral bone

Patellar Dislocation

- Females > males
- High Q-angle, laxity
- Average age 20 yo
- 50% dislocators had patella alta
- Most from sports
- Few had abnormal physical exam, contradicting typical fat adolescent girl who dislocates with minimal trauma (Atkin et al., 2000)
- Usually lateral dislocation
- Twisting knee on planted foot

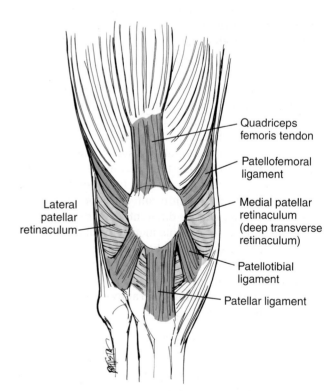

Anterior knee showing the patellar retinaculum. The superficial portion of the joint capsule interweaves with the retinaculum. The retinaculum has distinct thickenings, the patellofemoral and patellotibial ligaments.

- Strong quad contraction on valgus knee with externally rotated tibia
- If fat in joint, think osteochondral fracture (LFC or medial patellar facet, in 50% of dislocations)
- Reduce by manipulation in full extension

ANATOMY

- Medial patellofemoral ligament (MPFL) is critical injured structure in dislocation
  - In layer II, superficial to capsule but *deep to vastus medialis oblique (VMO)
  - From anterior femoral epicondyle to superomedial patella, fusing with undersurface of VMO tendon
- Usually avulsion off femur
- Bassett sign–tender over medial epicondyle

NATURAL HISTORY

- <14 yo–60% recur
- >19 yo—30% recur
- >20 yo—rare recurrence
- 15%–45% recurrence after first time dislocation (Hughston and Deese, 1988)
- MRI to rule out loose bodies

References

Atkin DM, et al. Characteristics of patients with primary acute lateral patellar dislocation and their recovery within the first 6 months of injury. Am J Sports Med 2000; 28(4):472–479.

Hughston JC, Deese M. Medial subluxation of the patella as a complication of lateral retinacular release. Am J Sports Med 1988; 16(4)383–388.

Patellar Tendonitis (Jumper's Knee)

- Degeneration at tendon insertion site—65% inferior pole patella, 25% superior pole, 10% tibial tubercle
- X-Ray studies
- Fragmentation of pole of patella
- Periosteal radiation at anterior patellar surface
- Tendon calcification
- Consider surgical débridement for chronic pain during and after activity

Patellofemoral Pain

PATELLAR SUBLUXATION

- Subluxators usually have ligament laxity and high Q-angle, ± traumatic dislocation
- Q-angle is anterior superior iliac spine (ASIS) to center of patella to tibia tubercle
- Patella engages trochlea with knee flexion
- "J" sign—patellar lateral excursion at terminal extension

*MERCHANT VIEW

- Knee in 45 degrees flexion
- Central ridge of patella should lie at or medial to bisector of the trochlear angle
- Tilt hard to see with Merchant view, better with Laurin

NONOPERATIVE

- Patella-stabilizing brace
- Strengthen VMO
- PF contact lowest at 0–30 degrees so should quad strengthen at this short arc
- Isotonic better than isometric

OPERATIVE

- Arthroscopic lateral release
- Take lateral retinaculum, vastus lateralis obliquus, distal patellotibial band
- Anteromedialization of tibial tubercle to correct Q-angle.
- Cannot do transfer until skeleton mature
- Proximal medial patella must be OK because increases load there

PATELLAR TILT

- Also known as lateral compression syndrome due to tight lateral retinaculum
- Diffuse anterior knee pain, worst over lateral retinaculum at flexion
- Inability to raise lateral facet to horizontal on examination
- *-Laurin view with 20 degrees knee flexion
- Line along lateral facet versus line connecting anterior aspects of medial and lateral trochlea
- If normal, this angle opens laterally
- If tilt, parallel or opens medially
- CT allows axial cuts at less than 20 degrees of flexion where patella is most likely to be unstable
- CT can determine excess lateralization of tibial tubercle

REHAB

Open Chain

- End segment free
- Axis of motion distal to joint
- Muscle action concentric
- Straight leg raising (SLR), sitting knee extension

Closed Chain

- End segment fixed
- Axis of motion proimal and distal to joint

- Muscle concentric, eccentric, and isometric
- More functional
- Muscle contraction synergistic
- Normal proprioception feedbacks used
- Squat, leg press, step exercises
- No PF joint contact at 0–10 degrees, least at 0–30 degrees
- Open chain may cause less joint compression
- VMO EMG activity lowest at 0–30 degrees and greatest at 60–90 degrees
- Improved patellar congruence as knee is flexed

Anterior Cruciate Ligament (ACL)

PATHOPHYSIOLOGY

- Most common in noncontact sports with plant-pivot or stop-jump
- "Pop," effusion within few hours
- 50% have meniscal tear also
  - Lateral most common in acute tear
  - Medial most common in chronic tear
- Post horn medial meniscus becomes primary restraint to anterior translation in ACL-deficient knee
- Lachman is most accurate test for diagnosis of acute tear in acute setting

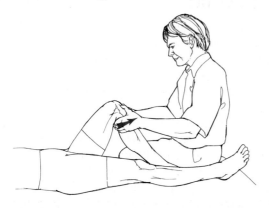

Anterior drawer test to assess the integrity of the ACL.

- Bone bruise on middle third of lateral femoral condyle and posterior third of lateral plateau (valgus load when clipped)

NATURAL HISTORY

- Deficient ACL leads to rotatory instability, which is what leads to disability
- Reason to operate may be to prevent meniscal tears caused by recurrent instability instead of future osteoarthritis (OA)?
- 92% of nonoperative patients had some degree of disability, which was worse if other concomitant injury

and did not get better with time (Fetto and Marshall, 1980)

- Compared x-ray view of normal knee to *symptomatic ACL deficient knee with 6.5-yr follow-up. 36% OA with increasing rate with longer follow-up. Postmeniscectomy knees had worst outcomes (Sherman et al., 1988).
- 292 ACL injuries over 12-yr period. 62% able to function well without ACL. Patients who underwent reconstruction had higher level of OA seen on x-ray and bone scan (Daniel et al., 1994)
- Is natural history of OA due to ACL or to cartilage and/or meniscal injury/resection?
- Unclear if ACL reconstruction changes the natural history

GRAFTS

Hamstring (HS) versus Bone Patellar Tendon Bone (BPTB) versus Allograft

- BPTB with greater initial tensile strength, greater collagen bulk, and more secure fixation
- BPTB tensile strength increases 30% by twisting 90 degrees
- BPTB with 30% anterior knee pain using older rehab techniques, but 25% of patients with chronic ACL deficiency also have PF knee pain
- HS easier to harvest and less risk of patellofemoral pain but weaker fixation
- Allograft with no donor site morbidity, smaller incision, faster but <1/million HIV, irradiation >2.5 cGy loses mechanical strength, and may have graft rejection with widening of bone tunnels
- Patellar tendon graft strength decreases to 20% of original at 6 wk, <50% at 1 yr

TREATMENT

Indication for Reconstruction

- Category 1 athlete (basketball, volleyball)
- >5 hr of athletics/wk
- KT 1,000 >5 mm from other side
- Concomitant meniscal tear
- Safe in skeletal age >14 or girls menstruating for 2 yr
- Partial tear
  - With 50% of fibers torn, half of those will go on to complete tear
  - Observe those 50% tears if Lachman, pivot, and functionally OK
- Repair best after full motion restored usually 3–6 wk postinjury to prevent arthrofibrosis
- Visualization of posterior compartment useful to see meniscal root avulsions
- Most common complication is anterior femoral tunnel

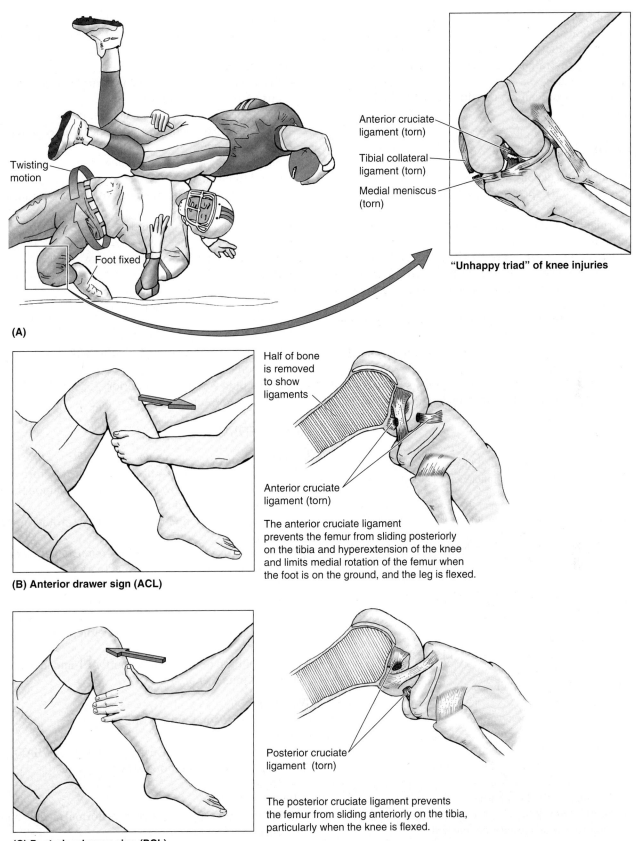

Twisting motion

Foot fixed

(A)

Anterior cruciate ligament (torn)

Tibial collateral ligament (torn)

Medial meniscus (torn)

"Unhappy triad" of knee injuries

(B) Anterior drawer sign (ACL)

Half of bone is removed to show ligaments

Anterior cruciate ligament (torn)

The anterior cruciate ligament prevents the femur from sliding posteriorly on the tibia and hyperextension of the knee and limits medial rotation of the femur when the foot is on the ground, and the leg is flexed.

(C) Posterior drawer sign (PCL)

Posterior cruciate ligament (torn)

The posterior cruciate ligament prevents the femur from sliding anteriorly on the tibia, particularly when the knee is flexed.

Knee joint injuries: torn ligaments, ACL ruptures, PCL ruptures. (From Moore KL, Dalley AF II. Clinical Oriented Anatomy, 4th ed. Philadelphia: Lippincott Williams & Wilkins; 1999.)

- Should be at intersection of Blumensaat and posterior lateral femoral condyle. Tibial tunnel should be a distal continuation of Blumensaat in extended knee
- Centralized straight graft leads to pivoting with normal Lachman
- Cyclops lesion can occur with anterior tibial tunnel placement

REHAB

- Quad control usually at 2 wk demonstrated by straight leg raise (SLR), then open up brace to allow ~50 degrees flexion
- Normal nonantalgic gait at 4–6 wk, then remove crutches
- Good motion, quad control, and normal gait usually at 6 wk, then discontinue brace and give neoprene sleeve
- In another month, able to ascend stairs (work up from small to larger step)
- At ~3 mo, able to descend stairs, then allow running
- Serial KTs postop and 3 mo
- Back to cutting sports no earlier than 6 mo, usually when full strength
- Hop test (hop a distance on one foot) symmetry between operative and normal leg is good test for full-strength return

References

Fetto JF, Marshall JL. The natural history and diagnosis of anterior cruciate ligament insufficiency. Clin Orthop Relat Res 1980; (147):29–38.

Sherman MF, et al. A clinical and radiographical analysis of 127 anterior cruciate insufficient knees. Clin Orthop Relat Res 1988; 227:229–237.

Daniel DM, et al. Fate of the ACL-injured patient. A prospective outcome study. Am J Sports Med 1994; 22(5):632–644.

ACL—ARTHROSCOPIC PROCEDURE TRANSTIBIAL TECHNIQUE

- Flexion bend at knee
- Examination under anesthesia (EUA)
- Diagnostic arthroscopy
- Meniscal débride/repair
- Graft harvest/prep
  - 10 mm osteotome as guide
  - Tibia tubercle triangular
  - Patella trapezoidal, keep <6 mm
  - Longer tibial plug for femoral side
  - 10 mm for femoral drill hole
  - 11 mm for tibial drill hole
  - Graft 30 mm, plugs 25 mm each
  - Tendo-osseous junctions marked
  - Ticron no. 5 for tibial plug
- Open 2.5 cm medial metaphyseal flare window on tibia, anterior to medial collateral ligament (MCL)

- Notchplasty to at least 20 mm wide
  - Shaver pointed away from posterior cruciate ligament (PCL)
- Tibial tunnel
  - Place pin posterior of anterior horn of lateral meniscus within ACL stump site
  - Angle 50–55 degrees, tunnel 45 × 11 mm
  - With knee extended, pin should clear intercondylar apex by 4 mm
  - Smooth intra-articular entrance
- Femoral tunnel
  - 7-mm guide, 10-mm reamer with 5-mm radius—leaves 2 mm cortex
  - Aim for 10 o'clock in right knee
  - Drill/ream with knee in 90 degrees flex
  - Femoral tunnel 30–35 mm × 10 mm
- Graft placement
  - Push in technique
  - Plugs oriented in coronal plane
  - Cortex of femoral plug posterior
  - Screw anteriorly on cancellous
  - Rock test—pull to rock patient in bed
  - Tension in near full extension
  - Tibial plug with cortex anterior
  - Tibial screw anterior also

ACL—PEDIATRIC

Evaluation

- See fracture, pediatrics—tibial eminence fracture
- Midsubstance tears now felt to be more common than tibial eminence avulsion fracture
- "Pop," more likely if element of contact, rotation, or deceleration
- Natural history similar to adults—recurrent episodes of instability and risk of meniscal tears
- Stress views to rule out physial injury
- 70 children with hemarthrosis scoped
- ~50% had ACL tears, 60% of those were partial tears
- Younger children tended to have either meniscal or ACL tear
- Older children tended to have both ACL and meniscal tears (Stanitski et al., 1993)

Treatment

- Nonoperative for Tanner 1 or 2
- Phase I
  - Progressive weight bearing as tolerated (WBAT)
  - Regain range of motion (ROM)
  - 10 days
- Phase II
  - Physical therapy (PT) to restore normal muscle balance
  - 6 wk
- Phase III
  - Low/moderate-demand sports

- High-demand sports if low/moderate sports tolerated
- Indications for surgery
  - Functional instability with activities of daily living (ADLs)
  - Unable to comply with activity modifications
  - Near skeletal maturity
- Physial-sparing reconstruction
  - Usually for Tanner 1s
  - Patellar or hamstring autograft that is left attached to the tibia distally and snuck under the transverse meniscal ligament, under femoral, over the top position, and sewed/stapled to lateral femoral periosteum
- Partial transphysial reconstruction
  - Usually for Tanner 2
  - Tibial physis violated
  - Around femoral over the top position and sewed to lateral femoral periosteum
- Complete transphyseal reconstruction
  - Usually for Tanner 3
  - Essentially same as adults

References

Stanitski CL, et al. Observations on acute knee hemarthrosis in children and adolescents. J Pediatr Orthop 1993; 13(4):506–510.

Posterior Cruciate Ligament

- Anterolateral stronger, tight in flexion
- Meniscofemoral ligaments of Humphrey (anterior) and Wrisberg (posterior) are secondary restraint to posterior instability
- PCL primary restraint in 90 degrees of flexion
- PL corner primary restraint to varus and ER at 30 degrees flexion
- Same neurovascular supply as ACL
- Increased pressure in PF and medial joints with PCL cut; seen on bone scan
- Posterior drawer
  - Recreate the 1-cm stepoff between medial femoral condyle and medial plateau and then push posteriorly
  - I—<1 cm drawer
  - II—1 cm drawer (loses stepoff)
  - III—>1 cm drawer
- Quad active test
- I and II usually respond to nonoperative therapy. Rehab with ROM, Q strengthening, back to athletics in 6–8 wk
- III usually has PL corner injury also, will likely require surgery, especially if bone scan positive
- 40% of PCL injuries are isolated
- Rehab preoperation to get ROM

MRI

- To assess location of injury
- Soft tissue avulsion off femur
- Bony avulsion off tibia

PRIMARY REPAIR

- In acute avulsion off MFC

RECONSTRUCTION

- Anatomic
- Nonisometric
- Reconstruct only anterolateral band
- Inlay versus onlay
- Consider posterior tibial slope

INDICATIONS

- Drawer >10 mm, symptomatic, failed PT, chronic
- Bone scan positive
- Acute bony avulsion (easy to fix, fix within 2 wk, great results)

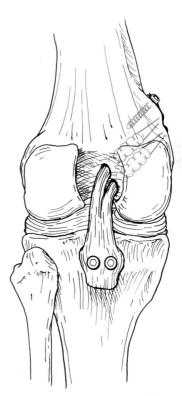

Two-tailed separate bundle reconstruction of the femoral posterior cruciate ligament (PCL) origin combined with the tibial inlay technique for PCL reconstruction. (From Bucholz RW, Heckman JD. Rockwood & Green's Fractures in Adults, 5th ed. Philadelphia: Lippincott, Williams & Wilkins; 2001.)

Posterolateral Corner

ANATOMY

- At all angles, PLc is primary restraint against varus/ER
- PLc cut alone results in small increased posterior translation at all angles but maximum at 30 degrees. Increased varus and increased ER at all angles, maximum at 30 degrees
- At all angles, PCL is primary restraint against posterior translation
- PCL cut alone results in increased posterior translation at all angles, maximum at 90 degrees. No increase in varus or ER at any angle
- At <30 degrees, isolated sections of PLc or PCL caused same posterior translation
- When PCL is cut after PLc is cut, a large increase in posterior translation and varus rotation resulted at all angles. At >30 degrees, external rotation of the tibia also increased (Gollehon et al., 1987; Veltri and Warren, 1994)
- LCL, popliteus, popliteofibular, and arcuate ligaments are most important

PHYSICAL EXAMINATION

- Prefer prone ER test and varus stress test
- Increased posterior translation, ER and varus at 30 degrees that decreases at 90 degrees indicates isolated injury to PLc
- Pain and instability in extension
- Peroneal nerve symptoms
- Usually along with ACL and/or PCL injury

IMAGING

- X-ray view with arcuate fibular head fracture, Segond fracture, or avulsion off Gerdy
- Anteromedial femoral condyle bruise with PLc combined with cruciate injury

TREATMENT

*Acute
- Reconstruct cruciate injury
  - Must fix PCL, but ACL OK not to fix
- Direct open lateral approach
- LCL
  - Direct repair
  - Advancement and recession
  - Augmentation
  - Reconstruction with central biceps tendon
- Address both tibial and fibular attachments of popliteus

- Achilles split allograft with bone in femur and two tendon ends in tibula and fibula to address both simultaneously
- *-Chronic and varus
  - Proximal valgus tibial osteotomy
  - PL reconstruction later
- *-Chronic and valgus
  - Patellar tendon or Achilles allograft is often required for repair
- If PCL and PLc, repair both because the repairs protect each other
- If ACL and PLc, repair PLc first, then ACL later. Repairing ACL causes stiffness. Not repairing PLc will cause ACL repair to fail
- Best results if direct repair within 3 wk of acute injury (Covey, 2001)

References

Gollehon DL, et al. The role of the posterolateral and cruciate ligaments in the stability of the human knee. A biomechanical study. J Bone Joint Surg Am 1987; 69(2):233–242.

Veltri DM, Warren RF. Anatomy, biomechanics, and physical findings in posterolateral knee instability. Clin Sports Med 1994; 13:599–614.

Covey DC. Injuries of the posterolateral corner of the knee. J Bone Joint Surg Am 2001; 83-A(1):106–118.

Chondral Defects

- 75% water, 10% type II collagen, 10% proteoglycans
- Few natural history studies

ACUTE CARTILAGE INJURY

- Rotational force
- Usually on weight-bearing portion of medial femoral condyle (MFC)
- Presents like meniscal tear
- Poor function with progressive chondral injury more likely in ACL-deficient post partial meniscectomy knee versus stable post partial meniscectomy knee
- Nondisplacement lesions before physial closure will likely heal
- Reparative versus restorative treatment
- Treatment in context of meniscal loss or transplant

OPTIONS

- Arthroscopic débridement
- Abrasion arthroplasty
  - Superficial, not to marrow
  - Response from cells in joint
- Microfracture
  - Awl to enter subchondral source of mesenchymal cells
  - Steadman—75% improved at 7 yr

- Partial weight bearing (PWB) and continuous passive motion (CPM) 6–8 wk
- Periosteal/perichondrial grafts
  - Chondrogenesis from cambium
- Autologous chondrocyte implantation (ACI)
  - Healing from cambium or chondrocytes?— conflicting animal studies
  - Younger, active
  - Isolated, femoral, 2–4 cm^2
- Autograft
  - Limited donor site tissue
  - Collapse, migration of dowels
- Allograft
  - For very large defects
- Synthetic matrices

TREATMENT BASED ON

- Acute versus chronic
- Age, skeletal maturity
- Size (2 cm^2)
- Bone attached?
- Location
- If bone attached, fixation ± bone grafting
- If large, ACI or osteochondral allograft
- If bone defect also, osteochondral allograft or mosaicplasty
- If small, older, abrasion/microfracture

High Tibial Osteotomy (HTO)

- 60% load medial, 40% lateral
- Typical varus deformity
- Valgus deformity in rheumatoid arthritis (RA), which may be contraindication for HTO
- Normal mechanical axis just medial to center
- Women less likely to accept necessary deformity
- Must rule out PF joint osteoarthritis
- Must have motion because patients lose some motion with surgery
- May treat ACL also if concomitant deficiency
- Medial or lateral shoe wedges

MEDIAL OPENING TECHNIQUE

- Midline incision
- Subperiosteal elevation off crest, heading medially until fibers of MCL seen
- Langenbeck behind patellar tendon
- Hohman around posteromedial tibia
- Saw at just around level of patellar tendon insertion, not violating posterior or lateral cortex fully
- Thin osteotome to break posterior cortex and crank open

- Flatten 4.5 mm locking T-plate to allow valgus after locked in
- Fix plateau to plate, crank open, then fix shaft to plate
- Non weight bearing (NWB) postop
- Opening wedge tends to accentuate posterior slope while closing wedge tends to lessen it

LATERAL CLOSING TECHNIQUE

- Curved incision along lateral tibial crest from lateral femoral condyle to fibula head
- Bend knee to keep nerve posterior and relax ITB
- Disrupt tibia-fibia joint with osteotome
- Resect medial/superior fibula head to give space for when fibula migrates superiorly but watch out for common peroneal nerve and leave LCL and biceps attached
- Release anterior compartment from proximal tibia, do fasciotomy
- Spinal needles to mark joint lines using flurorscopic imaging
- Lateral to medial tibial pins 1 cm distal to tibial joint line and proximal to tubercle, with no tilt in sagittal plane
- Measure pin length to determine depth of cut
- Protect patellar tendon and posterior nerve, cut at least 2 cm distal to joint line, avoid complete tibial transection
- Cut medially, aiming down away from joint surface to avoid plateau fracture
- Idea that 1 mm equals 1-degree correction is only true for very small tibia (57 mm) wide and will usually cause undercorrection
- Remove wedge with osteotome and towel clip, use it for bone grafting
- Over drill and set proximal screws
- Drilling medial cortex may help close osteotomy
- Close osteotomy by extending knee

Hip Pain in Athlete

DIFFERENTIAL DIAGNOSIS

- Hip subluxation
- History of developmental dislocation of the hip (DDH)
- Stress fracture
- Transient osteoporosis
  - Along with pregnancy
- Chondral lesion
- Labral tear
- Sports hernia
- Piriformis syndrome
  - Compression of sciatic nerve
- Inguinal hernia
- Abdominal/pelvic causes

Sports Hernia

- Ice hockey and soccer
- Primary adductor tightness leading to anterior pelvic tilt, causing strain of rectus abdominis
- Pain with crunches, resisted adduction

Labral Tear

- Anterior tear causes pain when flexion, ER, abduction to extend, IR, adduction
- Posterior tear causes pain with flexion, IR, posterior-directed load

DIFFERENTIAL DIAGNOSIS BY PHYSICAL EXAM

- OA—pain with flexion/adduction and loss of rotation prone
- Anterior labral tear—pain with flexion/adduction and axial load.
- Iliopsoas—pain with resisted flexion
- Adductor—pain with figure four

HIP SNAPPING (COXA SALTANS)

- Intra-articular causes
  - Synovial chondromatosis
  - Loose bodies
  - Exostosis
  - Hip subluxation
- Extra-articular causes
  - Iliotibial band (ITB) over greater trochanter (GT)
  - Iliopsoas (IP) over anterior femoral head
  - IP over iliopectineal eminence
  - iliofemoral ligament over femoral head
  - long head biceps over ischemic tubercle
- ITB over GT
  - flex hip from adduction and extend position
  - Ober test to see if ITB tight
- IP over anterior femoral head
  - Hip taken from flexion, abduction, ER to exension, adduction, IR: tendon moves lateral to medial
  - Iliopsoas live bursography for diagnosis
  - Fractionally lengthen IP if conservative measures fail via modified iliofemoral approach (Dobbs, et al. 2002)

Reference

Dobbs MB, et al. Surgical correction of the snapping iliopsoas tendon in adolescents. J Bone Joint Surg Am 2002; 84A(3): 420–424.

Anatomy of Shoulder

- Layer I
  - Deltoid
  - Pectoris major
  - Fascia, cephalic vein
- Layer II
  - Clavicopectoral fascia
  - Coracoacromial ligament
  - Conjoined tendon
  - Pectoris minor
- Layer III
  - Subdeltoid bursa
  - Rotator cuff muscles
  - Suprascapular nerve bundle
- Layer IV
  - Glenohumeral capsule
  - Coracohumeral ligament (CHL)
  - Long head biceps
  - Inferior glenohumeral ligament complex (LC)
  - Primary stabilizer for anterior and inferior translation in abduction*
  - Anterior and posterior band with axillary pouch to form hammock
  - Tightens in ER and IR for anterior and posterior stability
  - The major glenohumeral stabilizer
  - More important as UE abducts
  - Prevents inferior translation at 45 degrees abduction
  - Posterior band IGHLC and posterior capsule, and rotator interval prevent posterior translation
  - Medial glenohumeral ligament (MGHL)
  - Drapes obliquely over subscapularis
  - Limits ER of adducted humerus
  - Secondary stabilizer for inferior translation in adduction
  - Stabilizer for anterior translation in 60- to 90-degree abduction
  - In only 60%–80% of people
  - Superior Glenohumeral Ligament (SGHL) and CHL
    - Between biceps and subscapular tendons
    - Primary stabilization to inferior translation in adduction*
    - Secondary stabilization to post translation in flexed, adducted, internally rotated humerus
    - Stabilization for anterior translation in <60-degree abduction
    - Limits ER of adducted humerus
    - SGHL from supraglenoid tubercle to rotator interval to blend with CHL and insert into lesser tuber
    - Both in >90% of people
- Labrum
  - Fibrocartilaginous "meniscus"
  - Chock-block prevents abnormal motion
  - Anchor for IGHLC
  - Intimately associated with capsule
  - Loosely attached to glenoid on superior, anterior-superior like meniscus

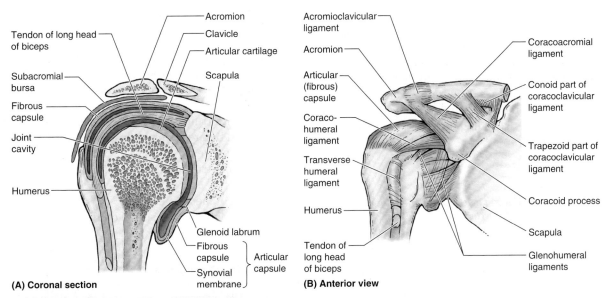

(A) Coronal section

Tendon of long head of biceps — Acromion — Clavicle — Articular cartilage — Scapula — Subacromial bursa — Fibrous capsule — Joint cavity — Humerus — Glenoid labrum — Fibrous capsule — Synovial membrane } Articular capsule

(B) Anterior view

Acromioclavicular ligament — Acromion — Articular (fibrous) capsule — Coraco-humeral ligament — Transverse humeral ligament — Humerus — Tendon of long head of biceps — Coracoacromial ligament — Conoid part of coracoclavicular ligament — Trapezoid part of coracoclavicular ligament — Coracoid process — Scapula — Glenohumeral ligaments

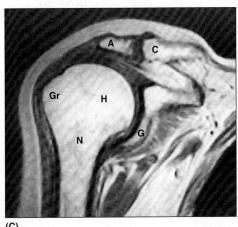

(C)

Glenohumeral joint. **A:** Coronal section of the shoulder region illustrating the articulating bones, the articular capsule and cartilage, and the subacromial bursa. **B:** Drawing of an anterior view of a dissection of the acromioclavicular (AC), coracohumeral, and glenohumeral ligaments. The glenohumeral ligaments strengthen the anterior aspect of the capsule of the glenohumeral joint, and the coracohumeral ligament strengthens the capsule superiorly. **C:** Coronal MRI of the right glenohumeral and AC joints. A, acromion; C, clavicle; Gr, greater tubercle of humerus; H, head of humerus; G, glenoid cavity; N, surgical neck of humerus. (Courtesy of Dr. W. Kucharczyk, Chair of Medical Imaging and Clinical Director of Tri-Hospital Resonance Centre, Toronto, Ontario, Canada). (From Moore KL, Dalley AF II. Clinical Oriented Anatomy, 4th ed. Philadelphia: Lippincott Williams & Wilkins; 1999.)

- Firmly attached inferiorly like fibrous extension of cartilage
- Quadrilateral space (axillary nerve, posterior humeral circumflex artery)
  - Trapezius minor superiorly
  - Trapezius major (confluent with latissimus dorsi)
  - Long head triceps
  - Humerus
- Triangular space (radial nerve, deep brachial artery)
  - Trapezius major (with latissimust dorsi) superiorly
  - Humerus
  - Long head triceps
  - (Inferior to quad space)
- Biomechanics
  - Glenohumeral to scapulothoracic motion in abduction is generally 2:1. More glenohumeral at beginning and more scapulothoracic at end of abduction
  - Joint reaction force 0.4 times BW at 60 degrees abduction, 0.9 times BW at 90 degrees abduction

- At 0 degrees abduction, joint reaction force is at lower glenoid; at 30–60 degrees, force is at upper glenoid; at 60 degrees, force is at center
- Bony
  - Scapula has 17 muscle insertions
  - Scapula is inclined 30 degrees anterior to coronal plane
  - Humeral head retroverted 30 degrees, neck-shaft angle 130 degrees, glenoid retroverted 5 degrees
  - Glenoid and humeral head have size mismatch but same radius of curvature
  - At any position only one-third head covered by glenoid
  - Glenoid is pear shaped
  - Joint most congruent with abduction
- Miscellaneous
  - Disc in AC joint incomplete but disc in sternoclavicular (SC) joint is complete
  - Clavicle first to ossify, last to fuse
  - Postcapsule is thinnest
  - Capsule has two times surface area of humeral head

- Latissimus dorsi and trapezius major internally rotate shoulder because attachments are anterior (miss between two majors)
- musculocutaneous nerve enters back of conjoined tendon ~5 cm distal to coracoid (3–8 cm)
- Axillary nerve passes 5 cm from acromion
- Humeral head blood supply from *anterior humeral circumflex via ascending branch of Laing found in bicipital groove

Reference

Cooper DE, et al. Supporting layers of the glenohumeral joint. An anatomic study. Clin Orthop Relat Res 1993; 289:144–155.

ANATOMY OF SHOULDER—NERVES

- Axillary nerve
  - Terminal branch of posterior cord
  - Crosses lateral border of subscapularis
  - Joins posterior humeral circumflex artery to exit quad space
  - Posterior trunk supplies teres minor and posterior deltoid before terminating as superior lateral cutaneous nerve
  - Anterior trunk supplies mid and anterior deltoid
- Musculocutaneous nerves
  - Terminal branch of lateral cord

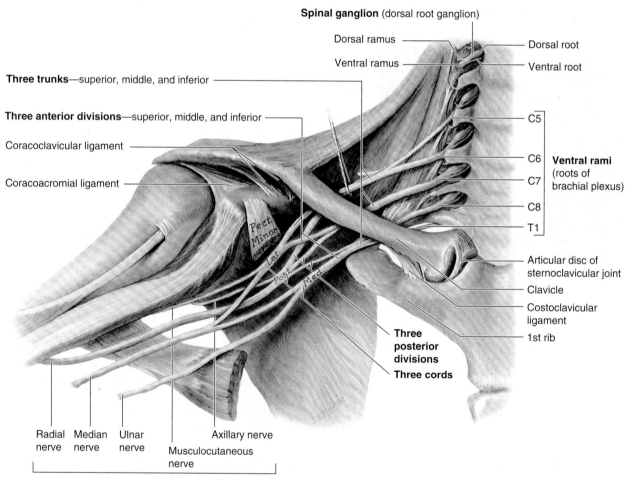

Formation of the brachial plexus. This large nerve network provides innervation to the upper limb and shoulder region. The brachial plexus is formed by the ventral rami of the 5th through 8th cervical nerves and the greater part of the ramus of the 1st thoracic nerve (the roots of the brachial plexus). Small contributions may be made by the 4th cervical and 2nd thoracic nerves. Observe the merging and continuation of certain roots of the plexus to three trunks, the separation of each trunk into anterior and posterior divisions, the union of the divisions to form three cords, and the derivation of the main terminal branches from the cords. (From Moore KL, Dalley AF II. Clinical Oriented Anatomy, 4th ed. Philadelphia: Lippincott Williams & Wilkins; 1999.)

- Enters deep surface of coracobrachialis from 3–8 cm distal to coracoid
  - Gets biceps, brachialis, and coracobrachialis, then becomes lateral antebrachial cutaneous nerve
- Suprascapular nerves
  - From upper trunk
  - Passes through suprascapular notch, then supplies supraspinatus
  - Passes through spinoglenoid notch to supply infraspinatus

Shoulder Physical Exam

- Inspection
- Palpation
- Range of motion
  - Society of Shoulder and Elbow Surgeons recommendations
  - Elevation in plane of scapula
  - ER in adduction and 90-degree abduction
  - IR based on thoracic vertebra
  - (Supine controls scapula)
- Strength
- Neurovascular exam

BLOCK TO ER (ACTIVE = PASSIVE) DIFFERENTIAL DIAGNOSIS:

- Posterior dislocation
- Adhesive capsulitis
- Osteoarthritis

WRIGHT (MODIFIED ADSON)

- UE extended, abducted, externally rotated and neck extended, rotated to opposite side causes reproduction of symptoms and loss of pulse

ROOS TEST

- Both UE in abduction and ER with rapid closing/opening of hands cause symptoms

GLENOHUMERAL TRANSLATION

- Translates up slope beyond normal, 1+
- Over the rim, comes back, 2+
- Remains dislocated, 3+

SULCUS SIGN

- 1+ to 3+ by 1-, 2-, 3-cm translation of head from lateral acromion
- 3+ pathognomonic of MDI

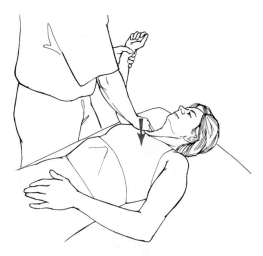

Relocation test. The humerus is often sitting slightly anterior in the glenoid fossa owing to rounded-shoulders posture or previous injury. This test ensures that the humerus is seated properly.

GENERALIZED LAXITY

- Thumb to forearm volar flexion
- Index finger metacarpophalangeal (MCP) hyperextension
- Elbow and knee hyperextension
- Apprehension test
- Jobe relocation test
- Subscapular lift-off test
- Bring arm to maximum IR (with hand near buttock)
- Normal if patient able to maintain position when MD releases hand
- Positive if cannot maintain IR and hand cannot be kept off spine without extending elbow
- Gerber subscapular belly test
- Have patient put hand/wrist flat and arm in maximum IR, elbows sticking out
  - Ask patient to press belly
  - If subscapularis strong, elbow does not drop back
  - If weak, elbow drops back behind trunk and shoulder extends rather than internally rotates

IMPINGEMENT SIGN

- Passive elevation beyond 90 degrees
- Hawkins test
- Forceful IR of the shoulder with arm flexed 90 degrees and adducted
- Neer test
- Forceful flexion of adducted and internally rotated shoulder with pain at 90–100 degrees
- Impingement test.
  - Impinge signs relieved with subacromial lidocaine
  - Most sensitive and specific

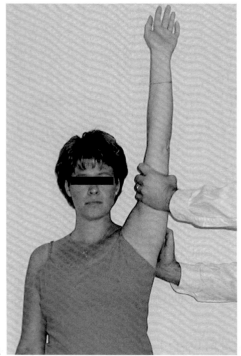

A

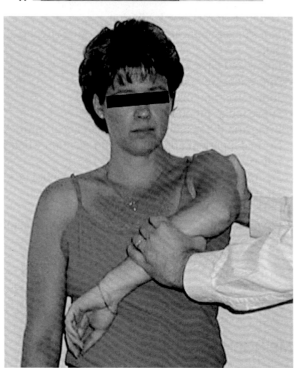

B

Arthroscopic acromioplasty and mini-open rotator cuff repair. **A:** The classic impingement sign occurs as the shoulder is placed in the position of maximum forward elevation, reproducing the patient's pain. **B:** Impingement of the greater tuberosity on the coracoacromial ligament occurs when the shoulder is forward-flexed to 90 degrees and internally rotated, reproducing the patient's pain. (From Koval KJ, Zuckerman JD. Atlas of Orthopaedic Surgery: A Multimedial Reference. Philadelphia: Lippincott Williams & Wilkins, 2004.

- Crossed adduction test
  - Horizontal adduction causes pain over AC joint
  - Relieved with lidocaine to AC joint
- Obrien active compression test
  - 100% sensitive, 98.5% specific for labral pathology
  - Elbew extended, shoulder flexed 90 degrees, maximum pronated, adducted 15 degrees, resisted elevation—places biceps on stretch and in contact with anterior superior labrum, which causes deep anterior pain and weakness
  - Relieved with supination
  - Pain must be deep, not AC, not biceps
- Yergason test
  - Resisted supination with elbow flexed
- Speed test
  - Resisted forward elevation with forearm supinated, elbow extended
- Spurling test
  - Lateral flexion and extension with compression causes pain to tilted side

Shoulder X-ray Studies

TRUE AP

- Beam fanned 30–45 degrees laterally to show glenohumeral (GH) joint in true profile.
- Film on back of scapula
- Can do with arm in neutral to get another view in addition to trauma AP in IR (sling position)

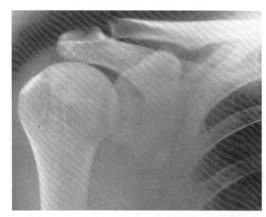

Explanation of why the AC joint is poorly visualized on routine shoulder x-ray views: When the exposure usually used to take the shoulder films is decreased by two-thirds, the AC joint is well visualized. However, the inferior corner of the AC joint is superimposed on the acromion process. (From Bucholz RW, Heckman JD. Rockwood & Green's Fractures in Adults, 5th ed. Philadelphia: Lippincott, Williams & Wilkins; 2001.)

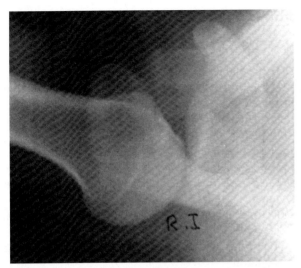

Axillary x-ray film reveals an acute posterior subluxation of the glenohumeral joint. (From Bucholz RW, Heckman JD. Rockwood & Green's Fractures in Adults, 5th ed. Baltimore: Lippincott, Williams & Wilkins; 2001.)

AXILLARY LATERAL

- Abduction 70–90 degrees
- Can do without abduction by using foam block to forward flex in sling
- Better at looking at posterior glenoid than West Point, i.e., in OA

WEST POINT

- Like axillary except with patient prone and beam angled 25 degrees in coronal and sagittal planes
- Anterior inferior glenoid rim
- Can see LT because arm in 90 degrees abduction and neutral rotation

STRYKER NOTCH

- Patient supine with hand on head, beam shoots A to P with 10 degrees cephalic tilt
- Can see coracoid well
- Evaluations for Hill-Sachs lesion
- AP view in IR also sees Hill-Sachs lesion

GARTH

- True AP with 45 degree caudad tilt
- Also sees anterior-inferior glenoid

ZANCA

- AC joint with 10-degree cephalic tilt
- AC joint arthritis or osteolysis

HOBBS

- Posteroanterior of sternoclavicular joint with patient slumped over cassette, resting on elbows

SERENDIPITY (ROCKWOOD)

- Sternoclavicular joint in supine patient with 40-degree cephalic tilt

SUPRASPINATUS OUTLET

- Scapula-Y with 10-degree caudal angle
- Acromion shape in impingement
  - (Bigliani—flat, curved, hooked)
- Acromion thickness in impingement
  - (Snyder—<8 mm, 8–12, >12 mm)

30-DEGREE CAUDAL TILT VIEW (ROCKWOOD)

- To see subacromial spurs

BICIPITAL GROOVE VIEW

- Supine with UE externally rotated, AP with beam aimed 15 degrees medially

Shoulder MRI

SYSTEMATIC APPROACH

- Infraspinatus, teres minor tendons
- Supraspinatus
- AC joint
- Joint orientation, subluxation, evaluate for Hill Sachs Lesion (H-S)
- Atrophy
- Subscapular, biceps tendons
- Labrum
- Capsule, MGHL
- Cartilage
- Axial for capsulolabrum, AC joint, subscapularis, biceps, cartilage, Hill Sachs Lesion (HS)
- Oblique coronal for SLAP, RTC
- Oblique sagittal for muscle atrophy and acromion shape
- Hill-Sachs is at level of coracoid or above
- Bandlike MGHL outside of labrum
- Sublabral foramen, Buford complex
- Rotator interval at MGHL, coracoid level

RTC TEAR

- Best seen on oblique coronal proton density (PD; balanced sequence between T1 and T2)
- Prove it is RTC by seeing fluid where cuff should be on T2
- Magic angle (55 degrees with magnet beam) occurs only with T1 or PD, not on T2. Thus, tear on T2 is real.
- Look for muscle atrophy on oblique sagittals
- On oblique coronal, look for teres minor, which is large, bipennate, and just superior to quadrangular space
- On oblique coronal, supraspinatus is on top of cut that is center of glenoid and muscle is cigar-shaped
- Infraspinatus is more posterior and superior to bipennate teres minor
  1. Normal
     - Usually low signal on all sequences
     - High-signal T1, no brighter on T2 at critical zone (2 cm from attachment)
       - Volume-averaged peritendon fat
       - Myxoid degeneration, "tendinopathy"
       - Magic angle effect
       - Calcium deposits
  2. Tendonitis ± partial tear
     - High-signal T1, brighter on T2
     - Little or no fluid in subacromial bursa
     - Bursal versus articular versus complex
  3. Cuff tear
     - Tendon disruption seen
     - High signal on T1 and T2 at critical zone
     - Large fluid in subacromial bursa

LABRUM

- Normally low signal
- Anterior larger than posterior
- Tear seen by high signal in labrum thus hard to see tear if no effusion
- Differential diagnosis—attachment of GH ligaments can mimic tear but line is intermediate signal so one must see high-signal joint fluid inside labrum to call a real tear
- Low signal ovoid mass anterior to anterior glenoid at the base of coracoid is torn anterior labrum that is retracted superiorly (GLOM, glenoid labrum ovoid mass)

BICEPS TENDON

- Can be impinged by acromion
- Fluid in sheath can just be fluid from GH joint
- If tendon enlarged or signal within tendon, then can call tendonitis
- If it becomes posterior to subscapularis, there must be a subscapular tear

Acromioclavicular (AC) Joint Injury

ANATOMY

- Diarthrodial joint
- At 24 yr, hyaline cartilage at distal clavicle becomes fibrocartilage
- Intra-articular disc usually incomplete
  - Typically degenerates with age
  - Nonfunctional by 40 yr
  - With upper extremity (UE) elevation, clavicle rotates up 45 degrees, AC joint rotates only 5 degrees
- Dynamic stabilizers
  - Deltoid: suspends arm from acromion (ACR) and clavicle
  - Trapezius: suspends ACR and clavicle from axial skeleton
- Static stabilizers
  - AC ligaments: anterior/posterior/inferior/superior
  - Superior strongest
  - Resists anterior/posterior (AP) translation
- Coracoclavicular ligaments: very strong
  - Conoid—medial
  - Trapezoid—lateral
    - Resists vertical translation

CLASSIFICATION

- Type I
  - Partial tear AC ligaments/sprain
- Type II
  - AC torn, CC intact
  - Same CC distance as other side
- Type III
  - Complete AC and CC tear
  - Up to two times CC distance
  - Radiographic study controversial
  - Classically no benefit from surgery (Phillips et al., 1998) though now more controversial
- Type IV
  - AC and CC tear
  - Clavicle pierces/traps posteriorly
- Type V
  - Complete ligamentous and muscle separation from clavicle, which is cephalad displaced
  - >Two times CC distance compared with other side
- Type VI
  - Clavicle below coracoid
  - No visible damage

IMAGING

- Stress views for I–III
- Need axillary view for suspected IV

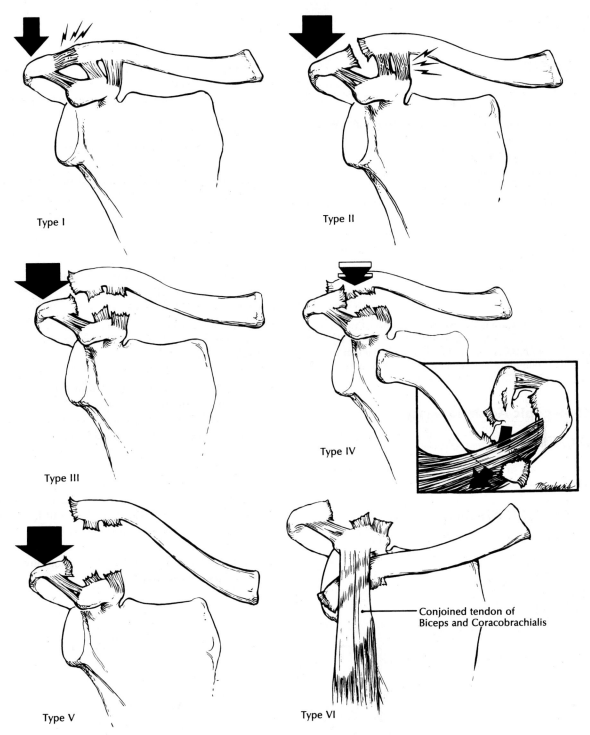

Type I

Type II

Type III

Type IV

Type V

Type VI — Conjoined tendon of Biceps and Coracobrachialis

Schematic drawings of the classification of ligamentous injuries to the AC joint. **Top left:** In the type I injury a mild force applied to the point of the shoulder does not disrupt either the AC or the coracoclavicular ligaments. **Top right:** A moderate to heavy force applied to the point of the shoulder will disrupt the AC ligaments, but the coracoclavicular ligaments remain intact (type II). **Center left:** When a severe force is applied to the point of the shoulder, both the AC and the coracoclavicular ligaments are disrupted (type III). **Center right:** In a type IV injury not only are the ligaments disrupted, but the distal end of the clavicle is also displaced posteriorly into or through the trapezius muscle. **Bottom left:** A violent force applied to the point of the shoulder not only ruptures the AC and coracoclavicular ligaments but also disrupts the muscle attachments and creates a major separation between the clavicle and the acromion (type V). **Bottom right:** This is an inferior dislocation of the distal clavicle in which the clavicle is inferior to the coracoid process and posterior to the biceps and coracobrachialis tendons. The AC and coracoclavicular ligaments are also disrupted (type VI). (From Bucholz RW, Heckman JD. Rockwood & Green's Fractures in Adults, 5th ed. Philadelphia: Lippincott, Williams & Wilkins; 2001.)

TREATMENT

- Conservative for I, II, ?III
- Acute surgery for IV, V, VI
- Coracoclavicular ligament reconstruction (Weaver and Dunn, 1972)
  - Distal clavicle resected
  - Coracoacromial ligament swung up to recreate CC ligament
  - PDS suture looped around coracoid and clavicle to augment graft
- Transacromial intramedial device
- Distal clavicle excision alone
- Arthroscopic assisted AC reconstruction using soft tissue graft

References

Phillips AM, et al. Acromioclavicular dislocation. Conservative or surgical therapy. Clin Orthop Relat Res 1998; (353):10–17.
Weaver JK, Dunn HK. Treatment of acromioclavicular injuries, especially complete acromioclavicular separation. J Bone Joint Surg Am 1972; 54(6):1187–1194.

Arthroscopic Acromioplasty

INDICATIONS

- Impingement syndrome with hook or down-sloped anterior acromion and partial RTC tear

CONTRAINDICATIONS

- Presence of full RTC tear because results of acromioplasty and RTC repair much better versus acromioplasty alone

- Sitting or lateral decubitus
- Posterior portal
  - 2 cm inferior and medial to posterolateral acromion corner
- Posterolateral portal
  - 2 cm lateral to posterolateral corner
- Anterior portal
  - 2 cm inferior and medial to anterolateral corner of acromion but lateral to coracoid process
- Lateral portal
  - 2 cm lateral to lateral acromion
- Distend joint with saline
- Scope through posterior portal
- Anterior portal for outflow, instruments
- Glenohumeral cartilage
- Glenohumeral ligaments
- Biceps anchor attachment
- Anterior and posterior capsular tissue
- Deep surface RTC
- Intra-articular biceps tendon
- Trocar to break subacromial adhesions
- Camera into posterior portal
- Orient by seeing medial and lateral borders of anterior acromion and coracoacromial ligament
- Coracoacromial ligament resected from medial to lateral with Bovie
- As ligament removed from anterior attachment, red fibers of deltoid seen above deep deltoid fascia
- Undersurface of anterior acromion outlined
- Acromioplasty begun laterally, sweeping in anteroposterior direction
- Shave medially until you see acromial joint
- More bleeders medially

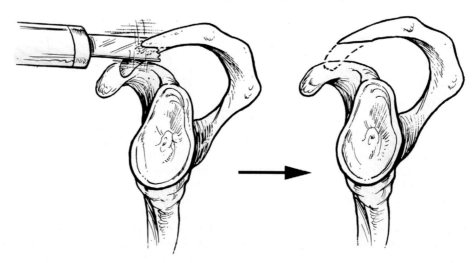

Acromioplasty and rotator cuff repair. Instruments used to facilitate open rotator cuff tear include (left to right): angled self-retaining retractors, deltoid retractor, large rasp, small rasp, flat Darrach elevators (two), and humeral head/"ring"/retractors (two). (From Koval KJ, Zuckerman JD. Atlas of Orthopaedic Surgery: A Multimedial Reference. Philadelphia: Lippincott Williams & Wilkins; 2004.)

RESULTS

- 8-yr follow-up on all Hospital for Special Surgery (HSS) arthroscopic subacromial decompression (SADs)
- 102 cases 1984–1988, 83 available for follow-up
- 81% good to excellent
- 16 failures, 13 required more surgery
- All RTC tears at operation were débrided (Stephens et al., 1998)

CATEGORIES OF FAILURES

- Diagnostic error
  - Missing early degenerative joint disease (DJD)
  - Missing instability
- Surgical error
  - Taking too much or too little bone
- Decompress AC joint only if symptoms
- Rotator cuff pathology
  - ? complete and repair partial tears that are 50% thick
  - 3 of 11 with asymptomatic partial cuff tears at index case required revision; 2 for full tear, the third refused surgery
  - 2 of 17 patients with full cuff tear at index procedure went on to repairs
  - Only 3 of 54 patients (6%) with clean cuff at SAD went on to full cuff tears

Reference

Stephens SR, et al. Arthroscopic acromioplasty: a 6- to 10-year follow-up. Arthroscopy 1998; 14(4):382–388.

Adhesive Capsulitis

CLASSIFICATION

- Primary idiopathic
  - Capsular thickening and contracture
  - Global motion loss in all planes
  - Resolves over 1–3 yr
  - In diabetes mellitus (DM), can be bilateral
  - Responds to PT
- Secondary
  - Contracture can be capsular, extracapsular, or between tissue planes
  - Motion loss in one or more planes
  - Postsurgical
  - Posttraumatic, rotator cuff (RTC) tear, OA

DIFFERENTIAL DIAGNOSIS

- Posterior dislocation
- RTC rupture
- Severe impingement

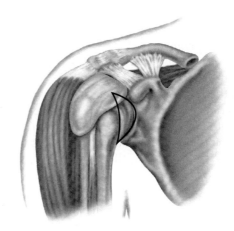

Adhesive capsulitis (frozen shoulder). Adhesive capsulitis refers to a mysterious fibrosis of the glenohumeral joint capsule, manifested by diffuse, dull, aching pain in the shoulder and progressive restriction of active and passive range of motion but usually no localized tenderness. The condition is usually unilateral and occurs in persons aged 50 to 70 years. There is often an antecedent painful disorder of the shoulder or possibly another condition (such as myocardial infarction) that has decreased shoulder movements. The course is chronic, lasting months to years, but the disorder often resolves spontaneously, at least partially. (From Bickley LS, Szilagyi P. Bates' Guide to Physical Examination and History Taking, 8th ed. Philadelphia: Lippincott Williams & Wilkins; 2003.)

- Cervical arthritis
- Pancoast tumor

EVALUATION

- Block to motion, active = passive
- For RTC disease, only active lost
- Medial scapular pain due to increased scapulothoracic motion

CLINICAL STAGES

- Pain—gradual onset, diffuse
- Stiff—gradually decreasing ROM
- Thawing—slow return of motion

Neviaser Arthroscopic Stages
- Stage I
  - Patchy fibrinous synovitis
  - Mainly in dependent fold
  - No contracture
- Stage II
  - Capsular contracture
  - Fibrinous adhesions
  - Synovitis

- Stage III
  - Increasing contracture
  - Resolving synovitis
- Stage IV
  - Severe capsular contraction
  - No other intra-articular process
- Arthrogram > loss of axillary recess but does not correlate with motion loss
- Limitation of external rotation (ER) to less than neutral leads to early osteoarthritis

TREATMENT

- First line is PT/stretching
- Do not treat primary adhesive capsulitis during painful phase. Wait until pain is only at end of motion

Closed Manipulation

- First line for primary or secondary (unless extraarticular cause known, in which case, one must open)
- Externally rotate adducted arm first to clear greater trochanter (GT), then flex, then abduct, then externally rotate and internally rotate abducted arm, then internally rotate adducted arm (Neviaser)

Arthroscopic Release with Manipulation

- For primary that failed closed manipulation
- For secondary adhesive capsulitis where cause is principally capsular
- Release sequentially
  - Interval release from biceps to subscapularis
  - Anterior-inferior capsule to 5 o-clock (subscapularis safe between capsule and axillary nerve)
  - Posterior capsule (for more internal rotation [IR] in abduction) (take at glenoid rim to protect infraspinatus)

Open Release

- Free up all layers
- Release rotator interval
- Z-plasty subscapularis as needed
- Protect axillary nerve. and release posteriorly from inferior to superior

Reference

Warner JJ. Frozen shoulder: diagnosis and management. J Am Acad Orthop Surg 1997; 5(3):130–140.

Rotator Cuff Disease

PATHOPHYSIOLOGY

Three Stages

- I. Edema/hemorrhage
  - <25 yo

- Reversible
- Conservative measures
- II. Fibrosis/tendinitis
  - 25–40 yo
  - Activity-related pain
  - PT ± surgery
- III. Bone spurs/tendon rupture
  - >40 yo
  - Progressive disability
  - Acromioplasty, RTC repair
    (Neer, 1972)

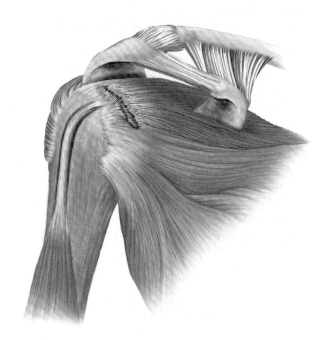

Anatomy and injuries of the shoulder. Rotator cuff tear. Partial tear. (Asset provided by Anatomical Chart Co.)

- RTC disease may be primary event leading to superior migration and impingement
- Neer—95% of RTC tears are due to impingement
- Hooked acromion in 80% RTC tears
- In young athletes, must rule out instability with functional impingement
- Most partial-thickness tears are on undersurface
- Distal 2 cm of supraspinatus (SS) is most common site of tear, also site with low blood supply
- Tears either crescent, U, or L
- One-third of cadavers >70 yo have RTC tear
- MRIs in old find asymptomatic tears
- Asymptomatic cuff tear diagnosis by ultrasound (US) has 50% chance of getting symptomatic in 2.8 yr
- Acromial shape (flat, curved, hooked) is age independent but presence of anteroinferior acromial spur is age dependent, indicating that shape is not result of cuff disease

- Partial-thickness tears usually more painful with resisted motion than full-thickness
- Stiffness limits passive range of motion (PROM) and causes pain at end of motion and difficulty sleeping
- Isolated SS tear will cause weakness only with elevation in plane of scapula with humerus internally rotated

Os Acromiale
- Must identify before acromioplasty
- Seen on axillary lateral
- Ossification centers
  - Preacromion
  - Meta-acromion
  - Mesoacromion
  - Basiacromion
- Ossification failure most common between MTA and MSA
- Patients with os acromiale who are decompressed feel better initially but by 6 mo symptome return, requiring os excision

IMAGING
- US 85% accurate to diagnose tear

TREATMENT
Observation
- >46 patients, 2.5-yr follow-up. Full-thickness tear, treat with home program of gentle stretch and strengthening. Supraspinal tear only in 60%; 59% got better, 11% same, 30% worsened (Goldberg et al., 2001)
- Try not to inject first visit because relief will make people avoid rehab
- RTC strengthening depresses humeral head, creating more space
  - Do not do RTC strengthening with thumb down; supinate arm instead

SAD Alone for RTC Tear
- 84% better at 2 yr
- By 4 yr only 62% better

Open RTC Repair
- 90% success
- Must take down deltoid

SAD, Miniopen Repair
- Scope incision extended
- Must retract deltoid carefully
- No need to débride GT to cancellous bone

- Double row increased surface area and 10% increased strength in goats
- Modified Mason-Allen stitch
- 94% success at 4 yr

Arthroscopic Repair
- 94% success at >4yrs
- Less postoperative pain

Massive RTC Repair
- Maintain coracoacromial (CA) ligament** if débride
- Check X-ray view for elevated head. If acromiohumeral distance <5 cm, then cuff is not repairable. These can just be débrided
- Check MR for fatty infiltration of muscle. If so, no repair
- L tear retracts to U tear. Fix into L shape by marginal convergence
- Muscle transfers—lats, pects
- Outcome is good if heals but high rate of re-tears

Results
- 105 open repairs, 5-yr follow-up
- Postoperative function versus status of cuff via US
- 80% of SS-only repairs still intact
- 57% of SS + infraspinatus (IS) repairs intact
- 32% of SS + IS + subscapular repairs intact
- Overall, only 65% still intact
- Most patients happy and good function
- Intact better function and flexion than large recurrent defects
- Function related to size of recurrent defect
- If intact at follow-up, did not matter if originally had larger tear (Harryman et al., 1991)

Postop Rehab
- Sling for 3 wk
- *PROM only until 4–6 wk. Restrict some ER depending on repair. Usually forward flexion and ER to 0 degrees
- Active-assistive range of motion (AAROM) at >6 wk
- Strengthen at 12 wk
- Full recovery at only 1 yr
- Manipulation under anesthesia (MUA) is not useful for stiffness after RTC repair, must scope lysis of adhesions (LOA)
- Single-tendon repair with 20% recurrence and double-tendon repair with 50% recurrence at 5 yr

References
Neer CS 2nd. Anterior acromioplasty for the chronic impingement syndrome in the shoulder: a preliminary report. J Bone Joint Surg Am 1972; 54(1):41–50.

Goldberg BA, et al. Outcome of nonoperative management of full-thickness rotator cuff tears. Clin Orthop Relat Res 2001; (382):99–107.

Harryman DT 2nd, et al. Repairs of the rotator cuff. Correlation of functional results with integrity of the cuff. J Bone Joint Surg Am 1991; 73(7):982–989.

Subscapularis Tear

ISOLATED TEAR

Gerber et al., 1996
- Forceful ER of adducted arm
- Weakness in tasks requiring IR, i.e., reaching for wallet
- Physical exam
  - Passive ER increased
  - Lift-off test with UE in maximum IR
  - Belly press test
- Repair recommended

IRREPARABLE TEAR

Resh et al., 2000
- Superior half to two-thirds of pectoralis major routed behind conjoined tendon and short head of biceps to LT

References

Resch H, et al. Transfer of the pectoralis major muscle for the treatment of the irreparable rupture of the subscapularis tendon. J Bone Joint Surg Am 2000; 82:372.

Gerber C, et al. Isolated rupture of the subscapularis tendon. J Bone Joint Surg Am 1996; 78:1015–1023.

Scapular Winging

MEDIAL

- Serratus anterior/long thoracic
- Usually traumatic traction injury
- Usually responds to rehab
- Can be due to shoulder pathology
- Impingement can be made worse by winging as acromion is brought down

LATERAL

- Cranial nerve (CN) XI, trapezius
- Usually iatrogenic from lymph node (LN) biopsy
- Treatment is by levator scapula and rhomboid transfer

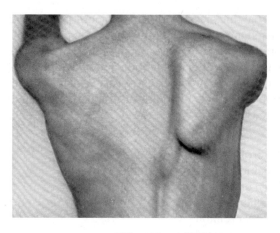

Winged scapula

Paralysis of serratus anterior. When the serratus anterior is paralyzed because of injury to the long thoracic nerve, the medial border of the scapula moves laterally and posteriorly and hangs away from the thoracic wall. This gives the scapula the appearance of a wing, especially when the person leans on his or her hand, presses the upper limb against a wall, or raises the arm—consequently the term *winged scapula*. In addition, the arm cannot be abducted above the horizontal position because the serratus anterior is unable to rotate the glenoid cavity superiorly (face upward) to allow complete abduction of the arm. Although protected when the limbs are at one's sides, the long thoracic nerve is exceptional in that it courses on the superficial aspect of the serratus anterior, which it supplies. Thus, when the limbs are elevated—as in a knife fight—the nerve is especially vulnerable. (From Moore KL, Agur A. Essential Clinical Anatomy, 2nd ed. Philadelphia: Lippincott Williams & Wilkins; 2002.)

Internal Impingement

- Overhead thrower
- Contact between the RTC undersurface and the posterosuperior glenoid rim
- Fraying of undersurface cuff and posterosuperior labrum

MR FINDINGS

- Posterior glenoid/labral hyperostosis, remodeling, seen above equator

Shoulder Dislocation

- Most common dislocated joint
- Mechanical ER and extension
- Anteroposterior, axillary, West Point, Stryker notch
- Bankart anteroinferior labral avulsion with plastic deformation of capsule

- RTC torn/avulsed in GT fracture if >40 yo (Neviaser, et al., 1988)
- Glenoid rim fracture
- Posterolateral Hill-Sachs impaction fracture
- 10% axillary nerve neurapraxia, rule out RTC tear
- Rowe maneuver—longitudinal traction with flexion and internal derotation

RECURRENCE

- 90% recurrence in patients <20 yo with conservative measures
- 500 shoulders with average 5-yr follow-up on 300 shoulders (Rowe, 1956)
- Overall ~60% recurrence
- <20 yo—83%
- 20–40 yo—63%
- >40 yo—16%
- 573 patients with follow-up on 101 shoulders
- >Overall 50% recurrence (McLaughlin and Cavallaro, 1950)
- <20 yo—90%
- 20–40 yo—60%
- >40 yo—10%
- 124 patients with 5-yr follow-up (Simonet and Cofield, 1988)
- Overall 33% recurrence
- <20 yo—66%
- 20–40 yo—40%
- >40 yo—0%
- Acute dislocation scope findings (Baker, et al., 1990)
  - Capsule tear only—13%
  - Capsule and partial labrum tear—24%
  - Capsule and labrum detached—63%
- HAGL (humeral avulsion of GH ligament) can also be seen
- Capsule tear requires surgery
- West Point cadets <24 yo (Taylor and Arciero, 1997)
  - Scope within 10 days of first dislocation
  - 63 patients chose scope, 53 patients nonoperative
  - 61/63 (97%) had Perthes-Bankart
  - 57/63 (90%) with Hill-Sachs
  - 48/53 (91%) of nonoperative developed instability
  - Only 12% of scope choice developed instability
- 95 anteriors for patients older than 60 yo (Gumina and Postacchini, 1992)
- 60% with RTC tear
- 20% with recurrent dislocation
- RTC tear in 100% of the recurrent dislocations
- Surgery successful in all except patients with multiple dislocations and RTC tear who had only the cuff repaired

References

Neviaser RJ, et al. Concurrent rupture of the rotator cuff and anterior dislocation of the shoulder in the older patient. J Bone Joint Surg Am 1988; 70(9):1308–1311.

McLaughlin HL, Cavallaro WU. Primary anterior dislocation of the shoulder. Am J Surg 1950; 80(6):615–621.

Rowe CR. Prognosis in dislocations of the shoulder. J Bone Joint Surg Am 1956; 38-A(5):957–977.

Simonet WT, Cofield RH. Prognosis in anterior shoulder dislocations. Am J Sports Med 1984; 12(1):19–24.

Baker CL, et al. Arthroscopic evaluation of acute initial anterior shoulder dislocation. Am J Sports Med 18: 1990;

Taylor DC, Arciero RA. Pathologic changes associated with shoulder dislocations. Arthroscopic and physical examination findings in first-time, traumatic anterior dislocations. Am J Sports Med 1997; 25:306–311.

Gumina S, Postacchini F. Anterior dislocation of the shoulder in elderly patients. J Bone Joint Surg Br 1997; 79(4):540–543.

Shoulder Dislocation: Complications

- Recurrent instability
  - 80%–90% at 20 yo
  - 10%–15% after 40 yo
  - Higher in men
  - Higher after low energy injury
  - Low recurrence rate with GT fracture
- Humerus fractures
- Small risk of anatomic neck fracture with reduction of subcoracoid dislocation with GT fracture
- Glenoid fracture
- RC tears: risk rises with age
  - 30% at >40 yo
  - 80% at >80 yo
- Vascular injury
  - More common in elderly
  - More in high-energy injury
  - More in forceful reduction
  - More in reduction of old dislocation
  - Rupture, tThrombosis, tear
  - Transfer—vein graft, not ligation
- Neural injury
  - Axillary: 5%–30% incidence
  - Light touch testing—unreliable
  - May cause delayed recovery
  - Any other brachial plexus nerve
  - EMG is reliable test 3–4 wk postinjury
    - Rule out RTC tear
- 4 wk sling for young
- 2 wk sling for older
- Open labral repair >95% success
- Open currently better results compared with scope
- Inferior dislocations
- Luxatio erecta
- Hyperabducted
- Neurovascular injury common

- Late vascular thrombosis
- Shorter sling time

Shoulder Instability—Anterior

STATIC RESTRAINTS

- Articular anatomy
- Glenoid labrum
- Negative pressure, joint fluid adhesion
- Capsule/GH ligaments
- Dynamic Restraints
- Rotator cuff
- (Cuff attachments into capsule)
- Biceps tendon
- Scapulothoracic motion
  - Deltoid, trapezial, rhomboid, pectoral, latissimal

BIOMECHANICS

- Isolated lesion of anterosuperior labrum without destabilizing biceps anchor does not lead to instability
- Joint compressive force (from RTC) more important to stability than negative joint pressure and glenohumeral ligaments
- Degree
- Direction—most common is subcoracoid
- Frequency
- Cause—96% traumatic, +family history
- Normal humeral head moves only 1 mm from center of glenoid
- AMBRI (*a*traumatic, *m*ultidirectional, *b*ilateral instability that often responds to *r*ehabilitation, but in case of surgery *i*nferior capsule shift is indicated) versus TUBS (Matsen)
  - Rehab 80% success with AMBRI
  - Rehab 16% success with TUBS
  - AMBRI: if surgery, open Bankart with capsular shift required

PATHOLOGIC LESIONS

- Hill-Sachs: posterolateral humeral head
- Bankart: capsule and labrum sheared off anteriorly
- Bony glenoid injury
- Subscapular lengthening and capsular release for IR contracture status post anterior stabilization

Shoulder Instability—Multidirectional (MD)

PATHOPHYSIOLOGY

- Loose redundant inferior pouch that extends anteriorly and posteriorly
- Large RTC interval along with inferior instability

Classic MD Instability

- Young, sedentary
- Generalized laxity
- Since childhood with minimum trauma
- Often bilateral, frequent, transient
- Dislocations reduced without doctor
- Large inferior pouch, usually no Bankart

Acquired MD Instability

- Overhead activity athlete
- Repetitive microtrauma
- Milder generalized laxity that allows patient to excel in sport
- After frank traumatic dislocation
- Capsule redundancy, usually with Bankart

Classification (Pagnani & Warren)

- Type I
  - Dislocates all three directions
- Type II
  - Anterior and inferior dislocation, inferoposterior subluxation
- Type III
  - Posterior and inferior dislocation, inferoanterior subluxation
- Type IV
  - Anterior and posterior dislocation, no inferior translation

HISTORY AND PHYSICAL EXAMINATION

- Anterior: symptoms with overhead activity
- Posterior: pushing open big door
- Inferior: carrying luggage, nerve symptoms
- Multidirectional: continuous vague ache, feeling of heaviness
- Unidirectional: infrequent, intense episodes of pain
- Sulcus sign positive if patient's sulcus seen and felt and symptoms reproduced
- Ulnar nerve symptoms from plexus traction
- Decreased scapular abduction and ER with arm progressively abducted
- At EUA, up to 50% translation is normal

TREATMENT

Rehab

- Immobilization useless in second dislocation or for first dislocation of atraumatic multidirectional instability (MDI)
- Rehab better for atraumatic MDI
- Rehab 6–12 mo greater than 80 percent success
- Arthroscopy (little role in MDI)

- Especially not useful in atraumatic
- Cannot fully address capsule laxity
- Cannot address RTC interval
- Open stabilization
  - Goal for stable joint by reducing capsule volume while maintaining motion
  - Surgical approach from side of greatest instability but anterior approach can tighten globally
  - Anterior-inferior capsular shift
- 40 patients with T-plasty modification of Bankart repair for acquired MDI, primarily anterior instability (Altchek et al., 1991)
- 36 from dislocations
- Three-fourths no laxity in opposite side
- Half had no generalized laxity
- 38 had Bankart
- 24 had Hill-Sachs
- Results 95% excellent at 2 yr
- Oblique subscapular tendon incision
- If interval large, use it to examine joint for Bankart
- If large interval with no Bankart, incorporate interval into lateral based L-plasty and shift capsule superolaterally
- If large interval with Bankart, use medial based L-plasty and shift superomedially
- If no Bankart, technically easier to do lateral capsular shift of Neer
- If interval normal, view labrum via oblique capsulotomy proximal to IGHLC and do medial or lateral T-capsulotomy based on presence of Bankart
- Anterior H-plasty for extreme inferior instability

Reference
Altchek DW, et al. T-plasty modification of the Bankart procedure for multidirectional instability of the anterior and inferior types. J Bone Joint Surg Am 1991; 73(1):105–112.

Shoulder Instability—Posterior

PATHOPHYSIOLOGY

- 2%–4% of shoulder instability

Anatomic Factors
- Circle theory where anterosuperior capsule damage is needed to allow posterior dislocation
- Glenoid retroversion >10 degrees (normal is 5 degrees)
- Humeral head retroversion >40 degrees
- Hypoplastic glenoid
- Generalized laxity
- Acute posterior dislocation
- Mechanism is flexion, adduction, IR
- Fall on outstretched hand

- Most common due to electric shock, seizure, ethyl alcohol (EtOH)
- Unable to externally rotate
- Missed acutely 50% of the time
- Presents adduction and internally rotated
- Along with lesser tubercle fracture**
- 50% with impaction fracture between articular margin and lesser tubercle
- Rowe sign—unable to fully supinate forearm with shoulder flexed forward
- Reduce by lateral traction to unlock bony notch, then externally rotate to relax posterior capsule, and posterior pressure to head. Arm then gently abducted in external rotation

IMAGING
- X-ray view signs
  - Reverse Hill-Sachs
  - Vacant glenoid sign on AP
  - >6 mm rim sign on AP (distance between anterior glenoid and head)
  - Cystic sign (head appears cystic due to increased IR)

TREATMENT
- Immobilize 4–6 wk in slight extension and ER, then PT to emphasize ER strengthening
- Recurrence ~40% overall, more recurrence in patients <20 yo
- PT more effective for patients with laxity and repetitive microtrauma compared to patients with macrotrauma

Arthroscopicic Repair—Suretac
- Indications
  - Acute traumatic posterior dislocation/subluxation
  - Detached posterior or superior capsule/labrum
  - Good tissue quality
  - Reattachment will restore stability

Glenoid Osteotomy
- 17 patients atraumatic post instability, 5 yr follow-up
- All with normal capsule/labrum
- 81% good/excellent
- 25% postop DJD
  (Graichen et al., 1999)

Biceps Tendon Transfer
- Posterior capsule repair and biceps tendon rerouted around posterior neck and inserted into post
- Glenoid (Boyd and Sisk, 1972)
- >67% success (Hawkins et al., 1984)

Posterior Capsulorrhaphy Alone

- Indications
- No bony glenoid defect
- Substantial posterior capsule and infraspinatus
- Horizontal or vertical incision
- Split infra tendon vertically
- Medial based T-capsulotomy
- Labrum may be partially detached by frank reverse Bankart (rare)
- Capsule advanced medially and superiorly (if inferior laxity)
- Repair capsule to labrum or to bone if labrum detached
- If inferior laxity, may need to convert T to H to obliterate pouch
- Lateral infra tendon sutured to glenoid and medial infra tendon advanced laterally
- Immobilize in neutral rotation, slight extension
- Sports in 9–12 mo

Posterior Capsulorrhaphy with Bone Block

- Indications
- Deficient glenoid
- Laxity and poor posterior tissues
- 15 × 30 mm graft from scapular spine
- Screw across two cortices of glenoid
- Do capsule repair first
- Graft in posteroinferior quadrant
- Avoid bony impingement
- 24 patients average 20 yo with posterior subluxation
- 5-yr follow-up
- 16 patients had PT: 63% success
- 11 patients had surgery (posterior capsulorrhaphy ± bone block): 91% success (Fronek et al., 1989)
- 6 sports injury, 4 accidents
- 8 of 11 had posterior labral vertical tear
- All patients had ligamentous laxity
- In PT group, minor trauma and more compliant patients had better results
- In surgery group, most return to sports but at lower level

CHRONIC LOCKED POSTERIOR DISLOCATION

Hawkins et al., 1987

- Bony defect <20%, dislocation <6 wk
  - Closed reduction
- Bony defect <45%, dislocation <6 mo
  - Tubercle/subscapular transfer to defect
- Bony defect >50%, dislocation >6 mo
  - Hemiarthroplasty with head in neutral version

Recurrent Posterior Subluxation

- Subluxation does *not* progress to dislocation
- Compared with pain, instability is secondary

- Pain can be anterior and/or posterior
- Apprehension very uncommon
- Habitual subluxators: psychological
- Voluntary subluxators do so by position or by firing certain movements
- Involuntary subluxators along with high forces of "follow-through" sports
- Some patients are MDI status post prior to anterior tightening
- 90% of patients with clicking
- Secondary RTC impingement
- Loss of IR in 90 degrees of abduction
- Be careful to examine for MDI

References

Graichen H, et al. Effectiveness of glenoid osteotomy in atraumatic posterior instability of the shoulder associated with excessive retroversion and flatness of the glenoid. Int Orthop 1999; 23(2):95–99.

Boyd HB, Sisk TD. Recurrent posterior dislocation of the shoulder. J Bone Joint Surg Am 1972; 54(4):779–786.

Hawkins RJ, et al. Recurrent posterior instability (subluxation) of the shoulder. J Bone Joint Surg Am 1984; 66(2):169–174.

Fronek J, et al. Posterior subluxation of the glenohumeral joint. J Bone Joint Surg Am 1989; 71(2):205–216.

Hawkins RJ, et al. Locked posterior dislocation of the shoulder. J Bone Joint Surg Am 1987; 69(1):9–18.

Anterior Instability—Arthroscopic Repairs

- Débridement not effective
- Indications—recurrent posttraumatic unidirectional anterior instability
- "Drive through" sign—scope easily passed into anteroinferior joint cavity due to inferior pouch laxity

TRANSGLENOID SUTURE (MORGAN)

- 40% failure rate
- Cartilage damage
- Drilling leads to suprascapular nerve injury
- Tying over infraspinatus muscle

CANNULATED SURETAC (WARREN)

- Biodegradable device
- Direct visualization for repair
- For TUBS (*t*raumatic, *u*nidirectional instability and *B*ankart lesion that often requires *s*urgery) with discrete Bankart and intact capsule
- Allows only minimal capsule shift
- Cannot close rotator interval
- Not for contact athletes

Anterior Instability—Open Repairs

HELFET-BRISTOW PROCEDURE

- Coracoid process transfer
- Screw fixation
- Effective subscapular tenodesis

MAGNUSON-STACK

- Transfer of subscapularis from lesser trochanter (LT) to greater trochanter (GT) across biceps

NICOLA

- Long head biceps used as checkrein

PUTTI-PLATT

- Plication of subscapular tendon

BONE BLOCKS

- Latarjet procedure as separate options

OPEN BANKART

- Anterior approach
- Bankart enlarged, strip medially
- Anchors at 2, 4, 6 o'clock for right shoulder
- Suture inside out through capsule

CAPSULAR SHIFT

- Capsular shift only for recurrent anterior subluxation
- If no RTC interval capsular defect, then use lateral based T-capsulotomy.
- If RTC interval defect, incorporate it into upside-down L-capsulotomy
- Check laxity by finger in axillary pouch
- Inferior capsule shifted superiorly
  - 45–60 degrees abduction
  - 25–45 degrees ER
  - 10 degrees flexion
- Superior capsule flapped inferiorly
  - 0 degrees abduction
  - 25–45 degrees ER
- After shift, should get:
  - 90 degrees abduction
  - 25–45 degrees ER
  - 1+ drawer in 45 degrees abduction, neutral
  - 0 drawer in ER, more abduction

Shoulder Arthroscopy—Operative Pearls

- No subacromial injection because once bursa is distended, it is difficult to get into subacromial space
- No injection into joint, just portal sites
- Horizontal lateral incision
- For access to AC joint:
- Put posterior portal higher and more lateral (1 cm down and medial to posterolateral corner of acromion)
- Anterior portal just lateral to AC joint
- Shaver through anterior portal, view with camera through lateral portal
- Distal clavicle should become obliquely slanted posteriorly and inferomedially after resection, because first place to make contact in adduction is posterior AC joint
- Take more clavicle posteriorly because acromion gets wider posteriorly
- Superior ligaments most important and attach 15 mm from AC joint so can take 1 cm usually

SLAP (SUPERIOR LABRAL TEARS ANTERIOR TO POSTERIOR)

- Wilmington portal at anterolateral acromial corner at edge of bone through RTC interval for anchor placement

BANKART

- Two anterior portals, using spinal needle to see if portal can get you to pathology
  - Superior portal for gray suture management as high as possible under biceps
  - Inferior portal as low as possible just on top of subscapularis for purple cannula for anchor placement, suture tying
- Mitek placed into articular cartilage to get more perpendicular to glenoid
- Spectrum suture (right- or left-handed) passer (looks like corkscrew) to pass PDS loop through ligament/labrum complex (loop at tip of passer)
- Usually three anchors
- Outside, put one arm of Mitek suture through loop to pull it through tissue, then tie
- Close interval by pushing loop of FiberWire through bottom of hole, then leaving loop in joint, backing up pointy grasper out of joint, pushing it through the other side of the hole, then grabbing the loop out cannula. The suture is then tied blindly.

SAD/RTC REPAIR

- Pump pressure up to 60
- Make posterior portal higher

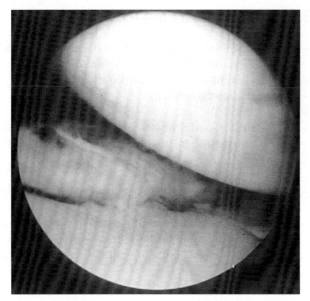

Arthroscopic view of a detached anterior labrum (Bankart lesion). (From Bucholz RW, Heckman JD. Rockwood & Green's Fractures in Adults, 5th ed. Philadelphia: Lippincott, Williams & Wilkins; 2001.)

- For SAD, facet where resected bone meets native bone is OK if >1 cm back. Otherwise, it impinges.
- To get to subacromion, point toward anterolateral corner. At about the crotch of the drawing (middle of acromion), there is a veil that you must pass
- Inspect CA ligament—degeneration and tattering indicate impingement
- Push ArthroCare against ligament instead of peeling it off
- Have constant outflow to allow higher pressures
- Ensure high lateral portal and adduct shoulder to allow more vertical anchor placement
- Higher lateral portal is better for anchor, but it makes acromioplasty harder, so split difference
- Clear white lateral corkscrew cannula
- Pull three sutures out front, leave one in clear cannula
- Move gray cannula laterally, more posterior, for suture management as needed. Can also put grasper in through here to pull on cuff while sutures tied
- More medial anchors at articular margin to mattress sutures. Expressew through cuff posteriorly first.
- Lateral anchors into cortical bone of GT and simple bites through these, forming a pseudo double row.

CAPSULAR SHIFT

- Use elevator to separate capsule from subscapularis
- Detach humeral attachment of MGHL

- Push penetrator through capsule, through inferior ligament, and leave loop in joint. Pull penetrator back off capsule and repenetrate superiorly, then pull entire loop through
- Tie knot blindly inside cannula, outside of capsule, anterior to subscapularis

SLAP Lesions

- First reported by Andrews in 1985
- Occurs with acceleration phase in overhead athletes
- Begins posteriorly, extends anteriorly
- Lesions that destabilize biceps anchor lead to subtle joint instability
- Symptoms from increasing joint translation, catching of unstable labrum

CLASSIFICATION

- SLAP coined by Snyder (Snyder et al. 1990)
- Type I
  - Fraying labrum, intact anchor
  - Arthroscopic débridement
- Type II
  - Detached labral-biceps anchor
  - Scope/open anchor stabilization
- Type III
  - Bucket-handle tear of superior labrum
  - Biceps intact
  - Arthroscopic debridement
- Type IV
  - Bucket-handle tear of superior labrum into biceps tendon (which becomes unstable)
  - If <30% tendon involved and older patient, tendon may be excised with bucket tear
  - If >30% tendon or smaller tear in younger patient, then perform tenodesis on biceps with excision of bucket tear
- Type V (Maffet et al., 1995)
  - Bankart continues superiorly to include biceps anchor
  - Bankart repair and anchor repair
- Type VI
  - Type II SLAP with unstable flap tear of superior labrum
  - Flap débridement and anchor repair
- Type VII
  - Labral-biceps anchor detachment extends anteriorly to include MGHL
  - MGHL and anchor repair
  - Commonly with other pathology that must be treated
  - 40% partial or full RTC tear

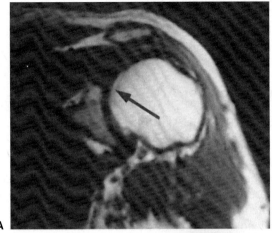

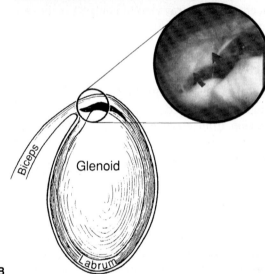

A so-called SLAP lesion of the long head biceps tendon origin and superior glenoid labrum as seen on magnetic resonance imaging (MRI) and arthroscopic examinations. SLAP, superior labrum anterior-posterior. (From Bucholz RW, Heckman JD. Rockwood & Green's Fractures in Adults, 5th ed. Philadelphia: Lippincott, Williams & Wilkins; 2001.)

- 15% anterior instability**
- 15% humeral head chondromalacia
- 10% AC joint arthrosis

DIFFERENTIAL DIAGNOSIS

- Sublabral recess or foramen
  - Physiologic superior labral detachment—seen in 70% of normal patients
  - True SLAPs have concomitant capsular injury and high signal in labrum
- Buford complex
  - Absent anterior-posterior labrum with cordlike MGHL instead

TREATMENT

- 22 patients with type II or IV SLAPs fixed with Suretac
- 2-yr follow-up
- 86% satisfactory results
- 12 of 13 overhead athletes back to prior level of play
- Two-thirds of failures had concomitant SAD (Pagnani et al., 1995)

References

Snyder SJ, et al. SLAP lesions of the shoulder. Arthroscopy 1990; 6:274–279.
Maffet MW, et al. Superior labrum-biceps tendon complex lesions of the shoulder. Am J Sports Med 1995; 23:93–98.
Pagnani MJ, et al. Arthroscopic fixation of superior labral lesions using a biodegradable implant: a preliminary report. Arthroscopy 1995; 11:194–198.

Suprascapular Neuropathy

- Suprascapular notch
  - Supraspinatus and infraspinatus affected
- Spinoglenoid notch
  - Only infraspinatus affected
  - Along with labral tear and ganglion
- Volleyball players
- Conservative measures
- Surgery for failures, address intra-articular pathology

Thoracic Outlet Syndrome

- Neurogenic
  - More common
- Vascular
  - Athlete with developed muscles, bruit
- Clinical exam for diagnosis
- Maneuver with loss of pulse and reproduction of symptoms
  - Adson maneuver
  - Hyperabduction

WRIGHT (MODIFIED ADSON)

- UE extended, abducted, externally rotated, and neck extended, rotated to opposite side—reproduction of symptoms and loss of pulse

ROOS TEST

- Both UE in abduction and ER with rapid closing/opening of hands leads to symptoms

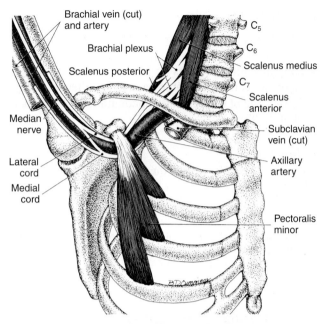

Thoracic outlet syndrome. (Reprinted with permission from Travell JG, Simons DG. Myofascial Pain and Dysfunction: The Trigger Point Manual, vol 1: The Upper Extremities, 1st ed. Baltimore: Williams & Wilkins; 1983.)

- Postural exercises for rhomboids, levator scapula
- Surgery rare unless cervical rib
- Reduction mammoplasty to reduce load on chest wall
- Between anterior and middle scalenes, clavicle, and first rib

Throwing Phases

WIND-UP

- Flexion

EARLY COCKING

- Deltoid, RTC
- Abduction, ER

LATE COCKING

- Deltoid, RTC, inferior capsule
- Begins with foot contact

ACCELERATION

- All tissues stressed
- Hand velocity 7,000 degrees/sec

FOLLOW-THROUGH

- Posterior capsule
- (Deceleration—RTC stressed)

Total Shoulder Arthroplasty

CONTRAINDICATIONS

- Loss of deltoid function
- Inability to reconstruct RTC
- Constrained, semiconstrained with hooded glenoid (prevents superior migration in RTC deficiency), and unconstrained
- Glenoid usually cemented and about 40% end up with lucent lines on x-ray view but only 8% of those needed revision

TECHNIQUE

- Check passive ER with EUA to see if subscapularis lengthening needed
- Incision from clavicle to deltoid insertion, passing over coracoid
- Cephalic vein taken laterally
- Take more pectoralis major off in patient with IR contracture, putting finger behind pectoralis and using Bovie
- Clavicle-pectoralis fascia taken just lateral to conjoined tendon (short head of biceps) to access anterior humeral circumflex artery and subscapularis
- Can take part of CA ligament to see
- Conjoined tendon partially detached 1 cm distal to coracoid to release tension off musculocutaneous nerve
- Find bicep and follow it proximally to find rotator interval and to find LT
- Palpate axillary nerve by hooking finger under subscapularis
- If passive ER adequate, take subscapularis and capsule 1 cm medial to insertion on LT; tag before incising
- If need to lengthen subscapularis, take it off subperiosteally from LT with capsule and repair it to osteotomy site when surgery done
- Caudal extension of subscapularis marked by three sisters (anterior humeral circumflex artery, veins)
- Put arm in ER to take axillary nerve Away, then take anterior inferior capsule to 6 o'clock
- Bent Hohmann or Darrach retractors under supraspinatus and under inferior neck
- ER, adduction, extend to deliver head. If hard, release more inferior capsule
- Excise inferior osteophytes with o-tome to expose entire head, then cut head in 30-degree retroversion

- Ream stem canal with retroversion in mind (keel should be 8 mm posterior to biceps groove)
- Keep trial in place while working on glenoid to avoid fracture and bleeding
- Repair cuff as needed after head removed
- Check whether glenoid orientation is normal by preop CT
- Fukuda or two-prong Anspach or T-handled Bankart retractor to posterior glenoid
- Small Darrach to posterosuperior glenoid
- Can saw off stem metaphysis that sticks out of Fukuda hole
- Bankart retractor to anterior glenoid
- Burr to find central glenoid canal and to normalize eroded glenoid surface
- Watch out for posterior blowout with burr, using curette to sound hole
- Can use angled reamer to avoid going too posteriorly
- Be careful taking out Fukuda after cementing in glenoid
- Ideal height is top of head just above GT to avoid impingement
- Recreate normal head size and offset
- Construction should allow 50% translation in AP and superior-inferior planes and 90-degree abduction, 70–80 degrees IR in 90-degrees abduction
- Subscapularis repaired to allow 40 degrees ER

REHABILITATION

- PROM as tested at end of surgery
- Assisted pulley exercises at 4 wk
- Isometrics at 6 wk
- Light weights at 12 wk

RESULTS

- 95% pain relief
- OA and avascular necrosis (AVN) get better motion
- Neer prosthesis 75% 10-yr survival
- Rheumatoid arthritis (RA) Neer prosthesis 92% at 11 yr
- Most common complication is instability
  - Define direction
  - Define anatomic problem
  - Component position
  - Release contractures
  - Plicate capsular laxity
  - Establish cuff integrity
  - Cofield—modest results (Sanchez-Sotelo et al., 2003)
- Mismatch >5.5 mm between head and glenoid along with less glenoid radiolucency
- Pitfalls
- Inadequate exposure

- Not addressing concomitant pathology
- Malpositioning
- Malsizing
- Inadequate soft tissue tension, instability
- Subscapular rupture
- Two-thirds abnormal subscapular function (shirt tucking, belly press) (Qureshi et al., 2003)
- Keel versus Peg
- Keel has more radiolucency
- Pegs have more superior-inferior stability
- Keel has more anterior-posterior stability

References

Sanchez-Sotelo J, et al. Instability after shoulder arthroplasty: results of surgical treatment. J Bone Joint Surg Am 2003; 85-A(4):622–631.
Qureshi S, et al. Subscapularis function after total shoulder replacement: results with lesser tuberosity osteotomy. J Shoulder Elbow Surg 2003; 17:68–71.

TOTAL SHOULDER ARTHROPLASTY: OPERATIVE PEARLS

- Retract cephalic vein medially to avoid avulsion from subclavian
- When coming around proximal humerus subdeltoid, put Cobb under clavipectoral fascia to protect axillary nerve and vessels when Biomet retractor put in
- Bovie three sisters
- Cut horizontal hole in subscapularis above three sisters and free up capsule
- Elevate subscapularis off glenoid and also anteriorly behind conjoint tendon
- Extend rotator interval to get more length
- Head cut
- Clear soft tissue out off glenoid
- Glenoid cemented before humerus reamed
- T-handled Bankart retractor to posterior glenoid
- Anspach anteriorly
- Burr central hole, then circular reamer
- Extend hole into rectangle, not going wider to allow press fit of keel into slot
- Intramedullary (IM) finder lateral and posterior
- Press fit stem so do not put down last broach all the way
- Mersilene for subscapular repair to osteotomy site if subscapularis taken off bone
- Do not close RTC interval too tight

TOTAL SHOULDER ARTHROPLASTY INDICATIONS

Osteoarthritis

- Anterior-inferior osteophyte on humeral neck
- Loss of ER, loss of subscapularis excursion
- Inferior capsular contracture

- Posterior erosion, osteophytes
- RTC tear only 1%–5%
- Posterior subluxation with flexion
- Posterior joint line tenderness
- Diagnostic injection

RA

- Glenoid and humeral head with cysts
- Anterior and central erosions
- RTC tear in 40%, many more with RTC attrition
- Poorly localized pain
- Glenohumeral motion lost more than scapulothoracic motion
- Total shoulder arthroplasty (TSA) predictable pain relief versus hemi

AVN

- Hemi may erode glenoid
- Modular better for these patients
- When glenoid preserved, then pain predominates, with loss of AROM leading to loss of PROM

Posttraumatic DJD

- CT to check greater tuberosity position
- MRI to evaluate RTC

Cuff Arthropathy

- Irreparable RTC tear
- Osteopenia/collapse of head
- Superior and anterior subluxation
- Without RTC, head elevates with abduction and causes edge loading of glenoid component via rocking horse effect and subsequent loosening
- Consider humeral head only
- Atrophy of supraspinatus and infraspinatus
- Weak in flexion, ER, abduction

Distal Biceps Rupture

- Middle aged
- Lifting with elbow extended

ANATOMY

- Lateral antebrachial cutaneous nerve exits deep fascia at level of muscle-tendon junction of biceps, between biceps and brachialis

NATURAL HISTORY

- Nonoperative
  - 30% flexion strength loss
  - 40% supination strength loss (Morrey et al., 1985)

OPERATIVE TECHNIQUES

- Two-incision technique
  - A benefit is that it avoids radial nerve damage from anterior approach
  - Stripping off ulna led to heterotopic ossification (HO)

RESULTS

- 10 athletes >40 yo, two incision
- All return to full unlimited sports
- Avoid HO by small posterior muscle splitting approach avoiding periosteal elevation of ulna
- Repaired dominant arm
  - Normal supinator endurance and strength
  - 20% decrease in flexion endurance, normal strength
- Repaired nondominant arm
  - Normal supinator endurance, 25% decreased strength
  - Normal flexion endurance and strength (D'Alessandro et al., 1993)

References

Morrey BF, et al. Rupture of the distal tendon of the biceps brachii. J Bone Joint Surg Am 1985; 67(3):418–421.

D'Alessandro DF, et al. Repair of distal biceps tendon ruptures in athletes. Am J Sports Med 1993; 21(1):114–119.

Elbow Arthroscopy

- Most common indications for elbow scope are synovectomy and loose body
- Flex elbow 90 degrees and insufflate 30 mL via lateral needle. This is most important way to prevent injury to radial nerve.* Needle goes between radial head, distal humerus, and olecranon
- Needle for anterolateral portal with free backflow to confirm intra-articular
- Cut skin, then dissect to fascia
- Aim trocar into center of joint
- Establish anteromedial portal using Wissinger rod technique (push scope/cannula to medial capsule, remove camera, push rod through cannula to tent skin, cut down on rod, put cannula over rod)

LATERAL PORTALS

Direct Lateral (Soft Spot Portal)*

- Also known as inferior posterolateral
- Cartilage and posterior antebrachial cutaneous nerve at risk
- Sees radial head, capitellum, trochlear notch, olecranon

Distal Anterolateral (Standard Anterolateral)

- Originally described by Andrews/Carson
- 2 cm distal, 2 cm anterior to lateral epicondyle
- Also described as 1 cm distal, 3 cm anterior to lateral epicondyle
- At risk are:
  - Radial nerve (posterior interosseous nerve [PIN])
  - Lateral antebrachial cutaneous nerve
- Sees anterior compartment
- This is the standard diagnostic portal

Proximal Anterolateral* (Superolateral)

- Described by Day and Field
- 2 cm proximal, 1 cm anterior to lateral epicondyle
- Same view and risk as distal anterior-lateral
- This portal farthest from radial nerve of all anterolateral portals. Brachialis used as safety buffer
- Sees coronoid, trochlea, capsular insertion on distal humerus

Midanterolateral

- 2 cm directly anterior to lateral epicondyle
- Also described as just proximal and 1 cm anterior to palpable radiocapitellar joint

MEDIAL PORTALS

Proximal Anteromedial* (Superomedial)

- 2 cm proximal to medial epicondyle and 1–2 cm anterior to medial intermuscular septum
- Directed toward radial head
- At risk are:
  - Ulnar nerve, med nerve, brachial artery
  - Medial antebrachial cutaneous nerve
- Sees radiocapitellar joint

Distal Anteromedial (Anteromedial)

- 2 cm distal, 2 cm anterior to medial epicondyle
- Same view as proximal anteromedial except higher neurovascular risk

POSTERIOR

Posterocentral (Straight Posterior)

- 2–4 cm above olecranon
- Ulnar nerve at risk
- Sees posterior-lateral and posterior-medial gutters

Posterolateral

- 2–4 cm proximal to olecranon, lateral to triceps
- Posterior antebrach cutaneous nerve at risk
- Sees posterolateral gutter

Elbow MCL Injury

ANATOMY

- Anterior MCL from lateral two-thirds of the anteroinferior medial epicondyle to sublime tubercle on medial aspect of coronoid
- Posterior bundle less distinct
- Transverse bundle originates and inserts on ulna
- flexor carpi ulnaris (FCU) and flexor digitorum superficialis (FDS) overlie MCL
- Internerve plane between FCU and FDS
- Innervation begins for FCU and FDS 1–3 cm distal to sublime
- Ulnar nerve courses over posterior MCL
- Ulnar nerve does not overlie anterior MCL but crosses over at sublime tubercle
- Ulnar nerve can thus be safely retracted posteriorly
- Primary restraint to valgus stress at functional ROM 20–120 degrees
- Greatest laxity at 70 degrees when aMCL sectioned

PATHOPHYSIOLOGY

- Valgus extension overload peaks at late cocking/early acceleration
- 90% are acute rupture of chronically attenuated ligament

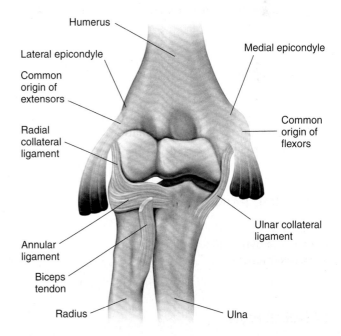

Right elbow joint, radius, and ulna—anterior view, showing the ligaments. (From Premkumar K. The Massage Connection Anatomy and Physiology. Philadelphia: Lippincott Williams & Wilkins; 2004.)

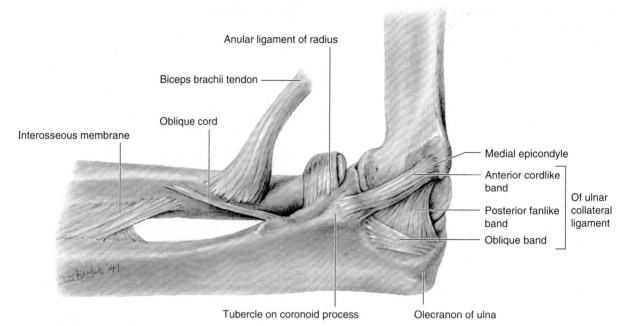

Ulnar (medial) collateral ligament. The anterior band, a strong, round cord, is taut when the elbow joint is extended; the posterior band is a weak, fanlike ligament that is taut in flexion of the joint; the oblique fibers merely deepen the socket for the trochlea of the humerus. (From Moore KL, Dalley AF II. Clinical Oriented Anatomy, 4th ed. Philadelphia: Lippincott Williams & Wilkins; 1999.)

- Leads to impingement at superomedial corner of olecranon and compression at radiocapite joint
- Bad prognosis if posteromedial spur and radiocapitate OA

MEDIAL PAIN

- MCL
- Ulnar nerve (three zones, no electromyogram [EMG])
- Flexor-pronator (pain with pronation)
- Posteromedial spur

ANTERIOR PAIN

- Distal biceps tendonitis
- Pronator syndrome
- Stress fracture

LATERAL PAIN

- Tennis elbow
- PIN syndrome
- Posterolateral rotatory instability (PLRI)
- Osteochondritis dissecans (OCD) capitellum

PHYSICAL EXAMINATION

- Valgus/varus stress in maximum pronation and 20-degree flexion because unable to valgus stress at ideal position, which is 70–90 degrees: positive if symptoms reproduced or laxity felt
- Valgus extension overload test for posteromedial impingement: quickly extend fully while valgus loading
- Partial tears do not produce laxity
- Milking maneuver
- 40% ulnar nerve symptoms but neurologic changes rare
- Loss of extension frequent

X-RAY STUDIES

- Oblique axial at 110 degrees flexion shows posteromedial spur
- At HSS, no stress x-rays
- MRI at HSS without articular contrast
  - Seen best on coronals

ARTHROSCOPIC TEST (ANDREWS)

- Cannot visualize ligament well
- Anterolateral portal view and valgus stress at 70 degrees: joint gapping 3 mm is pathologic

- Does not gap until entire anterior MCL sectioned (Field and Altchek)
  - Thus, patients may have pain from chronic partial tear but have negative scope. For these, must open and look at ligament and reconstruct if injured
- Loose bodies common

REMEDY—REHABILITATION

- Strengthen shoulder and flexion-pronation
- Good results in true acute injury in nonthrowing athlete
- 42% success in throwers

REMEDY—REPAIR

- May be OK in true acute tear
- Poor results from poor tissue in chronic injury

REMEDY—RECONSTRUCTION

- Palmaris or gracilis
- Andrews
  - Elevation of flexor pronator mass without detachment (as done originally by Jobe)
  - Subcutaneous (Sub-Q) instead of submuscular ulnar nerve transposition
  - Figure eight tendon graft
  - 81% of 59 patients back to play at previous level, 3-yr follow-up
- Altchek (docking procedure)
  - Expose via FCU splitting
  - Antebrachial cutaneous nerve of medial nerve
  - No ulnar nerve transposition needed
  - Safe zone
  - Single (vs. three) humeral tunnel
  - First limb of graft docked in humerus while it is tensioned
  - Brace for 6 wk
  - Full motion and begin PT at 6 wk
  - Tossing at 4 mo
  - Flat ground pitch at 6 mo
  - Mound pitch at 7 mo
  - Competitive pitching at 9 mo
  - 97% of 31 patients to previous level with 2.6-yr follow-up

Concussions

- Grades
  - I—transient confusion, dizzy, headache, memory loss, no loss of consciousness (LOC)
  - II—LOC <5 min or posttraumatic amnesia >30 min
  - III—positive LOC >5 min or posttraumatic amnesia >24 hr, assume cervical spine injury and treat accordingly, admit, offer referral to neurologist prior
- Evaluate three Cs
  - Cognition
  - Coordination
  - Cranial nerves
- Visual changes, progressive headache, neurologic deficits, intractable nausea and vomiting require imaging

Reference

Putukian M. The acute symptoms of sports related concussion: diagnosis and onfield management. Clin Sports Med 2011; 30(1):49–61.

Runner—Leg Pain Differential Diagnosis

MEDIAL TIBIAL STRESS SYNDROME (SHIN SPLINTS)

- Periosteal inflammation of soleus, posterior tibial muscle
- Tender medial border distal one-third tibia
- Pain resisted plantar flexion or inversion
- X-ray view normal
- Bone scan with increasing linear uptake in posteromedial tibia
- MRI—diffuse edema
- Relative rest
- Cross-training
- Muscle rehab if tight/weak
- Periosteal stripping if pain >1 yr

EXERTIONAL COMPARTMENT SYNDROME

- "Third lap syndrome"
- Usually anterolateral, occasional posteriors
- Muscle can increase in volume 20% during exercise
- Consistently reproducible dull ache
- Usually bilateral, but one worse
- Pain persists for hours after workout
- Weak, numb, paresthesia can occur
- Physical exam rarely diagnostic unless symptoms unilateral
- Measure pressures
- Decompress

STRESS FRACTURES

- Pain on exertion
- Vague, insidious
- Usually recent change in activity level, surface, shoes
- Symptoms usually subside with rest
- Tender to palpation most common finding

- X-ray view negative for 3 wk
- Bone scan can exclude diagnosis
- MR or CT if bone scan positive to define anatomy

POPLITEAL ARTERY ENTRAPMENT SYNDROME

- Abnormal relationship between popliteal artery and muscle/fascia

- Repeated compression with trauma to wall leads to localized atherosclerosis, leading progressively to arterial thrombosis
- 85% male, average age 28 yo
- Bilateral in 25%
- Exercise-induced leg pain
- Decreased pulse with knee hyperextended, foot dorsiflexed

CHAPTER 3

Pediatrics

Peter D. Fabricant, Kristin K. Warner, Daniel W. Green

General Pediatric Medicine
  Intravenous Fluid (IVF) Rates per Hour
  Meds
Development
  Growth Plates: Two Growth Centers
  Bone Age
  Milestones
Congenital Disorders
  Brachial Plexus Obstetric Palsy
  Congenital Pseudoarthrosis of the Clavicle
  Prune Belly Syndrome
  Amniotic Band Syndrome
Skeletal Dysplasias
  Achondroplasia
  Hypochondroplasia
  Pseudoachondroplasia
  Cleidocranial Dysplasia
  Diastrophic Dysplasia
  Engelmann-Camurati
  Metaphysial Chondrodysplasia: Schmid, Jansen
    McKusick
  Multiple Epiphyseal Dysplasia (MED)
  Spondyloepiphyseal Dysplasia
  Kniest Dysplasia
  Trevor Disease
  Trigger Terms
Genetics/Syndromes
  Apert
  Arthrogryposis
  Ehlers-Danlos
  Marfan Syndrome
  Juvenile Rheumatoid Arthritis
  Larsen Syndrome
  Neurofibromatosis (NF; von Recklinghausen
    Disease)
  Noonan Syndrome
  Osteogenesis Imperfecta
  Prader-Willi
  Rett syndrome

  Sandifer
  Trisomy 21 (Down Syndrome)
  Turner
Muscular Dystrophies
  Becker Muscular Dystrophy
  Facioscapulohumeral Dystrophy
  Duchenne Muscular Dystrophy
  Spinal Muscular Atrophy
Neuromuscular Disorders
  Cerebral Palsy
  Charcot-Marie-Tooth (CMT)
  Friedreich Ataxia
Metabolic Disorders
  Caffey Disease
  Gaucher Disease
  Homocystinuria
  Menkes Kinky Hair Syndrome
  Mucopolysaccharidoses
  Niemann-Pick Disease
Infection
  Discitis
  Kasser Disease (Chronic Recurrent
    Osteomyelitis)
  Osteomyelitis
  Septic Arthritis
  Transient Synovitis
Spine
  Back Pain in Children
  Myelomeningocele (MMC)
  Sacroiliitis
  Torticollis, Congenital Muscular
Upper Extremity
  Trigger Thumb
Hip
  Coxa Vara
  Developmental Dysplasia of the Hip
  Legg-Calvé-Perthes
  Slipped Capital Femoral Epiphysis
    (SCFE)

Thigh, Knee, Leg
Blount Disease
Discoid Meniscus
Femoral Anteversion
Fibular Hemimelia
Classification
Genu Valgum
In-Toeing
Internal Tibial Torsion
Leg Length Discrepancy (LLD)
Limping Child
Foot/Ankle
Accessory Navicular
Calcaneovalgus Foot
Cavus Foot
Club Foot (Congenital Talipes Equinovarus)
Congenital Vertical Talus
Curly Toe
Delta Phalanx
Flexible Flatfoot
Hallux Valgus
Metatarsus Adductus
Overlapping Fifth Toe
Subungual Exostosis
Tarsal Coalition

General Pediatric Medicine

INTRAVENOUS FLUID (IVF) RATES PER HOUR

- 4 mL/kg for 1st 10 kg
- 2 mL/kg for 2nd 10 kg
- 1 mL/kg for each kg after 2nd 10 kg
- Shorthand for children >20 kg: May add 40 to weight (in kg) for IVF Rate (mL/hr)

MEDS

- Codeine 0.5–1.0 mg/kg orally (PO) Q4–6h
- Morphine sulfate 0.1 mg/kg PO Q3–4h; 0.1–0.2 mg/kg subcutaneous (SC)/intramuscular (IM)/IV Q2–4h
- Tylenol 15 mg/kg PO/rectally (PR) Q4–6h (maximum 4 g/day)
- Ancef 50–100 mg/kg/day; IV divided in q8h, max dose 6 g/day

Development

GROWTH PLATES: TWO GROWTH CENTERS

Physis (Horizontal): Three Zones
- Reserve zone: cells store lipids, glycogen, and proteoglycan aggregates for growth and matrix production. (Lysosomal storage diseases)

- Proliferative zone: longitudinal growth, cell proliferation, and matrix production. Presence of proteoglycans inhibits calcification. (Achondroplasia)
- Hypertrophic zone: maturation, degeneration, and provisional calcification. Chondrocytes enlarge, accumulate calcium, and die. Osteoblasts then use these cartilage cells as scaffolding for bone formation. (Mucopolysaccharide diseases, enchondromas, slipped capital femoral epiphysis [SCFE])

Spherical
- Epiphyseal growth. Same arrangement, less organized.

BONE AGE

- Females (Short Hand Method, based on Gruelich and Pyle)
  - 10 years old—hook of hamate appears
  - 11 years old—thumb sesamoid appears
  - 12 years old—distal radius physis capping
  - 13 years old—thumb distal phalanx physis closes
  - 13.5 years old—II–V distal phalanx, thumb MC physes close
  - 14 years old—II–V proximal phalanx physes close
  - 15 years old—II–V metacarpal physes close
  - 16 years old—distal ulna physes close
  - 17 years old—distal radius physis closes
- For males, add 2 yr (approximately)

Reference
Heyworth B, Osei D, Fabricant PD, Schneider R, Widmann RF, Green DW, Doyle S, Scher DM. A New, Validated Shorthand Method for Determining Bone Age. 2011. [In Press].

MILESTONES

- 3 mo—head control
- 4 mo—rolls front to back
- 6 mo—sits unsupported
- 9 mo—pulls to stand
- 12 mo—walks alone
- 18 mo—handedness
- 2 yr—knows full name

Congenital Disorders

BRACHIAL PLEXUS OBSTETRIC PALSY

- Approximately 2/1,000 births per year in the United States. Results from brachial plexus stretching or contusion. Increased risk with large babies, forceps delivery, breech position, shoulder dystocia, and prolonged labor

- Three presentations:
  - Erb Duchenne palsy: C5, 6. "Waiter's tip." Deficit in deltoid, rotator cuff (RTC), elbow flexors, and wrist/hand extensors. Best prognosis
  - Klumpke: C8, T1. Deficit in wrist flexors, intrinsics. Horner syndrome
  - Total plexus: C5–T1. Flaccid arm. Sensory and motor function involved
  - Predictors of poor prognosis include Horner's (ptosis, miosis, ahydrosis) and nerve root avulsion Worst prognosis

CONGENITAL PSEUDOARTHROSIS OF THE CLAVICLE

- Failure of the (typically right side) medial and lateral ossification centers to unite. Open reduction and internal fixation (ORIF) for cosmetic deformities or functional disabilities
- Typically nontender over pseudarthrosis
- Differential diagnosis includes cleidocranial dysplasia

PRUNE BELLY SYNDROME

- 1/40,000 live births
- Strong male predominance
- Intrauterine obstruction leading to oligohydramnios. Orthopaedic manifestations include developmental dislocation of the hip (DDH), clubfeet, metatarsus adductus, congenital vertical talus, scoliosis, and muscular torticollis

AMNIOTIC BAND SYNDROME

- Also known as congenital constriction band or Streeter constriction band.
- 1/5,000–10,000 births
- Clinical manifestations: upper extremity affected more often than lower. Distal extremity most frequently involved
  - Most common cause of congenital transverse amputations
  - Clubfeet
  - Terminal limb malformations
  - Acrosyndactyly or simple syndactyly
  - Hypoplastic or absent nail beds
  - Neurovascular impairment distal to band
  - Leg length discrepancies greater than 2.5 cm
  - Craniofacial abnormalities
  - Impaired venous and lymphatic drainage
- Treatment:
  - Superficial, asymptomatic: no treatment
  - Deeper, neurovascular impairment: excise band, close with z-plasties, fasciotomies as needed
- Retrospective study of 55 patients with this syndrome, most common clinical feature was multiple extremity involvement. Malformations included constriction bands, clubfoot, intrauterine amputations, syndactyly, and acrosyndactyly; 38/55 patients had leg-length discrepancies (>2.5 cm) (Askins and Ger, 1988)

Reference

Askins G, Ger E. Congenital constriction band syndrome. J Pediatr Orthop 1988; 8:461–466.

Skeletal Dysplasias

- 1/3,000–5,000 births. Most with spontaneous mutations
- Proportionate dwarfism: limbs and trunk with normal proportions but are unusually small
- Authors review the literature on spinal disorders in dwarfism and report on 80 cases (Bethem et al., 1981)

Reference

Bethem D, et al. Spinal disorders of dwarfism. Review of the literature and report of eighty cases. J Bone Joint Surg Am 1981; 63:1412–1425.

ACHONDROPLASIA

- Most common skeletal dysplasia
- Most common short limb dwarf*, rhizomelic
- 1/30,000 births
- Autosomal dominant (AD), 80% spontaneous mutation
- Associated with advanced paternal age
- Etiology:
  - Fibroblast growth factor receptor (FGFR)-3 mutation
  - Abnormal *enchondral bone formation
  - Failure in *proliferative zone of physis
  - Quantitative, not qualitative, cartilage defect
- Manifestations
  - Anatomic/physiologic
    - Normal trunk, short limbs (rhizomelic)
    - Coxa valga
    - *Genu varum in half but little osteoarthritis (OA)
    - Fibula overgrowth (partial membranous ossification)
    - *Frontal bossing, button nose, small nasal bridge, midface hypoplasia
    - Trident hands: increased space between 3rd and 4th digits
    - Hypotonia in first year of life
    - Radial head subluxation
    - Radial or tibial *bowing
  - Developmental
    - Delayed walking
    - Normal speech, normal intelligence

- Radiographic
  - Delayed appearance of growth plates
  - Champagne glass pelvic outlet view due to short iliac wings
  - Metaphysial flaring ("inverted V" distal femoral physis)
- Spine manifestations
  - Thoracolumbar kyphosis is a common spinal deformity (T12, L1 apical wedging)
    - Onset before walking. 90% resolve with walking age
  - Spinal stenosis due to short thick pedicles, narrow interpedicular distance (at C, T, and L spine). Most common cause of disability
    - Lumbar symptoms (neurogenic claudication) onset in late adolescence.
    - Cervical symptoms (myelopathy) onset in middle adulthood
    - Herniated nucleus pulposus (HNP) into stenotic canal can cause sudden paraplegia or cauda equina
  - Scoliosis: in one-third but mild (usually <30 degrees), treatment rare
  - Small foramen magnum
    - May cause apnea, quadriparesis, clumsy gait, poor endurance
- Treatment
  - Genu varum
    - Bracing ineffective
    - Fibular epiphysiodesis, high tibial osteotomy (HTO) if lateral thrust
  - Kyphosis
    - Bracing: if persists >2 y/o or when kyphosis >30 degrees
    - Surgery: anterior/posterior spinal fusion (A/PSF) indicated for kyphosis >60 degrees

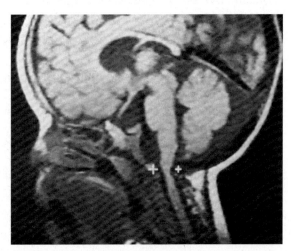

Magnetic resonance image (MRI) of a child with achondroplasia shows stenosis at the foramen magnum. (Courtesy of George S. Bassett, MD)

after age 5 y/o, even without neurologic symptoms. Decompress for buckling ligamentun flavum
  - Foramen magnum: early decompression if symptoms
- Authors report femoral lengthening improves lumbar hyperlordosis and reduces the symptoms of spinal stenosis in patients with achondroplasia (Gomez et al., 2001)

Reference

Gomez P, et al. Lumbar canal stenosis in achondroplasia. Prevention and prevention of lumbosacral lordosis [in Spaniosh]. An Esp Pediatr 2001; 54:126–131.

HYPOCHONDROPLASIA

- Etiology:
  - Insulinlike growth factor receptor (IGFR)-1 defect in some
  - Defect in tyrosine kinase domain of FGFR-3 in some (vs. transmembrane domain in achondroplasia)
- Manifestations
  - Mild short limb dwarf
  - Findings similar to achondroplasia but no midface hypoplasia, taller

PSEUDOACHONDROPLASIA

- Etiology
  - Cartilage oligomeric matrix protein gene (COMP)
  - AD, 1/250,000 live births
- Manifestations
  - Clinically similar to achondroplasia and spondyloepiphyseal dysplasia (SED)
    - Normal facies (in contrast to achondroplasia)
  - *Loose joints
  - *Premature OA (unlike achondroplasia)
  - *Cervical instability (unlike achondroplasia)
    - Fuse if symptomatic or atlantodens interval (ADI) >5 mm
  - Metaphyseal flaring, delayed/fragmented epiphyseal ossification
  - Femoral head abnormalities (resemble Legg-Calvé-Perthes disease [LCPD])
  - Knee varus, valgus ("windswept")
  - Lower leg bowing
  - Scoliosis with increased lumbar lordosis
    - Normal interpedicular distances

CLEIDOCRANIAL DYSPLASIA

- Proportionate dwarf
- AD. Abnormal CBFA (core-binding factor Alpha subunit 1) gene

- Defect in *intramembranous ossification
- Clinical manifestations
  - Clavicle deficient laterally or totally
  - Persistent fontanelles
  - Frontal bossing
  - Widened sutures
  - *Delayed pubic symphysis ossification
  - *Coxa vara
  - Short stature (especially females)
  - Undeveloped distal phalanges
  - Wormian bone
- Review of orthopaedic and other abnormalities associated with cleidocranial dysplasia and management recommendations (Cooper, 2001)
- Review of clinical manifestations of the disorder and three individuals with 8q22 rearrangements (Brueton et al., 1992)

References

Cooper S. A natural history of cleidocranial dysplasia. Am J Med Genet 2001; 104:1–6.
Brueton L, et al. Apparent cleidocranial dysplasia associated with abnormalities of 8q22 in three individuals. Am J Med Genet 1992; 43:612–618.

DIASTROPHIC DYSPLASIA

- Autosomal recessive. Mutation of *sulfate transport gene on chromosome 5
- Undersulfation of proteoglycan causes impaired cartilage properties
- Severe "twisted" dwarf
- Severe rhizomelic (proximal) limb shortening
- Normal intelligence
- No abnormalities of the heart or kidney
- Clinical manifestations
  - *Hitchhiker's thumb
  - *Rigid bilateral clubfoot
  - *Cleft palate in 60%
  - *Cauliflower ears in 80%
  - Short widely abducted 1st MC
  - Severe joint contractures
  - Hip flexion contractures, deformed epiphysis, early OA
  - Knee flexion contractures, valgus, patellar subluxation
  - Tracheomalacia (uncommon but can be fatal)
  - Spine abnormalities
  - Cervical kyphosis leads to quadriplegia
  - Atlantoaxial instability rare
  - *Thoracolumbar (TL) kyphosis/kyphoscoliosis in 83%
  - Early bracing
  - Lumbar lordosis

- Report on total hip arthroplasty (THA) in patients with diastrophic dysplasia. Good implant survival, improved Harris hip score (Helenius et al., 2003)
- Review on spinal manifestations in patients with diastrophic dysplasia (Poussa et al., 1991)

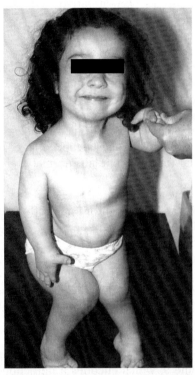

A 5-year-old girl with diastrophic dysplasia. Note prominent cheeks, circumoral fullness, equinovarus feet, valgus knees with flexion contracture, and abducted or "hitchhiker" thumbs. (From Morrissy RT, and Weinstein SL. Lovell and Winter's Pediatric Orthopaedics Sixth Edition Philadelphia: Lippincott Williams & Wilkins, 2006 with permission.)

References

Helenius I, et al. Total hip arthroplasty in diastrophic dysplasia. J Bone Joint Surg Am 2003; 85-A(3):441–447.
Poussa M, et al. The spine in diastrophic dysplasia. Spine 1991; 16:881–887.

ENGELMANN-CAMURATI

- Progressive diaphysial dysplasia.
- AD
- Clinical manifestations
  - *Late walkers due to muscle weakness
  - *Symmetric cortical thickening of long bones
  - Most common tibia, femur, and humerus
  - Leg length discrepancy (LLD) is common

- Treatment
  - Symptomatic treatment with nonsteroidal anti-inflammatory drugs (NSAIDs)
  - Steroids for refractory cases

METAPHYSIAL CHONDRODYSPLASIA: SCHMID, JANSEN MCKUSICK

Abnormal physes (proliferative and hypertrophic zones), normal epiphyses
Three types:
- Schmid
- More common, less severe, delayed diagnosis
- AD. Mutation in type X collagen
- Clinical manifestations
  - Short limb dwarf, normal intelligence
  - *Coxa vara, *genu varum, bowed legs
- Radiographs: wide physis, cupped/flared metaphysic
- *Similar to rickets but labs normal
- Jansen
  - Most severe, rare
  - AD. Mutation in receptor for parathyroid hormone (PTH)/PTH-related peptide
  - Clinical manifestations
    - Hypercalcemia
    - Short limb dwarf, mentally retarded (MR)
    - *Wide eyes, micrognathia, frontal bossing
    - Monkey-like stance, flexion contractures
    - Bulbous metaphyseal expansions
- McKusick (cartilage hair dysplasia)
  - Autosomal recessive (AR). RMRP gene on chromosome 9, which encodes a mitochondrial RNA-processing enzyme
  - Clinical manifestation
    - Brittle fine hair
    - Odontoid hypoplasia, atlantoaxial (AA) instability
    - Ankle deformity due to fibular overgrowth
    - Abnormal immune response to chickenpox
    - Immune deficiency, neutropenia, lymphopenia
    - Gastrointestinal (GI) malabsorption, anemia
  - Increased risk for cancer

MULTIPLE EPIPHYSEAL DYSPLASIA (MED)

- Short limbed disproportionate dwarf
- AD. Cartilage oligomeric matrix protein (COMP) (pseudoachondroplasia) and COL9 mutations
- Mild form (Ribbing). Severe form (Fairbanks)
- Must differentiate from spondyloepiphyseal dysplasia (SED).
- Clinical manifestations
  - *Does not manifest until 5–14 y/o
  - Irregular proximal femur (may be confused with Perthes)
  - Short stunted metacarpals, metatarsals
  - Valgus knees
  - *Waddling gait, *early OA
- Radiographs
  - Flattened femoral condyles
  - Irregular delayed ossification at multiple epiphyseal centers
  - *Double layer patella on lateral xray
  - Get spine, hand, ankle x-ray views to rule out
- Differential diagnosis: LCPD
  - MED is bilateral and symmetric
  - MED has early acetabular changes
  - MED has no metaphyseal cysts
- Review of avascular necrosis in the hip in patients with MED (McKenzie et al., 1989)

Reference

Mackenzie W, et al. Avascular necrosis of the hip in multiple epiphyseal dysplasia. J Pediatr Orthop 1989, 9:666–671.

SPONDYLOEPIPHYSEAL DYSPLASIA

- Two forms (congenita, tarda)
- Distinguished from multiple epiphyseal dysplasia (MED) by spine involvement
- Congenita
  - Defect in type II collagen
  - AD, clinically heterogeneous. Most cases sporadic
  - Clinical manifestations
    - Short trunked dwarf
    - Vertebral flattening/scoliosis causes short trunk
    - Rhizomelic short extremities
    - Classically present with hip pain, coxalgic gait
    - Flattened facies, *cleft palate
    - *Retinal detachment, myopia
    - *Odontoid hypoplasia
    - *Platyspondyly, vertebral beaking, *lordosis, scoliosis
    - Coxa vara universal (like cleidocranial)
    - Genu valgum
  - Radiographic
    - Affects proliferative zone of epiphyseal centers
    - Delayed appearance of epiphysis
  - Treatment
    - PSF if symptomatic or ADI >8 mm
    - Hips: Valgus extension osteotomy
    - Knees: Osteotomy for severe genu varum
    - Arthroplasties for hip and knee OA
- Tarda
  - X-linked recessive
  - Late manifestations (age 8–10 y/o)
  - *DDH, premature OA
- Differentiate from bilateral Perthes (note changes in other epiphyses with SED)

- *Kyphosis, thick vertebrae, scoliosis (treat like idiopathic scoliosis)

KNIEST DYSPLASIA

- "Milder form of SED"
- Short trunk, disproportionate dwarf
- AD
- Clinical manifestations
  - Joint stiffness, contractures
  - Scoliosis, kyphosis
  - Respiratory problems, *cleft palate
  - Retinal detachment, *myopia
  - Otitis media, *hearing loss
  - Early *hip OA
  - Clubfoot
- Radiographs
  - Osteopenia
  - "Dumbbell" femurs
  - Platyspondyly
  - Hypoplastic pelvis and spine
- Pathology
  - "Swiss cheese" physes

TREVOR DISEASE

- Epiphyseal osteochondroma
- Dysplasia epiphysealis hemimelica
- Most common at knee
- Partial excision, later osteotomies
- Recurrence common

TRIGGER TERMS

- Premature OA
  - SED, MED
  - Kneist
  - Pseudoachondroplasia
- Atlantoaxial instability
  - SED, Kneist
  - McKusick
  - Pseudoachondroplasia
  - Morquio
  - Down syndrome
- Cervical kyphosis
  - Larsen
  - Diastrophic dysplasia
- TL kyphosis
  - Achondroplasia
  - Morquio
- Coxa vara
  - Cleidocranial
  - Metaphysial
  - SED, MED
- Coxa valga
  - Achondroplasia

- Genu varum
  - Achondroplasia
  - Metaphysial chondrodysplasia
- Genu valgum
  - SED congenital
  - MED
  - Diastrophic dysplasia
- Rigid clubfoot
  - Diastrophic dysplasia
- Trident hand
  - Achondroplasia
- Hitchhiker thumb
  - Diastrophic dysplasia
- Bullet metacarpals
  - Mucopolysaccharidosis
- Retinal detachment
  - Kneist
  - SED
- Cataracts
  - Chondrodysplasia punctata
- Cleft palate
  - SED congenital
  - Diastrophic dysplasia
- Hearing loss
  - Kneist
- Cauliflower ear
  - Diastrophic dysplasia
- Proportionate dwarfism
  - Cleidocranial dysplasia
  - Mucopolysaccharidoses
- Disproportionate dwarfism
  - Short trunk
    - Kneist
    - SED
    - Metatropic
  - Short limb
    - Diastrophic dysplasia
    - Metaphyseal dysplasia
    - Hypochondroplasia
    - Pseudoachondroplasia
    - MED
  - Rhizomelic (proximal)
    - Achondroplasia
  - Mesomelic (middle)
  - Acromelic (distal)

Genetics/Syndromes

APERT

- Acrocephaly (craniosynostosis)
- Hypertelorism
- Bilateral complex syndactyly with synphalangism
- Delta thumb proximal phalanx

- Along with c-spine fusions, atlanto-occipital fusions, butterfly vertebra in 71%
  - Most commonly involves C5-C6
  - Cervical fusions progress with age
  - Intubation may be difficult
- Literature review of all extremity anomalies in patients with Apert with report of results of 68 patients (Upton, 1991)

Reference

Upton J. Apert bibliography. Clin Plast Surg 1991; 18:417–431.

ARTHROGRYPOSIS

- Two or more rigid joints, *nonprogressive
- Oligohydramnios or viral etiology
- Three major groups and approximately 150 forms of arthrogryposis
  - Group I—all four extremities involved
  - Amyoplasia (arthrogryposis multiplex congenita)
  - Most common form, 1/3,000
  - Negative family history (not genetic)
  - Decrease in anterior horn cells
  - Clinical manifestations
    - Motor function lost, sensation maintained
    - Multiple characteristic joint contractures
    - Normal facies, normal intelligence
    - No visceral abnormalities
    - Scoliosis in one-third (C-shaped neuromuscular)
    - Waiter-tip upper extremity (UE) (shoulder adduction/IR, elbow extension, wrist flexion/ulnar deviation)
    - Goal 90 degrees passive elbow flexion
    - Initial manipulation/casting of elbow
    - If <90 degrees passive flexion at elbow, posterior capsulotomy and triceps lengthening at 2 y/o
    - If passive flexion >90 degrees but no active, tendon transfer (many options)
    - Consider osteotomy >4 y/o for activities of daily living (ADLs)
    - Leave one elbow in extension
  - Knee contractures
    - Extension contracture typical, usually responds to physical therapy (PT)
    - Flexion contracture possible, surgery if >30 degrees
    - Correct prior to hip reduction
    - Take hamstring (HS), posterior cruciate ligament (PCL), posterior capsule, ± femoral shortening
  - Flexion deformity can recur with growth when femoral extension osteotomies are performed. The recurrence rate is higher at the end of growth. (Delbello and Watts, 1996)
  - Teratologic hip dislocations
    - Usually treatment (tx) at <1 y/o
    - Surgical tx of unilateral dislocation is indicated
    - Treatment of bilateral dislocation is controversial
  - Clubfeet, congenital vertical talus (CVT)
    - Goal stiff plantigrade foot
    - Poor response to manipulation/cast
    - Usually operate >1 y/o (after knees/hips)
    - Initially treated with extensive circumferential release
    - Recurrence may require salvage with *talectomy
    - CVT is less common than clubfoot in arthrogryposis multiplex congenita (AMC), consider diagnosis of distal arthrogryposis or multiple pterygia syndrome
- Group II—distal arthrogryposis
  - Distal arthrogryposis syndrome
    - AD
    - Predominantly affects hands/feet
    - Clubfoot
    - Better response to manipulation/cast than AMC
    - Congenital vertical talus
    - Adducted thumbs/web space thickening
    - Metacarpophalangeal (MCP), proximal interphalangeal (PIP) flexion contractures
    - Ulnar deviation of fingers
  - Group III–pterygia syndromes (skin webs)
- Summary of treatment options for upper extremity involvement in arthrogryposis (Bennett et al., 1985)

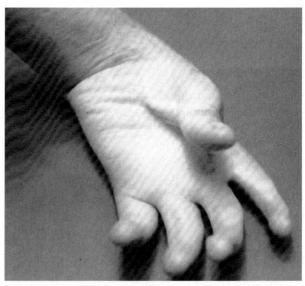

Distal arthrogryposis. Characteristic hand is the result of ulnar deviation at the metacarpophalangeal joints. Notice the deeply cupped palm and webbing of the MCP joint of the thumb. (From Morrissy RT, and Weinstein SL. Lovell and Winter's Pediatric Orthopaedics Sixth Edition Philadelphia: Lippincott Williams & Wilkins, 2006 with permission.)

References

DelBello DA, Watts HG. Distal femoral extension osteotomy for knee flexion contracture in patients with arthrogryposis. J Pediatr Orthop 1996; 16:122–126.

Bennett J, et al. Surgical management of arthrogryposis in the upper extremity. J Pediatr Orthop 1985; 5:281–286.

EHLERS-DANLOS

General

– Heterogeneous connective tissue disorder involving collagen synthesis
– Nine types, various inheritance patterns

Clinical Manifestations

– Scoliosis
– Clubfoot
– Joint laxity
– Muscle hypotonia
– Hyperextensible skin
– Cigarette paper scars (atrophic)
– Easy bruising
– Vascular and visceral spontaneous ruptures

Types of Ehlers-Danlos (Nine Types)

I—Gravis

– Most common and least disabling
– Scoliosis
– Joint laxity, pes planus
– Clubfoot, DDH, OA
– Hyperextensible skin
– "Cigarette paper" scars
– Poor wound healing

II—Mitis

– Similar to I, less severe
– Joint laxity (especially small joints)

II—Hypermobility

– Marked joint laxity (multidirectional instability (MDI) of the shoulder, patellar subluxation)
– Early OA
– Scoliosis
– No scarring

IV—Vascular

– Minimal joint hypermobility
– Hands/feet prematurely aged
– Vascular fragility, visceral ruptures
– Thin skin, not hyperextensible

V–X-linked Type

– Rare, similar to I, II, III
– Joint laxity

VI—Ocular Scoliotic

– Joint laxity
– Kyphoscoliosis
– Muscle hypotonia
– Ocular fragility
– Hyperextensible skin
– Arterial rupture, easy bruising

VII—Arthrochalasis Multiplex Congenita

– Autosomal dominant, *seen by orthopedics
– Bilateral DDH
– Joint laxity/dislocations
– Bone fragility
– Tendon contractures (Achilles, foot extension)
– Clubfoot
– Diffuse muscle hypotonia
– Short stature in VII A, B
– Blue sclera in VII C
– Skin elasticity ± fragility
– Easy bruising

VIII—Periodontitis

– Periodontal disease, early tooth loss
– Joint laxity
– Skin elasticity/fragility, easy bruising

X—Fibronectin Abnormality

– Mild, similar to II and III
– Platelet dysfunction, poor clotting

Treatment

– PT, orthotics
– Avoid contact sports
– Avoid surgery—bad skin, bleeds
– Soft tissue procedures ultimately fail
– Arthrodesis preferred to arthroplasty
– Scoliosis treatment like idiopathic
– 28% of children with EDS had aortic root dilation (Wenstrup et al., 2002)

Reference

Wenstrup RJ, et al. Prevalence of aortic root dilation in Ehlers-Danlos syndrome. Genet Med 2002; 4:112–117.

MARFAN SYNDROME

General

– Fibrillin* defect, chromosome 15
– AD. incomplete penetrance, variable expression, 1/2 are new mutations
– Males = females

Differential Diagnosis

– Congenital contractural arachnodactyly
– Homocystinuria
– Stickler syndrome

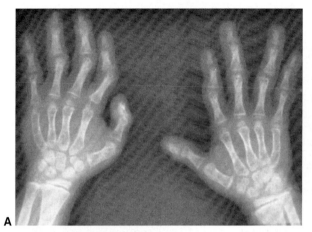

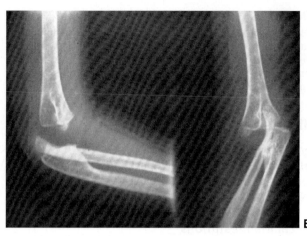

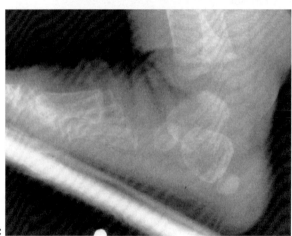

Characteristic roentgenograms of a 4-year-old patient with Larsen syndrome. **A:** The hands show more carpal centers and interphalangeal joint subluxations than is normal. **B:** The elbow demonstrates total dislocation but full functional ability. **C:** The foot has an abnormal os calcis containing two ossification centers. (A and B from Goldberg MJ. The dysmorphic child: an orthopedic perspective. New York: Raven Press, 1987, with permission.) (C from Morrissy RT, and Weinstein SL. Lovell and Winter's Pediatric Orthopaedics Sixth Edition Philadelphia: Lippincott Williams & Wilkins, 2006 with permission.)

Clinical Manifestations

Musculoskeletal
- Flatfoot, long toes
- Arachnodactyly
    - Walker-Murdoch sign
        - Overlap of thumb and fifth finger when grasping opposite wrist
    - Steinberg sign
        - Thumb in fist extends beyond ulnar border of hand
- Ligamentous laxity, patellar subluxation
    - Carter-Wilkinson signs of laxity/Beighton Criteria
        - MCP hyperdorsiflexion
        - Thumb to forearm
        - Elbow hyperextension
        - Knee hyperextension
        - Palms touch floor with straight knee forward bend
- Genu recurvatum
- Protrusio acetabuli
    - Differential diagnosis
        - Osteogenesis imperfecta (OI)
        - JRA
        - Marfan

- Dolichostenomelia (long extremities)
    - Reduced upper:lower segment ratio
    - Top of head to pubis symph to feet
    - 0.93 is normal at maturity, 1.6 at birth
    - <0.85 in Marfan
    - Arm span:height >1.05
- Pectus excavatum (more than carinatum)
- High arched palate
- *Spine*
    - Single right thoracic or double right thoracic/left lumbar (RT/LL)
    - Thoracic lordoscoliosis
    - TL junction kyphosis
    - C-spine spared

Ocular
- Myopia, retinal detachment
- Ectopia lentic (superior lens disloc)
- (Inferior lens dislocation for homocystinuria)

Cardiovascular
- Aortic dilatation
- Aortic regurgitation
- Mitral valve prolapse

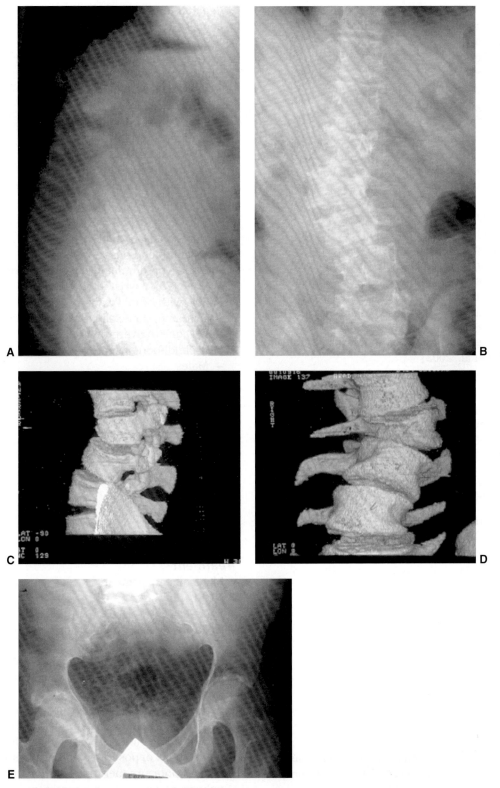

Scoliosis **(A, B)** and protrusio of the hips **(E)** in a patient with Marfan syndrome.
C, D: Deformity of the apical vertebrae is shown in a three-dimensional reconstruction of a computerized tomographic scan image. (Courtesy of Chris Reily, MD, Vancouver, British Columbia, Canada.)

Treatment

- Cardiac screening for aortic root dilatation
    - Yearly echo
    - Beta-blockers
    - Surgery for aortic root >5 cm
    - High mortality from dissection
- Ophthalmologic screening
- Protrusio acetabuli
    - Triradiate epiphysiodesis (Steel)
- Scoliosis
    - Needs preoperative echo
    - Role of bracing is limited (Sponseller et al., 2000)
        - 83% failure of bracing for <45 degrees
        - Follow closely for progression (accelerated compared with idiopathic scoliosis)
        - Early surgical intervention when indicated
        - Pedicle screw fixation or anterior instrumentation can be performed. Be aware of dural ectasias
        - Wait until >4 y/o because patient may die from cardiac causes before then
- Review of current concepts in Marfan syndrome (Giampietro et al., 2002)

References

Sponseller PD, et al. Results of brace treatment of scoliosis in Marfan syndrome. Spine 2000; 25:2350–2354.
Giampietro PF, et al. Marfan syndrome: orthopedic and genetic review. Curr Opin Pediatr 2002; 14:35–41.

JUVENILE RHEUMATOID ARTHRITIS

Diagnostic Criteria

- Onset <16 y/o
- Persistent arthritis >6 wk
- Exclude other types of childhood arthritis

Systemic Still Disease (10%–20%)

- Females:males, 1:1
- Clinical manifestations
    - Fever, rash, malaise
    - Lymphadenopathy, hepatosplenomegaly
    - Pericardial and pleural effusions
    - Muscle atrophy
    - Initially, arthralgia only with daily fevers
    - Within months, symmetric arthritis occur
    - Facet fusion (most common spine finding), asymptomatic Possible increased ADI—usually no pain and no neurologic deficit
    - Basilar invagination (rare)
- Rheumatoid factor (RF) and antinuclear antibody (ANA) negative
- 25% go on to chronic severe arthritis whereas the rest go into remission

Polyarticular (30%–40%)

- Females > males, 3:1
- Worse prognosis
- Frequently develop adult rheumatoid arthritis (RA)
- Clinical manifestations
    - Five or more joints
    - Mild systemic symptoms
    - Loss of mandible
    - Symmetric small joint arthritis
- 20% rheumatoid factor (RF) positive
- High rate of surgical intervention
- 50% go on to chronic destructive arthritis

Pauciarticular (45%–50%)

- ≤Four joints, two subtypes
- Early childhood onset
    - Female predominance; well appearing
    - Knee (75%), wrist, elbow, ankles
    - 50% with iridocyclitis
    - *Slitlamp, especially if ANA positive
    - LLD due to overgrowth
- Late childhood onset
    - Males
    - Many HLA-B27 positive
    - Hips and sacroiliac (SI) joints

Differential Diagnosis

- Acute reactive arthritis
    - 7–21 days after strep infection
    - Less iridocyclitis
- Lyme disease
- Septic arthritis
  Acute rheumatic fever

Treatment

- Medical management
- Night splinting
- Synovectomy
- Arthrodesis/arthroplasty (for severe)
- Twice yearly slitlamp exam
- Review of the immunologic abnormalities in juvenile arthritis and their associated clinical manifestations (Miller, 1993)
- Classic description of JRA presentation (Still, 1990)
- Results of total knee arthroplasty (TKA) in patients with juvenile rheumatoid arthritis (JRA) showed increased risk of post op infection and stiffness in presence of poor preoperative function, multiple joint involvement and poor preoperative function (Parvizi et al., 2003)

References

Miller JJ III. Psychosocial factors related to rheumatic diseases in childhood. J Rheumatol Suppl 1993; 38:1–11.

Still GF. On a form of chronic joint disease in children. 1896. Clin Orthop Relat Res 1990; (259):4–10.

Parvizi J, et al. Total knee arthroplasty in young patients with juvenile rheumatoid arthritis. J Bone Joint Surg Am 2003; 85-A(6):1090–1094.

LARSEN SYNDROME

- AD or AR
- 40% mortality in first yr (respiratory failure)
- Clinical manifestations
    - Bilateral congenital knee dislocations (tibia anterior, anterior cruciate ligament [ACL] absent)
    - Multiple upper and lower extremity joint dislocations
    - Scoliosis, *cervical kyphosis
    - Bilateral clubfeet
    - Equinovarus, equinovalgus, skewfoot
    - Flattened facies, hypertelorism
- Treatment
    - UE dislocations rarely require treatment
- Knee dislocations
    - Rarely respond to conservative treatment
    - Surgical reduction as early as 3–4 mo
    - Treat before or simultaneous with hips
    - Often need long-term orthoses
- Hip dislocations
    - Treatment of bilateral dislocations is controversial
    - Treatment knees first or at same time
    - Resistant to conservative treatment
    - High rate redislocation/revision surgery
- Clubfoot
    - Cast until knee deformity corrected
    - Less residual deformity with surgical treatment
    - May need ankle orthosis for instability
- Cervical kyphosis/instability
    - Assessed and treated before general anesthesia

NEUROFIBROMATOSIS (NF; VON RECKLINGHAUSEN DISEASE)

- AD disorder of neural crests
- Half are new mutations
- 5%–15% will develop central nervous system (CNS) malignancy
- Two types
    - Coast of California smooth café-au-laits
    - Subneurofibromas
    - CNS tumors
    - NF1 has many associated orthopaedic problems, NF2 does not

NF I—Peripheral

- Mutation in neurofibromin (chromosome 17), a tumor suppressor

- 1:4,000
- Most common single gene disorder in humans

Diagnostic Criteria (Two of Seven)

- ≥Six café-au-lait spots (smooth borders)
- ≥Two neurofibromas or one plexiform NF
- Multiple axillary/inguinal freckles
- Osseous lesions (sphenoid dysplasia, cortical thinning)
- Optic glioma
- ≥Two Lisch nodules by slitlamp
- First-degree relative with NF

Clinical Manifestations

- Spine
    - Most common site of involvement
    - Cervical kyphosis or atlanto-axial instability
    - Dystrophic or nondystrophic scoliosis
    - Dystrophic scoliosis with short, sharp thoracic kyphoscoliosis
    - MRI all patients for dural ectasia, meningoceles, "dumbbell" tumors

Congenital Tibial Dysplasia

- Tibial anterolateral bowing/*congenital pseudoarthrosis (1%–2% of NF1 patients)
- (vs. anteromedial bow in fibular hemimelia or posteromedial in physiologic)
- Nondysplastic (type I) with anterolateral bow, increased bone density, sclerosis of medullary canal
- Dysplastic (type II)
    - Type IIA with failure of tubularization
    - Type IIB with cystic prefracture or canal enlargement from previous fracture
    - Type IIC with frank pseudarthrosis, "sucked candy" narrowing of fragment ends

Other Orthopedic Manifestations

- Segmental hypertrophy with overlying soft tissue elephantiasis, hemangioma
- Cystic bone lesions resembling nonossifying fibromas (NOFs)
- Subperiosteal bone proliferation (usually initiated by minor trauma causing subperiosteal hemorrhage, "doughnut sign" on bone scan caused by microcalcification at periphery of subperiosteal hemorrhage)

Radiographic Findings

Spine

- Vertebral scalloping, wedging
- Enlarged foramina
- Penciling of transverse processes (TPs) or ribs
- Severe apical rotation
- Short tight curves
- Paraspinal mass

Extremities
- Cystic bone lesions resembling NOFs
- Congenital tibial dysplasia
- Subperiosteal bone proliferation

Treatment
Spine
- Bracing fails
- *A/PSF (pseudarthrosis rate unacceptable with PSF alone)
- Nondystrophic scoliosis behaves like adolescent, treated like adolescent

Tibial Dysplasia
- Osteotomies for correction are contraindicated (concern about healing)
- Initial treatment—contact brace to prevent fracture Nonhealing fracture—excise/graft/IM rod (Williams technique—transankle stabilization with Rush rod)
- Other options—vascular fibula graft or Ilizarov
- After two or three failed surgeries: Symes amputation

NF II—Central
- Bilateral acoustic neuromas
- Chromosome 22 (schwannoma)
- 1:40,000

Differential Diagnosis
- Jaffe-Campanacci Syndrome
  - Multiple NOFs with café-au-laits
- McCune-Albright syndrome
  - NF, polyostotic fibrous dysplasia, precocious puberty
- Review of 91 patients with spinal deformity and neurofibromatosis reports that nondystrophic curves can modulate into dystrophic curves before the age of 7 y/o (Durrani et al., 2000)
- Study of surgical correction of dystrophic spinal curves in patients with neurofibromatosis demonstrating that failure of the posterior instrumentation and fusion alone was 53% and failure of combined posterior and anterior fusion was 23% (Parisini, 1999)

References
Durrani AA, et al. Modulation of spinal deformities in patients with neurofibromatosis type 1. Spine 2000; 25:69–75.
Parisini P, et al. Surgical correction of dystrophic spinal curves in neurofibromatosis. A review of 56 patients. Spine 1999; 24:2247–2253.

NOONAN SYNDROME
- *Male predominance, normal sexual genotype
- Short stature
- Web neck
- Cubitus valgus
- Malignant hyperthermia
- Review of Noonan syndrome with description of associated malignant hyperthermia (Allanson, 1987)

Reference
Allanson JE. Noonan Syndrome. J Med Genet 1987; 24:9–13.

OSTEOGENESIS IMPERFECTA

General
- 1:25 000, males = females
- Disorder of type I collagen (vs. type II—diastrophic dysplasia)
- Can confirm diagnosis with skin biopsy/fibroblast count

Clinical Manifestations
- Bone fragility
- Frequent fractures
  - Heal but do not remodel
  - Bowing of long bones
  - Distal femur tends to varus postfracture
  - Vertebral compression fractures (codfish vertebrae)
- Short stature
- Defective teeth
- Hearing defects
- Blue sclera, tympanum
- Basilar impression in 25%
- Scoliosis in 50%

Silence Classification
Type I (quantitative defect)
- Autosomal Dominant
- 50% loss of production of type I collagen
- Mild, normal looking
- Blue sclera, hearing loss
- Fracture onset at preschool
- Standard fracture care

Type II (quantitative and qualitative defect)
- AR, AD, or mosaic
- Unstable collagen triple helix
- Dark blue sclera
- Intrauterine fractures
- Concertina femur
- Beaded ribs
- *Perinatal death

Type III (qualtitative defect)
- AD or AR
- Abnormal type 1 collagen
- Severe. Rare
- Extreme short stature

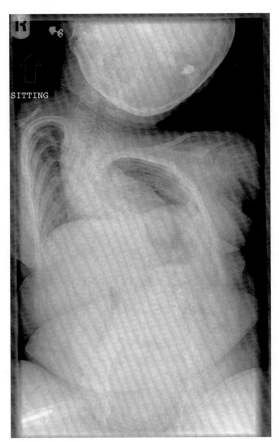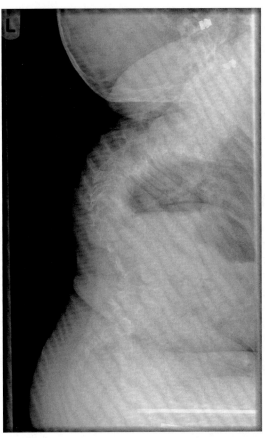

Osteogenesis imperfecta (OI). Marked spinal deformity in a 5-year-old girl with severe OI. (From Morrissy RT, and Weinstein SL. Lovell and Winter's Pediatric Orthopaedics Sixth Edition Philadelphia: Lippincott Williams & Wilkins, 2006 with permission.)

- Fractures from birth heal readily
- Progressive deformity
- Sclerae less blue with age
- Hearing loss

Type IV (qualtitative defect)
- Autosomal dominant
- Shortened pro alpha chains
- Moderate severity
- Bone fragility, long bone bowing
- Sclerae and hearing are normal
- A: teeth involved
- B: teeth not involved

Radiographic Findings
- Rhinal cortices, osteopenia
- Femur bowing with anterior stress fracture
- Mild acetabular *protrusio
- Wormian bones: Intrasutural bones that lie between cranial sutures and are more brittle in Osteogenesis patients

Treatment
- Bracing of extremities early
- Closed fracture treatment for <2 y/o
- Surgical indications
  - Surgical intervention deferred until child pulls-to-stand
  - Recurrent fractures (two or three fractures)
  - Progressive angulation deformity
  - >40-degree angulation predisposes to fractures
  - Once a rod, always a rod
- Surgical options
  - IM rods to prevent deformity and recurrent fracture (risk possible physial injury)
  - IM fixation superior to plates/screws, which dislodge from weakened bone
  - Rush rods, multiple exchanges
  - Fassier-Duval telescoping rods
  - Sofield osteotomies ("shish kebab")
    - Usually wait until 5 y/o
  - Scoliosis treatment
    - Bracing not used (bone plasticity)
    - Surgery for curve >40–50 degrees

– Comprehensive review of classification, biochemistry and orthopaedic management (Marini, 1988)
– Review of current knowledge of mutations of OI (Cole, 2002)

References

Marini JC. Osteogenesis imperfecta: comprehensive management. Adv Pediatr 1988; 35:391–426.
Cole WG. Advances in osteogenesis imperfecta. Clin Orthop Relat Res 2002; 401:6–16.
Zeitlin L. Modern approach to children with osteogenesis imperfecta. J Pediatr Ortho B 2003; 12:77–87.

PRADER-WILLI

– Mutation in chromosome 15
– Floppy hypotonic infant
– Mental retardation
– *Insatiable appetite, obesity pica
– *Hypoplastic genitalia
– Scoliosis, hip dysplasia, growth retardation common
– Review of the syndrome including orthopaedic manifestations and management options (Cassidy, 1984)

Reference

Cassidy SB. Prader-Willi Syndrome. Curr Probl Pediatr 1984; 14:1–55.

RETT SYNDROME

– *Female predominance at 6–18 mo
– *Progressive impairment
– *Stereotactic hand movements (hand wringing)
– Unibrow, hirsutism
– Present with developmental delay like cerebral palsy (CP)
– Spasticity, joint contractures
– Treatment like in CP
– C-shaped progressive scoliosis in majority of cases
– A/PSF for curve >40 degrees
– Upper thoracic to pelvis
– Description of orthopaedic manifestations in nine patients with Rett syndrome: scoliosis, lower extremity contracture, and coxa valga (Guidera et al., 1991)

Reference

Guidera KJ, et al. Orthopaedic manifestations of Rett syndrome. J Pediatr Orthop 1991; 11:204–208.

SANDIFER

– Gastroesophageal reflux disease (GERD), often with hiatal hernia
– Torticollis (likely an attempt to decrease discomfort from reflux)
– Clinical presentation
  – Presents in infancy

– Torticollis (sternocleidomastoid muscle [SCM] not tight, short)
– Dystonic movements, tics
– Vomiting, failure to thrive
– Recurrent respiratory disease
– Dysphagia
– Imaging
  – X-ray c-spine to rule out anomalies
  – Upper gastrointestinal (UGI) series to diagnose hiatal hernia and GERD
  – Esophageal pH studies may be needed
– Treatment
  – Medical first
  – Fundoplication
– Dystonia goes away after GERD treated

TRISOMY 21 (DOWN SYNDROME)

– Most common chromosomal abnormality
– 1/660 live births

Clinical Manifestations

Medical
– Hearing loss 50%
– *50% congenital heart defects
– GI malformations 5%–7% (duodenal atresia)
– Leukemia in 1%
– Hypothyroidism (SCFE), diabetes mellitus (DM), JRA
– Premature aging (Alzheimer-like dementia in fourth decade)

Orthopaedic Delayed Ambulation (2–3 y/o)
– Ligament laxity, hypotonia 50% with idiopathic-like scoliosis
– Half scoliosis, idiopathic type
– Flat acetabulum, flared iliac wings on x-ray view can make diagnosis before chromosome analysis

Hip Instability
– In 4.5% of children
– Not congenital, usually acquired
– Natural history
  – Stable as infant
  – Dislocatable in childhood
  – Habitual dislocation (2–10 y/o)
  – Fixed subluxation or dislocation (10–25 y/o)
  – Treatment: surgery before dislocation is fixed
  – Soft tissue and bony procedures to stabilize

Atlantoaxial Instability
– 15%–25% atlantoaxial instability
– May also have atlanto-occipital instability
– May be asymptomatic, symptomatic, progressive, or catastrophic
– Present with change in motor milestones

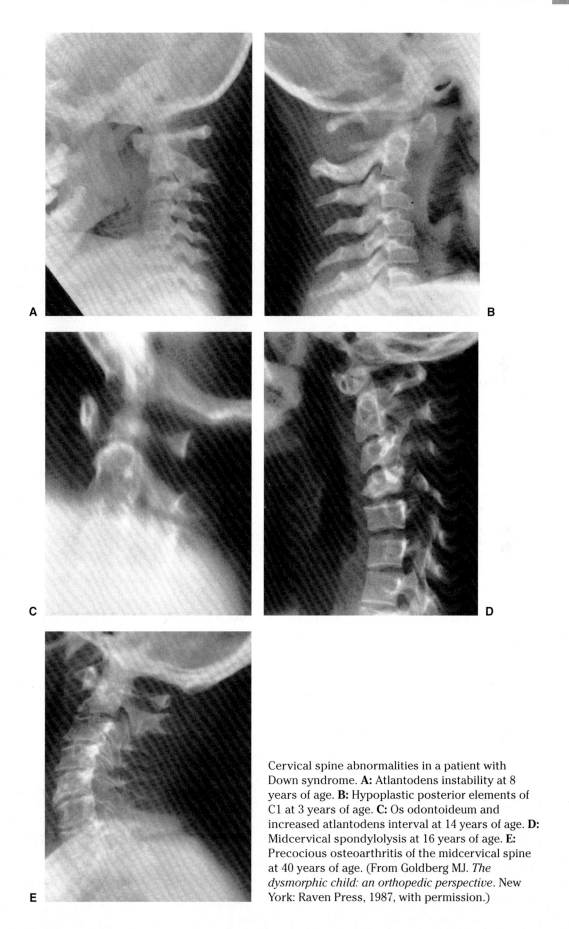

Cervical spine abnormalities in a patient with Down syndrome. **A:** Atlantodens instability at 8 years of age. **B:** Hypoplastic posterior elements of C1 at 3 years of age. **C:** Os odontoideum and increased atlantodens interval at 14 years of age. **D:** Midcervical spondylolysis at 16 years of age. **E:** Precocious osteoarthritis of the midcervical spine at 40 years of age. (From Goldberg MJ. *The dysmorphic child: an orthopedic perspective.* New York: Raven Press, 1987, with permission.)

- Screen with flexion/extension x-ray views
- Screen every 1–2 yr, beginning at ~5 y/o
- Discourage neck stressing activities in all patients
- If unstable without symptoms, ADI <10 mm
  - Forbid neck-stressing activities
  - Yearly follow-up
  - No evidence that bracing helps
- *Indications for surgery
  - Any instability along with myelopathy
  - ADI >10 mm with or without symptoms
  - Progressive instability
- Complication rate for C1-C2 fusion is significant

Foot Deformity
- Metatarsus primus varus, pes planus, planovalgus
- Related to ligamentous laxity
- Treatment with well-fitting shoes
- Surgery rarely indicated for foot

Patellar Instability
- Occurs in up to one-third
- Can progress to chronic patellar dislocation, valgus external rotation (ER) force across the knee, and eventually to femoral-tibial subluxation
- Initial treatment: brace/observe
- PT difficult
- If progressive, consider surgery
- Risk recurrence due to laxity
- Distal realignment with Galeazzi procedure (semi-tendinosus through drill hole in distal patella), lateral release, medial plication, or combination.
- Avoid bony realignment until after skeletal maturity
- Postoperative casting/long-term knee/ankle/foot orthosis (KAFO)
- Study of 15 Down syndrome patients who underwent upper cervical spine arthrodesis; 11 had 23 major complications including nonunion, loss of reduction, neurologic deterioration, late subaxial instability, infection, wound dehiscence (Doyle et al., 1996)
- Radiographic review of 32 patients with down syndrome from 1970–1983. The average atlantodens interval increased and instability developed in seven patients (Burke et al., 2003)
- Reports that children with Down syndrome can participate in athletics if their orthopedic problems are appropriately managed (Winell and Burke, 2003)

References

Doyle JS, et al. Complications and long-term outcomes of upper cervical spine arthrodesis in patients with Down syndrome. Spine 1996; 1223–1231.

Burke SW, et al. Chronic atlantoaxial instability in Down syndrome. J Bone Joint Surg Am 1985; 67:1356–1360.

Winell J, Burke SW. Sports participation of children with Down syndrome. Orthop Clin North Am 2003; 34:439–443.

TURNER

- Female, 45XO
- 1/2,500 phenotypic females
- Clinical manifestations
  - Short stature
  - Sexual infantilism
  - Broad chest
  - Micrognathia
  - Drooping eyelids
  - Low-set ears
  - Osteoporosis (due to low estrogen)
  - Web neck
  - Cubitus valgus
  - Short fourth, fifth metacarpals
  - Genu valgum—usually no treatment
  - One-third cardiac, two-thirds renal abnormalities
  - Malignant hyperthermia with anesthesia
- Hormone treatment can worsen scoliosis
- Review of clinical manifestations and management of patients with Turner syndrome (Batch, 2002)

Reference

Batch J. Turner syndrome in childhood and adolescence. Best Pract Res Clin Endocrinol Metab 2002; 16:465–482.

Muscular Dystrophies

BECKER MUSCULAR DYSTROPHY

- X-link recessive, abnormality in quantity and quality of dystrophin
- Color blind
- Compared to Duchenne
  - Less severe, later onset
  - Slower progression, longer life span

FACIOSCAPULOHUMERAL DYSTROPHY

- *AD. Mutation in chromosome 4

Clinical Manifestations
- Weak face, shoulder, and upper extremity
- Glenohumeral muscles spared compared to scapulothoracic muscles
- Severe scapular *winging
- Normal creatine phosphokinase (CPK)

Treatment
- Scapulothoracic arthrodesis restores functional flexion and abduction

DUCHENNE MUSCULAR DYSTROPHY

- X-link recessive
- Most common neuromuscular disorder in children (50/million)

Pathology
- Complete absence of dystrophin
- Necrosis, connective tissue infiltration
- High CPK (50–100 times normal)
- DNA testing can diagnose 65%

Clinical Manifestations
- Calf pseudohypertrophy
- Gower maneuver compensates for weak gluteus maximus and quads
- Gait with increased lumbar lordosis, increased hip flexion, increased ankle plantarflexion ground rotation force produced by toe walking causes extension moment at knee, keeping center of gravity anterior to knee, compensating for weak quad

Scoliosis
- 95% incidence of progressive scoliosis
- Rarely develops while patient ambulatory
- After wheelchair bound, 10-degree increase per yr (Kurz et al., 1983)
- Each 10-degree increase in T curve decreases forced vital capacity (FVC) by 4%
- Each year of age after wheelchair bound decreases FVC by 4%

Natural History
- Late walkers, difficulty with walking at 3 y/o
- Lose ambulation age 10 y/o, wheelchair bound at 15 y/o, then become obese
- KAFO and contraction release can delay ambulation loss 2–4 yr
- Death in early adulthood due to pulmonary insufficiency
- Tracheostomy/mechanical vent are late treatment options

Treatment
Knee Flexion Contractures
- Hamstring lengthening if adequate strength
- Night ankle-foot orthosis (AFO) to prevent equinus (not for ambulation)
- Achilles/post tibial tenotomy for equinovarus with post tibial transfer to dorsal midfoot
- KAFO may be necessary after tenotomy
- Early postoperative mobilization to retain strength
- Risk of malignant hyperthermia with anesthesia

Scoliosis
- Bracing contraindicated
- Spinal stabilization maintains pulmonary function, prolongs life (Galasko et al., 1992)
- Fuse before scoliosis becomes severe
- Scoliosis >20 degrees
- FVC still >40%

- Usually 11–13 y/o
- PSF with instrumentation is treatment of choice
- Fusion to pelvis debatable (Mubarak recommends if pelvic obliquity >10 degrees)
- Anterior surgery not recommended because of limited pulmonary reserves
- Mobilize rapidly after surgery
  - Study of wheelchair bound patients with DMD who underwent Luque segmental instrumentation and fusion. Twelve were instrumented to the sacropelvis, ten to L5. The authors recommend instrumentation from T2-3 to L5 in patients treated early with curves of 20 degrees or more and if FVD is more than 40% (Mubarak et al. 1993)
  - Detailed review of the current treatment and research on Duchenne muscular dystrophy (Sussman, 2002)

References
Kurz LT, et al. Creation of scoliosis and pulmonary function in Duchenne muscular dystrophy. J Pediatr Orthop 1983; 3:347–353.

Galasko CS, et al. Spinal stabilisation in Duchenne muscular dystrophy. J Bone Joint Surg Br 1992; 74:210–214

Mubarak SJ, et al. Spinal fusion in Duchenne muscular dystrophy-fixation and fusion to the sacropelvis? J Pediatr Orthop 1993; 13:752–757.

Sussman M. Duchenne muscular dystrophy. J Am Acad Orthop Surg 2002; 10:138–151.

SPINAL MUSCULAR ATROPHY

General
- Autosomal recessive.
- 1/20,000 live births
- 95% along with deletion of survival motor neuron (SMN) gene on chromosome 5
- In absence of SMN, apoptosis persists in fetus
- Loss of anterior horn cells
- Progressive muscle weakness from normal growth exceeding reserve
- DNA testing preferred over muscle biopsy
- Normal intelligence

Three Types
Type I—Acute Werdnig-Hoffman Disease
- Marked weakness, hypotonia
- Appears by 6 mo
- Death by 2 y/o from respiratory failure

Type II—Chronic Werdnig-Hoffman Disease
- Onset between 6 mo and 2 y/o
- Scoliosis universal, usually by age 3 yr
- Never walk
- Achieve independent sitting and head control
- Dislocation of one or both hips by age 10 yr
- Lives to 40s

Type IIIa
- Onset before age 3 yr
- Usually loses ability to walk in adolescence
- Life expectancy may be normal

Type IIIb—Kugelberg-Welander Disease
- Onset after age 3 yr
- Remain adult ambulators
- Normal life span

Treatment
- Progressive hip subluxation in type II
  - Temporarily symptomatic
  - Does not influence function in nonwalker
  - Surgery not indicated in most patients
- Scoliosis (all II, most IIIa)
  - Thoracolumbar "C" and single R thoracic curves are most common
  - Thoracolumbosacral orthosis (TLSO) brace 20–40 degrees
  - PSF for >40 degrees
  - Add ASF to prevent crankshaft in younger patients
- Fuse to pelvis if obliquity present

Neuromuscular Disorders

CEREBRAL PALSY

General
- Brain matures at 2–3 y/o (? when myelination complete)
- Neurons form at 12–30 wk prenatally and never after that
- *Encephalopathy is static, nonprogressive, but disease manifestations change with growth
- Affects strength, tone, control
- Etiology—lesion of the immature brain
  - TORCH (*t*oxoplasmosis, *o*ther infections, *r*ubella, *c*ytomegalovirus infection, and *h*erpes simplex) infection
  - Prematurity
  - Anoxia, bleed, meningitis
  - Low birth weight
  - Teratologic agents
- 1–7/1,000 live births
- 10% postnatal
- 12 times more common in twin pregnancies
- Review of the natural history, pathophysiology, and the role of surgery in the cerebral palsy patient (Kerr Graham and Selber, 2003)

Reference
Kerr Graham H, Selber P. Musculoskeletal aspects of cerebral palsy. J Bone Joint Surg Br 2003; 85:157–166.

Neuropathic Patterns
Spastic (80%)
- Lesion in pyramid/corticospinal tract
- Increased tone and hyperreflexia
- Velocity dependent resistance
- Joint contractures common
- Most common, most amenable to orthopedic surgery
- MR more common with spastic patients than ataxic or athetoid

Athetoid
- Duskiness from extrapyramidal lesion (midbrain, basal ganglia, subset Ingram)
- Purposeless, slow, writhing
- Along with erythroblastosis fetalis and kernicterus*
- Joint contractures uncommon
- Tendon lengthening unpredictable

Ataxic
- Cerebellar lesion, uncommon
- Disturbance of coordinated movement
- Wide-based gait, mild tremor

Mixed
Anatomic Patterns
Quadriplegia
- Usually from severe hypoxia
- All four extremities
- Lower IQ, higher mortality
- Diagnosis MR if IQ <50 (average IQ 100)
- Only 20% with spastic quadriplegia ever walk
- Scoliosis in two-thirds of spastic quadriplegic patients

Diplegia (50%)
- Spastic diplegia along with prematurity and low birth weight
- Periventricular leukomalacia/hemorrhage* (more common in prematurity) causes diplegia because leg corticospinal tracts run closest to ventricles
- Both lower extremities worse than upper
- Strabismus common
  Usually walk, often normal IQ

Hemiplegia
- Often due to focal traumatic, vascular, or infectious lesion
- One side, upper worse than lower
- Early handedness
- Walk, may present with toe-walking only
- *Seizure disorder most common with this type

Presentation
- First finding is mother saying something is wrong with baby

- First clinical sign is hypotonia (lack of myelin blocks abnormal spastic signals)
- Diagnosed at average of 9 mo (depends on neuropathic pattern)
- Spastic diplegia 8–10 mo
- Hemiplegia 20–24 mo
- Athetosis >24 mo

Ambulation Prognosis

- Degree of spasticity most important
- No sitting balance by 2 y/o = poor prognosis
- Ambulation ability plateaus at 7 y/o

Bleck Criteria

- Assess seven primitive reflexes in child >1 y/o
- Persistent primitive reflexes or absent postural reflexes given 1 point each
- 0/7 good prognosis for ambulation
- 1/7 "guarded"
- 2/7 poor prognosis
- 95% accurate

Reflexes: Primitive (Bad If Present)

- Asymmetric tonic reflex
  - Turn head to one side
  - UE and lower extremity (LE) of that side extend
  - UE and LE of other side flex
- "Fencing position"
  - Head turns to one side with ipsilateral arm outstretched and contralateral arm bends at the elbow
  - Disappears 6 mo
- Neck-righting
  - Turn head to one side
  - Trunk and limbs follow head
  - Disappears at 10 mo
- Extensor thrust
  - Hold under arms
  - Then touch feet to floor
  - Abnormal = leg extension (disappears by 2 mo)
  - Normal = leg flexion
- Symmetric tonic neck
  - Crawling position
  - Flexed neck causes UE flexion, LE extension
  - Extended neck causes UE extension, LE flexion
  - Disappears 6 mo
- Moro startle
  - Sudden extension of neck or jarring table causes spread and extension of UEs
  - Disappears at 4–6 mo

Reflexes: Postural (Bad If Absent)

- Foot placement (stepping)
- Persists until 3–4 y/o
- Parachute reflex
  - Normally appears at 1 yr, stays until adult

- Drop slightly to simulate fall causes extended UEs to "brace fall"
- May be one sided in hemiplegia
- Life expectancy (Eyman et al., 1990)
  - 100,000 Californians with developmental disabilities who received state services from 1984 to 1987
  - Three subgroups, all retarded, incontinent
  - Future life expectancy
  - Immobile, tubefeed—5 yr
  - Immobile, assisted feed—8 yr
  - Mobile, assisted feed—23 yr

Reference

Eyman RK, et al. The life expectancy of profoundly handicapped people with mental retardation. N Engl J Med 1990; 323:584–589.

Treatment

- Functional Priorities
  - Communication
  - ADLs
  - Mobility
  - Walking

Nonoperative

- Bracing
- Wheelchair: total body orthosis
- Botox for dynamic deformity
  - Presynaptic block of acetylcholine release at neuromuscular junction
  - Max dose 12 units per Kg (Max 400 units)
  - Decreases spasticity for 3–6 mo
- Intrathecal baclofen
  - Decreases LE spasticity

Selective Dorsal Rhizotomy

- Afferent fibers in dorsal rootlets of spinal nerves that carry stimulatory imputs from muscle spindles
- Best candidate is 3–8 y/o, diplegic, pure spastic, ambulator, intelligent enough to cooperate with extensive postoperative PT
- Contraindications: athetosis, ataxia, rigidity, weakness, contractures
- No postoperative sensory deficits
- Decreased spasticity only

Surgery (in General)

- >3 y/o spastic patients with voluntary motor
  - Wait for mature gait pattern
  - Until patient can do postoperative PT
  - Address multiple problems at same operation
  - Exception for <3 y/o is hip at risk
  - Abduction <45 degrees
  - Partial uncovering of head
  - **See CP hip/LE/UE/spine sections for more details

CP—Hip
- Spectrum of hip pathology
- Subluxation (usually painless)

Clinical Manifestations
- Spasticity
- Instability with progressive subluxation in 15% of spastic patients, 25–50% of spastic quadriplegic patients
- Dislocation (50% painful)
- Abduction <30 degrees, flexion contracture >20–25 degrees

Natural History
- Hips normal at birth, dysplasia and subluxation by 2–4 yr, frank dislocation at 7 yr

Causative Factors
- Adductor spasticity > head erodes lateral acetabular > acetabular dysplasia > head migrates laterally > head steeple-shaped

Physical Exam
- Difficult to detect hip abnormalities due to spasticity/contractures
- Thomas or Staheli test for flexion contracture
- Hyperlordosis, crouch gait with hip flexion contracture
- Reduced abduction with adductor spasticity
- Increased prone hip IR with fem anteversion
- Ober test for ITB tightness

Radiographs
- *Yearly anteroposterior (AP) pelvis in spastic quadriplegic patients and nonambulatory diplegic patients
- Break in Shenton line
- Decrease in capital epiphyseal angle
- Increase in acetabular index
- Migration index of Reimers
  - Percent of head that lies outside bounds of lateral acetabulum
- Normally 80% covered, 20% index
- If <50% covered patient may require femoral or pelvic osteotomy to appropriately reduce the hip

Treatment
- Goals: stable painless hip needed to walk, sit, perform perineal care

Soft Tissue Releases for Hip at Risk or Early Subluxation
- Indications
  - <4 y/o
  - Decreased hip abduction with early subluxation
  - <30% migration index
- Adductor + psoas tenotomy
  - Adductor alone leads to recurrent sublux
  - If mild with abduction of 35–45 degrees, percutaneous adductor longus tenotomy

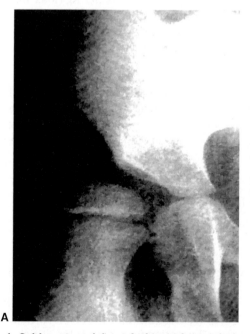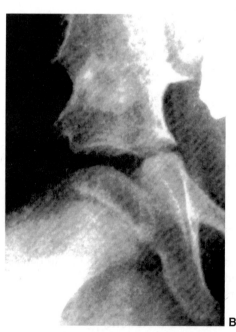

A: Subluxation of the right hip with acetabular dysplasia. **B:** Result after varization and derotation osteotomies of the proximal femur and Albee pelvic osteotomy. (From Morrissy RT, and Weinstein SL. Lovell and Winter's Pediatric Orthopaedics Sixth Edition Philadelphia: Lippincott Williams & Wilkins, 2006 with permission.)

- If severe with abduction <35 degrees, open release of longus, gracilis, ± brevis, ± treatment of these tendons to ischium
- If psoas flexion contracture >20–25 degrees
- In nonambulatory
    - Anterior incision over joint
    - Take anterior tensor fascia lata (TFL), straight head RF
    - Take psoas tendon beneath iliacus
- In ambulatory
    - Anterior intrapelvic approach
    - Psoas recession over pelvic brim
    - This preserves flexor strength
- 60% success, subluxation prevented
- 40% recurrence of subluxation due to chronic spasm, scoliosis, and pelvic obliquity

Osteotomies for Subluxation
- Indications
    - 3–8 y/o
    - 30%–50% migration index
- Treatment
    - Usually varus reduction osteotomy (VRO) with tenotomies
    - Can take internal rotation (IR)/abduction x-ray before VRO to assess hip location after proposed osteotomy
    - Psoas cut from lesser trochanter (LT) during VRO
    - Goal of derotation is ER two times IR
    - Goal of varization 125 degrees
    - Add pelvic osteotomy if
        - Acetabular index >25 degrees
        - >8 y/o
        - >50% migration index
        - 80% success with these guidelines
        - Usually post acetabular deficiency
        - If <9 y/o with unilateral symptoms, do bilateral osteotomy

Treatment of Dislocation
- If <1 yr ago, <9 y/o with open triradiate and head physis, joint not significantly degenerated, then
- Anterior open reduction with tenotomy
- Proximal femoral shortening VRO
- ± Acetabuloplasty
- Before surgery for dislocation, must address pelvic obliquity, contralateral hip abduction contracture
- If dislocation >1 yr ago and painless, no surgery required
- Salvage later if painful, interfering with care

Salvage of Painful Chronic Hip Dislocations
- Resection arthroplasty
    - Proximal one-third femoral resection with soft tissue interposition arthroplasty of Castle and Schnei-

der (Castle and Schneider, 1978) better than standard Girdlestone
- Level of resection can be estimated by the inferior aspect of the ischium
- Total hip replacement (THR) (Buly et al., 1993)
    - 19 THRs, postoperative spica
    - 95% pain relief, better function
    - 86% 10-yr implant survivorship
- Arthrodesis
- No good position for sitting and supine

References
Castle ME, Schneider C. Proximal femoral resection—interposition arthroplasty. J Bone Joint Surg Am 1978; 60: 1051–1054.
Buly RL, et al. Total hip arthroplasty in Cerebral Palsy. Long-term follow-up results. Clin Orthop Relat Res 1993; 296:148.

CP—Lower Extremity
General
- Spasticity leads to shortened muscle-tendon unit
- Muscle-tendon unit fails to keep pace with bone growth
- Ultimately develop joint contractures
- Frequently multiple LE procedures together

Clinical Manifestations
Hip Flexion Contracture
- Thomas test
- Release when contracture >20–25 degrees
- In ambulatory patient, release of entire iliopsoas (IP) may prevent stair climbing. Do psoas recession over pelvic brim without iliacus

Hip Adduction Contracture
- Limited hip abduction on exam
- Adductor longus tenotomy ± gracilis myotomy
- In ambulatory patient, avoid anterior branch obturator neurectomy (leads to broad-based gait with hip hyperabduction)

Hip IR Deformity
- Due to femoral anteversion or gluteus medius spasticity
- Increased femoral anteversion
- Derotational osteotomy
- Timing = timing of other LE surgery
- ER of distal fragment tightens medial HS
- Usually need medial HS release as well
- Gluteus medius spasticity
- Steel gluteus medius/minimus transfer to anterolateral proximal femur
    - Risk Trendelenburg gait postoperatively
    - Need 20 degrees passive ER preoperation

Hip Subluxation/Dislocation
- See CP hip section

Knee Flexion Deformity
- Along with hip flexion, crouch gait, or (rarely) excess ankle dorsiflexion
- Spasticity more common than true capsular contracture
- Medial hamstring usually the cause
- HS release when short latency response (SLR) <70 degrees, popliteal angle from vertical >45 degrees, or >15 degrees flexion contracture at stance
- Incise semimembranous fascia at two levels
- Lengthen or tenotomize semitendinosus (ST), gracilis
- ± Lateral HS aponeurotic lengthening
- Must recognize/treat other deformities
- If ankle equinus not addressed, leads to genu recurvatum
- If hip flexion contracture not addressed, leads to hip flexion and lordosis may get worse because HS is hip extensor
- If quad/HS cospastic, HS release alone can lead to stiff knee gait with poor foot clearance in swing and circumduction

RF Spasticity/Stiff Knee Gait
- Ely test (prone knee flexion causes hip flexion)
- RF spasticity limits knee flexion during swing phase, makes it hard to clear foot
- Distal rectus transfer to sartorius or iliotibial band (ITB) indicated for
  - Stiff knee gait with <80% of motion, hamstring-rectus cospasticity, rectus active through *entire gait cycle
  - Excess knee flexion through stance, stiff knee during swing, and RF activity in swing
  - Do not do if other quad muscles have decreased activity during stance because then will not be able to support standing
  - Improves knee flexion during swing by 15 degrees and improves foot clearance
  - Improves stride length, velocity, and knee range of motion (ROM) but only short-term

External Tibial Torsion
- Usually along with excess femoral anteversion, pes planovalgus
- Unstable base of support, compromised push-off power
- Supramalleolar derotational tibia/fibula osteotomy with crossed smooth Steinmann pins or plate/screws

Equinus
- Uncommon without varus or valgus
- Due to overactivity of gastrocnemius (G), soleus (S), or both

- Treatment
  - PT, brace
  - Botox for spasticity only, will only weaken if contracture
  - G aponeurosis lengthening (Volpius) alone causes less push-off weakness but ? higher recurrence (≤48%)

Tendo-Achilles Lengthening (TAL)
- Z-lengthening with repair
- Hoke triple cut and slide, open or percutaneous
- White double cut (DAMP)
- Distal anterior cut
- Proximal medial cut
- Weight bearing (WB) SLC for 6 wk, walk as soon as possible
- Complications of surgery
  - Recurrence inversely related to age
  - 25% recurrence if <4 y/o
  - Almost 0% recur if >8 y/o
  - If Achilles overlengthened
    - Dorsiflexion (DF) during single leg stance
    - Iatrogenic calcaneus deformity
    - Crouched gait
    - TAL can cause crouched posture if HS, IP contracture not addressed
    - Avoid TAL in athetosis because calcaneal deformity results

Equinovalgus
- Most common foot deformity in spastic diplegia (followed by equinovarus and calcaneus)
- Gastrocnemius soleus (GS) spastic, weak posttibial, overpull of peroneals
- Planovalgus along with hallux valgus, external tibial torsion, femoral adduction, femoral internal rotation
- Deformity usually in subtalar joint but must rule out ankle as source of valgus
- Treatment
  - If mild/supple AFO or UCBL (University of California Berkley Lab) ± peroneus brevis (PB) lengthening (peroneus longus [PL] lengthening causes excess varus)
  - If supple, calcaneal lateral lengthening with medial plication and peroneal lengthening (Mosca) preserves subtalar motion and supports talus
  - In both supple and rigid, consider calcaneal medial slide
  - If severe, consider Grice extra-articular subtalar arthrodesis (iliac homograft in sinus tarsi, results improved with screw to secure corrected talocalcaneal relationship)
  - Triple arthrodesis for rigid deformity in >12–13 y/o nonwalker with shoeing problems or painful ambulatory
- No treatment for painless nonambulator

Equinovarus
- *Usually in spastic hemiplegic
- Due to tibial posterior* or tibial anterior overactivity, peroneal weakness, tight heel cord
- Confusion test for tibial anterior versus posterior tibial
    - Flex hip versus resistance
    - In CP children, tibialis anterior will fire
    - If foot supinates while tibialis anterior fires, then tibial anterior may cause equivarus
    - Hindfoot varus, persistent varus in stance and swing: posterior tibial
    - Forefoot supination, hindfoot varus in swing only: tibial anterior
    - Treatment
        - Intramuscular or step-cut lengthening of posterior tibial corrects dynamic equivarus but results inconsistent
        - Complete tenotomy or transfer of posterior tibial leads to excess valgus, should not be done
        - Posterior tibial transfer to dorsum of foot okay for nonspastic patients but causes calcaneovalgus in CP
        - *If deformity supple, tibialis posterior lengthening/split treatment to PB ± TAL
        - *If hindfoot varus rigid, then calcaneal lateral closing wedge osteotomy or slide + tibial posterior lengthening or split treatment + TAL
        - If tibial anterior overactive (less common), split tibial anterior treatment to cuboid

Dorsal Bunion
- Overpull of ankle dorsiflexors causes flexion deformity of metatarsophalangeal (MTP) hallux
- McKay dorsal treatment of flexor hallices brevis (FHB)

Bracing
Solid AFO
- Standard rigid orthotic for correctable equinus spasticity

Ground Reaction AFO
- Like solid AFO except has additional bar on anterior proximal tibia and foot plate may have 2–3 degrees of plantarflexion on it
- This treats crouched gait (with calcaneus deformity) because after you "toe strike," anterior proximal tibial bar will be forced posteriorly, giving extension force to knee
- Restores plantarflexion—knee extension couple
- Contraindication in fixed knee flexion contracture

Hinged AFO (with Plantarflexion Stop)
- No spring loads
- Has hinge that does not allow plantarflexion beyond neutral but allows active dorsiflexion

- Allows heel strike
- For minimally involved patients who can actively dorsiflex ankle

CP—Upper Extremity
General
- Seen in patients with hemiplegia, spastic quads
- Only 5% of CP patients benefit from UE surgery
- Must have normal sensation for surgery
- High motivation and fair-to-good motor control improve outcome

Clinical Manifestations
- Shoulder IR, adduction contracture
- Elbow flexion, pronation
- Wrist flexor spasticity/ulnar deviation
- Hand deformities
    - Claw hand
    - Finger flexion
    - Swan neck deformities

Treatment
Shoulder IR/Adduction Contracture
- Surgery rarely indicated
- If good hand function but impaired hand placement due to shoulder, subscapular release/pectoralis lengthening ± humeral derotational osteotomy

Elbow Flexion Contracture
- Resect lacertus fibrosis
- Fractional lengthening if brachialis, biceps
- Release brachioradialis origin
- If severe, biceps step-cut lengthening and anterior capsulotomy

Pronation Deformity
- Distal release of pronator teres

Wrist Flexor Spasticity
- Flexor carpi ulnaris (FCU) or flexor carpi radialis (FCR) lengthening if finger extension good, spasticity mild
- Flexor pronator release from medial epicondyle if spastic wrist and fingers flexed (nonspecific release)
- FCU to extensor carpi radialis brevis (ECRB) if poor wrist extension, poor grasp, active finger extension
- FCU to extensor digitorum communis (EDC) if adequate grasp, poor release
- FCR lengthening with pronator teres transfer improves wrist ext

Wrist Ulnar Deviation
- Due to overactivity/volar displacement of extensor carpi ulnaris (ECU)
- Split transfer of ECU to ECRB

Claw Hand with Wrist Flexion, MCP Extension
- Usually due to imbalance between wrist flexion/ extension
- FCR or FCU to ECRB

Finger Flexion Deformity
- If mild (can extend fingers with wrist flexed), circumferential flexor digitorum superficialis/profundus (FDS/FDP) aponeurosis release in proximal one-third forearm
- If severe, sublimis to profundus treatment
- Proximal row carpectomy can gain soft tissue length

Swan-Neck Deformities
- Mild, correct wrist flexion ± splinting
- Severe requires complex surgery

Thumb-in-palm Deformity
- Redirection of extensor pollicis longus (EPL) through first dorsal compartment improves abduction and MCP extension
- Review of treatment principles of managing hand deformities in patients with CP. Emphasis is placed on providing a balanced grasp and release, a reasonable range of pronation and supination, and sufficient strength of the hand (Golder, 1988)

Reference

Golder JL. Surgical reconstruction on the upper extremity in cerebral palsy. Hand Clin 1988; 4:223–265.

CP—Spine
- Neuromuscular scoliosis
  - In 25% of CP
  - Highest risk in spastic quadriplegic patients (65%)
  - Worse in nonambulator
  - Low risk in hemiplegic patients
  - Longer curves, often to pelvis earlier, progressive beyond maturity
- Natural history
  - Progression and loss of function
  - CP adults progress at 0.8 degrees/yr for curvature <50 degrees at maturity versus 1.4 degrees/yr for curvature >50 degrees (Thometz and Simon, 1988)
  - Institutionalized CP patients with >45 degrees scoliosis and those without scoliosis compared
  - Scoliosis patients had worse pelvis and hip deformities and needed more modified wheelchairs
  - No difference in decubitus, highest functional level, O_2 saturation, pulse (Kalen et al., 1992)
  - Institutionalized CP patients with 35-degree fused scoliosis versus 76 degrees unfused
  - No difference in pain, decubitus, function, need for pulmonary medications, nurse hours (Cassidy et al., 1994)

References

Thometz JG, Simon SR. Progression of scoliosis after skeletal maturity in institutionalized adults who have cerebral palsy. J Bone Joint Surg Am 1988; 70:1290–1296.

Kalen V, et al. Untreated scoliosis in severe cerebral palsy. J Pediatr Orthop 1992; 12:337–340.

Cassidy C, et al. A reassessment of spinal stabilization in severe cerebral palsy. J Pediatr Orthop 1994; 14:731–739.

Types

Type 1 (Ambulators)
- Like idiopathic pattern
- Single or double, no pelvic obliquity

Type 2 (Nonwalkers)
- Long TL or L curve
- Pelvis higher on concave side
- With lumbosacral (LS) fractional curve or with sacrum part of curve

Treatment
- Observe for 25–30 degrees
- Brace >30 degrees but stops progression in only 15%, may be useful to slow progress and delay surgery
- PSF for >50 degrees because progresses at any age and affects sitting
  - Fuse from upper T to L5 or pelvis to prevent proximal kyphosis
  - Fuse pelvis if obliquity >10 degrees on sitting x-ray view compared to L4 or L5, nonambulatory
- ASF only if more correction needed
  - Curve does not correct to <50 degrees on bending x-ray view
  - To level pelvis if obliquity is severe
  - To release anterior tether of kyphosis
  - Improve respiratory function
  - Decrease pseudarthrosis rate
- Reduction in spasticity seen following selective dorsal rhizotomy (SDR) (McLaughlin et al., 2002)
- Overview of gait analysis and its use in CP patients (Gage, 1995) (DeLuca et al., 1997)
- Overview of operative treatment strategies of spinal deformities in CP (including traction, anterior/posterior fusion, fusion to pelvis) (Lonstein et al., 1983)

References

Lonstein JE, Akbarnia A. Operative treatment of spinal deformities in patients with cerebral palsy or mental retardation. An analysis of one hundred and seven cases. J Bone Joint Surg Am 1983; 65(1):43–55.

McLaughlin J, et al. Selective dorsal rhizotomy: meta-analysis of three randomized controlled trials. Dev Med Child Neurol 2002; 44:17–25.

Gage JR. Gait analysis: principles and applications. Emphasis on its use in cerebral palsy. J Bone Joint Surg Am 1995; 1995;77:1607-1623.

DeLuca PA, et al. Alterations in surgical decision making in patients with cerebral palsy based on three-dimensional gait analysis. J Pediatr Orthop 1997; 17:608–614.

CHARCOT-MARIE-TOOTH (CMT)

- Hereditary motor sensory neuropathy
- Demyelinating disease of peripheral nerves
- Abnormal electrodiagnostic studies
- Nerve biopsy shows endoneurial fibrosis (onion bulb)
- Seven types, first three involve children

IA—Hypertrophic CMT
- AD, *can be diagnosed by DNA testing
- Duplication of peripheral myelin protein
- Onset in second decade

Clinical Manifestations
- "Stork legs"
- Absent deep tendon reflexes
- Diminished distal sensation

- Foot weakness—plantar intrinsics (first), peroneals, and tibialis anterior leads to cavovarus and claw toes
- Cavus foot caused by relative weakness of tibialis anterior and peroneus brevis; overdrive of peroneus longus causes flexion of first ray which drives cavus deformity
- Hand involvement—intrinsic wasting, intrinsic minus deformity
- Acquired hip dysplasia in 6%–8% of Hereditary Sensory and Motor Neuropathy (HSMN) (more common in type I than II), usually asymptomatic
- Scoliosis in 10%
- Slow nerve conduction velocities (NCVs), prolonged distal latencies

Treatment
- Cavovarus foot
  - Soft tissue releases/transfers when young and supple
  - Plantar release
  - PT transfer to middorsum

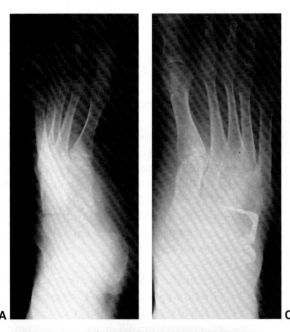
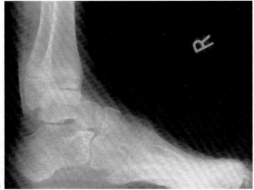
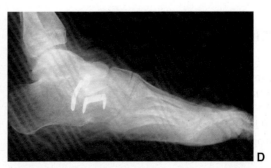

A: Anteroposterior radiograph of severe cavovarus deformity of the right foot in a 14-year-old boy with Charcot-Marie-Tooth disease, in standing posture. B: Lateral radiograph demonstrates a varus hindfoot and midfoot, and a plantar flexed first metatarsal. C: Postoperative anteroposterior radiograph, taken in standing posture, following a Ryerson triple arthrodesis, soft tissue balancing, and correction of his claw toe deformities. D: Lateral radiograph showing markedly improved alignment. (From Morrissy RT, and Weinstein SL. Lovell and Winter's Pediatric Orthopaedics Sixth Edition Philadelphia: Lippincott Williams & Wilkins, 2006 with permission.)

– Jones procedure—extensor hallucis longus (EHL) transfer to first metatarsal (MT) neck to help dorsiflex first MT, + great toe IP fusion
– If becoming rigid (Coleman block test)
– MT and calcaneus osteotomies
– Avoid triple arthrodesis if possible

II—Neuronal CMT
– Variable inheritance
– Onset third or fourth decade
– Presents with cavovarus foot
– Normal reflexes
– Less weakness
– Mildly abnormal NCVs

III—Dejerine-Sottas Disease
– AR
– Onset in infancy, delayed ambulation
– Pes cavus, foot drop
– Stocking-glove dysesthesia
– Spinal deformities
– Wheelchair by third/fourth decade
– More severe NCV disturbances
– Discussion of mutations in 10 genes linked to subtypes of CMT (Berger et al., 2002)
– Improvement in foot scores and radiographs in 15 feet treated with combined calcaneal and metatarsal osteotomies (Sammarco and Taylor, 2001)
– Evaluation of 30 triple arthrodeses performed in 16 patients with CMT on average 21 years post-operatively. 14 rated poor, 9 fair, 5 good, 2 excellent. 6 went on to have ankle arthrodesis. Authors recommend triple arthrodesis for most severe foot deformities in CMT only (Westmore and Drennan, 1989)

References
Berger P, et al. Molecular cell biology of Charcot-Marie-Tooth disease. Neurogenetics 2002; 4:1–15.
Sammarco GJ, Taylor R. Cavovarus foot treated with combined calcaneus and metatarsal osteotomies. Foot Ankle Int 2001; 22:19–30.
Westmore RS, Drennan JC. Long-term results of triple arthrodesis in Charcot-Marie-Tooth disease. J Bone Joint Surg Am 1989; 71:417–422.

FRIEDREICH ATAXIA

General
– Most common inherited ataxia
– Autosomal recessive. Mutation in frataxin (chromosome 9)
– 1:50,000 live births
– Slow progressive spinocerebellar degeneration
– Motor and sensory defects

Natural History
– Onset 7–15 y/o
– Loss of ambulation in 20s due to ataxia (not weakness)
– Death in 40s due to hypertrophic cardiomyopathy (HCM)

Clinical Manifestations
– Staggering wide-based gait (ataxia)
– Dysarthria, areflexia, pos Babinski
– Nystagmus
– Cavus foot, LE weakness
– Loss of position, vibratory sense
– Scoliosis
– DM, hypertrophic cardiomyopathy

Treatment
Cavovarus
– Orthotics ineffective
– Plantar release/tendon transfers ± MT and calcaneus osteotomies if flexible
– Triple arthrodesis if rigid

Scoliosis
– Does not behave like neuromuscular scoliosis
– Natural history, treatment similar to idiopathic scoliosis
– No correlation between muscle weakness and curve progression
– Curve progression correlates with age at disease onset and age at scoliosis diagnosis
– Thirty-three patients with FA were followed for an average of 6 years for evaluation of muscular strength assessment. Weakness usually manifested in hip extension first, followed by lower extremity weakness. Patients began using a wheelchair at 18 y/o and were unable to ambulate at 20.5 y/o (Beauchamp et al., 1995)
– Natural history study (Labelle et al., 1986)
  – *100% of patients had >10-degree curve
  – 66% had hyperkyphosis
  – Progressive in >60 degrees, onset before 10 y/o
  – Stays <40 degrees, onset after 10 y/o
  – Bracing of limited value, poorly tolerated
  – Observe <40 degrees
  – Observe or surgery 40–60 degrees
  – PSF for >60 degrees

References
Beauchamp M, et al. Natural history of muscle weakness in Friedreich's ataxia and its relation to loss of ambulation. Clin Orthop Relat Res 1995; (311):270–275.
Labelle H, et al. Natural history of scoliosis in Friedreich's ataxia. J Bone Joint Surg Am 1986; 68:564–572.

Metabolic Disorders

CAFFEY DISEASE

- Infantile cortical hyperostosis
- Follows febrile illness in 0–9-mo-old children

Clinical Manifestations
- Afebrile or febrile
- Soft tissue swelling
- Can affect any bone except vertebrae and phalanges
- Mandibular involvement characteristic
- Ulna most commonly involved extremity bone
- Erythrocyte sedimentation rate (ESR) and alkaline phosphatase often elevated
- Cultures negative
- Spontaneous recovery 2–3 mo

Differential Diagnosis
- Trauma
- Child abuse
- Progressive diaphysial dysplasia
- Infection
- Scurvy
- Hypervitaminosis A

Radiographs
- Cortical thickening
- Periosteal reaction

Treatment
- NSAIDs

GAUCHER DISEASE

General
- Lysosomal storage disease
- Common in Ashkenazi Jews
- Autosomal recessive. Mutation in beta-glucocerebrosidase
- Cerebroside build-up in reticuloendothelial cells

Clinical Manifestations
- *Bone crisis
- Hepatosplenomegaly/marrow replacement leads to pancytopenia
- AVN
- Pathologic Fracture

Radiographic Findings
- Osteopenia, moth-eaten trabeculae
- Pathologic femoral neck, spine fractures
- *Femoral head necrosis (differential diagnosis MED, Perthes)
- *Erlenmeyer flask distal femur

Pathology
Treatment
- Enzyme replacement is available as one form of management
- Fractures largely managed conservatively

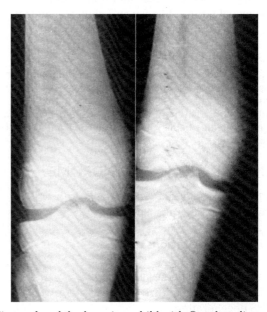

Radiographs of the knee in a child with Gaucher disease. Note the typical flaring of the distal femoral metaphysis, or Erlenmeyer flask deformity. (Photo courtesy of Henry J. Mankin, MD)

HOMOCYSTINURIA

General
- Autosomal recessive. Deficient cystathionine beta-synthase
  - Defective methionine metabolism
  - Accumulation of homocysteine

Clinical Manifestations
- Marfanoid habitus
  - Arachnodactyly
  - Dolichostenomelia
  - Pectus excavatum
- Unlike Marfan
  - Seizures, retarded
  - Inferior (vs. superior) lens dislocation
  - *Osteoporosis
  - Cavus foot
  - Joint tightness
- Scoliosis (up to one-third)
- Progressive kyphosis
- Spontaneous thrombosis, cardiac events

Diagnosis
- Cyanide-nitroprusside test of urine
- Multivitamins (MVI) may suppress positive test
  - must do amino acid assay if on MVI

Treatment
- Vitamin B6 and decrease methionine in diet
- Review of natural history and clinical manifestations of homocystinuria (Mudd et al., 1985).

References
Boers GH. Homocystinuria versus Marfan's syndrome: the therapeutic relevance of the differential diagnosis. Neth J Med 1984; 27:206–212.
Mudd SH, et al. The natural history of homocystinuria due to cystathionine beta-synthase deficiency. Am J Hum Genet 1985; 37:1–31.

MENKES KINKY HAIR SYNDROME

- X-linked recessive
- Defective copper absorption

Clinical Manifestations
- Newborn male
- Characteristic sparse kinky hair
- Profound failure to thrive
- CNS degeneration
- Periosteal reactions
- *Can present with metaphysial corner fractures
- May be confused with abuse or rickets

MUCOPOLYSACCHARIDOSES

General
- Proportionate dwarfism
- Due to hydrolase enzyme deficiency
  Diagnose with complex sugars in urine

Morquio Disease
- AR, proportionate dwarf
- Most common form of mucopolysaccharidosis
- *Keratan sulfate in urine
- Presents at ~2 y/o with
  - Waddling gait
  - Knock-knees
  - Thoracic kyphosis
  - *Cloudy cornea
  - *Normal intelligence

Radiographic Changes
- *Thick skull, wide ribs
- Vertebrae with anterior beaking
- Wide flat pelvis
- Unossified femoral heads
- *Bullet shaped metacarpals
- *C1–C2 instability

- Due to dens hypoplasia
- Can cause myelopathy
- May need C1–C2 fusion

Reference
Dalvie S, et al. Mobile thoracolumbar gibbus in Morquio type A: the cause of paraparesis and its management. J Pediatr Orthop B 2001; 10:328–330.

Hurler Syndrome
- AR
- *Most severe, worst prognosis
- Dermatan/heparan sulfate in urine
- Mental retardation, cloudy cornea
- Carpal tunnel syndrome, joint contractures

Hunter Syndrome
- *Sex-linked recessive
- Dermatan/heparan sulfate in urine
- Mental retardation, clear cornea
- Joint contractures, extension defecits
- Surgical correction rare

Sanfilippo Syndrome
(White et al.)
- AR
- *Heparan sulfate in urine
- Normal until 2 y/o
- Mental retardation, clear cornea
- Hip osteonecrosis, carpal tunnel, scoliosis, trigger digits

NIEMANN-PICK DISEASE

- "Niem picks nose with sphinger"
- Autosomal recessive, sphingomyelinase defect
- Sphingomyelin (phospholipid) accumulates in reticoendothelial system
- Common in Ashkenazi Jews
- Marrow expansion, cortical thinning
- Coxa valga (Link B, et al.)

Infection

DISCITIS

General
- Clinical continuum of bacterial or viral (milder) infection of vertebral body that spreads into disc
- Most common cause of back pain in young child
- Typical patient 2–7 y/o

Clinical Presentation
- Most commonly persistent with back pain, malaise, fever

- One-third of patients 1–3 y/o present with failure to walk
- 3–8 y/o can present with abdominal pain if T8–L1
- Loss of lumbar lordosis and tight HS
- Positive SLR
- Tender to palpation/paravertebral muscle spasm
- Loss of spinal flexibility/reluctance to bend
- Pseudo Gower sign

Laboratory Evaluation
- 90% with high ESR
- 10% with high white blood cell count (WBC), 40% with high-normal WBC
- 41% blood culture positive
- 67% biopsy positive
- Biopsies usually not done in children because not much better at getting bug than blood culture
- Most common bug is *Staphylococcus aureus*

Imaging
- X-ray view is negative for up to 1 mo
- Disc space narrowing
- Erosion or sclerosis of end plate
- Bone scan if normal x-ray but high ESR
  - Hot within 5 days of symptom onset
  - Increased uptake across involved disc
- MRI to rule out abscess
- Able to differentiate osteomyelitis (OM)/discitis from epidural abscess, which is operative
- Can distinguish pyogenic OM from tuberculosis (TB) (TB spares disc)

Treatment (Controversial)
- IV antibiotics shorten symptoms and reduce risk of long-term sequelae
  - 73% excellent relief by 2–4 days
  - 82% excellent relief by 2–3 wk
  - Monitor treatment by checking ESR and C-reactive protein (CRP)
  - CRP should decrease by 5 days
  - ESR can take >2 wk to come down
  - Recommends 6 days of Ancef or nafcillin, then 6 weeks of oral antibiotics (Ring et al., 1995)

Reference
Ring D, et al. Pyogenic infectious spondylitis in children: the convergence of discitis and vertebral osteomyelitis. J Pediatr Orthop 1995; 15:652–660.

KASSER DISEASE (CHRONIC RECURRENT OSTEOMYELITIS)
- Multifocal, nonpyogenic, inflammatory bony lesions with prolonged fluctuating course
- Blood and lesion cultures negative

- Etiology unknown
- Benign and self-limiting
- Must rule out infection with negative cultures prior to withholding antibiotics
- Treatment with NSAIDs

OSTEOMYELITIS
- In neonate
  - Vessels from metaphysis cross into epiphysis
  - Bacteria localize in cartilaginous epiphysis
  - Infection causes destruction, impaired growth
  - By 3–4 mo, separate epiphyseal blood supply
  - Physis acts as barrier when formed
- In children
  - Metaphyseal arterial loops empty into sinuses leading to stasis, turbulence
  - Bacteria lodge in area beneath physis
  - Trauma to metaphysis can predispose to infection from normal daily low-grade bacteremia (rabbit study)
  - Infection starts in metaphysis
  - Hip, shoulder, distal fibula, radiocapitate metaphyses are intra-articular; OM can lead to septic arthritis
  - Child's periosteum is thick, easily separated from bone by pus, not easily penetrated by infection
  - As periosteum elevated, cortical blood supply impaired and necrosis/sequestrum may develop
  - Elevated periosteum (blood supply from overlying muscle) lays down new bone to form involucrum

Differential Diagnosis
- Trauma, CRP can be elevated
- Leukemia (30% present with bone pain)
- Neoplasm (metastatic neuroblastoma, epidermal growth (EG), Ewings)
- Bone infarct (sickle cell, Gaucher)

Laboratory Findings
White Blood Count
- Elevation in 25%, abnormal differential in 65%

Erythrocyte Sedimentation Rate
- Elevated in 90%
- Less reliable in first 48 hours
- Unreliable in anemia, sickle cell, steroid
- ESR lower than in septic arthritis

C-Reactive Protein
- Increased in 1–2 days, decreases faster than ESR

Blood Cultures
- Positive in 30%–50%

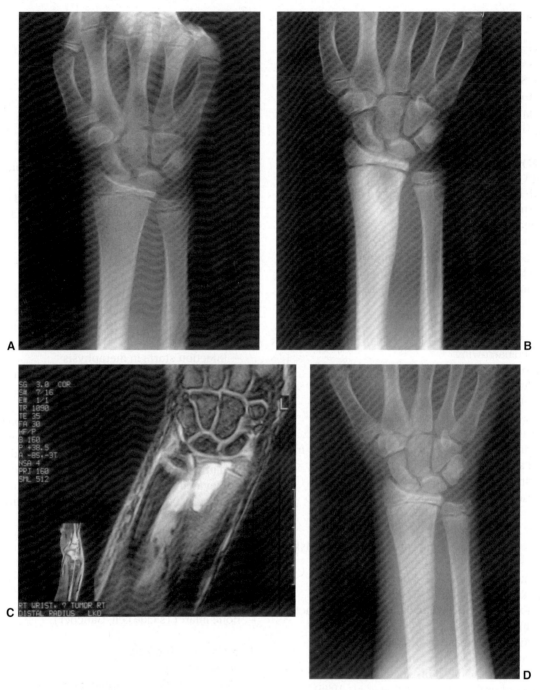

A: 12-year-old boy was struck in the distal radius by a hockey puck. Initial radiographs were negative, and the patient's symptoms completely resolved over 2 weeks. **B:** Two months later, the patient experienced increasing pain and swelling. Radiographs were repeated and demonstrated a lytic lesion with a sclerotic margin that appeared to cross the physis consistent with osteomyelitis. **C:** T2-weighted magnetic resonance imaging (MRI) suggested the diagnosis of infection that crossed the distal radial physis with cortical breach and adjacent soft-tissue abscess. **D:** Irrigation and debridement of purulent material was performed, and cultures obtained at surgery confirmed *S. aureus* osteomyelitis. To reduce risk of persistent infection and to reduce the likelihood of physeal arrest, no bone graft was placed. Two years after surgery, the bone defect has healed, there is no evidence of infection, and the distal radial physis is growing normally. (From Morrissy RT, and Weinstein SL. Lovell and Winter's Pediatric Orthopaedics Sixth Edition Philadelphia: Lippincott Williams & Wilkins, 2006 with permission.)

Bone Aspiration
- Positive in 50%–70%
- Pus rarely found with symptoms <3 days

Radiology
- Less than 5 days soft tissue swelling, obliteration of fat planes
- Greater than 5–7 days
  - Resorption of bone
  - Periosteal new bone
  - Involucrum (bone formed beneath elevated periosteum, surrounding sequestrum)
  - Sequestrum (necrotic bone often with denser surrounding bone)

Bone Scan
- Tc bone scan used to identify site; indium scan specific to WBCs/infection
- Must differentiate early OM metaphysial changes from normal large uptake in physis
- Sensitivity/specificity approximately 90% each
- Cold scan can be due to necrosis from subperiosteal abscess
- Bone aspiration does not affect bone scan

MRI
- (Mazur et al., 1995)
- Sensitivity 97%
- Specificity 92%
- Good anatomic detail (especially useful in axial skeleton)
- Low signal T1, high signal T2 due to marrow edema, hyperemia, purulence
- Brodie abscess (subacute osteomyelitis)—cystic within medullary canal, high signal on T2, surrounded by sclerotic bone
- Disadvantages are cost, frequent need for sedation in children

Reference
Mazur et al. Usefulness of magnetic resonance imaging for the diagnosis of acute musculoskeletal infections in children. J Pediatr Orthop, 1995; 15:144–147.

Organisms
- *S. aureus* most common overall
- Neonates—Guillain-Barré syndrome (GBS): empiric cefotaxime
- 6 mo–4 y/o—*Haemophilus influenzae*: empiric Ancef
  - Incidence of *H. influenzae* nearly 0% due to vaccination
  - Foot, sneaker, nail: think *Pseudomonas*

Treatment
- IV antibiotics after cultures drawn
- Follow CRP for resolution with treatment
- Switch to oral antibiotics when symptoms resolve
- Usual course 4–6 wks
- Surgical débridement (indications controversial)
  - Aspiration of pus (= subperiosteal abscess)
  - Failure to improve within 36–48 hr

SEPTIC ARTHRITIS

General
- Two times incidence of osteomyelitis
- Can get septic joint from osteomyelitis in neonates
- In older children, occurs when metaphysis is intra-articular
- Knee metaphysis is extra-articular
- Hip, shoulder, distal fibula, radiocapitate metaphysis are intra-articular

Differential Diagnosis of Acutely Swollen/Painful Joint
- Toxic synovitis
- JRA
- Henoch-Schönlein purpura
- Nonthrombocytopenic purpura
- Abdominal pain, nephritis
- Arthritis (knee/ankle, periarticular swelling leads to effusion, tenderness)
- Lyme disease
- Acute rheumatic fever
- Large joints, migratory
- Group A strep infection 2 wk prior (Kocher and Kasser, 1999)
  - 300 children who were aspirated
  - Four predictors
    - Temperature >38.5°C
    - Inability to weight bear
    - ESR >40
    - WBC >12
    - 0 predictors—<0.2% septic arthritis
    - 1 predictor—3%: observe, admit?
    - 2 predictors—40%: aspirate in radiology
    - 3 predictors—93%: aspirate in OR
    - 4 predictors—99.6%: aspirate in OR

Reference
Kocher, Kasser. Differentiating between septic arthritis and transient synovitis of the hip in children; evidence-based clinical prediction algorithm. J Bone Joint Surg Am 1999; 81:1662–1670.

Laboratory Workup
- *Complete blood count (CBC), ESR/CRP, Lyme, RF, ANA, ASLO
- WBC increases in only 25%–35%, left shift in 50%–70%
- ESR increases in 90% within 2–3 days, peaks day 3–5, normal in 2–4 wk

- ESR less reliable—48 hours
- ESR unreliable in inflammatory conditions, anemia or sickle cell
- CRP rises in 6 hr, peaks in 36–50 hr, drops sooner than ESR, normal in 1 wk
- CRP falls to normal with successful treatment
- Blood culture positive in 30%–50%
- Joint aspiration
  - Gram stain positive in approximately one-third
  - Culture positive in 65%
  - Synovial WBCs, Percentage of polymorphonuclear leukocytes
    - Normal: <200, <25%
    - Trauma: <5,000, <25% (many red blood cells [RBCs])
    - Toxic synovitis: 5–15 K, <25%
    - Adult rheumatic fever: 10–15 K, 50%
    - JRA: 15–80 K, 75%
    - Septic joint: >50 K, 80%
- If aspiration consistent with infection, then incision and drainage (I&D)

Radiographic Findings
Bone Scan
- Bone scan 90% sensitive/specific for osteomyelitis and septic joint but cannot differentiate between the two
- Cannot differentiate between infectious and noninfectious arthritis
- Increased uptake both sides of joint in septic joint
- Cold scan means dead bone
- Joint aspiration before bone scan does not change results but changes MRI results

MRI
- Decreased marrow signal on T1 because fat replaced by inflammatory cells, edema
- Increased signal on T2 (fluid)

Organisms
- <12 mo—staph, GBS: first-generation cephalosporin
- 6 mo–5 yr—staph, *H. influenzae*: second, third generation
- 5–12 y/o—*S. Aureus*: first-generation cephalosporin
- 12–18 y/o—*S. aureus*, gonococcus: oxytetracycline/ cephalosporin
- Culture synovial fluid on chocolate agar, and take urethral swab if suspect gonorrhea
- Incidence of *H. influenzae* near 0% now because of vaccination
- If *H. influenza* diagnosed, then lumbar puncture should be performed. 30% of *H influenza* infections associated with meningitis

- Lyme septic arthritis in endemic areas. Fever, CRP and WBCs lower than in bacterial septic arthritis. Obtain Lyme titers.

Neonate
- First 28 days of life
- premie and c-section are risk factors
- Usually OM and septic joint together
- Usually hematogenous
- In premie, usually *S. aureus* or gram negative, 40% in multiple sites
- In healthy, *usually GBS, *single site
- ESR and CRP unreliable
- Bone scan most sensitive for diagnosis

SI Joint
- FABER test
- MRI to localize and diagnose abscess
- Aspirate only if atypical and no response to antibiotics
- Surgery only if needed for biopsy or if abscess
- Treat with antibiotics like osteomyelitis

TRANSIENT SYNOVITIS

General
- Acute monoarticular hip or knee pain, limp, decreased ROM in nonill patient
- Most common cause of childhood hip pain
- 3% risk for each child to have it once
- Males > females = 2:1
- Less common in blacks
- Pathology = nonpyogenic synovitis
- Transient mild decrease in vascular perfusion to femoral head in early stages, resolves

Natural History
- Gradual, complete resolution over days to weeks
- Average duration is 10 days but may persist for up to 8 weeks
- 67% <1 wk, 88% <4 wk
- Recurrence in 4%–17%
  - Ipsilateral or contralateral
  - Most likely to recur within 6 mo
- >2 mm coxa magna noted but asymptomatic, no long-term DJD

Differential Diagnosis
- Transient synovitis is a diagnosis of exclusion
- Septic arthritis, TB arthritis, osteomyelitis
- JRA
- Acute rheumatic fever
- Poststrep reactive arthritis
  - 2–4 wk after group A strep infection
  - Joint symptoms may be migratory
  - Associated with a transient rash
- Legg-Calvé-Perthes disease

- SCFE
- Tumor

Presentation
- Usually 3–8 y/o
- Temperature >38°C
- Never bilateral
- Hip flexed, externally rotated
- Decreased ROM, especially abduction, IR
- 70% associated with upper respiratory infection (URI)
- 17%–30% associated with trauma

Laboratory Findings
- *CBC, ESR/CRP, Lyme, RF, ANA, ASLO
- WBC 10–14
- ESR ~20
- Urinalysis (UA), blood culture, tuberculin skin test, rheumatoid factor (RF) within normal limits
- Aspiration: 1–5 mL fluid, culture negative
- 43% with high systemic interferon (IFN) levels
- 95% with high IFN in joint fluid

Radiographic Findings
- Effusion causes displacement of muscle shadows of IP, obturator internus, gluteus medius
- Inflammation causes loss of intermuscular fat planes
- X-ray views debatable, ? due to positioning

Ultrasound (US)
- Joint effusion in ~70%
- 30% symptomatic patients have no effusion
- Average resolution of effusion in 9 days (with average symptom resolution in 5 days in same series)

Bone Scan—No Clear Role
Treatment
- Bedrest until pain resolves and motion improves
- Failure to rest will prolong symptoms
- NSAIDS (avoid ASA to prevent concomitant Reye's syndrome)
- If asymptomatic limp persists, continue bedrest in non-ambulatory patients or PWB with crutches in capable patients

Spine

BACK PAIN IN CHILDREN

General
- Incidence of LBP in adolescents 10–30%
- Severe pain nearly always along with pathology
- Diagnosis can be made in up to 84% if > -6bwk of symptoms
- Differential Diagnosis <10 y/o

- Discitis/OM (see Discitis)
- EG, leukemia, neuroblastoma, astrocytoma
- Idiopathic juvenile osteoporosis

Differential Diagnosis >10 y/o
- spondylolysis, listhesis
- Scheuermann
- HNP
- Apophysial ring fracture
- Osteoblastoma, osteoid osteoma, osteosarcoma, lymphoma, Aneursymal bone cyst (ABC)
- Psychogenic, conversion, overuse

History
- Age
- Nature of pain (intermittent, unrelenting, night)
- Fever, weight loss
- Activities, sports

Physical Exam
- Non-idiopathic Scoliosis (osteoid osteoma, osteoblastoma)
- Pain with hyperextension (spondylolysis)
- Asymmetric abduction reflexes (syringomyelia)
- Clonus/Babinski (abnormal cord/cord compression)
- Hamstring tightness: measure popliteal angles (nl. <50 degrees)

Workup
- Radiographs if >4 wks of symptoms or <4 y/o
- Bone scan if normal x-ray, normal neurologic exam
- Single photon emission computed tomography (SPECT) for lysis suspicion
- CBC, ESR, CRP
- MRI if abnormal neurologic exam, abnormal labs

Leukemia
- Back pain is presenting complaint in 6% of acute lymphocytic leukemia (ALL)
- Best screening test is CBC for high platelets and abnormal morphology white cells
- Bone marrow aspiration is diagnostic

HNP in Children
- Rare, usually in 10–18 y/o
- Usually caused by trauma
- Presents with back pain, sciatica (rarely below knee), +SLR
- If below knee, think epidural abscess or tumor
- Most common radiographic finding is nonstructural scoliosis
- MRI shows HNP
- Associated with presence of congenital transitional vertebra at L5 or S1

Apophyseal Ring Fracture
- Fracture between body and apophysis (normally fuses at age 18 yr)
- Most common at inferior apophysis of L4
- Apophysis is displaced posteriorly with disc
- Most commonly seen in teenage boy weight lifter
- Usually acute or repetitive hyperextension
- Signs, symptoms similar to HNP
- Sciatica rarely below knee
- Lateral radiograph shows triangular opacity posterior to vertebral body
- CT is study of choice
- Treat with laminotomy, removal of bone/cartilage fragment

Idiopathic Juvenile Osteoporosis
- Usually <10 y/o
- One-third present with back pain
- One-third present with long bone pain due to metaphysial compression fractures
- Vertebrae always abnormal on radiograph
  - Progressive height loss
  - Multiple growth arrest lines
  - Symmetric biconcavity
- Labs normal
- Dual energy x-ray absorptiometry (DEXA) shows decreased bone density
- Osteoporosis is self-limiting, spinal changes are reversible

Tumor versus Infection on MRI
- Pyogenic infection does not cross discs.
  - Discitis starts in endplate and may spread to adjacent VB but osteomyelitis does not cross into discs.
- TB: osteomyelitis without discitis
- Metastatic malignancy goes to vascular-rich VB, not in avascular disc

MYELOMENINGOCELE (MMC)

General
- 1:1,000 (in U.S., 0.15% in whites, 0.04% in blacks)
- Risk increased to 5% with one affected child
- One-third with *latex hypersensitivity
- In utero diagnosis
- High alpha-fetoprotein (AFP) (normal AFP gone after 16 wk)
- Ultrasound

Etiology (Variable)
- Multifactorial
- Chromosome abnormality or single gene abnormality
- Usually have other birth defects
- Teratogens (valproic acid)
- *Deficiency of folate

Prevention
- 0.4 mg folate/day for all women of child bearing age
- 4 mg folate/day for high-risk women

Natural History
- 90%–100% death without treatment
- Early sac closure and ventriculoperitoneal (VP) shunt to prevent meningitis and death
- May see progressive neurologic degeneration with increasing level of paralysis
- Must recognize/treat hydrocephaly, hydrosyringomyelia, Arnold-Chiari, tethered cord
- High infection rate, chronic urinary tract infections (UTIs)
- Lower level better orthopedically but worse genitourinary (GU) problems
- Need neurosurgery, orthopedic, urology follow-up

Spectrum of Defects
- Spina bifida occulta
  - Lack of fusion of spinous process
  - Most common in L5 and S1
  - 10% of adults
  - No neurologic abnormalities
- Meningocoele
  - Cyst only with meninges
  - No neurologic deficits
  - Neurosurgery to close, no other treatment
- Myelomeningocoele
  - Abnormal neural elements part of sac
  - Peripheral neurologic deficits common
  - CNS abnormality common (Arnold-Chiari, 90% with hydrocephalus)
  - Can cause tethered cord
- Lipomeningocoele
  - Meningeal sac with lipoma associated with sacral nerves
  - Neurology normal at birth but worsens
- Rachischisis
  - No skin or sac
  - Muscle, bone, neural exposed
  - Dysplastic cord
- Sacral agenesis
  - Associated with maternal DM
  - Increased congenital abnormalities
  - Spine to pelvis fusion
  - Levels—based on lowest fracture level

Level of Defect (lowest intact level)
Thoracic
- No hip or LE activity
- No fixed deformities, no dislocations
- Posture due to gravity

- Hip ER, knee flexion, ankle equinovarus/valgus
- Completely neurogenic bladder with low pressures and minimal GU problem

L1, L2
- Strong hip flexion, moderate adductors
- Hips flexed, adducted
- Hip and knee flexion contracture

L3
- Normal hip flexion and adduction power
- Quad almost normal
- Hips flexed/adducted, knees extended
- Feet flaccid

L4
- Normal quad power
- Tibial anterior power leads to feet varus and calcaneus
- Hip abductor weakness
- Hips flexed/adducted, knees extended

L5
- Hip adductors, HS, posterior tibia working
- Hips flexed, knees flexed, feet calcaneus

Sacral
- Hip extension/abduction, HS working
- Hip and knee flexed, feet variable
- *Congenital problems versus developmental problems due to muscle imbalance

Mental Status
- Change in mental status: rule out central nervous system involvement
  - Syrinx
  - Tethered cord
  - Hydrocephalus
- MRI of brain and spine.

Ambulation

L1 level	0%–5% ambulate	HKAFO/RGO
L2	10% ambulate	HKAFO/RGO
L3	50%–60% ambulate	KAFO
L4	80% ambulate	AFO

HKAFO, hip, knee, ankle, foot orthosis

Hip
- Congenital dislocations can happen at any level but developmental subluxation/dislocation most common at *L3/L4
- Valgus neck due to weak abductors
- Acetabular dysplasia due to abnormal forces

- Pelvic obliquity from scoliosis leads to dislocation on higher side
- Unilateral dislocation usually painless but leads to pelvic obliquity which leads to pressure sore on one tuberosity
- If unilateral dislocated, close reduce or dislocate other hip to gain symmetry, even if patient is a T level (not necessarily osteotomies)
- operative treatment indicated only if patient can get hip flexion to >90 because sitting requirements are straight spine and hip flexion >90 degrees
- Thoracic levels
  - Hips rarely dislocated due to no motor function
  - Hip surgery avoided due to painless deformity
  - Can walk even if dislocated but most T levels in wheelchair at 8–9 y/o because of energy expenditure
- L1–L2 levels
  - IP and adduction contracture lead to dislocations
  - Hip flexors cause pitching forward with walking
  - Need orthosis crossing hips to provide stability for ambulation
  - PT with ROM is key, then releases
  - If ROM okay, dislocated hip does not cause functional loss
  - IP transfer contraindicated (can lead to extension contracture and increased disability)
  - May walk into young adulthood
- L3–L5 levels
  - Sensate to below knee
  - *Hip dislocation most common at L3/L4
  - Flexors and adductors overpower
  - Natural history is progressive dysplasia and dislocation
  - IP transfer to greater trochanter (GT) maintains hip reduction, decreases hip flexion contracture, may adversely affect walking
  - Quad function is key to ambulation
  - 50% of L4s walk
- Hip treatment according to level
  - Nonambulators: no surgery
  - Ambulator with bilateral involvement: no surgery
  - Ambulator with unilateral involvement: questionable surgery
  - L2 or higher: no surgery
  - L5: always surgery
  - L3 bilateral: no surgery
  - L3 unilateral or L4 bilateral: controversial
  - L4 unilateral: VRO ± acetabular osteotomy, soft tissue release, capsule placation
  - Tendon transfers
    - IP transfer to GT via hole in pelvis (Sharrard procedure)—contraindicated in high lumbar, consider in mid/low lumbar
    - Adductors to ischial tuber

Knees

- Most high lumbars require orthosis for stability
- With L4–L5, usually sufficient motor to control knee
- Congenital dislocations at any level
- Serial casting to get flexion
- Once a little flexed, increase flexion with Pavlik
- Extension contracture occurs with breech (knees extended, HS displaces anterior to knee) and midlumbar (+quad, no HS)
- PT
  - Quadriceps VY lengthening (Curtis)
- Flexion contracture
  - Gastrocnemius or HS spasticity in some
  - Co-contraction of HS and quad during stance leads to persistent knee flexion
  - PT when <1.5–2 y/o
  - If >20–30 degrees, Hamstring release should considered
  - HS lengthening (if voluntary control) versus sectioning
  - Resect gastrocnemius origin
  - ± Posterior capsulotomy
  - ± Partial or complete ACL resection
  - ± Extension osteotomy
- Valgus, rotational deformities
  - Due to tight ITB
  - Section the distal iliotibial band
  - If fixed, distal femoral osteotomy

Foot

- Almost all MMC patients need treatment of feet
- Deformity, weakness, spasticity
- *Goal is often flaccid, braceable foot
- *Lack protective sensation, so monitor pressure points in brace
- Clubfoot (>50%)
  - Most common congenital foot deformity in MMC
  - Presents in all levels
  - Most are rigid, require surgery
  - Complete circumferential subtalar release (resect rather than lengthen spastic tendons)
  - Often requires talectomy
  - "Pistol grip" calcaneus deformity
    - L4/L5 because dorsi > plantar
  - Along with cavus (forefoot equinus)
  - Problems with shoes, heel sores
  - <5 y/o, transfer or release tibialis anterior
  - Transfer to heel via interosseous (IO) membrane
  - Treat if strong toe extension to counteract
  - >5 y/o, often need calcaneus osteotomy
  - Cavus from tight plantar structures, do plantar release
- Calcaneovalgus
  - In L5 level
  - Release tibia anterior and peroneal

- Peroneal transfer to heel
- Calcaneovarus
  - Posterior tibial transfer to heel
- Cavus
  - Usually in sacral levels
  - Usually with claw toes
  - Weak GS (calcaneus), intrinsics (claw toes)
  - Strong PL (plantarflex first MT), tibia anterior (pull up midfoot), toe extension (hyperextend MTP joints), toe flexors (flex IP joints)
  - Goal plantigrade braceable foot
  - AFO
  - Plantar release ± tarsal/MT osteotomies ± calcaneus osteotomy
- Valgus
  - Find cause of valgus first by x-ray studies
  - Do not do subtalar fusion if cause of valgus is short fibula
  - If fibula short, do supramalleolar osteotomy
  - Avoid subtalar and triple arthrodesis
  - In insensate foot leads to Charcot changes in other joints
  - *Do not do this in MMC children
- Fractures
  - Common, present like infection
  - Mistaken for Osteogenic sarcoma (OGS)
  - Conservative treatment—abundant callus

Myelomeningocoele—Spine

Scoliosis

- 10% congenital, 90% neuromuscular
- Presents early (2–3 y/o), often severe by age 7 yr
- Incidence varies by level
  - 100% in T, 85% >45 degrees
  - 90% in L1, 85% in L2
  - 80% in L3, 60% in L4
  - 35% in L5, 5% in sacral
- High-level paraplegia or asymptomatic paralysis ± spastic hemiplegia leads to C-shaped curve, pelvic obliquity
- Usually flexible
- Hyperlordosis from hip flexion contracture
- Imaging
  - X-ray view at 1 y/o, then annually (sitting if possible)
  - If progressive scoliosis, MRI head and C/T/L spine to rule out hydrocephalus, Arnold-Chiari, syrinx, tethered cord, dermoid cyst
- Treatment
  - Correct neurologic problems first
  - if <30 degrees and balanced, observe
  - If unbalanced or >30 degrees, progression certain
  - if <7 y/o and curve supple, brace for <50 degrees to delay surgery until maturity
  - Watch for brace pressure sores

- Surgically treat while curve small, correctable to <20-degree lumbar curve and <15-degree pelvic obliquity
  - Pseudarthrosis 75% with ASF or PSF alone but 20% with A/PSF
  - Pelvic obliquity <15 degrees rarely interferes with balance or walking
  - Fuse to sacrum in thoracic, high lumbar levels
  - Spare lumbosacral joint in low lumbar and sacral levels if spine can be aligned satisfactorily (especially if walkers)
  - Residual pelvic obliquity between 15 degrees and 35 degrees can be corrected with bilateral posterior iliac osteotomy (if sitting difficulty or ischial ulcers)
  - Treat hip flexion contractures prior to surgery for scoliosis
- Kyphosis (8%–15%)
  - Braces often unable to fit
  - Average 80 degrees at birth
  - Progresses 8 degrees/yr
  - MMC with hydrocephalus most severe kyphosis
  - Surgical treatment early (almost always progressive, delay causes increasing severity)
  - Surgical treatment complicated by young age, potential loss of spine growth
- Hydrocephalus (70%–90%)
  - Most common cause of sudden function change

SACROILIITIS

- Limp, pain with weight bearing
- Patient prefers prone with hip and knee extended
- Positive FABER test (pain with flexion, abduction, ER of hip)—also known as the Patrick test
- Radiographic studies: MRI is study of choice

TORTICOLLIS, CONGENITAL MUSCULAR

General
- Congenital deformity
- Contracture of the sternocleidomastoid muscle
  - Compartment syndrome of SCM
- Associated with "molding disorders"
  - 20% have DDH or metatarsus adductus
  - Breech presentation
- Positive family inheritance

Differential Diagnosis
- Retropharyngeal infection
- Cervical spine abnormalities
- *Ophthalmologic abnormalities
- Tumors of posterior fossa
- Sandifer syndrome (GERD)
- C1–C2 rotatory subluxation

Clinical Presentation
- Presents at a few weeks of life with mass (75% on right side)
- Mass disappears and SCM remains contracted at 4–6 mo
- Head tilt to ipsilateral side, turn to contralateral side
- Contrast to cock-robin for atlantoaxial rotatory instability

Evaluation
- Check hips for DDH
- C-spine x-ray view to rule out bony deformity

Treatment
- Up to 90% resolve with passive stretching
- Surgery if deformity persists after 12 mo
- SCM release (unipolar or bipolar) versus Z-plasty
- If deformity persists, skull and facial abnormalities can occur (plagiocephaly) (skull finishes development at age 3 yr)
- If untreated may result in progressive C–T scoliosis due to unilateral tether and cervical spondylosis
- Review of 57 patients followed up for mean of 18.9 years. If torticollis lasted beyond 1 year of age, unlikely to resolve spontaneously or to respond to nonsurgical management. Children treated within the first year of life had better outcomes than those who were not (Canale et al., 1982)

Reference
Canale ST, et al. Congenital muscular torticollis. A long-term follow-up. J Bone Joint Surg Am 1982; 64(6): 810–816.

Upper Extremity

TRIGGER THUMB

Differential Diagnosis
- Congenital extensor deficiency where thumb MP joint flexed (vs. trigger thumb, which causes locked flexion of IP joint)
- CP

Article
- (Dinham and Meggitt, 1974)
- Retrospective on 131 thumbs in newborns
- Newborns
  - Observed only
  - 30% resolve at 1 yr
- 6–30 mo
  - Observed for 6 mo
  - 12% resolve in that time
- >3 y/o
  - Surgery
  - Delayed operation left no residual flexion contracture provided surgery done before age 4 yr

Reference

Dinham JM, Meggitt BF. Trigger thumbs in children. A review of the natural history and indications for treatment in 105 patients. J Bone Joint Surg Br 1974; 56:153–155.

Hip

COXA VARA

– Decrease in femoral neck-shaft angle

Congenital

– Embryonic limb bud abnormal
– Minimal progression with growth
– Associated with proximal femoral focal deficiency (PFFD), short femur
– Multiple epiphyseal dysplasia, Spondyloepiphyseal dysplasia, cleidocranial dysplasia, metaphyseal dysplasia

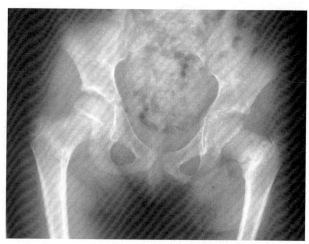

The radiographic appearance of acquired coxa vara in a 7-year-old girl who had an intertrochanteric left hip fracture. (From Morrissy RT, and Weinstein SL. Lovell and Winter's Pediatric Orthopaedics Sixth Edition Philadelphia: Lippincott Williams & Wilkins, 2006 with permission.)

Acquired

– Slipped capital femoral epiphysis, Perthes
– Rickets, fibrous dysplasia
– Traumatic physis closure

Developmental

– Normal at birth, progressive with growth
– No associated muscular-skeletal abnormalities
– 1:25,000
– Males = females
– 30%–50% bilateral

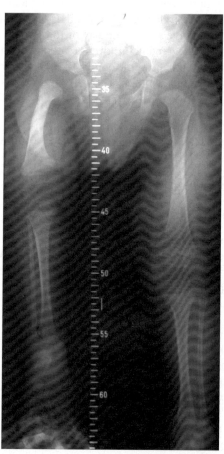

Congenital coxa vara in an 18-month-old child with a congenital short femur. (From Morrissy RT, and Weinstein SL. Lovell and Winter's Pediatric Orthopaedics Sixth Edition Philadelphia: Lippincott Williams & Wilkins, 2006 with permission.)

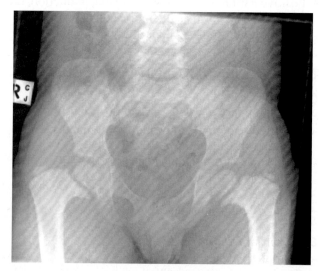

Radiographic appearance of developmental coxa vara in a 3-year-old child. (From Morrissy RT, and Weinstein SL. Lovell and Winter's Pediatric Orthopaedics Sixth Edition Philadelphia: Lippincott Williams & Wilkins, 2006 with permission.)

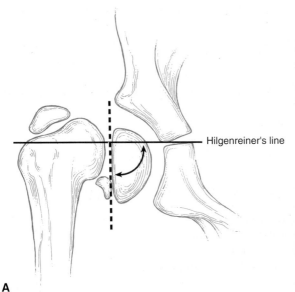
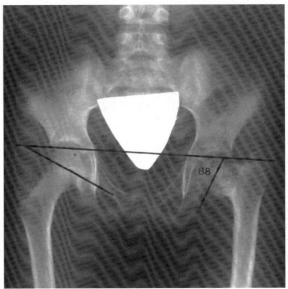

A

B

Hilgenreiner's line

Hilgenreiner-epiphyseal (H-E) angle. **A:** The H-E angle is the angle between Hilgenreiner's line and a line drawn parallel to the capital femoral physis. **B:** H-E angle of 68 degrees in a patient with developmental coxa vara. (From Morrissy RT, and Weinstein SL. Lovell and Winter's Pediatric Orthopaedics Sixth Edition Philadelphia: Lippincott Williams & Wilkins, 2006 with permission.)

– AD in some patients
– Primary ossification defect in inferior femoral neck → fatigue of local dystrophic bone and progressive coxa vara
– Infantile coxa vara may develop in patients with normal radiographs at 1 year old. (Amstutz, 1970)

Reference

Amstutz HC. Developmental (infantile) coxa vara—a distinct entity. Report of two patients with previously normal roentgenograms. Clin Orthop Relat Res 1970; 72:242–247.

Pathology
– Similar to Blount and Schmid metaphysial dysplasia

Clinical Presentation
– Presents between walking and 6 y/o
– Painless limp (unilateral) or waddling gait (bilateral)
– LLD
– Decreased abduction and internal rotation
– Along with decreased femoral anteversion
– Functionally weak abductors

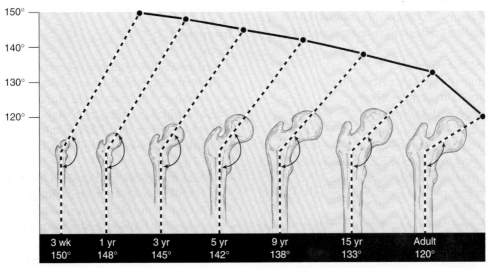

| 3 wk | 1 yr | 3 yr | 5 yr | 9 yr | 15 yr | Adult |
| 150° | 148° | 145° | 142° | 138° | 133° | 120° |

Evolution of the neck-shaft angle in the normal hip. (From Morrissy RT, and Weinstein SL. Lovell and Winter's Pediatric Orthopaedics Sixth Edition Philadelphia: Lippincott Williams & Wilkins, 2006 with permission.)

Natural History
- Depends on degree of deformity (Weinstein et al., 1984)
  - If Hilgenreiner-epiphyseal angle <45 degrees, more likely to heal femoral neck defect, not progress
  - 45–60 degrees, grey zone (watch closely)
  - >60 degrees, deformity progresses

Reference
Weinstein JN, et al. Congenital coxa vara. A retrospective congenital view. J Pediatr Orthop 1984; 4:70–77.

Radiographs
- Decreased neck-shaft angle
- More vertical proximal femoral physis
  - Hilgenreiner-epiphyseal angle (normal <25 degrees)
  - Triangular ossification defect in inferomedial femoral neck
  - Inferior physis may be widened with triangle of dystrophic bone interposed. This may appear as a radiolucent inverted "Y"
  - Coxa breva: structural shortening of the femur

Treatment
- Nonsurgical spicas and traction do not work
- Surgical goals
  - Correct varus, LLD
  - Establish mechanics of abductors
  - Make epiphyseal plate more horizontal
- Operative indications
  - Neck-shaft angle <100 degrees
  - Hilgenreiner-epiphyseal angle >60 degrees
  - HEA 45–60 grey zone, osteotomy if child limps
  - Progression of deformity
  - OR when operative criteria met, not based on age because waiting leads to dysplastic changes

Valgus Rotational Osteotomies
- Langenskiöld intertrochanteric osteotomy
- Borden subtrochanteric osteotomy
- Pauwels Y-shaped osteotomy
- Concomitant adduction tenotomy
- Overcorrect to >160 degrees
- Goal of surgery is to decrease HEA to <35–40, correct anteversion, re-tension abductors
- Make Hilgenreiner-physial angle <38 degrees (Carroll and Coleman, 1997)
  - If <38 degrees, 95% had no recurrence during growth. If >40 degrees, 93% require revision for recurrence
- Distal/lateral greater trochanter transfer may be done to restore abductor mechanics
- Results

- Metaphysis defect closes by 3–6 mo postop if osteotomy done correctly
- Premature closure of physis by 12–24 months postop seen in 50%–90% and can be a source of LLD and recurrent varus
- Proximal femur contributes 13% to LE growth

Reference
Carroll K, Coleman S. Coxa vara: surgical outcomes of valgus osteotomies. J Pediatr Orthop 1997; 17:220–224.

DEVELOPMENTAL DYSPLASIA OF THE HIP

Diagnosis
- Physical exam
  - Barlow
    - Dislocation maneuver
    - Out the back
    - Flex, adduct hips, posterior pressure on hip joints
    - Palpable dislocation
  - Ortonlani
    - Reduction maneuver
    - Bring in
    - Abduct flexed hips, anterior pressure at hip joint
    - Palpable reduction
- Galleazi sign—Apparent femoral length discrepancy with hips flexed and knees together (Graf, 1984)
- Ultrasound until 6 months
- Normal alpha angle >60 degrees
- Radiographs at or after 6 months old
- Normal acetabular index is <20 degrees at 2 years old

Reference
Graf R. Fundamentals of sonographic diagnosis of infant hip dysplasia. J Pediatr Orthop 1984; 4:735–740.

Treatment
Pavlik
- *<6 mo (>50% failure in >6 mo old)
- Prevents hip extension and adduction
- Contraindicated in muscle imbalance (CP, MMC) and joint stiffness (arthrogryposis)
- Can be used for dysplasia, subluxation, or dislocation
- Pavlik for 1–2 wk can reduce an irreducible dislocation if <6 mo old
- Give at most 3 wk for Pavlik to locate hips to prevent Pavlik disease (posterior cartilage deformity due to constant subluxation and rubbing)
- Position: 90–100 degrees of hip flexion, 35–75 degrees of hip abduction
- Repeat ultrasound within 2 weeks after Pavlik applied
- Duration of Pavlik is usually 3 months. First 6 weeks, full time

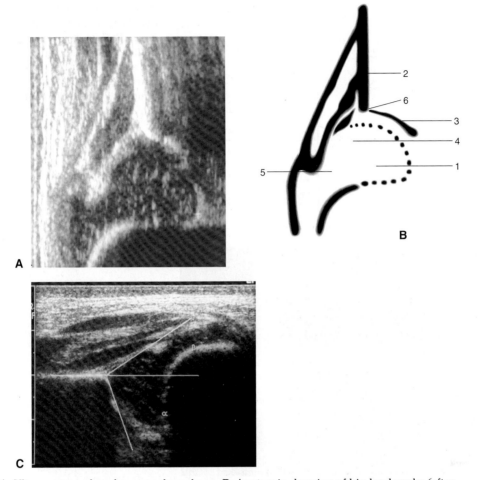

A: Ultrasonography of a normal newborn. **B:** Anatomic drawing of hip landmarks (after Graf): 1, femoral head; 2, iliac limb; 3, bony acetabular roof; 4, acetabular labrum; 5, joint capsule; 6, osseous rim. **C:** The α and β angles are identified on this ultrasonograph of a newborn. (From Morrissy RT, and Weinstein SL. Lovell and Winter's Pediatric Orthopaedics Sixth Edition Philadelphia: Lippincott Williams & Wilkins, 2006 with permission.)

- Follow patients until skeletal maturity
- Complications of Pavlik
  - Avascular necrosis (AVN)
    - Disastrous, due to too much abduction
    - Compression of medial circumflex between IP and pectineus
  - Femoral nerve palsy from hyperflexion
  - Inferior dislocation from hyperflexion
  - Brachial plexus palsy from shoulder straps

Results/Prognosis with Pavlik
- DDH at birth >90% normal at 6 wk without treatment
- <6 mo + Barlow—Pavlik 90% success
- <6 mo + Ortolani—Pavlik 80% success
- >6 mo old—Pavlik <50% success (not recommended)
- Barlow (Lerman and Kasser, 2001)
  - 137 hips treated with Pavlik

- Assessed risk factors for failure in 26 hips
- Clinical exam and initial low α angle were risk factors for failure
- 6/6 hips that were initially irreducible and coverage <20% failed
- Bilateral, male, older age was associated with no difference in failure of reduction

Reference
Lerman JA, Kasser J. Early failure of Pavlik harness treatment for developmental hip dysplasia: clinical and ultrasound and predictors. Pediatr Orthop 2001; 21:348–353.

Closed Reduction (CR)
- Indication in >6 mo or failed >3 wk of Pavlik
- By 3 mo, contracture has developed with *loss of abduction

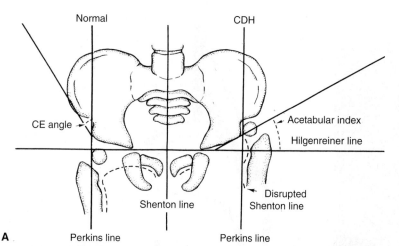

A: Radiographic parameters. CDH, congenital dysplasia of the hip; CE Angle, center-edge angle. **B:** Center-edge angle of Wiberg. C, Center of the femoral head; E, bony edge of the acetabulum; G, gravity line. (From Morrissy RT, and Weinstein SL. Lovell and Winter's Pediatric Orthopaedics Sixth Edition Philadelphia: Lippincott Williams & Wilkins, 2006 with permission.)

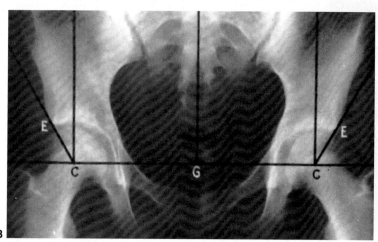

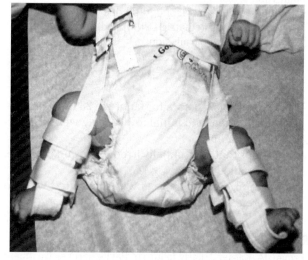

Newborn with bilateral hip dislocations in a Pavlik harness. Appropriately applied, the harness prevents hip extension and adduction which can lead to redislocation, but allows further flexion and abduction, which lead to reduction and stabilization. (From Morrissy RT, and Weinstein SL. Lovell and Winter's Pediatric Orthopaedics Sixth Edition Philadelphia: Lippincott Williams & Wilkins, 2006 with permission.)

- Examination under anesthesia (EUA), closed reduction, arthrogram to confirm reduction, spica (3 mo to 1 y/o)
- Forceful reduction leads to AVN
- Routine adductor tenotomy
- Percutaneous adduction tenotomy with closed reduction-increases safe zone of Ramsey

Arthrogram: medial dye pool must be <5 mm

- Spica with flexion in position of stability and limited abduction (wide abduction along with proximal femoral growth disturbance)
- Reduction must be anatomic with <60 degrees abduction
- CT or MRI <1 hr after arthrogram to look for posterior subluxation in spica
- Spica for 12 wk then full-time brace for 2–3 mo, then night brace until acetabular development normal
- Spica position
  - "Human position" of Salter/Dubos
  - Flexion 90–100 degrees
  - Abduction 45 degrees, no greater than 60 degrees

- Prognosis depends on
  - Timing
  - Degree of subluxation (Tonnis classification)
  - Nonossified cartilage head is more susceptible to AVN from reduction; thus, although AVN rate increases with waiting longer to perform CR, younger patients may have worse involvement of the head when AVN does occur
  - AVN diagnosis made after growth spurt

Blocks to Concentric Reduction
- Intra-articular
  - Pulvinar
  - Hypertrophied ligamentum teres
  - Transverse acetabular ligament
  - Capsular
    - Constricted anteromedial capsule
    - Inverted or hypertrophied labrum/limbus
  - Extra-articular
    - Contracted adductus longus, iliopsoas
- Treated only those infants with persistent subluxation at 2 wk of age; no difference in outcome (Sampath et al., 2003)
- Follow-up of 152 hips in 119 patients, growth disturbance of proximal femur in 60%, 17 THA by age of 35. Function tended to deteriorate over time for all patients (Malvitz and Weinstein, 1994)

References
Sampath JS, et al. Splintage in developmental dysplasia of the hip: How low can we go? J Pediatr Orthop 2003; 23:352–355.
Malvitz TA, Weinstein SL. Closed reduction for congenital dysplasia of the hip. Functional and radiographic results after an average of thirty years. J Bone Joint Surg Am 1994; 76(12): 1777–1792.

Open Reduction
- Indicated in 6 mo–2 y/o if failed safe concentric CR (persistent subluxation, soft tissue interposition/not concentric, only stable in extreme abduction)
- In <2 y/o rarely need secondary femoral/acetabular procedure
- ± Traction
- ± Femoral shortening if excess tension
- Open reduction via anterior Smith Petersen
- "Bikini" incision
- Between sartorius and TFL, then between rectus femoris and gluteus medius
- Most versatile (can plicate capsule, can do pelvic osteotomy through same incision)
- Medial approach
  - Above or below brevis
  - Capsule cannot be plicated, thus reduction depends on cast
  - IP* and transverse acetabular ligament* can be cut

- Medial femoral circumflex artery crosses field
- Can perform bilateral at same OR

Open Reduction, Femoral Shortening
- Virtually all >2 y/o need open reduction
  - In >2 y/o, routine femoral shortening has supplanted traction as adjunct to open reduction
  - Study showed 54% AVN and 32% redislocation in >3 y/o treated with skeletal traction, open reduction (Schoenecker and Strecker, 1984)
- Derotation and varus correction can be performed with shortening

Reference
Schoenecker PL, Strecker WB. Congenital dislocation of the hip in children. Comparison of the effects of femoral shortening and of skeletal traction in treatment. J Bone Joint Surg Am 1984; 66: 21–27.

LEGG-CALVÉ-PERTHES
General
- 4–8 y/o
- M:F = 4:1
- Along with attention deficit hyperactivity disorder (ADHD)
- Older parents, poor, urban
- Osteonecrosis of proximal femoral epiphysis
- Etiology
  - Ischemia (femoral head supply differs based on age)
  - Hypothyroid
  - Hypercoagulability (antitrypsin)
- 75% with coagulation abnormal (protein C, S deficiency)

Clinical Presentation
- *Painless Trendelenburg limp
- Knee, medial thigh pain
- **Decreased IR and Abduction
- Appears like LLD due to adduction contracture
- 10% bilateral, in different stages
- Small stature
- Synovitis, effusion

Radiographs
- X-ray view sufficient to diagnose and follow
- May need x-ray view of both hips/knee/wrist/spine to differentiate from other diagnoses
- *90% with delayed bone age average 21 mo
- MRI/bone scan add little to management
  - MRI may be too sensitive, picking up transient ischemic episodes

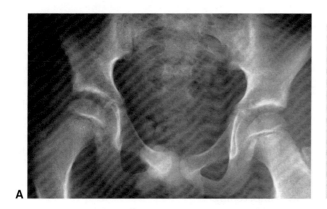
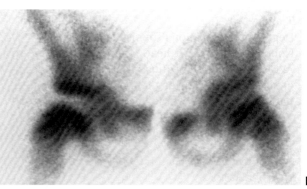

An 8-year-old boy with right hip pain. **A:** Anteroposterior radiograph demonstrates a slight increase in width and medial joint space; the femoral ossific nucleus is slightly smaller than the one on the opposite side. **B:** Technetium 99 radionuclide scan demonstrates decreased uptake in the entire right femoral head, with increased vascularity in the neck. (From Morrissy RT, and Weinstein SL. Lovell and Winter's Pediatric Orthopaedics Sixth Edition Philadelphia: Lippincott Williams & Wilkins, 2006 with permission.)

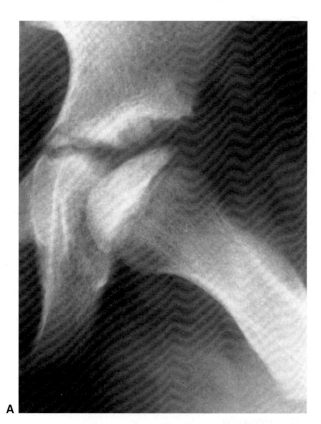
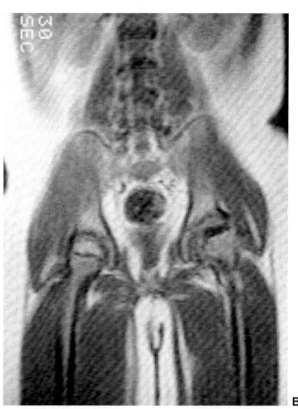

A 6-year-old boy with Catterall group 3 disease in the early fragmentation stage. **A:** Plain radiograph shows apparent sparing of the posterior head. **B:** Magnetic resonance image demonstrates a complete absence of signal on the affected side. (Courtesy of Peter Scoles, MD, Case Western Reserve Medical School, Cleveland, Ohio.)

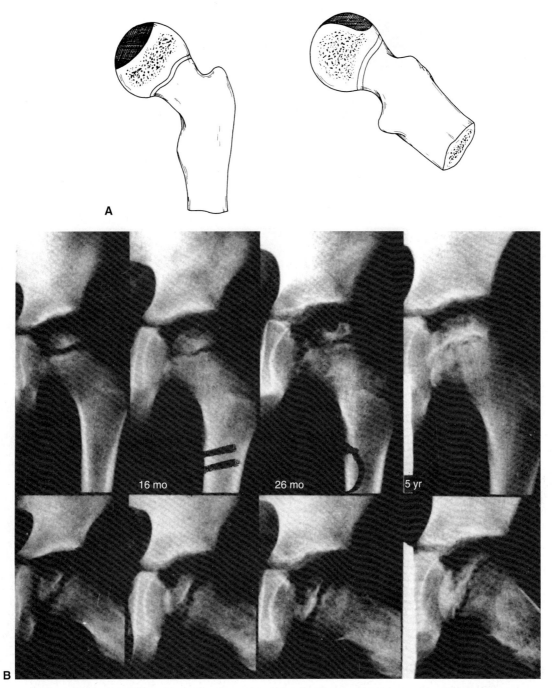

A: Catterall group 1 disease shows anterior femoral head involvement with no evidence of sequestrum, subchondral fracture line, or metaphyseal abnormalities. **B:** Catterall group 1 disease 1 week to 5 years after onset of symptoms. (From Morrissy RT, and Weinstein SL. Lovell and Winter's Pediatric Orthopaedics Sixth Edition Philadelphia: Lippincott Williams & Wilkins, 2006 with permission.)

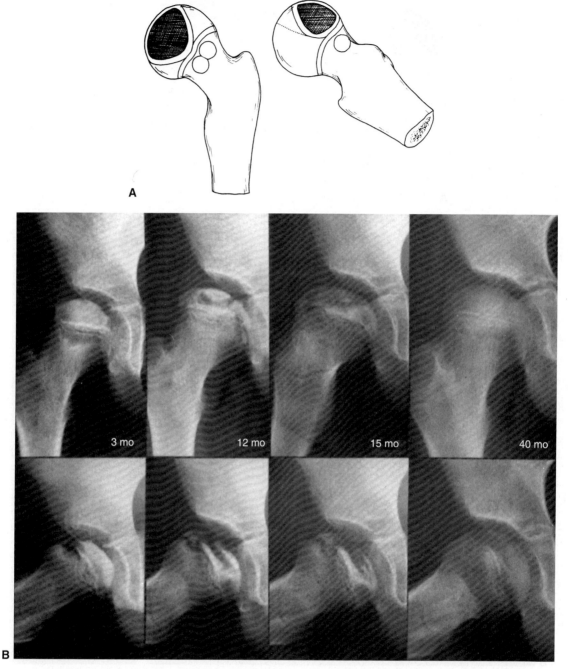

A: Catterall group 2 disease showing anterolateral involvement, sequestrum formation, and a clear junction between the involved and uninvolved areas. There are anterolateral metaphyseal lesions, and the subchondral fracture line is in the anterior half of the head. The lateral column is intact. **B:** Catterall group 2 disease. Three to 40 months after onset of symptoms, the lateral pillar is still intact. (From Morrissy RT, and Weinstein SL. Lovell and Winter's Pediatric Orthopaedics Sixth Edition Philadelphia: Lippincott Williams & Wilkins, 2006 with permission.)

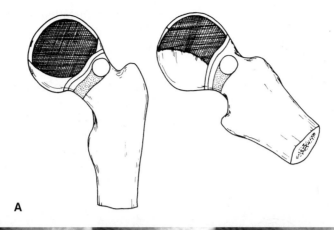

A

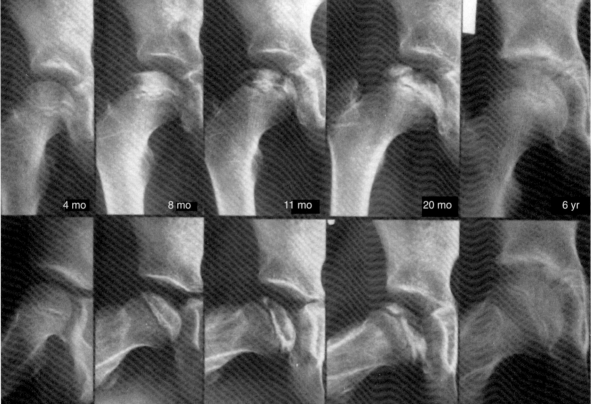

B

A: Catterall group 3 disease shows large sequestrum involving three-fourths of the femoral head. The junction between the involved and the uninvolved portions is sclerotic. Metaphyseal lesions are diffuse, particularly anterolaterally, and the subchondral fracture line extends to the posterior half of the epiphysis. The lateral column is involved. **B:** Catterall group 3 disease, 4 months to 6 years after symptom onset. Note the involvement of the lateral pillar, as well as the subchondral radiolucent zone on the radiograph taken 8 months after onset of symptoms. (From Morrissy RT, and Weinstein SL. Lovell and Winter's Pediatric Orthopaedics Sixth Edition Philadelphia: Lippincott Williams & Wilkins, 2006 with permission.)

Radiographic Differential Diagnosis
- SED, MED
- Hypothyroid
- Gaucher
- Trichorhinophalangeal syndrome
- Steroid use
- Meyer dysplasia (both hips same stage unlike LCPD)
- Septic arthritis

Catterall Head at Risk Signs
- Gage sign—"V" on lateral epiphysis
- Calcification lateral to epiphysis

- *Lateral subluxation of head
- Horizontal physis
- Metaphysial cyst

Radiographic Stages (Waldenstrom, 1917)
- Initial stage
    - Irregular physis, wider joint space
    - Radiolucencies
- Fragmentation stage
    - Bone replaced by vascular
    - Connective tissue

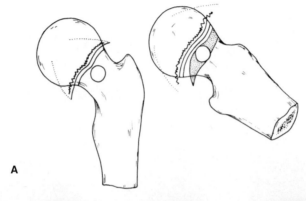

A

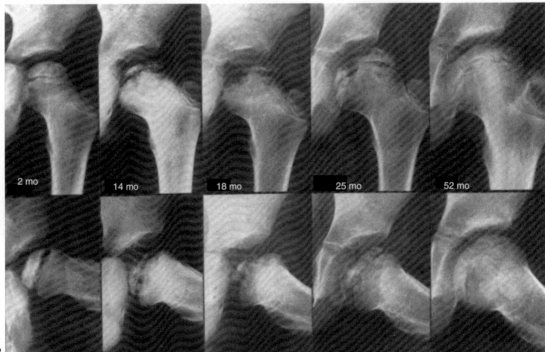

B

A: Catterall group 4 disease shows involvement of the whole head of the femur, with either diffuse or central metaphyseal lesions and with posterior remodeling of the epiphysis. **B:** Catterall group 4 disease, 2 months to 52 months after onset of symptoms. Note the stages: 14 months, fragmentation; 18 months, early reossification; 25 months, late reossification; 52 months, healed. Note also the growth-arrest line and evidence of reactivation of the growth plate along the femoral neck. (From Morrissy RT, and Weinstein SL. Lovell and Winter's Pediatric Orthopaedics Sixth Edition Philadelphia: Lippincott Williams & Wilkins, 2006 with permission.)

- Reossification stage
  - New bone formation
- Healed stage
  - Patients may have various forms of residual deformity

Classification

Catterall (Catterall, 1971)

I—25%, Only Anterior and Central
- No metaphyseal involvement. (adequate description)

II—50%, Anterolateral Involvement
- Medial and lateral pillars are intact

III—75%, Including Lateral Column
  Diffuse metaphyseal involvement

IV—100% of Head Involved
- III and IV with worse prognosis with lateral column
- Poor interobserver reliability
- Fragmentation appears at 6–8 mo

Reference
Catterall A. The natural history of Perthes' disease. J Bone Joint Surg Br 1971; 53: 37–53.

Salter-Thompson
- Extent of subchondral crescent
- A—<50% of head, lateral column okay
- B—>50% of head, lateral column involved

*Lateral Pillar (Herring et al., 1992)
- A—No involvement of lateral pillar; lateral pillar is radiographically normal; possible lucency and collapse in central and medial pillars, but full height of lateral pillar is maintained
- B—>50% of lateral pillar height is maintained; lateral pillar has some radiolucency, with maintenance of bone density at a height 50%–100% of original height of lateral head
- BC—>50% of lateral pillar height maintained, however width of lateral pillar decreased to 2–3 mm
- C—<50% of lateral pillar height is maintained; lateral pillar becomes more radiolucent, and any preserved bone is <50% of original height of lateral pillar

Reference
Herring JA, et al. The lateral pillar classification of Legg-Calvé-Perthes disease. J Pediatr Orthop 1992; 12:143–150.

Prognosis
(Gigante et al., 2002) and (McAndrew et al., 1984)

General
- *Age is key to prognosis
- Females = males (before, females felt to have poorer prognosis)
- Poor prognosis if
  - Bone age at onset >6
  - Lateral margin involvement

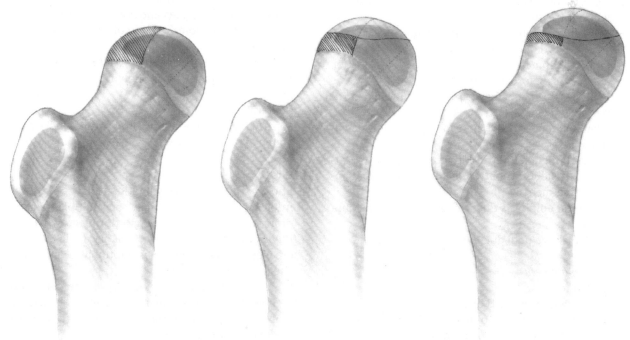

A　　　　　**B**　　　　　**C**

Lateral Pillar Classification. (From Morrissy RT, and Weinstein SL. Lovell and Winter's Pediatric Orthopaedics Sixth Edition Philadelphia: Lippincott Williams & Wilkins, 2006 with permission.)

- Herring C
- Herring B with bone age >6 yr
- Salter-Thompson B
- Catterall III and IV
- Prolonged limitation of hip ROM
- Loss of containment
- Lateral extrusion of >20% of head
- Incongruent hip at maturity
- Good prognosis if
  - Bone age <6 yr
  - Catterall I and II
  - Salter-Thompson A
  - Herring A
  - Herring B with bone age <6 yr
- 70% with partial physial arrest; leads to short and/or angulated neck
- After healing, little pain but limp persists
- Most have symptoms by age 40 yr

Residual Deformity
Stulberg (risk of OA based on x-ray view at maturity)
  - I—no deformity
  - II—coxa magna
  - III—oval head
  - IV—coxa plana (flat head)
  - V—incongruous joint

Treatment (Controversial)
- By age
  - <6 y/o bone age symptomatic only (will remodel without treatment)
  - 6–9 y/o symptomatic ± containment
  - >9 y/o—bad outcome regardless
- First principle is to maintain ROM—PT, NSAIDs for all comers, before containment
- Crutches do not change collapse (symptom control only)
- *Containment effective only in initial and fragmentation stage
- Hinge abduction from adduction contracture or lateral extrusion is a contraindication to any containment treatment
  - Lateral epiphysis does not slide under acetabulum
  - Medial dye pool due to distraction

Surgical Containment
- Indicated for
  - 8–9 y/o with Herring B or C
  - 6–8 y/o with Herring C or failed closed containment
  - Before containment surgery, hip must have
    - Free range of motion
    - Nearly round head
    - Congruent on arthrography
  - Adductor release

- Proximal femoral varus osteotomy ± derotation
- Limit varus to 20 degrees
- Resultant neck-shaft should be >110 degrees to prevent limb length discrepancy and abductor lurch
- ± Various pelvic osteotomies

Salvage for Late, Noncontainable
- Chiari osteotomy
- Shelf osteotomy
  - Valgus extension osteotomy for hinged abduction
  - Cheilectomy
- Comparison of outcomes between various methods of treatment with treatment recommendations (Herring, 1994)

References
Gigante C, et al. Prognostic value of Catterall and Herring classification in Legg-Calvé-Perthes disease: follow-up to skeletal maturity of 32 patients. J Pediatr Orthop 2002; 22:345–349.

McAndrew MP, Weinstein SL. A long term follow up of Legg-Calvé-Perthes disease. J Bone Joint Surg Am 1984; 66:860–869.

Herring JA. The treatment of Legg-Calvé-Perthes disease. A critical review of the literature. J Bone Joint Surg Am 1994; 76(3):448–458.

SLIPPED CAPITAL FEMORAL EPIPHYSIS (SCFE)

General
- Slip through *hypertrophic* zone of physis
- Neck externally rotates and comes anteriorly
- Most common adolescent hip disease
- 2:100,000
- Males > females, average 12-y/o female, 13.5-y/o male
- Commonly seen in black, Polynesian, fat, skeletally immature
- Bilateral in 20%–40%
- More likely for second side if first side diagnosed when young (11-y/o boy)

Etiology
- Etiology unknown, likely multifactorial
- Adolescent physis biologically susceptible (perichondral ring decreases in strength during growth)
- Physis becomes more vertical in adolescence: increased weight causes symptomatic mechanical shear
- If <10 y/o or >16 y/o: rule out hypothyroidism (<10% in height), hypogonadism, exogenous growth hormone, panhypopituitarism, history of radiotherapy (XRT) (Loder et al, 1995)
- In renal failure, fracture through *metaphysial spongiosa due to osseous effects of secondary hyperparathyroid (renal failure–associated SCFE is always bilateral, will not progress if PTH treated)

- 50% AVN, like acute physis fracture
- Only 50% satisfactory results

Stable
- *Weight bearing possible (with or without crutches)
- Medial metaphysis remodeling
- <3% AVN
- 96% satisfactory results

Chronic versus Acute (No Longer Used)
- Preslip—wide physis only
- Acute—symptoms <3 wk
- Chronic—symptoms >3 wk
- Acute on chronic

Reference
Loder RT, et al. Acute slipped capital femoral epiphysis: the importance of physial stability. J Bone Joint Surg Am 1993; 75(8):1134–1140.

Radiographic Findings
- AP/true or frog lateral
- Avoid frogleg in unstable
- Wide and irregular physis
- Blanch sign of Steel (double density of femoral head on femoral neck)
- Klein line along superior neck on AP does not intersect epiphysis
- Deeper acetabulum
- Decreased femoral anteversion
- Normalized Center edge Wiberg Angle

Radiographic Grading
- Percent slip on frog lateral
  - Mild, less than one-third
  - Moderate, one-third to one-half
  - Severe, more than one-half
- Southwick head-shaft angle on frogleg
  - Line perpendicular to physis versus line down shaft
  - Measure difference between affected and unaffected hips
  - <30 mild, 30–50 mod, >50 severe
  - If bilateral (cannot rely on difference), 12 degrees is average normal angle

Treatment
- Progression until physis closes is the rule
- At time of diagnosis, admit/bedrest until surgery for acute/unstable
- Surgery indicated to prevent progression, difficulty sitting, and OA
- Endocrine/systemic workup if <10 or >16
- Frequent x-ray monitoring of contralateral hip
- Prophylactic pinning of contralateral hip (controversial, consider with endocrinopathy)

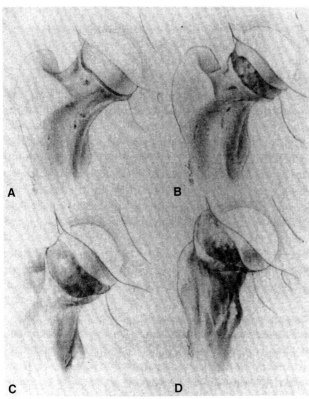

Pathoanatomy of SCFE is demonstrated. **A:** No displacement is seen. **B:** Rotation of the proximal femoral neck, with the femoral head (which is anchored in the acetabulum) posterior relative to the femoral neck. **C:** Progressive external rotation, with progressive posterior relation of the femoral head to the femoral neck. **D:** Proximal migration of the femoral neck due to the markedly posterior relation of the femoral head to the femoral neck. (From Morrissy RT. Principles of in situ fixation in chronic slipped capital femoral epiphysis. Instr Course Lect 1989;38:257–262, with permission.)

Reference
Loder RT, et al. Slipped capital femoral epiphysis associated with endocrine disorders. J Pediatr Orthop 1995; 15:349–356.

Clinical Presentation
- Hip pain
- 15% of children complain of only knee pain
- Coxalgic gait with foot externally rotated
- Classically loss of IR*, but loss of abduction and flexion also
- Increased ER with hip flexion

Classification
(Loder et al., 1993)

Unstable
- *Inability to bear weight
- Abrupt onset

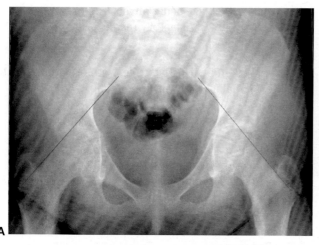
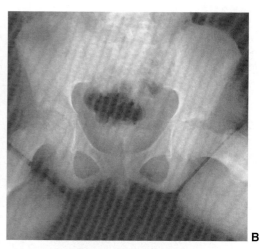

Radiographs of a 12-year-old boy with 3 months of hip pain show typical findings of a slipped capital femoral epiphysis (SCFE). **A:** Anteroposterior view demonstrates physeal widening, osteopenia, decreased epiphyseal height, increased metaphyseal-teardrop distance, and asymmetry of Klein's line. **B:** Although many of these features are seen on the anteroposterior view, the most striking feature is how much more easily the displacement is seen on the frog lateral view. The importance of obtaining lateral views when evaluating for SCFE cannot be overemphasized. (From Morrissy RT, and Weinstein SL. Lovell and Winter's Pediatric Orthopaedics Sixth Edition Philadelphia: Lippincott Williams & Wilkins, 2006 with permission.)

Surgical Intervention

- *One or two screws in situ is the recommended treatment
- Single-screw fixation in situ
  - 6.5–7.5 cannulated screw
  - Start on anterior femoral neck (FN), end in center of epiphysis
  - Safest for AVN and chondrolysis
  - Superoanterior quadrant: higher risk AVN
- Multiple pin fixation in situ
  - 30% more stiff with two screws
  - More pin penetration (iatrogenic cause of chondrolysis) and AVN
  - Some authors recommend two screws with unstable

Complications

- AVN
  - Howorth—no AVN in untreated stable SCFE
  - 50% in unstable
  - Pin penetration can occur as head with AVN collapses: remove and replace if physis still open
  - Reossification takes ~2 yr
  - Painful hips with AVN may require arthrodesis or total hip arthroplasty (THA)
- Chondrolysis (especially with spica or iatrogenic pin penetration)
- OA in 40% at 35-yr follow-up (pistol grip)

- Nonfunctional ROM/ER gait/impingement (anterior metaphysis impacts anterior acetabulum, leads to pain with sitting) (cam lesion)
  - May require realignment osteotomy before versus after physial closure
  - Subcapital cuneiform osteotomy (only if physis open, optimal correction at site of deformity, high AVN 12%–35%)
  - Intertrochanteric osteotomy (familiar, low AVN, farther from deformity)
  - Basilar neck osteotomy (splits difference)
- Decision analysis formula based on probabilities of achieving good long-term outcomes supports prophylactic pinning of the unslipped hip (Schultz et al., 2002)

References

Schultz WR, et al. Prophylactic pinning of the contralateral hip in slipped capital femoral epiphysis evaluation of long-term outcome for the contralateral hip with use of decision analysis. J Bone Joint Surg Am 2002; 84-A:1305–1314.

Thigh, Knee, Leg

BLOUNT DISEASE

General

- Most common cause of pathologic genu varum
- Disease of posterior medial tibial physis
- Associated with walking at early age

- Does not occur in nonwalker
- Hueter-Volkmann law—compression inhibits and tension stimulates bone growth (explains tibia vara and scoliosis)

Differential Diagnosis

- Physiologic varus (Salenius and Vankka, 1975)
  - 980 children, 1,500 exams
  - Maximum varus at birth—6 mo (15 degrees)
  - Neutral by age 2 y/o
  - Maximum valgus occurs at age 3–4 y/o (10 degrees)
  - Adult valgus of 7 degrees by age 6 y/o
  - Valgus needed to put feet under center of gravity for efficient gait
- Rickets, renal osteodystrophy
- OI, osteochondroma, trauma
- Bone dysplasia
  - Metaphysial chondrodysplasia
  - Achondroplasia
  - Focal fibrocartilaginous dysplasia

Reference

Salenuis P, Vankka E. The development of the tibiofemoral angle in children. J Bone Joint Surg Am 1975; 57:259–261.

Types

- Infantile tibia vara (<5 y/o)
  - Most common form
  - Bilateral 80%
  - Associated with internal tibial torsion
  - Common in African Americans, obesity, and females
  - Faster progression of varus
- Adolescent/late-onset tibia vara (>6 y/o)
  - Less severe, usually unilateral
  - Common in African Americans, obesity, and males
  - Associated with overgrowth of lateral femoral condyle
  - Subsequent distal femoral varus
  - Lateral distal femoral physis widens
  - Internal torsion not common

Physical Exam

- Acute angular deformity in Blount versus gentle curve of entire extremity in physiologic
- Associated with lateral thrust due to LCL laxity
- Oblique popliteal crease if distal femoral varus prominent

Radiographic Findings

- X-ray view if severe, <3 y/o, or unilateral to rule out Blount
- Metaphysial beaking
- Drennan metaphysis-diaphysis angle >11 degrees (Levine and Drennan, 1982)

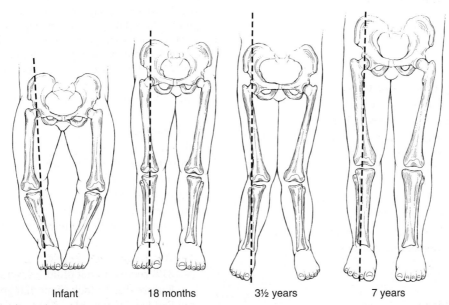

Infant   18 months   3½ years   7 years

Lower-limb alignment follows a predictable pattern. Infants typically have a gentle varus bow throughout the femur and tibia. By 18 to 24 months, the lower leg is nearly straight with a neutral mechanical axis. Valgus gradually develops and is most apparent between 3 and 4 years of age. By 7 years of age, the lower limb is in slight valgus and changes very little thereafter. Varus should not recur nor should valgus increase. (From Morrissy RT, and Weinstein SL. Lovell and Winter's Pediatric Orthopaedics Sixth Edition Philadelphia: Lippincott Williams & Wilkins, 2006 with permission.)

- Line perpendicular to shaft versus line connecting two beaks
- Predicts tibia vara in infants
- More reliable with older children
- With >11 degrees, false-positive rate 3%
- Epiphyseal-metaphyseal angle
  - Angle formed by the line through physis and line from midpoint of physis to tip of medial beak of the tibia

Reference

Levine AM, Drennan JC. Physiological bowing and tibia vara. The metaphyseal-diaphyseal angle in the measurement of bowleg deformities. J Bone Joint Surg Am 1982; 64(8):1158–1163.

Staging (Langenskiöld with Finnish, Infantile)

- I—Medial and distal beaking
  - Irregularity of entire metaphysis
  - <3 y/o
- II—Sharp depression of medial metaphysis
  - 2.5–4 y/o
- III—Deepening beak, steplike metaphysis
  - 4–6 y/o
- IV–Enlarged epiphysis that occupies medial metaphysial depression
  - 5–10 y/o
- V—Epiphyseal cleft looks like double epiphysis
  - Medial joint surface deformed
  - 9–11 y/o
- VI—Closure of medial physis
  - 10–13 y/o

Treatment of Infantile Tibia Vara

- Initiation of treatment (controversial)
  - Drennan angle >11 degrees as basis
  - Angles 9–16 degrees are generally treated if no tendency toward correction by 2 y/o
  - Based on age and stage
    - <18 mo, I–II: none
    - 18–24 mo, I–II: A-frame, night brace
    - 2–3 y/o, I–II: locked KAFO
    - 3–8 y/o, III–V: valgus rotational osteotomy
    - 3–8 y/o, VI: resect bony bridge

Bracing
- (H)KAFO, 23 hr/day
  - Fixed knee, ankle free, weight bearing
  - Worn ~1 yr until deformity corrected and medial physial growth reconstituted
  - Not viable option in >3 y/o
  - Must have open physis, compliant
  - 50%–80% success

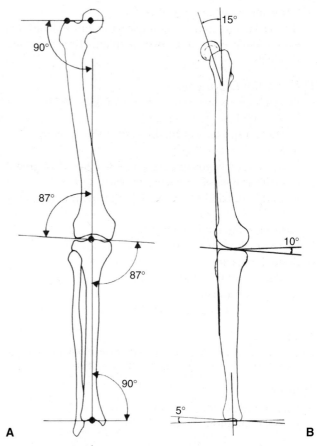

A: Frontal plane mechanical axis of the lower extremity consists of two components: colinear centers of the femoral head, knee joint, and ankle joint; and an almost perpendicular relation of the hip, knee, and ankle joints' orientation lines to the mechanical axis. **B:** Normal sagittal plane mechanical axis and joint orientation lines. (From Morrissy RT, and Weinstein SL. Lovell and Winter's Pediatric Orthopaedics Sixth Edition Philadelphia: Lippincott Williams & Wilkins, 2006 with permission.)

Surgical Intervention
- Indications
  - progressive despite brace
  - older than 3 y/o
  - large deformity
  - before age 5 y/o to prevent total physial arrest/permanent plate damage (Ferriter and Shapiro, 1987)
    - 76% recurrence if child >4.5 yr
    - 31% recurrence if child <4.5yrs
    - Failure due to lack of medial growth
    - Failure predictable >5 y/o, stages V and VI
    - Must address deformity *and* bar
- Proximal tibia-fibula osteotomy
  - Cut distal to tubercle
  - Correct rotation at same time
  - Normal LDFA and MPTA is 87 degrees
  - Limited internal fixation

- Bridge resection if <50%, >2 yr growth remaining; epiphysiodesis if not

Reference
Ferriter and Shapiro Infantile tibia vara: factors affecting outcome following proximal tibial osteotomy. J Pediatr Orthop 1987; 7:1–7.

Late-Onset Treatment
- Bracing not indicated
- Treat varus >10 degrees to prevent medial OA
- Consider hemiepiphysiodesis versus osteotomy
- Lateral staple hemiepiphysiodesis (Henderson et al., 1992)
  - Physis open, >18 mo growth left
  - Deformity not severe
  - Contraindicated if dynamic lateral thrust because of slow correction
  - Can staple lateral femur and lateral tibia
  - Curette and rotate bone-block
  - Average correction 14 degrees (7 degrees/yr)
  - Staple medial later if fully corrected
- Proximal tibial osteotomy
  - Transphysial or distal to physis
  - Indicated with closed physis or near maturity or severe deformity
  - Can correct torsion
  - Unilateral or circular external fixation versus internal fixation
  - Millis: oblique lateral–based closing wedge osteotomy that ends just near physis without need for translation, internally fixed
    - Goal is normal mechanical axis, level knee joint
    - Complications due to obesity
    - Hard exposure, hardware failure
    - Distal femur osteotomy if >5 degrees varus there

References
Henderson RC, et al. Adolescent tibia vara: alternatives for operative treatment. J Bone Joint Surg Am 1992; 74:342–350.

DISCOID MENISCUS
General
- 3%–5% in whites
- 15%–20% in Asians
- High incidence bilaterality
- Most involve lateral meniscus
- Meniscus is abnormal with mucoid degeneration

Clinical Presentation
- Classic symptoms pain/clicking/locking with loss of extension
- Unstable Watanabe type III causes snapping knee syndrome in younger children

- Older children present with tear of discoid menisci
  - Tears uncommon <10 y/o unless discoid
  - Most are longitudinal tears
  - Adolescent tears along with ligament tears (Stanitski et al., 1993)
    - Scoped kids with hemarthrosis
    - In 7–12 y/o, meniscal injury in 47%; 70% medial, 30% lateral
    - In 13–18 y/o, meniscal injury in 45%; 88% medial, 12% lateral
    - In 13–18 y/o, 36% of meniscal injuries were along with ACL tears

Reference
Stanitski CL, et al. Observations on acute knee hemarthrosis in children and adolescents. J Pediatr Orthop 1993; 13:506–510.

Radiographic Findings
- X-ray views
  - Widened lateral joint space
  - Squaring lateral femoral condyle
  - Cupping lateral tibial plateau
  - Lateral tibial spine hypoplasia
- MRI—>two bowties in 5-mm cuts
  - Can evaluate quality of meniscus tissue
  - Diagnose associated tears

Differential Diagnosis
- Osteochondrosis dissecans
- Patellofemoral pathology
- Intra-articular hemangioma (recurrent hemarthrosis in kids)

Watanabe Classification (1967)
- I – Complete
- II – Incomplete
- III - Wrisberg-ligament type
  - Posterior horn lacks capsular attachment
  - May present as unstable meniscus
  - Wrisberg ligament may cause meniscus to fall into the intracondylar notch during flexion and fall out of the notch during extension

Treatment
- Observation if no symptoms
- Stable meniscus
  - Partial meniscectomy to more normal shape
  - Saucerize central portion and leave 6–8 mm rim
  - Leaving less rim reduces rate of recurrent tear
- Unstable meniscus
  - Total excision (not recommended)
  - Saucerize/reattach
  - Allograft

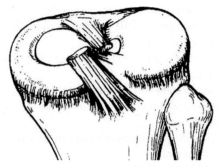

Type I. Intact meniscotibial ligaments. Entire tibial plateau covered. (From Morrissy RT, and Weinstein SL. Lovell and Winter's Pediatric Orthopaedics Sixth Edition Philadelphia: Lippincott Williams & Wilkins, 2006 with permission.)

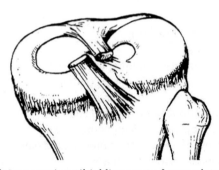

Type II. Intact meniscotibial ligaments. Incomplete tibial plateau covered. (From Morrissy RT, and Weinstein SL. Lovell and Winter's Pediatric Orthopaedics Sixth Edition Philadelphia: Lippincott Williams & Wilkins, 2006 with permission.)

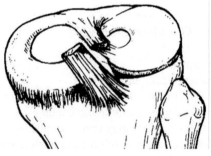

Type III. discoid meniscus with deficient peripheral attachments. (From Morrissy RT, and Weinstein SL. Lovell and Winter's Pediatric Orthopaedics Sixth Edition Philadelphia: Lippincott Williams & Wilkins, 2006 with permission.)

FEMORAL ANTEVERSION

General
- Usually 3–6 y/o
- Most common cause of in-toeing for >4 y/o
- Usually bilateral and symmetric
- Females > males
- Version is angle between transcervical and distal transcondylar axes
- Version 30 degrees (10–50) at birth due to flexed intrauterine position
- Version usually changes to normal 20 degrees (10–35) by age 10 y/o (Staheli et al., 1985)

Reference
Staheli LT, et al. Lower extremity rotational problems in children. Normal values to guide management. J Bone Joint Surg Am 1985; 67(1):39–47.

Physical Exam
- Prone hip ROM with IR >70° or ER <20°
- In-toeing gait
- Internal foot progression angle
- Patella internally rotated
- If along with external tibial torsion, may have patellofemoral problems

Treatment
- Splints/orthotics do not work
- Will get better on its own
- No functional significance of excess version.
- Surgery is only cosmetic

Derotational Osteotomy
Crider and Leber
- Distance between two marks on femur equals radius times desired rotational correction times a constant (0.017)
- Detach linea aspera to prevent tethering and translation instead of pure rotation
- Heavy 5/32-in. parallel pins into anterior femur proximal and distal to osteotomy used to determine amount of correction
- Insert seating chisel
- Transverse osteotomy at lesser trochanter
- Goal to get $ER = 2 \times IR$

FIBULAR HEMIMELIA

General
- Most common congenital deficiency of long bones
- Spectrum from hypoplasia to absence
- Ipsilateral tibia may be hypoplastic or normal
- Associated with
  - Proximal focal femoral deficiency
  - Coxa vara
  - *ACL deficiency, absent tibial spine
  - Knee valgus (short femur, lateral femoral condyle dysplasia)
  - Tibial anteromedial bowing
  - Lateral foot deficiencies
  - Equinovalgus foot
  - Ankle instability, *ball-in-socket ankle
  - Talocalcaneal coalition (Grogan et al., 1994)

- 54% talocalcaneal coalition on amputation path
- Only 15% talocalcaneal coalition on x-ray
- More common with both fib hemimelia and PFFD

CLASSIFICATION

- Achterman and Kalamchi
  - 1A, hypoplasia
  - 1B, proximal deficiency
  - 2, complete absence

References

Achterman C, Kalamchi A. Congenital Deficiency of the Fibula. JBJS Br 1969; 61-B (2):133–137.

Grogan DP, et al. Talocalcaneal coalition in patients who have fibular hemimelia or proximal femoral focal deficiency. A comparison of the radiographic and pathological findings. J Bone Joint Surg Am 1994; 76:1363–1370.

Treatment

- Decisions based on degree of foot deformity and limb shortening
- Shoe lift, bracing
- Syme or Boyd amputation at ~10 mo for
  - Complete absence *or*
  - Severe shortening *or*
  - Stiff, nonfunctional foot *or*
  - Expected LLD >16 cm and <3 rays
- Tibial lengthening
  - Partial absence

- Stable hip, knee, ankle
- Plantigrade foot
- Tibial growth inhibition <25%–30%
- Tendency for knee/ankle valgus and tibial bowing to recur
- Unstable ankles may require ankle arthrodesis
- Tibial lengthening is associated with multiple surgical interventions which may require prolonged/frequent hospitalizations

GENU VALGUM

General

- Appears at age 2 y/o
- Parents notice flat foot
- Maximum valgus of 8–10 degrees at 3–4 y/o
- Adult valgus of 5–7 degrees at 6–7 y/o

Differential Diagnosis

- Physiologic (typically symmetric)
- Idiopathic
- Metabolic—rickets
  - Similar timing as physiologic
  - More likely to progress
- Trauma
- Lateral femoral physial injury
  - Overgrowth medial proximal tibia
  - Proximal tibial Cozen fracture
- Dysplasias
- Chondroectodermal Ellis-van Creveld

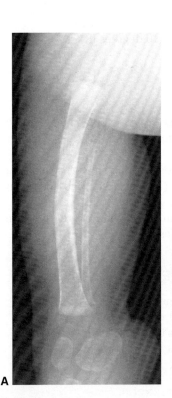 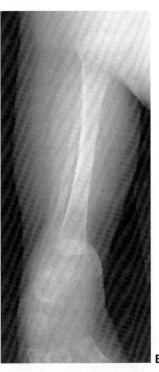

A, B: Type IB fibular deficiency (Achterman and Kalamchi), in which the proximal fibula is missing. This type is often associated with proximal focal deficiency, as in this child. (From Morrissy RT, and Weinstein SL. Lovell and Winter's Pediatric Orthopaedics Sixth Edition Philadelphia: Lippincott Williams & Wilkins, 2006 with permission.)

A   B

- Mucopolysaccharidosis
- SED tarda

Radiographs
- AP standing long-cassette x-ray BLE with patellae facing forward, without regard to foot position
- Indicated with excess femur-tibia angles when
  - Outside physiologic valgus age range
  - Asymmetric
  - <10% height
- Determining the mechanical axis of the tibia:
  - The proximal tibia is longitudinally divided into four parts
  - A positive value is applied to an axis that lies are lateral to the midline (Valgus)
  - Negative values are applied to an axis that lies medial to the midline (Varus)
  - Zone 1 is centered over the tibial spines
  - Zone 2 is within the tibial condyle
  - Zone 3 is beyond the cortex
  - *A normal mechanical axis falls within zone 1

Treatment
- Do not brace physiologic
- Valgus-correcting KAFO for <4 y/o with metabolic disorder
- Surgery deferred until 10–11 y/o

Hemiepiphysiodesis
- Stapling leads to rapid correction in young, uncertain growth resumption after staple removal
- Preferable for patients with 1–2 yr growth remaining
- Staple site of deformity, distal femoral most common
- Extraperiosteal insertion, prongs parallel to physis
- Cobalt/chromium staples with reinforced corners or hinged guided growth plate
- Does not work until about 6 mo after insertion because growth needed to produce pressure across physis
- After correction
  - Complete epiphysiodesis if near maturity
  - Remove if significant growth remains
  - Question rebound growth after removal
  - Unpredictable growth after removal if >24 mo or subperiosteal placement
  - Must follow patient until skeleton mature

Osteotomy
- Blade plate laterally or medially
- External fixation with immediate versus gradual correction

IN-TOEING

Differential Diagnosis
- Femoral anteversion
- Internal tibial torsion
- Metatarsus adductus

Physical Exam
- Foot progression angle
  - Nonspecific rotational abnormality
- Prone hip IR versus ER
  - Excess internal rotation with femoral anteversion
  - IR >70 degrees, ER <20 degrees
- Thigh foot angle
  - Normal 0–20°
  - >10 degrees IR with internal tibial torsion
- Transmalleolar angle
  - Abnormal with internal tibial torsion
- Heel bisector line
  - Normal between second and third toes
  - Lateral with metatarsus adductus
- Foot lateral border
  - Convex with metatarsus adductus

INTERNAL TIBIAL TORSION

General
- Usually presents at 1–2 y/o
- Most common cause of in-toeing for <4 y/o
- Associated with prone infant sleeping posture
- Natural history is of no arthritis, no correlation with tripping/clumsiness/functional disability
- Athletic ability does not correlate with position during walking although sprinters toe-in during running regardless of their walking style

Physical Exam
- In-toeing gait
- Internally rotated foot progression angle
- Thigh foot angle (TFA) >10 degrees IR

Treatment
- Sleep supine
- Bracing does not work
- Usually improved by age 3 y/o, resolved by age 10 y/o
- Surgery very rare but indicated for TFA >10 degrees IR
- Distal supramalleolar osteotomy slower healing but lower neurovascular (NV), physial, compartment complications
  - **All tibial osteotomies in children require concomitant fasciotomies

LEG LENGTH DISCREPANCY (LLD)

- White/Menelaus arithmetic method
  - Distal femur grows 1 cm/yr
  - Proximal tibia grows 0.6 cm/yr
  - Girls stop growing at 14
  - Boys stop growing at 16
  - Use calendar age

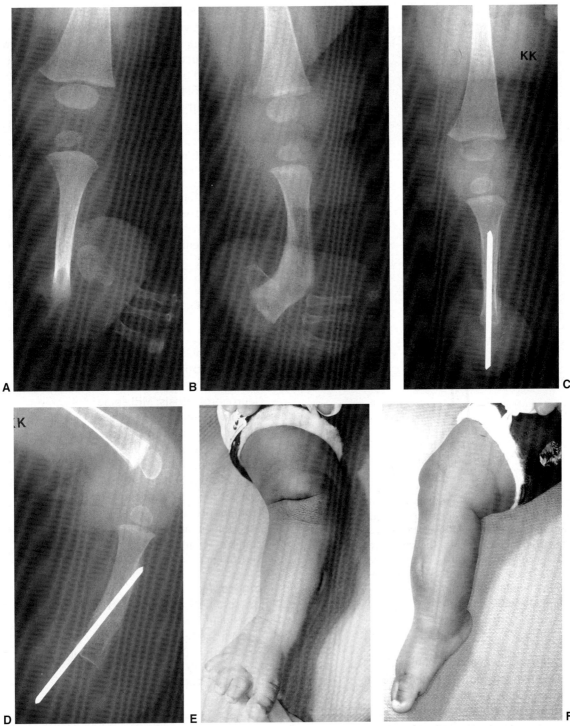

A, B: Anteroposterior and lateral radiographs of a type II fibular deficiency (Achterman and Kalamchi), in which the entire fibula is missing. Note the missing lateral rays of the foot and the severe angulation of the tibia. **C, D:** The limb, 6 weeks after Syme amputation and an anterior closing-wedge osteotomy of the tibia. Placing the pin through the anterior cortex of the proximal fragment provides rigid fixation, which is not obtained if the pin is simply passed up the medullary canal. The pin was removed in the office at the time of cast removal. **E, F:** The clinical appearance of the same deficiency at the time of surgery in another patient. Note the short tibial segment, the valgus knee and foot, and the dimple over the tibia. (From Morrissy RT, and Weinstein SL. Lovell and Winter's Pediatric Orthopaedics Sixth Edition Philadelphia: Lippincott Williams & Wilkins, 2006 with permission.)

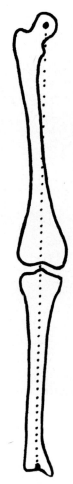

The mechanical axis is assessed on a standing, anteroposterior, long cassette radiograph that includes the hips and ankles. A line is constructed from the center of the femoral head to the center of the ankle. For consistent serial measurements, the knees are positioned with the patellae facing forward. (From Morrissy RT, and Weinstein SL. Lovell and Winter's Pediatric Orthopaedics Sixth Edition Philadelphia: Lippincott Williams & Wilkins, 2006 with permission.)

- Green/Anderson growth remaining
    - Limb length related to chronologic age to determine growth percentile
    - Another graph to show remaining growth of physes
    - Uses only most recent bone age
    - Moseley Straight Line (Moseley, 1977)
        - Distills Green/Anderson data into single graph
        - Draw vertical down from long leg line, then plot short leg on same vertical line
        - This leads to two differing sloped lines
        - Plot where this vertical line intersects current bone age
        - Over several times, draw best fit horizontal line to determine percentile of patient
        - When this horizontal line hits the age of maturity, draw it vertical to find expected LLD
    - Reference slopes for each of three epiphysiodesis procedures used to determine effects on growth by changing slope
    - Effect of lengthening will be a shift of the growth line without change in slope

Reference
Moseley CF. A straight-line graph for leg-length discrepancies. J Bone Joint Surg Am 1977; 59:174–179.

- Multiplier method
    - Formulae use multipliers to predict final limb length based on chronological age
    - For congenital or developmental LLD (Paley et al., 2000)

Reference
Paley D, et al. J Bone Joint Surg Am 2000; 82-A(10):1432–1436.

Etiology
- Limb hypoplasia syndromes
- Hemihypertrophy
    - Idiopathic—most
- Neurofibromatosis: MRI spine
    - Most common known cause
- *Wilms tumor: get renal ultrasound
- Klippel-Trenaunay-Weber
- Proteus syndrome
- Beckwith-Weidemann: get abdominal ultrasound, glucose, chromium analysis, AFP
- Trauma (premature arrest or overgrowth)
- Infection, inflammation
- Tumors—Ollier, MHE, fibular dysplasia
- Neurologic—MMC, CP

Radiographs
- Measure heel to ASIS (anterior superior iliac spine) to account for foot height
- Skeletal age by hand x-ray
- X-ray both hands in hemihypertrophy
- Accurate only to 12 mo
- Inaccurate before 6 y/o
- Scanogram
    - Center hip to medial femoral condyle (MFC) to tibial plafond
    - No magnification with scanogram
    - Terry—direct measure with tape better than drawing lines across
    - CT scanogram gives only 20% radiation of standard scanogram

Treatment
- 0–2 cm: shoe lift (1 cm inside shoe)
- 2–6 cm: shorten contralateral or lengthen

- >6 cm: lengthen ± contralateral shorten
- >20 cm: amputation, prosthesis
- Leave side with stiff or weak hip/knee shorter to allow clearance at swing
- If pelvis oblique, make functional length equal
- Do not shorten contralaterally if shorter leg has angular deformity
- Knee height disparity <4 cm is okay
- LLD not proven to cause lower back pain (LBP), OA
- Epiphysiodesis
    - Procedure of choice in growing child with normal axial alignment, sufficient data points, and predicted LLD 2–5 cm
    - Staples
        - Three medial, three lateral
        - Most common complication is extrusion
    - Blount or Phemister techniques
    - Canale percutaneous
        - No postoperative immobilization required
    - Femoral versus tibial shortening
        - Shorten no more than 5 cm in femur
        - Shorten no more than 3 cm in tibia
        - Tibia shortening rare because higher nerve complications, nonunion
            - Need for fasciotomy
            - Harder to internally fix
            - Leg muscles slower to adjust
        - Femoral shortening
            - If patient presents at maturity
            - Open/closed middiaphysis cut, nail
            - If shorten >10% weakness due to muscle tensioning
            - Proximal subtrochanteric cut/blade plate
- Leg lengthening
    - Higher complications than epiphysiodesis and shortening
    - Goal should be <10 cm femur, <7 cm tibia
    - Higher complications if <8 y/o or >14 y/o
    - Lengthening causes growth retardation
    - Percutaneous corticotomy, multiplanar (circular) or uniplanar (cantilever) external fixation
    - Uniplanar external fixation with lengthening in femur causes knee medialization
    - Can lengthen over nail with external fixation only during distraction period
    - Potential intramedullary sepsis
    - Distract 1 mm/day in increments of 0.25 mm
- Limb lengthening for LLD (Karger et al., 1993)
    - 83 limbs with lengthening of femur/Wagner, tibia/Wagner, tibia/Ilizarov
    - Overall 77% complication rate
    - No difference between tibia Wagner and tibia Ilizarov
    - 13% fracture, 47% angulation, 9% palsy
    - 20% pin, 13% deep infection

- Higher complication rate with femorals
    - 35% fracture, 49% angulation, 2% palsy
    - 27% pin, 12% deep infection
    - Higher poor results in femur (18%)
    - Higher complications if lengthen >25%
    - LLD and gait (Song et al., 1997)
- Gait, force plate of 35 children with LLD
- LLD <3% led to no compensations
- LLD <5.5% used compensations such as vault, circumduction, flexed knee to equalize work of two legs
- if LLD >5.5%, patients had to use toe-walking, longer leg had to do more work, and center of weight had more vertical displacement during gait

References
Karger C, et al. Lengthening of congenital lower limb deficiencies. Clin Orthop Relat Res 1993; (291):236–245.
Song KM, et al. The effect of limb-length discrepancy on gait. J Bone Joint Surg Am 1997; 79:1690–1698.

LIMPING CHILD
(Flynn et al., 2001; Kocher et al., 1999)
- Evaluation
    - CBC
    - ESR
    - CRP
    - RF
    - Lyme
    - Radiographs
    - Ultrasound/CT to rule out appendicitis if *right* hip pain
- Toddler (1–3 y/o)
    - Septic arthritis
    - Transient synovitis (3–8 y/o)
    - Toddler's fracture
    - Arthritis (JRA, Lyme)
    - Neoplasm (osteoid osteoma, leukemia)
    - Neuromuscular—CP, muscular dystrophy
    - Developmental—DDH, coxa vara
    - *Discitis
- Child (4–10 y/o)
    - Transient synovitis
    - Leg length discrepancy
    - LCPD
    - Discoid meniscus
- Adolescent (11–14 y/o)
    - SCFE
    - Tarsal coalition
    - Overuse syndromes
    - OCD
    - DDH
    - Sacroiliitis

References

Flynn JM, Widmann RF. The limping child: evaluation and diagnosis. J Am Acad Orthop Surg 2001; 9(2):89–98.

Kocher MS, et al. Differentiating between septic arthritis and transient synovitis of the hip in children: an evidence-based clinical prediction algorithm. J Bone Joint Surg Am 1999; 81(12):1662–1670

Proximal Femoral Focal Deficiency

General
- Short femur, defect between neck and shaft (PFFD defect in subtrochanteric region versus neck defect in coxa vara)
- Complete discontinuity or bridged by cartilage connection
- 15% bilateral
- Etiology unknown, possibly teratogenic (thalidomide)
- Associated anomalies
  - Most commonly associated with (75%) fibula hemimelia
  - ACL deficiency
  - Equinovalgus foot, lateral ray deficiency
  - Tarsal coalition

Clinical Presentation
- Short, bulky thigh
- Proximal limb flexed, abducted, externally rotated
- Knee near groin
- Foot at or above contralateral knee
- Hip/knee flexion contractures
- Knee has sagittal instability
- Trendelenburg gait secondary to dysplastic muscles
- LLD can be significant

Aitken Classification
- A—head present, normal acetabulum
  - *Cartilage connection between head/shaft
  - Ossifies eventually
  - Femur short with varus deformity
- B—hypoplastic femoral head present
  - Moderately dysplastic acetabulum
  - *No connection between head and shaft
- C—*Ossicle head
  - Severely dysplastic acetabulum
  - Proximal femur will not appear
  - Distal femur migrates proximally
- D—*Absent head, absent acetabulum
  - Very little femur at all
  - Distal metaphysis and epiphysis only

Treatment
- Limb lengthening if
  - Hip stable
  - No knee flexion contractures
  - Expected LLD much less than 20 cm
  - Foot plantigrade

- Proximal femoral valgus osteotomy
  - Correct coxa vara in type A
  - Achieve union in type B
  - With knee fusion + Syme/Boyd/Van Nes
- Knee fusion with Syme/Boyd amputation
  - Functional above knee amputation (AKA) Surgery usually at 2–3 y/o
  - Boyd (tibiocalcaneal fusion) saves heel pad but not much of an issue for children
  - Boyd gets extra length, but in PFFD stump usually too long (need stump to be 6 cm shorter than contralateral knee for AKA prosthesis with knee joint)
- Van Nes rotationplasty
  - Functional below knee amputation (BKA)
  - Less O_2 consumption
  - Wait until >7 y/o because derotates
  - Contraindicated with foot deformities, fibular deficiency
- Pelvic femoral fusion
  - Types C and D to gain hip stability
  - Knee functions as hip joint
- In bilateral PFFD
  - Preserve feet, avoid knee fusions
  - Usually nonoperative treatment

Tibial Bowing

Anterolateral: Congenital Pseudarthrosis
General
- Anterolateral bowing of tibia
- 1:190,000
- Usually unilateral
- Associated with NF in >50%
- Associated with tibial pseudarthrosis

Natural History
- Discovered at 1–2 y/o
- propensity for progression to pathologic fracture/nonunion by 3 y/o
- Delayed pseudarthrosis presenting at 3–5 y/o has better prognosis
- Anterolateral bowing along with duplication of hallux takes benign course like posteromedial bowing with LLD being only lasting sequelae

Treatment
- Clamshell brace to prevent fracture
- Electrical stimulation
  - 55%–85% union but still deformity
- IM rod with iliac crest bone graft (ICBG)
  - 80% union but still short
- Vascularized fibula autograft
  - From contralateral LE
  - 90%–95% union
  - Adds bone stock and length
  - Donor site morbidity (ankle valgus)

- Circular external fixation to compress nonunion
  - 90%–100% union
  - Can also lengthen through a proximal corticotomy
  - Refracture is a problem
- Amputation
  - Poorly defined indications (after three failed operations)
  - Boyd or Syme distal to pseudarthrosis
  - Amputation at pseudo site leads to bony spike

Posteromedial
General
- Congenital apex posteromedial bowing of middistal tib/fib
- Etiology most likely mechanical
- Associated with calcaneovalgus foot and LLD
- Not associated with pathologic fracture or pseudarthrosis

Natural History
- Dramatic improvement in 1 yr
- Bowing usually spontaneously resolves (especially posterior); medial bow may lead to persistent valgus
- Progressive LLD (growth inhibition even after bowing resolves)

Treatment
- Infant-passive stretching
- Serial casts for more severe
- AFO for inability to get plantigrade
- Corrective osteotomy rarely necessary, deferred until 2 y/o since natural history is resolution
- Contralateral epiphysiodesis for projected LLD up to 4–5 cm
- Ipsilateral leg lengthening for projected LLD >4 cm
- Bilevel osteotomy to lengthen proximally and correct deformity distally is ideal

Anteromedial
- Associated with fibular hemimelia (absent or deficient fibula)
- Good prognosis

Tibial Hemimelia
General
- May be part of inherited syndrome (AD)
- 1 in 1,000,000
- 30% bilateral
- Two-thirds with associated anomalies, mostly musculoskeletal (lobster claw hand)

Clinical Presentation
- Shortened or absent tibia
- Marked rigid equinovarus
- Knee instability

- Quad aplasia or weakness
  - Knee flexion contracture
- Preaxial (big toe) polydactyly
- Absent preaxial rays also seen

Classification (Kalamchi and Dawe)
- I—complete tibial absence
  - Jones Ia—no proximal tibia, no extensor
  - Jones Ib—unossified proximal tibial remnant, extensor mechanism intact
- II—absent distal tib, normal proximal articulation
- III—short tib, distal tibia-fibula diastasis

Treatment
- Active knee extension is key and implies active quad with insertion on tibia remnant
- Wider distal femoral condyles and better distal femoral epiphysis ossification are clues that proximal tibia is present but not yet ossified
- Type I—knee disarticulation
  - Consider Brown procedure (fibular centralization) if active extension, but most recommend against it
  - If type I concomitant with PFFD and short limb, fuse fibula to distal femur to increase lever arm for femoral segment
- Type II-A synostosis can be formed from the tibial remnant and fibula to improve length
  - Peform syme amputation following synostosis to allow for fitting with BKA prosthesis
  - Resect residual proximal fibula
- Type III
  - Foot is deformed, looks like clubfoot
  - Short tibia with varus foot can be reconstructed
- True ankle diastasis requires amputation

Foot/Ankle

ACCESSORY NAVICULAR

General
- Most common accessory bone of foot
- Congenital enlargement of medial navicular
- In 5%–15% of population
- Most are asymptomatic
- Frequently bilateral
- Associated with flexible flatfoot*

Clinical Manifestations
- Symptoms onset 8–14 y/o
- Can cause arch pain with overuse
- Tender over posterior tibial tendon (PTT) insertion at talonavicular (TN) joint
- Pain with resisted inversion

Radiographs
- Seen best on oblique view

Classification
- Type I
  - Small anatomically separate round or oval bone
  - Possibly a sesamoid within posterior tibial tendon
  - Rarely symptomatic
- Type II
  - Large ossicle at medial aspect of navicular
  - Connected by fibrocartilaginous plate (syndesmosis or synchondrosis)
  - Often fuses with navicular at maturity
  - Painful in adolescence
- Type III
  - Large horn-shaped navicular
  - Probably represents fusion of type II

Treatment
Conservative
- Reduce sports
- Shoe modification to avoid pressure on painful prominence
- Arch supports to limit pronation
- Temporary SLC/PWB for symptom relief
- Treat for >6 mo before surgery

Surgical
- Simple excision (recommended)
- Good/excellent results in 90%
- Kidner procedure
  - Excise accessory navicular
  - Advance PTT to support arch
  - Does not improve results over simple excision

CALCANEOVALGUS FOOT

General
- Benign, positional foot deformity
- Reported incidence highly variable (30%–50% of all live births vs. 1/1,000)
- Due to intrauterine packing

Clinical Manifestations
- Ankle dorsiflexed with limitation of passive plantarflexion
- Subtalar joint everted but flexible
- Forefoot can be plantarflexed on hindfoot to create longitudinal arch
- Dorsum of foot may contact tibia
- Different from CVT, which is fixed

Treatment
- Almost all correct spontaneously
- Passive stretching may help

CAVUS FOOT

General
- Fixed plantarflexion of forefoot
- Abnormally high arch
- Can cause abnormal hindfoot posture with weight bearing
- Initially various components are flexible, increasing severity and rigidity with time
- Two-thirds painful high arch with neuromuscular diagnosis
  - Half of those with Charcot-Marie-Tooth
- Calcaneocavus in polio, Myelomeningocele
- Due to gastrocnemius/soleus (G/S) paralysis
- Cavovarus in CMT, Friedrich ataxia
  - *PL overpowers tibialis anterior (plantar flexes first MT)
  - Tibialis posterior overpowers PB (inverts heel)
  - Windlass effect (EHL paradoxically plantarflexes first MT)
  - Tripod effect (heel varus with weight bearing)

Clinical Manifestations/Exam
- Calluses (first MT head/fifth MT base/dorsum of PIPs), pain
- <10 y/o may have high arch sitting that resolves with standing
- Forefoot with PF first MT, pronation, claw toes
- Midfoot with contracted plantar fascia, PF talonavicular or navicular cuneiform joints
- Hindfoot with flexible (forefoot driven) vs. rigid varus

Evaluation
- Evaluate non–weight bearing and in stance
- Evaluate hindfoot, midfoot, forefoot separately
- Coleman block test with heel and lateral forefoot on block to differentiate rigid and flexible hindfoot varus
- Evaluate spine, MR, NCV, DNA test
- Pediatric neurology consult

Radiographs
Standing Lateral
- Varus
  - Subtalar joint seen en fosse
  - Talocalcaneal angle decreased or parallel
- Calcaneus
  - Calcaneal pitch increased (normal 15–20 degrees)
  - Posterior tibiocalcaneal angle (normal 120–130 degrees)
- Cavus
  - Meary talus-first MT angle increased (normal 0–20 degrees)
  - Hibb calcaneal-first MT angle decreased (normal >150 degrees)

- Standing AP
  - Talocalcaneal parallelism
  - Kite talocalcaneal angle decreased (normal 20–40 degrees, <20 degrees indicates hindfoot varus)
  - Forefoot adductus

Treatment
- Correct all segmental deformities
- Balance deforming muscle forces
- Soft tissue procedures alone may be adequate in younger patients with flexible deformities
- Older patients with rigid structural deformities will likely require osteotomies
- Avoid fusion if possible
- Six classes of procedures
  - Plantar release
  - Tendon transfer
  - MT osteotomies (first or more)
  - Midfoot osteotomies (medial cuneiform to correct cavus)
  - Calcaneal osteotomies (corrects rigid hindfoot varus)
  - Triple arthrodesis (salvage)
- Flexible forefoot with flexible hindfoot
  - Young: plantar release, serial casting
- Rigid forefoot with flexible hindfoot
  - Older: plantar release, metatarsal or cuneiform osteotomy
- Rigid forefoot with rigid hindfoot
  - Plantar release, metatarsal or cuneiform osteotomy, Dwyer or lateral slide calcaneal osteotomy
  - Dorsal midfoot osteotomy or triple arthrodesis as second, third line
- Individualized second-stage tendon transfers
- Jones transfer of EHL to MT head for flexible claw toes

CLUB FOOT (CONGENITAL TALIPES EQUINOVARUS)

General
- Autosomal dominant with variable penetrance versus multifactorial
- 1:1,000 births
- 50% bilateral
- 33% twin concordance

Etiology
- Postural
  - Associated packaging abnormalities (torticollis, DDH)
- Syndromic
  - Rigid, resistant to nonoperative treatment

- Associated with constriction band syndrome, diastrophic dwarfism, Moebius, arthrogryposis, and Larsen syndrome.

Diagnosis
- Prenatal ultrasound at 16–20 weeks
  - 67% associated with other anomalies

Physical Exam
- Cavus: forefoot plantarflexed on hindfoot
- Adductus: forefoot adductus on midfoot
- Varus: subtalar joint varus deformity
- Equinus: hindfoot equinus

Radiographs
- Useful at 2–3 mo of age
- Weight bearing or forced dorsiflexion
  - Talar neck is deviated plantar and medial.
  - Subtalar joint is inverted, internally rotated, and plantarflexed around talocalcaneal ligament.
  - Anterior facet of calcaneus is tilted medially
  - Navicular comes near medial malleolus
  - Calcaneus rotates down and medial to become parallel to the talus in the AP and lateral views
  - Varus heel and midfoot adduction result in forefoot supination
- Lateral: parallel talocalcaneal line (not convergent)
  - Calcaneal pitch <35 degrees indicates hindfoot equinus
  - Meary angle (normal 0 degrees) assesses cavus
  - Tibial-talar angle (normal 90 degrees)
  - Tibial calcaneal (normal >90 degrees)
- AP: parallel talocalcaneal line (not divergent)
  - Kite talocalcaneal <20 degrees (normal 20–40 degrees) indicates hindfoot varus
  - Talus–first metatarsal angle (normal 180 degrees) measures forefoot adductus
  - Calcaneal-cuboid alignment.

Treatment
Serial Long Leg Casting (Ponseti)
Order of Correction: CAVE (Five to Six Casts)
- Cavus
- Adductus
- Varus
- Equinus: percutaneous Achilles tendon lengthening
- Casting is followed by abduction bracing, 23 hr/day for 3 months and then at night until age 3 or 4 y/o

Complications
Rocker bottom foot results from correction of equinus before varus (need to unlock midfoot first)
Bean foot results if hindfoot is everted before midfoot varus is corrected

Surgery
- Turco: medial incision, open subtalar joint, excess internal rotation of foot and hindfoot valgus
- Goldner: lengthen deltoid, do not circumferentially release subtalar joint
- Simons: circumferential release of subtalar joint (including IO ligament) and calcaneus-cuboid joint. Leads to gross instability
- Cincinnati incision: 1 cm proximal to posterior crease to avoid heel pad sloughing

CONGENITAL VERTICAL TALUS

General
- Congenital flat foot, rocker bottom foot, convex pes valgus
- AD with variable penetrance
- 50% bilateral
- Etiology muscle imbalance or intrauterine contracture
- Associated with
  - Arthrogryposis multiplex congenita
  - Myelomeningocele (10% with CVT)
  - Sacral agenesis, tethered cord
  - DDH, contralateral clubfoot
  - Neurofibromatosis, nail-patella syndrome
  - Trisomy 13, 14, 15, 19

Clinical Manifestations
- Four fixed components
  - Congenital fixed dorsolateral dislocation of talon-avicular joint
    - Longitudinal arch cannot be restored with passive manipulation
    - Talus medially rotated and in extreme plantarflexion
    - Talar head prominent/palpable on medial plantar surface
    - Patient bears weight on talar head, which causes callus
  - Calcaneus fixed in equinovalgus
  - Midfoot valgus
  - Forefoot dorsiflexed at midtarsal joint
- TA (tibialis anterior), EHL, EDL (extensor digitorum longus), PB, PL, Achilles contractures

Differential
- (CVT is rigid, unlike many of these)
  - Ligament ligamentous
  - Talipes calcaneovalgus
  - Flexible flatfoot
  - Tarsal coalition
  - Paralytic pes valgus
  - Congenital oblique talus (may respond to manipulation or more limited release)

Radiographs
- Lateral in maximum dorsiflexion (DF) shows fixed equinus of talus/hindfoot
- Lateral in maximum plantarflexion (PF) shows irreducible dislocation of talonavicular joint
- AP shows midfoot and hindfoot valgus with increased talocalcaneal angle >40 degrees (normal 20–40 degrees)
- Ossification of navicular occurs at 3 years old
- Lack of ossification limits visualization of navicular dorsal to talus

Treatment
- Establish underlying diagnosis before surgery
- Serial casting not expected to reduce talonavicular joint but stretches dorsal skin, tendons, NV structures
- OR at 12–18 mo
  - Cincinnati incision
  - Achilles, EHL, EDL, TA, PB lengthened
  - TN and subtalar capsules incised
  - Navicular reduced to talus, K-wired
  - Talocalcaneal joint reoriented, K-wired
  - K-wire through calcaneocuboid joint
  - Splint for 12 wk, AFO until patient walks
  - Salvage with navicular resection, subtalar or triple arthrodesis, or talectomy for recurrent deformity or late presenters

CURLY TOE

- Excess flexion/varus/rotation at IP joint
- Toe underlaps adjacent medial toe
- Most common at third toe
- AD
- Due to flexor digitorum longus (FDL) and/or flexor digitorum brevis (FDB) contracture
- Usually no pain, normal walking
- Treatment
  - Tenotomy of toe flexors 95% effective
  - Taping, stretching ineffective

Open flexor tenotomy (Ross and Menelaus, 1984)
- 62 children with flexor tenotomy average 10 y/o
- 5% failure due to incision crossing crease and subsequent contracture
- No abnormal extended posture
- No loss of flexor power
- Must prove preop that FDL resting length is too short

Surgical trial for curly toe (Hamer et al.,1993)
- 19 patients with bilateral curly toes, average 7 y/o
- Sides randomized to flexor tenotomy or flexor-to-extensor transfer, same incision used for both
- No Difference at 4 year follow-up

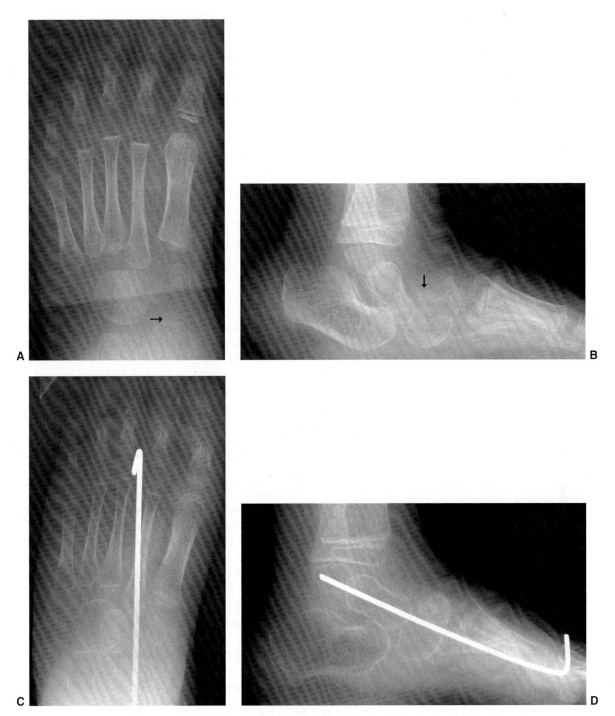

Radiographs before **(A, B)** and after **(C, D)** naviculectomy for congenital vertical talus in an older child. Arrow indicates the navicular. (From Morrissy RT, and Weinstein SL. Lovell and Winter's Pediatric Orthopaedics Sixth Edition Philadelphia: Lippincott Williams & Wilkins, 2006 with permission.)

References

Ross ER, Menelaus MB. Open flexor tenotomy for hammer toes and curly toes in childhood. J Bone Joint Surg Br 1984; 66:770–771.

Hamer AJ, et al. Surgery for curly toe deformity: a double-blind, randomized prospective trial. J Bone Joint Surg Br 1993; 75:662–663.

DELTA PHALANX

General

- Epiphysis extends along base of phalanx or metatarsal, up alongside of diaphysis, across distal physis
- May be familial
- In isolation or along with polysyndactyly, tarsal coalition, Apert syndrome, congenital hallux varus

Natural History

- Growth of abnormal epiphysis leads to short, wide, triangular phalanx
- Results in hallux varus if in great toe

Radiographs

- Not apparent on plain radiograph
- May have D-shaped MT (convex medial border of diaphysis)
- MRI—on plantar-medial surface

Treatment

- Osteotomy alone leads to recurrence
  Central physiolysis (Mubarak et al, 1993) JPO '93'
  - Resect abnormal longitudinal section
  - Interposition with PMMA or fat
  - Best results with surgery at 6 mo

Reference

Mubarak SJ, et al. Metatarsal epiphyseal bracket: treatment by central physiolysis. J Pediatr Orthop 1993; 13:5–8.

FLEXIBLE FLATFOOT

General

- Lack of accepted definitions, classifications, and nomenclature
- Most children and 20% of adults have it
- Higher incidence in shoe-wearing kids
- Arch increases during first decade
- Etiology is bony, ligamentous, or both
- Contributors to flexible flatfoot
  - Tight heel cord
  - Posterior tibial tendon weakness, rupture
  - Tight peroneals
  - External tibial torsion
  - Lax spring ligament
  - Short lateral column

Differential Diagnosis

- Accessory navicular
- PTT dysfunction
- Tarsal coalition (rigid flatfoot)

Clinical Presentation

- Often asymptomatic
- Diffuse activity-related pain (fatigue due to greater intrinsic muscle activity in flatfoot)
- If Achilles tight, may have pain at midstance and callus under talar head
- Tight Achilles prevents talus dorsiflexion
- Force transferred to talonavicular joint, which dorsiflexes with eversion

Physical Exam

- Flatfoot shape results from multiple altered relationships
- Valgus hindfoot
  - Midfoot sags with loss of long arch
  - Forefoot supinated in relation to hindfoot (may be revealed only when hindfoot valgus passively corrected)
  - Assess flexibility (ability to reverse malalignment of longitudinal arch and subtalar joint)
  - Subtalar mobility revealed by toe standing or Jack toe-raise test
  - Windlass action of plantar fascia mobilizes subtalar joint into inversion to create arch

Radiographs

- Lateral
  - Calcaneus plantarflexed, evaluated by calcaneal pitch (bottom of calcaneus vs. horizontal)
  - Talus plantarflexed, evaluated by talus-horizontal angle
  - Dorsiflexion of navicular on plantarflexed talar head
  - Meary talus-first MT angle to evaluate midfoot sag (normal 0–20 degrees, apex dorsal)
- AP
  - Navicular ossifies eccentrically (laterally first), making talonavicular joint hard to evaluate
  - Line from Talus to metarsal is unreliable for determining treatment of severity of flat foot

Treatment

- If flexible, no potential for disability unless along with Achilles contracture
- No benefit from inserts and shoe modifications to increase arch
- Inserts may help pain from intrinsic fatigue
- If painful and along with Achilles contracture
  - Soft insert, UCBL is standard
  - Firm insert will worsen symptoms
  - Program of cord stretching with subtalar complex inverted

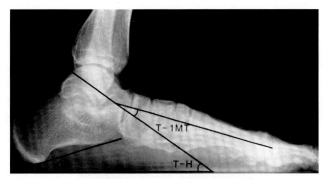

Weight-bearing lateral radiograph. The calcaneal pitch (CP) and the talus-horizontal angle (T-H) are the best measurements to assess valgus deformity of the hindfoot. The talus-first-metatarsal angle (T-1MT) is known as the Meary angle. A plantarflexed apex is seen in a valgus foot. (From Mosca VS. Calcaneal lengthening for valgus deformity of the hindfoot. Results in children who had severe, symptomatic flatfoot and skewfoot. J Bone Joint Surg Am 1995;77:500–512, with permission.)

- Surgery rarely indicated
    - Medial displacing calcaneal osteotomy improves valgus appearance, but does not correct subtalar malalignment
    - Evans/Mosca calcaneal lengthening with TAL corrects eversion of subtalar complex and avoids arthrodesis
    - Plantar-based closing wedge of medial cuneiform corrects forefoot supination
    - TAL corrects Achilles contracture
    - Ensure posterior tibial tendon functioning
    - Correct external tibial torsion in neuromuscular

HALLUX VALGUS

General
- Two-thirds bilateral
- 88% of operative cases are girls

Etiology
- Inheritance (two-thirds with positive family history)
- Metatarsus primus varus
    - Common in juvenile bunions
    - Intermetatarsal angle (IMA) >10 degrees
    - Oblique first MT-medial cuneiform joint
- Increased distal MT articular angle
    - Present in ~50% of juvenile bunions
    - Valgus deformity at distal first MT
    - MTP joint often congruent
    - Associated with long first MT, <10 y/o, positive family history
- Shoe wear (extrinsic)
- Ligamental laxity, pes planus
- Hypermobile first ray
- Spasticity (in CP)

Presentation in Children versus Adults
- Less severe
- Degenerative changes rare
- Proximal physis open
- Medial eminence less prominent
- No bursal thickening
- Intermetatarsal angle greater
- Hallux valgus angle less
- Increased distal metatarsal articular angle (DMAA) more common

Radiographs
- Standing AP and lateral of foot
- Intermetatarsal angle (normal <9 degrees)
- Slope of first MT-cuneiform joint
- Hallus valgus angle (normal <16 degrees)
- Congruency of MTP joint
- Distal MT articular angle (normal <15 degrees of valgus)
- First MT length, proximal physis
- Subluxation of sesamoids

Treatment
- Shoe modification for comfort
- Orthotics worsen deformity (Kilmartin et al., 1994)

Reference
Kilmartin TE, et al. A controlled prospective trial of a foot orthosis for juvenile hallux valgus. J Bone Joint Surg Br 1994; 76:10–14.

Surgery
- Procedure depends on IMA, DMMA, congruency of MTP joint, severity
- High recurrence rates in young patients
- Postpone revision surgery until maturity
- Distal soft tissue realignment (McBride)
    - Needed if MTP incongruent
    - Often fails if done alone
    - Risk AVN with medial *and* lateral release
- Distal metatarsal osteotomy
    - Chevron or Mitchell (step cut)
    - Does not address large IMA
- Basilar metatarsal osteotomy
    - Addresses increased IMA
    - Does not address increased DMMA
    - No AVN of MT head
    - Risk injury to first physis
- Medial cuneiform opening wedge
    - Corrects malaligned first MT-med cuneiform joint
    - Avoids first MT physis injury
- Double osteotomy
    - Indicated in severe HV with congruent MTP joint
    - Address increased IMA with proximal valgus osteotomy
    - Address increased DMAA with distal varus osteotomy

- First MT-cuneiform arthrodesis (Lapidus)
  - Indicated in first ray hypermobility
- MTP arthrodesis
  - Indicated in spasticity (CP) or RA

METATARSUS ADDUCTUS

General
- Forefoot adducted at tarsal-metatarsal (TMT) joint
- Most common congenital foot deformity
- Males = females
- 1:1,000
- Due to intrauterine packing versus muscle imbalance versus abnormal shaped medial cuneiform
- Associated with DDH, torticollis
- Seen in isolation or in conjunction with clubfoot or skewfoot

Natural History
- 85%–95% spontaneous resolution
- Spontaneous resolution seen up to 4 yr
- Results of treatment (Ponseti and Becker, 1966)
  - 379 children minimum 10-yr follow-up
  - Only 11% (rigid or partly flexible) needed casts
  - 90% of treated group good at 32-yr follow-up
- Hooked forefoot (Rushforth, 1978)
  - 130 feet, 7-yr follow-up with no treatment
  - 86% normal feet
  - 10% moderate deformity
  - 4% severe deformity
- Outcomes of treatment (Bleck, 1983)
  - 265 feet, 147 treated with cast
  - Better results if treated at 0–8 mo

References
Ponseti IV, Becker JR. Congenital metatarsus adductus: the results of treatment. J Bone Joint Surg Am 1966; 48:702–711.
Rushforth GF. The natural history of hooked forefoot. J Bone Joint Surg Am 1978; 60-B(4):530–532.
Bleck EE. Metatarsus aduncus: classification and relationship to outcomes of treatment. J Pediatr Orthop 1983; 3:2–9.

Physical Exam
- Lateral foot border convex, medial concave
- Prominent base of fifth MT
- Heel bisector (normal goes between toe 2 and 3)
- Check if actively corrects with peroneal stimulation
- Flexible passively overcorrects beyond normal bisector
- Partly flexible passively corrects to normal

Radiographs
- Usually not necessary or indicated for diagnosis in infants
- X-ray view shows normal talocalcaneal divergence (hindfoot normal, as opposed to skewfoot/clubfoot)
- Trapezoidal shape of medial cuneiform with obliquity of medial cuneiform-MT joint

- Calcaneus-fifth MT angle (normal = 0 degrees) correlates clinically with lateral foot border

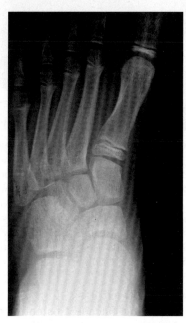

Metatarsus adductus in an older child with trapezoidal-shaped medial cuneiform. (From Cappello T, Mosca VS. Metatarsus adductus and skewfoot. (Foot Ankle Clin 1998:683, with permission.)

Treatment
- No treatment <6 mo of age, initiate <1 y/o
- Most common deformity after cast is pronated foot, so avoid excess valgus at hindfoot
- Surgery rarely indicated, poor results
  - If <2 y/o, distal abductor hallucis tendon release
  - If <6 y/o, can consider Heyman TMT capsulotomies, but high failure and complication rate
  - If >4 y/o and rigid, medial cuneiform opening wedge ± cuboid closing wedge ± multiple MT osteotomies

Serpentine Foot (Z-foot, Skewfoot)
- Along with residual metatarsus adductus
- Talonavicular lateral subluxation
- Hindfoot valgus and pronation
- Resistant to nonsurgical treatment

OVERLAPPING FIFTH TOE

General
- Bilateral 20%–33%
- Cause unknown, familial tendency

Clinical Presentation
- Present at birth
- Fifth toe is dorsally and proximally displaced, adducted, externally rotated

- IP joints are in full extension (toe not clawed)
- Skin in web space is malaligned
- Toe has active flexion/extension

Radiographs
- Dorsomedial subluxation of MTP joint

Treatment
- Stretching, taping not effective
- Surgery indicated in severe deformity, pain, calluses
- Butler procedure
  - Double racket-handle incision
  - Release of extensor tendon, capsule
  - Toe translated plantar-laterally
  - V-to-Y dorsally and a Y-to-V plantar-lateral

SUBUNGUAL EXOSTOSIS

- Benign bony growth on dorsomedial surface of distal phalanx
- Posttraumatic etiology
- Great toe most common location
- Females > males
- Adolescent with pain, toenail irritation
- Diagnose with lateral radiograph

Treatment
- Partial nail removal
- Longitudinal nail bed incision
- 11% recurrence rate

TARSAL COALITION

General
- Fibrous, cartilaginous, or bony connection between two or more tarsal bones

- Autosomal dominant
- Affects <1% of population
- >50% bilateral
- calcaneonavicular coalition most common, then middle facet talocalcaneal

Clinical Presentation
- Only 25% become symptomatic
- Onset of symptoms usually once bar ossifies
  - Talonavicular—age 3–5
  - Calcaneonavicular—age 8–12
  - Talocalcaneal—age 12–16
- Activity-related pain in sinus tarsi
- Possible peroneal spasm

Evaluation
- Rigid flatfoot (arch not restored with toe standing or Jack toe-raising test)
- Findings seen with bar ossification
  - Progressive hindfoot valgus
  - Flattening of longitudinal arch
  - Restricted subtalar motion

Differential Diagnosis
- Rigid flatfoot
- Tarsal coalition
- CVT
- JRA
- Chondral injury
- Old flexible flatfoot

Radiographs
- Calcaneonavicular coalition
  - Seen on oblique x-ray view
  - Anteater nose (elongated anterior process of calcaneus) on lateral

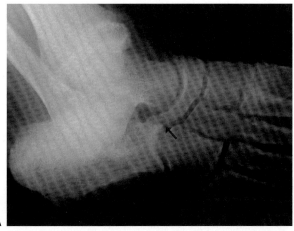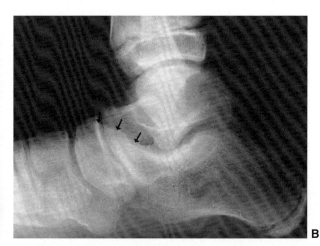

A: A calcaneonavicular coalition (arrow) is best seen on an oblique radiograph of the foot. **B:** Lateral radiograph demonstrating the anteater nose sign (arrows), indicating a calcaneonavicular coalition. (From Morrissy RT, and Weinstein SL. Lovell and Winter's Pediatric Orthopaedics Sixth Edition Philadelphia: Lippincott Williams & Wilkins, 2006 with permission.)

- Talocalcaneal coalition
  - Harris heel view shows irregular middle facet
  - C-sign on lateral (extending from talar dome through coalition compontnt of posterior talocalcaneal joint to sustentaculum)
  - Secondary x-ray view changes
    - Talar beaking (not degenerative)
    - Flat, broad lateral process of talus
    - Ball and socket ankle to compensate for stiff subtalar joint
- CT allows for confirmation of diagnosis
- CT also permits evaluation of additional joints for involvement

Treatment
- Only if symptomatic
- NSAIDS, orthotics
- Below knee walking cast (4–6 wk, twice)
- Surgery
  - Only for failed casting twice
  - Calcaneonavicular (<16 y/o, no DJD, no other coalitions), resect and interpose with EDB or fat (77% good/excellent)
  - Talocalcaneal bars
    - If <50% of joint involved and no OA, resect and interpose fat
    - If >50%, arthrosis, or pain after resection, then subtalar fusion or triple arthrodesis

CHAPTER 4

Trauma

Milton Little, Michael J. Gardner, Dean G. Lorich

General Principles
  Multitrauma
  Acute Respiratory Distress Syndrome
  Brain Injury
  Shock
Upper Extremity
  Clavicle Fracture
  Scapular Fractures
  Brachial Plexus Injury
  Proximal Humerus Fractures
  Humerus—Shaft
  Distal Humerus Fractures
  Capitellar Fracture
  Elbow Dislocation
  Monteggia Fracture
  Olecranon Fracture
  Radial Head Fractures
  Galeazzi Fracture
  Forearm Fractures
  Approaches
  Ulnar Shaft Fractures
  Distal Radius Fracture
Lower Extremity
  Pelvic Fractures
  Acetabular Fracture
  Hip Dislocation
  Femoral Head Fracture
  Hip Fracture—Femoral Neck
  Hip Fracture—Intertrochanteric
  Femoral Subtrochanteric Fracture
  Femoral Shaft Fracture
  Femur—Supracondylar Fracture
  Knee Dislocations
  Floating Knee
  Extensor Mechanism Injuries
  Patellar Fracture
  Tibial Plateau Fractures
  Tibial Shaft Fracture
  Pilon Fractures

  Ankle Fracture
  Ankle Fracture—Open
  Talus Fractures
  Calcaneus Fracture
  Subtalar Dislocation
  Lisfranc—Tarsometatarsal Fracture/Dislocation
  Fifth Metatarsal/Jones Fracture
  Navicular Fracture
  Cuboid Fracture
Pediatric Orthopaedic Trauma
  Conscious Sedation
  Pediatric Proximal Humerus Fractures
  Pediatric Elbow
  Pediatrics—Transphyseal Humerus Fracture
  Supracondylar Humerus Fractures
  Pediatrics—Radius and Ulnar Shaft Fractures
Pediatric Lower Extremity Injuries
  Pediatric Pelvic/Acetabular Fractures
  Pediatric Septic Hip
  Pediatric Hip Fractures and Dislocations
  Pediatric Femur Fractures
  Distal Femoral Epiphyseal Fractures
  Pediatrics—Tibial Eminence Fracture
  Pediatric Tibial Tubercle Fractures
  Pediatric Tibial Shaft Fractures
  Pediatric Ankle Fractures
  Pediatrics—Physeal Injuries

General Principles

MULTITRAUMA

Injury Severity Score
(Baker & Long 1974)
- Six organ systems considered
  - Soft tissue
  - Face
  - Head and neck
  - Chest

- Abdomen
- Extremity and/or pelvis
- Each graded on 6-point system
  - 1—minor
  - 2—moderate
  - 3—severe (non–life threatening)
  - 4—severe (life threatening)
  - 5—critical (survival uncertain)
  - 6—fatal (dead on arrival)
- Add squares of three highest scores to get Injury Severity Score (ISS)
- ISS >18 defines multi-injured
- Lethal Dose for 50% of Patients (LD50) depends on age and ISS score
  - 15–44: LD50 is ISS of 40
  - 45–64: LD50 is ISS of 29
  - >65: LD50 is ISS of 20
    - i.e., older patients require fewer injuries to cause mortality
  - Tornetta (1999)
    - ISS most closely correlates with mortality in patients >60 yr, not including slips/falls
    - Need for only orthopedic surgery associated with less mortality (Risk Ration [RR] 0.5) vs. need for general surgery (RR 2.5)
  - Pape (1994): Increased risk of
    - Death within 24 hr due to brain injury
    - Death in 2–7 days due to pulmonary failure
    - Death in >7 days due to systemic inflammatory response syndrome, multiorgan failure

Metabolic Response to Trauma
- Increased insulin secretion, hyperglycemia with increased peripheral resistance to insulin
- Increased aldosterone secretion
- Catabolism lasts several weeks
- Catacholamines stimulate lipase, leading to increased fatty acids for energy
- Decreased affinity of hemoglobin for oxygen via increased PCO_2 or decrease pH, allows release of oxygen into damaged tissues

Recommended Readings
Baker SP, et al. The injury severity score: a method for describing patients with multiple injuries and evaluating emergency care. J Trauma 1974;14:187–196.

Chawda MN, et al. Predicting outcome after multiple trauma; which scoring system? Injury 2004;35:347–358.

Osler T, et al. A modification of the injury severity score that both improves accuracy and simplifies scoring. J Trauma 1997;43:922–925.

Pape HC, et al. Postraumatic multiple organ failure–a report on clinical and autopsy findings. Shock 1994;2(3):228–234.

Tornetta P, 3rd, Mostafavi H, Riina J, Turen C, Reimer B, Levine R, et al. Morbidity and mortality in elderly trauma patients. J Trauma. 1999;46:702–706.

Fat Embolism Syndrome
- Inflammatory reaction to embolized fat globules and marrow contents
- Classic symptoms usually within 48 hr
  - Anxiety, confusion (mental status changes)
  - Tachycardia, hypoxemia
  - Petechiae
- These symptoms occur in 10% of patients with multiple fractures
- Ventilation support with positive end-expiratory pressure is the treatment of choice
- Long bone fracture stabilization minimizes ongoing insult
- Steroids, heparin, and dextran have not proven effective

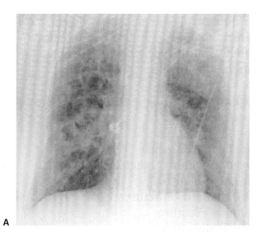

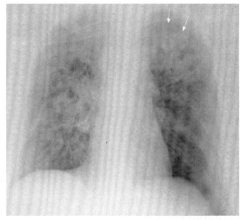

A 40-year-old man who developed a left pneumothorax while being ventilated for acute respiratory distress syndrome (ARDS). **A:** Baseline chest radiograph shows diffuse parenchymal airspace opacity compatible with ARDS. **B:** A chest radiograph obtained during respiratory deterioration shows a new lucency over the region of left hemidiaphragm (deep anterior sulcus). There is also increased depth of the lateral costophrenic sulcus. The thin white line of pneumothorax is evident superiorly (arrows). (From Crapo JD, et al., eds. Baum's Textbook of Pulmonary Diseases, 7th ed. Philadelphia, PA: Lippincott Williams & Wilkins; 2004.)

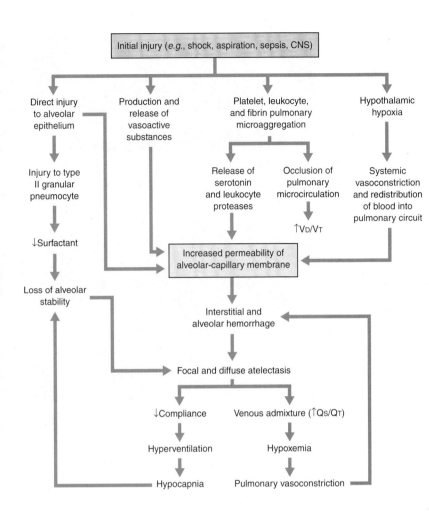

Pathogenesis of acute respiratory distress syndrome. (From Nettina SM. The Lippincott Manual of Nursing Practice, 7th ed. Philadelphia, PA: Lippincott Williams & Wilkins; 2001.)

ACUTE RESPIRATORY DISTRESS SYNDROME

- Refractory hypoxemia and diffuse infiltration on chest radiographs
- Decreased lung compliance and poor gas exchange
- Late sepsis, multiorgan failure, and high mortality
- Only one randomized prospective study of early vs. delayed stabilization of femur fracture
  - **Bone & Johnson (1989)**
    - 178 patients were divided into multiply injured and isolated femur fracture
    - In multiply injured (ISS >18), pulmonary complications (acute respiratory distress syndrome [ARDS], fat embolism syndrome, pneumonia) were higher, hospital and intensive care unit stay longer in delayed stabilization (>48 hr vs. <24 hr)
- Morshed and Colford (2009)
  - Recently published contrary data to the previously held standard
  - In a retrospective evaluation of multisystem trauma patients with femoral shaft fractures, they determined that delayed repair beyond 12 hr reduced mortality by 50%

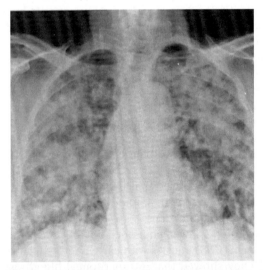

Fat embolism. Frontal chest radiograph made 3 days after a leg fracture demonstrates diffuse bilateral airspace consolidation due to alveolar hemorrhage and edema. Unlike cardiogenic pulmonary edema, the distribution in this patient is predominantly peripheral rather than central, and the heart is not enlarged. (From Eisenberg RL. An Atlas of Differential Diagnosis, 4th ed. Philadelphia, PA: Lippincott Williams & Wilkins; 2003.)

- The rate was significant in patients with head/neck injuries as well as abdominal injuries
- There was a trend toward better outcomes in patients with chest injuries, but this was not found to be significant

Recommended Readings

Bone LB, et al. Early versus delayed stabilization of femoral fractures. A prospective randomized study. J Bone Joint Surg Am 1989;71:336–340.

Bone L, Bucholz R. The management of fractures in the patient with multiple trauma. J Bone Joint Surg Am 1986;68: 945–949.

Lhowe DW, Hansen ST. Immediate nailing of open fractures of the femoral shaft. J Bone Joint Surg Am 1988;70(6): 812–820.

Morshed S, Colford JM. Delayed internal fixation of femoral shaft fracture reduces mortality among patients with multisystem trauma. J Bone Joint Surg Am 2009;91:3–13.

Pape HC, et al. Influences of different methods of intramedullary femoral nailing on lung function in patients with multiple trauma. J Trauma 1993;35(5):709–716.

BRAIN INJURY

- Primary
  - Concussion
  - Diffuse axonal injury
  - Disruptive (gunshot wound [GSW])
  - Skull fracture
- Secondary
  - Hypoxia from decreased perfusion
- Patients with significant head injury or Glasgow Coma Scale (GCS) <9 are more likely to experience hypotensive events after femur fracture fixation within 2 hr of injury compared to 24 hr after injury
- Femur fracture repair should be delayed until adequate fluid resuscitation has been performed to avoid hypoxia, hypotension, or low cerebral perfusion pressure
- Temporizing methods such as external fixation or traction pin placement can be performed to limit blood loss, improve pain control, and decrease risk of fat embolism
- Starr (1998) showed that delaying fracture stabilization associated with 45 times increase in risk of pulmonary complications
- The group showed no association of central nervous system (CNS) injuries with early fracture fixation
  - They showed that intraperitoneal blood loss, hypotension, decreased perfusion was worsened by the procedure
  - The group recommended external fixation for unstable, multi-injury patients
  - Patient should be stabilized by either external fixation to decrease further blood loss and prevent increased stress from definitive procedure

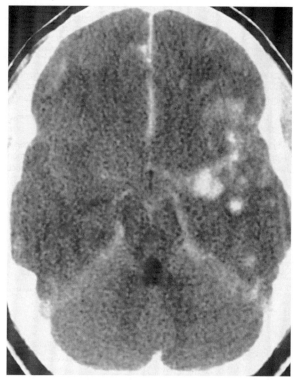

Cerebral contusion. This 16-year-old girl was comatose after being a passenger in a high-speed motor vehicle collision. A head computed tomography scan shows hemorrhagic contusion of the left temporal lobe, subdural hematoma along the tentorial margins, and effacement of the sulci throughout. The patient expired despite intensive medical management for increased intracranial pressure. (From Fleisher GR, Ludwig S, Baskin MN, eds. Atlas of Pediatric Emergency Medicine. Philadelphia, PA: Lippincott Williams & Wilkins; 2004.)

Glasgow Coma Scale

Eye Opening
- 4—spontaneous
- 3—response to speech
- 2—response to pain
- 1—none

Motor Response
- 6—obeys commands
- 5—purposeful response to pain
- 4—withdrawal to pain
- 3—flexion to pain
- 2—extension to pain
- 1—none

Verbal Response
- 5—oriented
- 4—confused
- 3—inappropriate

- 2—incomprehensible
- 1—none

Recommended Readings

Chesnut RM, et al. The role of secondary brain injury in determining outcome from severe head injury. J Trauma 1993;34:216–222.

Schmeling GJ, Schwab JP. Polytrauma care. The effect of head injuries and timing of skeletal fixation. Clin Orthop Relat Res 1995;(318):106–116.

Sarrafzadeh AS, et al. Secondary insults in severe head injury—do multiply injured patients do worse? Crit Care Med 2001;29:1116–1123.

Starr AJ, et al. Treatment of femur fracture with associated head injury. J Trauma 1998;12(1):38–45.

Townsend RN, et al. Timing fracture repair in patients with severe brain injury (Glasgow Coma Scale score <9). J Trauma 1998;44(6):977–983.

SHOCK

Causes of Hypotension

- 95% from hemorrhage
- Brain injury: loss of blood pressure (BP) regulation
- Neurogenic: loss of peripheral vascular resistance, no tachycardic response
- Hypothermia
- Myocardial infarction
- Mediastinal shock (tamponade, rupture of heart or aorta)
- Tachycardia is often first sign of shock, followed by increased diastolic pressure
    - 30% of blood volume can be lost before drop in systolic pressure

Treatment

- Initial treatment: 2 L of saline over 20 min
- Tachycardia and hypotension after the 2 L suggests ongoing bleeding and thus requires O negative blood transfusion or type specific transfusion
- Ratio of blood to fresh frozen plasma continues to be evaluated: Current recommendations are for 1.5/1 ratio during massive transfusion protocols to avoid hypocoagulative state

Hemorrhagic Shock

- Class I (up to 15% blood volume loss)
    - Heart rate (HR) 80, respiratory rate (RR) 14, systolic blood pressure (SBP) 120, urine output (UOP) 35
    - Fluids alone suffice
- Class II (20%–25% blood volume)
    - HR >100, RR 20, SBP 100, UOP 30
    - Fluids alone usually suffice
- Class III (30%–35%)
    - HR >120, RR 30, SBP 80, UOP 15
    - Mental status changes (confusion)
    - Fluids and blood required

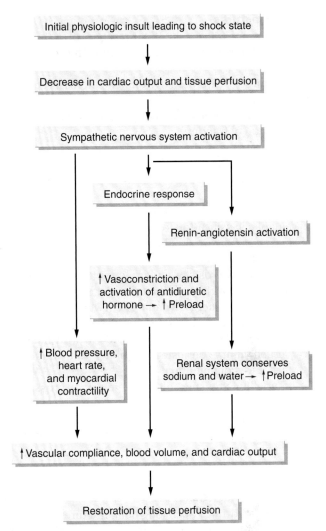

Compensatory mechanisms in shock. (Adapted with permission from Jones K. Shock. In: Clochesy JM, et al., eds. Critical Care Nursing, 2nd ed. Philadelphia, PA: WB Saunders; 1996.)

- Class IV (40%–50%)
    - Life threatening
    - HR >140, RR >35, SBP 50, no UOP
    - Lethargic
    - Fluids and blood required emergently

Recommended Readings

Blow O, et al. The golden hour and the silver day: detection and correction of occult hypoperfusion within 24 hours improves outcome from major trauma. J Trauma 1999;47: 964–969.

Moore FA, et al. The next generation in shock resuscitation. Lancet 2004;363:1988–1996.

Rixen D, Siegel JH. Metabolic correlates of oxygen debt predict post trauma early acute respiratory distress syndrome and the related cytokine response. J Trauma 2000;49: 392–403.

Open Fractures

- Soft tissue injuries in the presence of a fracture should be evaluated for continuity with the fracture site
- Exposure to external environment increases risk of infection
- Soft tissue/periosteal injury increases risk of nonunion of fracture
- Irrigation of wound removes initial fracture hematoma and osteoprogenitor cells
- Debridement should be performed prior to irrigation

Gustilo Anderson Classification

- Valuable classification for open fractures
- Final classification should not be performed until final debridement completed
- Late tissue necrosis or underlying soft tissue damage may further declare itself after serial debridements
    - Type I: Low energy: Wound <1 cm with simple transverse or short oblique fracture
    - Type II: Wound >1 cm and <10 cm with minimal crush injury, periosteal stripping, and moderate fracture comminution
    - Type III: Extensive soft tissue injury or gross contamination (farm injury)
    - Type IIIA: Large wound, high-energy mechanism, extensive contamination including any farm contamination
    - Type IIIB: Will require soft tissue flap coverage
    - Type IIIC: Extensive vascular injury requiring repair
- Gustilo & Anderson (1976)
    - Evaluated 1,025 open long bone fractures
    - Cephalosporins are the prophylactic antibiotic of choice in open fractures
    - Retrospective arm of the study showed the rate of infection in type III open fractures dropped to from 44% to 9% with the addition of cephalosporins
    - In 1984, the group separated the type III injuries into their current subtypes based on prognosis due to associated morbidity (soft tissue damage, vascular injury or severe contamination)
    - Rates of wound infection in the three subtypes: Type IIIA, 4%, IIIB, 52%; and IIIC, 42%
    - Rate of amputation: Type IIIA 0%, IIIB 16%, and IIIC 42%
    - They also suggested including an aminoglycoside in addition to a first-generation cephalosporin as prophylactic antibiotic
- Patzakis (1989)
    - Showed that the most important factor in preventing infection after an open fracture was early administration of antibiotics
    - Administration within 3 hr was associated with a rate of 4.7% vs 7.4 % for >3 hr
    - In contrast, time to surgery >12 hr vs. <12 hr infection (both 7%), delayed or primary closure, or

length of antibiotic administration did not alter the infection rate of infection

Management of Open Fractures

- First-generation cephalosporin should be initiated in all patients at presentation
- An aminoglycoside (gentamicin 3–5 mg/kg/day) should be added in grade III injuries
- Penicillin (PCN) should be added in farm contamination (PCN 2,000,000 units IV q4h)
- Any gross contamination should be removed in the emergency department
- Reduce the fracture early and apply saline-soaked dressing
- Plan for early debridement and irrigation in addition to preliminary stabilization
- There is no standard cutoff for timing to surgery
- Intraoperatively, extend wounds to allow for thorough debridement of devitalized tissue/exploration of the underlying soft tissues
- Any nonviable or devitalized bone should be removed to decrease foci of infection
- Marginal tissue may be maintained, as the patient should undergo redebridement in 48 hr
- Following thorough debridement, 9 L of normal saline should be utilized to irrigate the tissue using cystology tubing or other low-pressure mechanism (volume dependent on extent of injury)
- High-pressure pulse irrigators have been shown to further imbed bacteria in nonhuman studies
- Wounds with opposable edges should be closed tension free with the use of Donati-Allgower sutures if necessary
- If the wound size or edges precludes closure, consider a negative pressure, vacuum-assisted closure device
- External fixation is utilized in most high-grade open injuries with soft tissue injury requiring multiple debridements
- Care should be taken to avoid contaminated regions for insertion of external fixation pins
- External fixators may be maintained up to 2 wk before the risk of infection is increased following definitely open reduction internal fixation (ORIF)
- If fixator in place for >14 days, patient should have fixator pins removed for a total of 2 wk to minimize risk of deep infection
- Early stabilization of open tibial fractures has been shown to be safe and viable option in grade I through grade IIIB injuries if adequate soft tissue closure was performed
- Despite immediate stabilization, the patients should still undergo additional irrigation and debridement
- Femoral shaft fractures have also been shown to have successful results following immediate intramedullary nailing of grade I through grade III open fractures

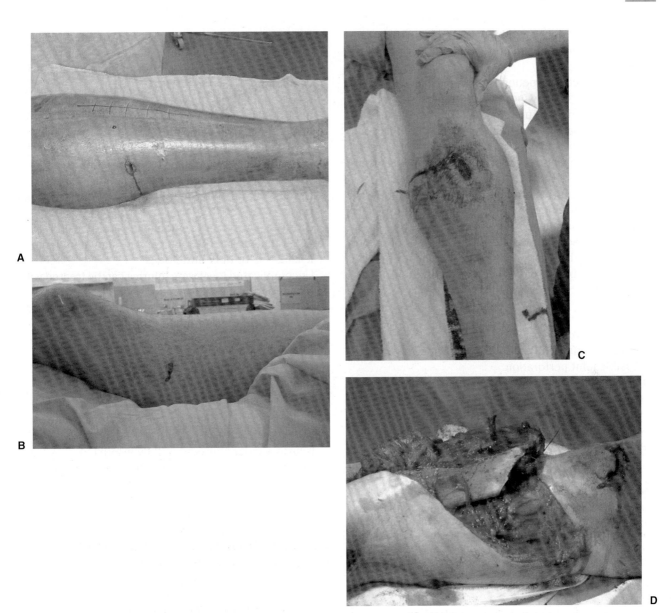

A. Gustilo type I open tibial shaft fracture with wound on the medial face of the tibia.
B. Gustilo type I open femoral shaft fracture. Note that many surgeons feel that because of the amount of energy required and the amount of soft tissue traversed for this injury to become open, most open femoral shaft fractures should be classified as type III injuries.
C. Gustilo type II open proximal tibial shaft fracture. **D.** Gustilo type III open tibial fracture prior to débridement, note the associated substantial periosteal stripping and severe muscle injury. (From Bucholz RW, Court- Brown CM, Heckman JD, et al. *Rockwood & Green's Fractures in Adults*, 7th ed. Philadelphia: Lippincott, Williams & Wilkins, 2010.)

- Immediate plating runs a higher risk of postoperative infection, nonunion and poor outcomes in open tibial fractures
- Soft tissue reconstruction is a crucial aspect of postoperative care following grade IIIB open fractures
- Proximal third fractures can be treated with either a medial or lateral gastrocnemius rotational flap followed by skin graft
- Middle third fractures are treated with a soleus rotational flap
- Distal third injuries are best treated with free tissue flaps with the donor site determined by the plastic surgeon performing coverage
- A vascularized fibula can be utilized in cases of severe bone loss with an associated fasciocutaneous pedicle to assist in both bony regeneration and soft tissue coverage

Traumatic Arthrotomies
- Wounds should explored after irrigation to evaluate possible joint perforation
- Unrecognized joint injury can predispose patient to septic arthritis
- Nord et al. (2009) showed that at least 155 cc of normal saline was necessary to detect 95% of 1-cm inferolateral knee arthrotomies

Recommended Readings

Gustilo RB, Anderson JT. Prevention of infection in the treatment of one thousand and twenty-five open fractures of long bones: retrospective and prospective analyses. J Bone Joint Surg Am 1976;58:4:453–458.

Nord RM, Quach T, Walsh M, Pereira D, Tejwani NC. Detection of Traumatic Arthrotomy of the Knee Using the Saline Solution Load Test. J Bone Joint Surg Am 2009;91(10):66–70.

Patzakis MJ, Wilkins J. Factors influencing infection rate in open fracture wounds. Clin Orthop Relat Res 1989;243:36–40.

Gunshot Wounds
- Gunshots are separated into low-velocity (<2,000 ft/sec) or high-velocity (>2,000 ft/sec) injuries
- **Low-velocity injuries**
  - Generally treated the same as closed injuries
  - Do not require immediate debridement, extraction of the bullet and
  - May not require operative intervention
- All gunshot victims should receive tetanus booster in those whose tetanus status is unknown or not up to date
- Those not previously immunized will require tetanus Immunoglobulin (IG)
- **High-velocity injuries**
  - Generally open with extensive soft tissue damage

- Require provisional stabilization after debridement and irrigation
- Gustilo-Anderson classification should be utilized for evaluation
- I—<1 cm
- II—1–10 cm
- III—>10 cm, high-velocity GSWs, crush, barnyard
  - A—Soft tissue coverage is maintained
  - B— Requires soft tissue reconstruction/free flap
  - C—Requires vascular reconstruction
- Grades I and II—Ancef/first-generation cephalosporin
- Grade III—Ancef and gentamicin should be utilized
- GSWs that violate the joint capsule should undergo at least 24–48 hr of IV antibiotics
- Uncomplicated low-grade injuries can be treated with 3 days of oral ciprofloxacin or cephalexin
- Extend wounds as necessary to allow for adequate debridement of surrounding soft tissues
- Debride wounds prior to irrigation to allow for removal of all foreign tissue

Physical Examination
- Patient should be evaluated carefully for entrance and exit wound
- Neurovascular status should be evaluated
- Rule out compartment syndrome in all injuries
- Care should be taken to evaluate injured compartments closely

Mangled Extremity Severity Score (MESS)
- Developed as a means of evaluating lower extremity injuries to delineate limb salvage from early amputation
- Based on retrospective evaluation of 25 patients with severe skeletal/soft tissue injuries of the lower extremity and applied prospectively to an additional 25 patients
- The MESS is determined by the 4 patient/injury categories shown below

Skeletal/Soft Tissue Injury
- 1—low-energy wound
- 2—medium energy, moderate crush
- 3—high-energy wound
- 4—massive crush

Shock
- 0—BP stable in field and emergency room
- 1—unstable in field, responds to IV fluid
- 2—BP <90, only responds to large IV fluid

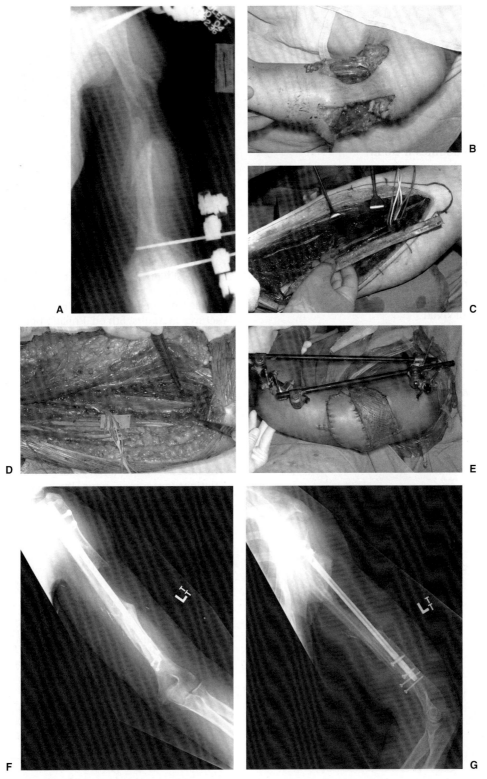

A, B. A 44-year-old woman sustained a gunshot wound to the left humerus resulting in a large entrance and exit wound (>15 cm each) with segmental bone loss of the humerus exceeding 10 cm in length. The fractures were temporarily stabilized with external fixation and the soft tissue defect addressed with an ipsilateral free latissimus dorsi flap. **C–E.** Once the soft tissues were stabilized, a free vascularized fibula was used to bridge the bony defect after an intramedullary nail had been placed. **F, G.** The fibula was incorporated into the proximal and distal ends of the humerus by 3 months, resulting in a salvaged and very functional upper extremity. (From Bucholz RW, Court- Brown CM, Heckman JD, et al. *Rockwood & Green's Fractures in Adults*, 7th ed. Philadelphia: Lippincott, Williams & Wilkins, 2010.)

Ischemia
- 0—no evidence of ischemia, pulses normal
- 1—decreased pulse, no evidence of ischemia
- 2—no Doppler, decreased refill, motor, numbness to touch
- 3—no Doppler, cool, no refill, no motor
- **Ischemia score doubles if >6 hr**

Age
- 0—<30 yr
- 1—30–50 yr
- 2—>50 yr
- Developed with 26 lower extremity open fractures with vascular compromise, then prospectively evaluated in 26 more limbs
- Maximum score 14
- <7—all limbs survived
- ≥7—all limbs amputated

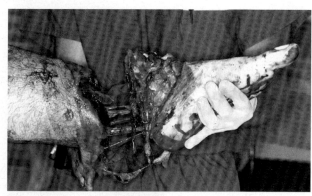

A type IIIC open tibial fracture. The extent of soft tissue crush and avulsion in this injury precludes limb salvage. However, if limb salvage were to be performed, vascular repair would be necessary for limb survival. (From Bucholz RW, Heckman JD, eds. Rockwood and Green's Fractures in Adults, 5th ed. Philadelphia, PA: Lippincott Williams & Wilkins; 2001.)

Relative Indications for Amputation
- Warm ischemia >6 hr
- No posterior tibial nerve function
- Severe ipsilateral foot trauma

Lower Extremity Amputation Prevention Study (LEAP)
- Evaluated similar injuries and outcomes
- Patient outcomes have been shown to be highly related to patient factors including socioeconomic

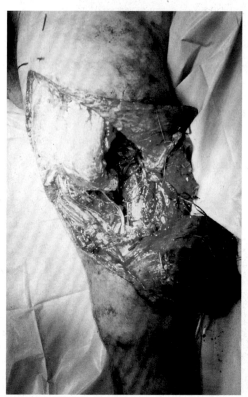

An occasional indication for cast brace treatment is a severely comminuted grade IIIB open fracture illustrated by this clinical photograph. Note that the bone fragments, which were completely detached from the soft tissue, were not removed from the fracture site but were left in situ after thorough debridement of the soft tissues. This prevented a gap from forming and added to the stability of the fracture. (From Bucholz RW, Heckman JD, eds. Rockwood and Green's Fractures in Adults, 5th ed. Philadelphia, PA: Lippincott Williams & Wilkins; 2001.)

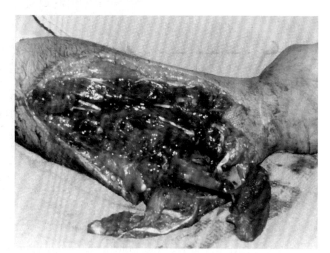

Open fracture of both bones of the forearm as a result of an industrial accident. The mechanism of injury was crush-avulsion. There has been extensive soft tissue damage with avulsion of much of the extensor musculature, ulnar nerve, and ulnar artery. Management of the soft tissue wound demands the restoration of underlying skeletal stability. (From Bucholz RW, Heckman JD, eds. Rockwood and Green's Fractures in Adults, 5th ed. Philadelphia, PA: Lippincott Williams & Wilkins; 2001.)

status, personal resources and demographics rather than the injury characteristics

Recommended Reading

Helfet DL, et al. Limb salvage versus amputation. Preliminary results of the Mangled Extremity Severity Score. Clin Orthop Relat Res 1990;256:80–86.

Acute Compartment Syndrome

- Acute orthopaedic emergency that can result from a fracture (69%), fracture fixation, fracture reduction, prolonged compression
- Results from increased pressure in an intramuscular compartment → inadequate perfusion of intracompartmental musculature and nerves
- Sequelae of missed compartment syndrome include muscular necrosis, neurologic deficits, infection, sepsis, and amputation
- Men <35 yr old are highest risk
- Care should be taken when casting pediatric patients
- Factors that decrease the risk of compartment syndrome in casting (Garfin 1991)
  - Univalve: Decrease pressure by 30%
  - Spreading the cast: Decreased pressure by 65%
  - Avoid wet Webril or Kerlix

Physical Exam

- Most sensitive diagnostic symptom is pain out of proportion
- Pain with passive stretch most sensitive test
- Pediatric patients should be monitored for increased pain medication requirements
- 5 Ps (pain, pulselessness, poikilothermia, parasthesias, paralysis) are late symptoms other than pain
- If the 5 Ps are seen, then the prognosis is poor

Diagnosis

- Stryker pressure monitor is utilized for measurement of the compartment pressures (CPs) within the at risk compartments
- All compartments should be tested within 5 cm of the fracture
- Low threshold should exist for checking pressures in patients with mental status changes, polytrauma/distracting injuries, or inability to verbalize their pain level
- If stryker pressure monitor not available and 18-gauge needle and arterial line setup can be utilized to measure compartments
- Fasciotomy indicated for delta P (diastolic minus CP) <30 (Whitesides); most sensitive diagnostic value
- Some use mean arterial pressure (MAP) minus CP [MAP = 2/3 (systole – diastole) + diastole]

- Matsen recommended fasciotomy for pressure >45 measured by continuous infusion technique
- Mubarek recommended fasciotomy for absolute pressure >30–35
- Need for fasciotomy is absolute indication for rigid stabilization of fracture
- Despite fasciotomy, renal function, creatine kinase, and myoglobin should be montiored closely

Lower Leg

- Four muscular compartments
- Most common site of compartment
- Compartments described below

Anterior

- Tibial anterior
- Extensor hallucis longus
- Extensor digitorum longus
- Peroneus tertius
- Anterior tibial artery and vein
- Deep peroneal nerve
- Foot drop, numb first web space

Lateral

- Peroneus longus
- Peroneus brevis
- Superficial peroneal nerve

Posterior Superficial

- Gastrocnemius
- Soleus
- Plantaris

Posterior Deep

- Tibialis posterior
- Flexor hallucis longus
- Flexor digitorum longus
- Popliteus
- Posterior tibial artery
- Tibial nerve
- Peroneal artery
- Rigid equinus, claw toes
- Lateral incision
  - Positioned midway between tibia and fibula
  - Identify intermuscular septum
  - Care must be taken to avoid the superficial peroneal nerve
  - The anterior and lateral compartments are then incised through the incision
- Posteromedially
  - Incision is made 2 cm posterior to the posterior border of the tibia
  - The saphenous vein and nerve should be avoided
  - Incise gastrocnemius-soleus fascia, retract posteriorly, then incise fascia over flexor digitorum longus

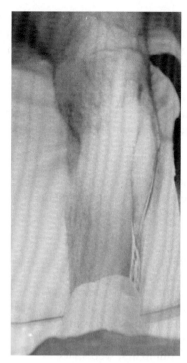

Double-incision fasciotomy in a patient who also required mid-foot amputation. (From Bucholz RW, Heckman JD, eds. Rockwood and Green's Fractures in Adults, 5th ed. Philadelphia, PA: Lippincott Williams & Wilkins; 2001.)

- Inspect tibia and posterior fascia, and elevate the compartment off the posterior surface of the tibia
- Must take soleus bridge if it extends more than halfway down tibia because it takes origin from tibia and fibula for entire proximal half of leg
- Detach bridge from tibia or fibula; be aware of the neurovascular bundle posteriorly
- Cut along anterior/lateral fascia to find plane between these two compartments
- Cut horizontally on superficial posterior/deep posterior fascia to find plane
- Wounds can be dressed with a vacuum-assisted dressing for later definitive closure or split-thickness skin graft

Recommended Readings

Cohen MS, Garfin SR, Hargens AR, Mubarak SJ. Acute compartment syndrome. Effect of dermotomy on fascial decompression in the leg. J Bone Joint Surg Br. 1991;73(2):287–290.
Matsen FA, Clawson DK. The deep posterior compartmental syndrome of the leg. J Bone Joint Surg Am 1975;57:34–39.

Hand
- The hand is composed of 10 compartments
  - Seven interossei (four dorsal and three volar)
  - Thenar
  - Hypothenar
  - Adductor pollicis

- Compartment syndrome results from blunt trauma, metacarpal fracture, air injection, infection, or reperfusion
- Adequate decompression can be performed with two dorsal incisions and decompression of any additional compartments based on measured pressures

Forearm
- Second most common location of compartment syndrome
- There are three compartments of the forearm (volar, dorsal, and mobile wad)
- Volkmann's contracture is a flexion deformity of the hand and forearm, which results from unrecognized forearm compartment syndrome

Forearm Fasciotomy
Volar Henry Approach
- Superficial wad and deep volar compartments must be released
- Incise from medial to biceps tendon to thenar crease
- Superficial fascia incised from proximally to elbow crease to across carpal tunnel
- Brachioradialis muscle and superficial radial nerve retracted laterally, flexor carpi radialis and radial artery retract medially, exposing the pronator teres, flexor digitorum profundus, flexor pollicis longus, pronator quadratus
- Decompress the fascia of each of these muscles individually

Dorsal Approach
- Incise from lateral epicondyle to mid pronated wrist
- Follow the Interval between the extensor digitorum communis and extensor carpi radialis brevis to fully decompress the compartment

Gluteal
- Associated with pelvic fractures and falls in the setting of antithrombotic agents
- Despite rarity, should not be overlooked

Thigh
- Uncommon source of compartment syndrome due to the size of the compartments
- Thigh compartments
  - Anterior (quadriceps)
  - Posterior (hamstrings)
  - Medial (adductors)
- Quadriceps compartment syndrome is more often secondary to intramedullary nailing of femur fractures

Fasciotomy
- Standard lateral incision followed by splitting the iliotibial band

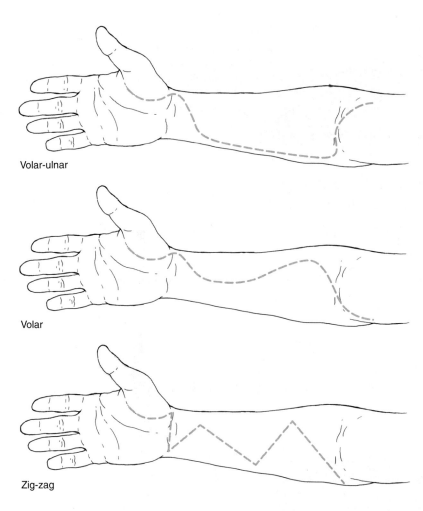

Volar-ulnar

Volar

Zig-zag

3 possible volar incisions for forearm fasciotomies. (From Bucholz RW, Heckman JD, eds. Rockwood and Green's Fractures in Adults, 5th ed. Philadelphia, PA: Lippincott Williams & Wilkins; 2001.)

- Anterior and posterior compartments should be opened
- A separate medial incision is necessary if the adductor CP is elevated

Foot
- Suspect compartment syndrome in crush injuries of the foot
- Composed of nine muscular compartments
  - Medial, lateral, central, and interosseous (IO) compartments
  - Central divided into two by transverse septum, superficial with flexor digitorum brevis and deep calcaneal compartment with quad plantae and lateral plantar nerve
  - This calcaneal compartment communicates with deep posterior leg compartment
- Sole sensation paramount and major reason for proceeding with fasciotomies

Fasciotomy
- Dorsal incision between the second and fourth metatarsals access the IO compartments and central compartment

- Medial and lateral compartments can also be accessed through those incisions
- Medial incision can be made to release the calcaneal compartment if necessary

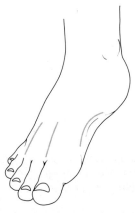

Recommended method of foot fasciotomy. Relative incision locations on the foot surface. (From Bucholz RW, Heckman JD, eds. Rockwood and Green's Fractures in Adults, 5th ed. Philadelphia, PA: Lippincott Williams & Wilkins; 2001, with permission.)

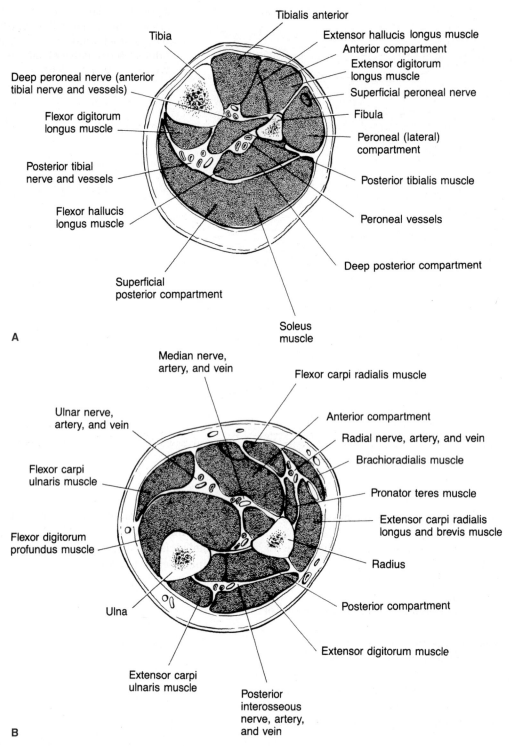

Compartments of the leg **(A)** and forearm **(B).** (From Harwood-Nuss A, et al. The Clinical Practice of Emergency Medicine, 3rd ed. Philadelphia, PA: Lippincott Williams & Wilkins; 2001, with permission.)

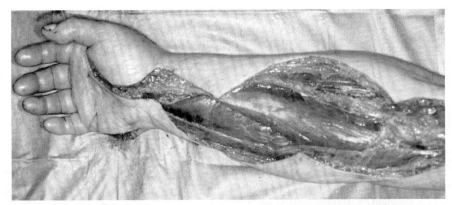

Volar incision for forearm compartment release. (From Bucholz RW, Heckman JD, eds. Rockwood and Green's Fractures in Adults, 5th ed. Philadelphia, PA: Lippincott Williams & Wilkins; 2001, with permission.)

Recommended Readings

Cohen MS, et al. Acute compartment syndrome. Effect of dermotomy on fascial decompression in the leg. J Bone Joint Surg Br 1991;73(2):287–290.

Garfin SR, Murbarak SJ. Quantification of intracompartmental pressure and volume under plaster casts. J Bone Joint Surg 1981;63(3): 449–453.

Matsen FA, et al. Diagnosis and management of compartmental syndromes. J Bone Joint Surg Am 1980;62:286–291.

McQueen MM, Court-Brown CM. Compartment monitoring in tibial fractures. The pressure threshold for decompression. J Bone Joint Surg Br 1996;78(1):99–104.

McQueen MM, et al. Acute compartment syndrome: who is at risk? J Bone Joint Surg Br 2000;82:200–203.

Mubarak SJ, et al. Double incision fasciotomy of the leg for decompression in compartment syndromes. J Bone Joint Surg (Am) 1977;59-A: 184–187.

Fracture Blisters

- Cleavage injury at dermal–epidermal junction
- Secondary to soft tissue swelling adjacent to fracture sites
- Worse in areas with decreased subcutaneous tissue
- Average time noted on clinical examination is 2.5 days postinjury
- May be serous or hemorrhagic
  - Serous:
    - Retained epithelial cells, leading to faster re-epithelialization
    - Serous blisters can be unroofed and treated with silvadene or aspirated
  - Hemorrhagic
    - Increased soft tissue injury
    - Increased risk of wound breakdown and need for soft tissue coverage at hemorrhagic blister sites

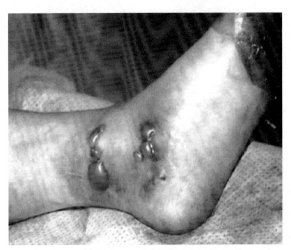

A photograph of a patient's ankle with a tibial plafond fracture taken 6 days after injury. The medial side of the ankle has dark, hemorrhagic fracture blisters, which represent a slightly deeper zone of injury than the white fracture blisters. (From Bucholz RW, Heckman JD, eds. Rockwood and Green's Fractures in Adults, 5th ed. Philadelphia, PA: Lippincott Williams & Wilkins; 2001, with permission.)

Recommended Readings

Koval K, et al. Tape blisters following hip surgery. A prospective, randomized study of two types of tape. J Bone Joint Surg Am 2003;85-A(10):1884–1887.

Giordano CP, Koval KJ. Treatment of fracture blisters: a prospective study of 53 cases. J Orthop Trauma 1995;9(2):171–176.

Fracture Healing Stages

Stage I—Immediate Response

- Fracture leads to hematoma formation
- Platelets release cytokines which stimulate vessel dilatation, cellular migration and angiogenesis

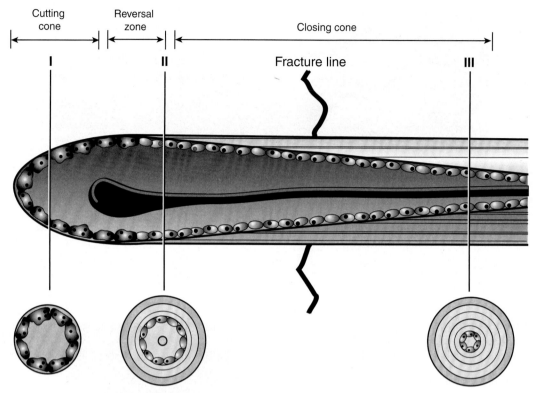

Primary bone healing utilizes an osteoclastic cutting cone crossing the fracture gap (I) followed by bone reconstitution by the trailing osteoblasts (II, III).

- Angiogenesis leads to maximum vascularity at 2 wk post injury
- Inflammation stimulates further influx of bone matrix proteins
- Hematoma is replaced by fibrovascular tissue and the acellular hematoma becomes granulation tissue
- Granulation tissue formation is promoted by micromotion at the fracture site and may be inhibited by smoking

Stage II—Soft Callus (Cartilage, Type II Collagen)
- Granulation tissue replaced by cartilage
- Osteoid formed by osteoblasts at periosteum (modulation: local bone cells activated)
- At fracture site, mesenchymal cells from hematoma differentiate into chondroblasts, osteoblasts, and fibroblasts to make soft callus
- Necrotic bone at fracture site resorbed
- Low oxygen and increased motion favors cartilage and granulation tissue formation rather than ossification

Stage III—Hard Callus, Healed (Bone, Type I Collagen)
- 4–8 wk
- Callus remodels via creeping substitution
- Controlled by Wolfe's law (based on strains)

- During repair of unstable fracture (enchondral ossification), osteoclasts form from circulating monocytes and marrow monocytic precursors
- Osteoblasts form from undifferentiated mesenchymal cells that migrate into the area

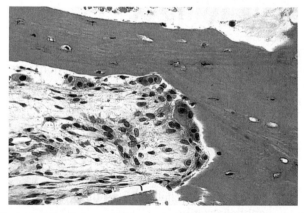

Basic multicellular unit (bone remodeling unit of Frost) of bone. Osteoclasts form the leading edge of the bone resorption ("the cutting cone"), and just behind them are mononuclear macrophages and osteoblasts. The newly created space is filled with a vascular loose connective tissue. (From Mills SE. Histology for Pathologists, 3rd ed. Philadelphia, PA: Lippincott Williams & Wilkins; 2007.)

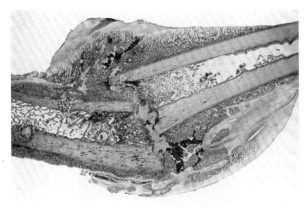

Light micrograph showing healing of a diaphyseal fracture under conditions of loading and motion. This femur fracture occurred in a pig that continued to use the limb for 3 weeks. Even though the fracture was not stabilized, it is healing. A large fracture callus consisting primarily of woven bone surrounds and unites the two fracture fragments. As the callus matures, it progressively stabilizes the fracture. Note that the fracture callus contains areas of mineralized and unmineralized cartilage. (From Bucholz RW, Heckman JD, eds. Rockwood and Green's Fractures in Adults, 5th ed. Philadelphia, PA: Lippincott Williams & Wilkins; 2001.)

Direct (Primary) Bone healing
- Fracture healing that results from rigid fixation
- Rigid fixation leads to fracture healing without the development of callus, granulation and the development of creeping substitution
- Fractures heal through the development of cutting cones (clusters of osteoclasts followed by osteoblasts) that extend across the fracture lines and deposit new bone
- Bone matrix enclosed osteocytes and blood vessels are formed in the setting of well formed lamellar bone across the fracture site

- Primary means of fracture healing in rigidly fixed fractures (i.e., both bone forearm fractures and humeral shaft fractures)
- In order for fractures to heal the strain across the fracture line must not surpass the tolerance of the tissue as described by Perren (1979)
- Increasing strain favors formation of cartilage and fibrous tissue rather than bone formation

Recommended Readings

Buckwalter JA, et al. Bone biology II. Formation, form, modeling and remodeling. J Bone Joint Surg 1995;77A:1276–1289.

Einhorn TA. The cell and molecular biology of fracture healing. Clin Orthop Relat Res 1998;(335 Suppl):S7–S21.

Perren SM. Physical and biological aspects of fracture healing with special reference to internal fixation. Clin Orthop Relat Res 1979; 138:175–196.

White AA, et al. The four biomechanical stages of fracture repair. J Bone Joint Surg 1977;59A:188–192.

Osteomyelitis—Adult

Background
- Infectious processes of the bone represent pathology that can result in severe disability and long-term morbidity
- Treatment is directed based on the depth and timing of the infection, in addition to the medical status of the patient
- Adequate cultures, organisms and treatment regimens are necessary for true eradication of the infection

Physical Exam
- Patients often present with a remote/acute history of trauma or operative intervention
- Recent systemic illness
- Report pain, swelling, or erythema at a previous operative site or the site of trauma

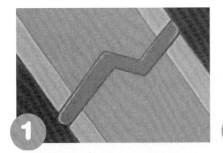

A broken bone starts to heal itself right away. The blood vessels send a protective material into the break. This helps new bone cells grow and stick together

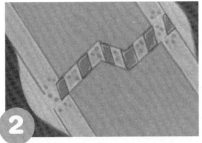

Next, a layer of hard bony material forms a lump around the break like a natural cast. This holds it together while the new bone cells make bone that grows into the break

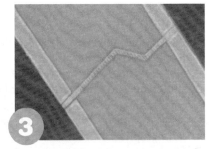

The bone fills in the break. The bump of bony tissue is bemoved by other bone cells. The bone is back in shape.

Healing broken bones. (From ACC Pediatric Image Collection, 2009-02-02 0850, Skeletal System, Anatomical Chart Company.)

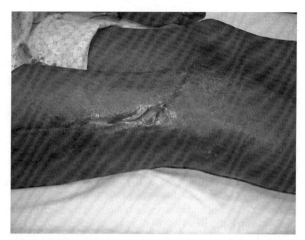

Typical appearance of a postoperative wound. The limb looks relatively benign. This patient had an extensive type III infection and had been treated with attempted debridement on several occasions before referral. Poor nutrition and nicotine use together with her previous multiple surgeries made her a B systemic/local host. (From Bucholz RW, Court-Brown CM, Heckman JD, et al. *Rockwood & Green's Fractures in Adults*, 7th ed. Philadelphia: Lippincott, Williams & Wilkins, 2010.)

- Timing of symptoms should be determined based on the history
- A complete medical history of the patient should be performed to rule out any concomitant cause of immunosuppression or factor that may contribute to an increased propensity for infection

Laboratory Evaluation
- Complete blood count
- Erythrocyte sedimentation rate (ESR): Elevated for up several weeks following infection and treatment
- C-reactive protein: Most sensitive measurement of acute infection as well as response to treatment
- Blood cultures can be performed initially to rule out septicemia or systemic illness

Imaging
- **Radiographs:** May take weeks before showing any signs of acute infection
  - In the setting of previous surgery, close attention should be paid to any broken hardware or lucencies surrounding screws or screw plate interfaces
  - 30%–50% matrix must be lost to see lytic lesion on radiographs
- **Bone scan:** sensitive but unspecific
  - Three phased bone scans increase specificity of the test
    - Flow = angiogram
    - Equilibrium—extracellular space
    - Delayed—osteoblast uptake

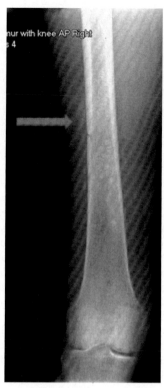

The arrow points to periosteal reaction. (From Bucholz RW, Court-Brown CM, Heckman JD, et al. *Rockwood & Green's Fractures in Adults*, 7th ed. Philadelphia: Lippincott, Williams & Wilkins, 2010.)

- All three phases are hot in cases of osteomyelitis (OM)
- **Indium white blood cell (WBC) scan**
  - Very sensitive for OM
  - Although extremely sensitive OM, may be less sensitive in chronic OM because response is mainly lymphocytic at that point and Indium scan labels neutrophils
- Magnetic resonance imaging (MRI): Provides evaluation of early marrow/bone changes treatment

Classification
- Classification previously based on timing of infection/ presentation
- Multiple factors must be considered in the evaluation of these patients
  - Time: acute/subacute/chronic
  - Source: hematogenous/exogenous
- Cierney described a classification that takes into account both patient and location, as shown below
  - Cierney's host types
    - A—normal, nonsmoker
    - B—mild systemic deficient, smoker
    - C—major nutritional, systemic disorder
  - Cierney's anatomic classification

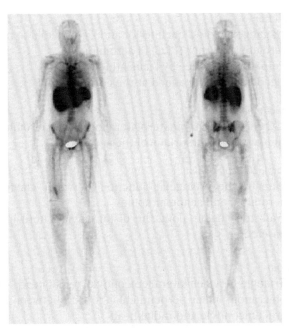

White cell scan of patient in Figure 24-6 demonstrating increased accumulation of tracer in distal femur. (From Bucholz RW, Court-Brown CM, Heckman JD, et al. *Rockwood & Green's Fractures in Adults*, 7th ed. Philadelphia: Lippincott, Williams & Wilkins, 2010.)

- Medullary (IM nail)
- Superficial (decubitus)
- Localized (mechanically stable)
- Diffuse (mechanically unstable)

Organisms
- 0–4 mo
  - Most common: *Staphylococcus aureus*, gram-negative bacilli, group B streptococcus
  - Oxacillin/nafcillin/vancomycin and a third-generation cephalosporin
- >4 yr
  - Most common: *S. aureus*, group A streptococcus, coliforms
  - Oxacillin/nafcillin/vancomycin/clindamycin
  - Add third-generation cephalosporin if Gram stain contains gram-negative organism
- >21 yr
  - Most common: *S. aureus*
  - Nafcillin/oxacillin/cefazolin (Ancef)/vancomycin
- IV drug abusers, hemodialysis—*Pseudomonas* > vancomycin + ciprofloxacin (Cipro)
- Sickle—*Salmonella* > ciprofloxacin (Cipro)
  - *S. aureus* still most common
- For patients previously or currently on antibiotics, think fungal
- Acute OM after open fracture or ORIF
  - Most common: *S. aureus, Pseudomonas*, coliform

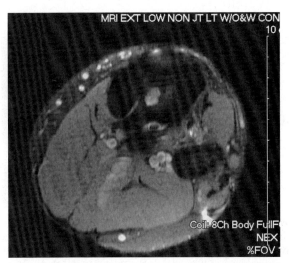

Magnetic resonance image of infected tibia with sinus tract leading to central sequestrum (white area in medullary canal). (From Bucholz RW, Court-Brown CM, Heckman JD, et al. *Rockwood & Green's Fractures in Adults*, 7th ed. Philadelphia: Lippincott, Williams & Wilkins, 2010.)

  - Nafcillin + ciprofloxacin (Cipro), or vancomycin + third-generation cephalosporin
  - Peripheral vascular disease and immunocompromised will likely be polymicrobial
- Chronic OM
  - Operative sample from multiple foci needed to get correct bug
  - Empiric treatment is not indicated
  - Most common: *S. aureus, Enterobacter, Pseudomonas*
- Subacute OM
  - Brodie's abscess may be present on radiographs: differential diagnosis includes Ewing's sarcoma
- Metaphyseal brodie's abscess must curetted to collect adequate culture sample
- Epiphyseal brodie's abscess
  - Differential diagnosis chondroblastoma
- Irrigation and debridement if purulence present
- Patient will likely require IV antibiotics for definitive treatments directed at cultures/sensitivities

Radiographic Changes
- Soft tissue swelling—early
- Osteopenia—10–14 days
- Involucrum—bone formed beneath elevated periosteum, surrounding sequestrum
- Sequestrum—necrotic bone often with denser surrounding bone
- Brodie's abscess—cystic within medullary canal, high signal on T2, surrounded by sclerotic bone

Surgical Indications
- Visible collection on imaging
- Debridement necessary to prevent further destruction

Involucrum   Living

Dead

The appearance of bone at debridement. Note that the living bone has a pinkish hue and a petechial appearance indicating vascularity. The surrounding bone is involucrum and is also vascular. Resection of the involucrum should be at the judgment of the surgeon. The dead bone is clearly avascular and requires resection. (From Bucholz RW, Court- Brown CM, Heckman JD, et al. *Rockwood & Green's Fractures in Adults*, 7th ed. Philadelphia: Lippincott, Williams & Wilkins, 2010.)

- Refractory cases which do not respond to antibiotic treatment
- Chronic OM may require debridement of dead, non-viable, bone and soft tissue to re-establish a healthy environment

Arthrocentesis/Injections
- Essential tool for evaluation of septic joints, traumatic arthrotomies, and performing pain-relieving injections

Aspirations
- Care must be taken to maintain sterility while performing arthrocentesis
    - Laboratories to send
        - Cell culture and Gram stain (small amount of sample required)
        - Cell count
        - Crystals

Injections
- Water-soluble steroids have shorter half-lives than water insoluble steroids
- Most soluble: celestone > depomedrol > kenalog
- Use soluble for acute traumatic injuries and insoluble for chronic injuries or arthritis

Shoulder
Anterior
- 18-gauge needle 1 cm lateral to coracoid
- Palpate the joint space by translating head anteriorly and posteriorly, entering joint with minimal resistance

Posterior
- 18-gauge needle 2 cm inferior and 2 cm medial to posterolateral corner (PLC) of acromion
- Palpate joint space by translating head
- Needle should be aimed at the coracoid

Subacromial Space
- 1–2 cm inferior to posterolateral or lateral acromion
- Aim at the undersurface of the acromion

Acromioclavicular Joint
- Palpate the triangular junction between clavicle, acromion, and scapular spine
- Walk the needle along the distal clavicle until joint entered

Elbow
- Triangle between lateral epicondyle, radial head, and olecranon; inject perpendicular to skin between lateral epicondyle and radial head

Wrist
- Palpate Lister's tubercle between the third and fourth dorsal compartment.
- Flex the wrist to distract the joint space

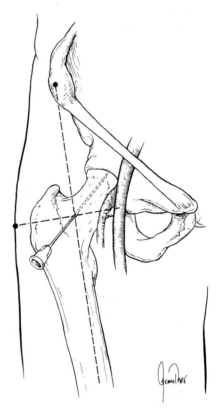

Right hip. (From Koopman WJ, Moreland LW, eds. Arthritis and Allied Conditions: A Textbook of Rheumatology, 15th ed. Philadelphia, PA: Lippincott Williams & Wilkins; 2005, with permission.)

- Hip aspirations should be performed under fluoroscopic guidance

Anterior Approach
- Visualize a line from anterior superior iliac spine (ASIS) to pubic tubercle
- Palpate the femoral artery along this line
- Entry point is 2–3 cm lateral to the femoral artery and 2–3 cm inferior to the ASIS to this point
- Aim needle posteromedial until palpating bone

Lateral Approach
- Palpate the greater trochanter (GT)
- Entry point is anterior and superior to trochlear tip
- Upon entering, slide medial and cephalad along femoral neck

Medial Approach
- Hip should be abducted, externally rotated and flexed
- Palpate the adductor tendon
- Needle should be inserted under the abductor tendon aiming superomedially until contacting the femoral neck

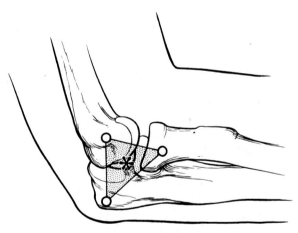

The landmarks for aspiration of the elbow joint are the radial head, lateral epicondyle, and tip of the olecranon. A needle inserted into the center of the triangle (asterisk) penetrates only the anconeus muscle and capsule before entering the joint. (From Bucholz RW, Heckman JD, eds. Rockwood and Green's Fractures in Adults, 5th ed. Philadelphia, PA: Lippincott Williams & Wilkins; 2001, with permission.)

Ankle
- Palapate the tibialis anterior
- Palapate the soft space just medial to the tibialis anterior while the foot is dorsiflexed.
- Aim the needle toward the center of the joint
- Care should be taken to avoid damage to the talar head

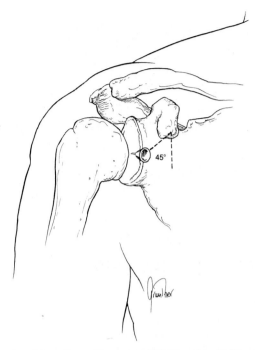

Right shoulder. (From Koopman WJ, Moreland LW, eds. Arthritis and Allied Conditions: A Textbook of Rheumatology, 15th ed. Philadelphia, PA: Lippincott Williams & Wilkins; 2005, with permission.)

- Insert the needle in line with the radius' dorsal tilt
- Palpate the space between fourth and fifth dorsal compartment (extensor digiti quinti tendon) or ulnar or radial to the sixth dorsal compartment (extensor carpi ulnaris tendon [ECU])
- Aim needle into the distracted joint space

Hip
- Anatomy can be remembered with the pneumonic NAVEL (femoral **N**erve, femoral **A**rtery, femoral **V**ein, **E**mpty space, **L**ymph nodes)

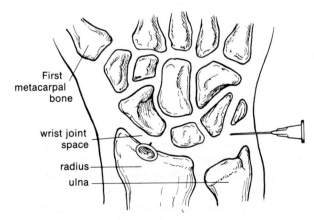

Right wrist. (From Koopman WJ, Moreland LW, eds. Arthritis and Allied Conditions: A Textbook of Rheumatology, 15th ed. Philadelphia, PA: Lippincott Williams & Wilkins; 2005, with permission.)

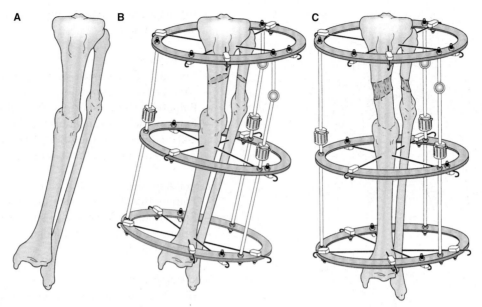

Malunion. **A:** Schematic depiction of malunited fractures of the tibia and fibula with unacceptable shortening and varus deformity. **B:** The use of the Ilizarov technique, proximal corticotomies, and appropriate positioning of external fixator rings with transfixation pins followed by gradual distraction (1 mm/day) and simultaneous correction of malunion. **C:** The angulation and shortening were both corrected, and healing of the histogenesis site has occurred. (From Mulholland MW, et al., eds. Greenfield's Surgery Scientific Principles and Practice, 4th ed. Philadelphia, PA: Lippincott Williams & Wilkins; 2006.)

Ring Fixator/Ilizarov Method

Background
- Additional means of fracture fixation in patients with soft tissue that precludes ORIF
- Fracture fixation performed through a combination of tensioned wires and 5-mm half pins
- Circular fixators in association with computerized alignment programs allow for correction of angular deformity in addition to acute fracture management
- All for distraction osteogenesis in patients with significant bone loss, or nonviable bone which must be excised
- Goal of application and treatment is to minimize periosteal stripping and limit disruption of fracture hematoma

Histology
- Fractures heal through intramembranous ossification, but compression can be applied across fracture sites utilizing the frame
- Fibrin hematoma, inflammatory cells during latency
- Vascular sinusoids formed via mesenchymal cell organization during start of distraction
- With continued distraction, becomes less vascular and fibrous tissue bridge forms
- Microcolumns of bone form, surrounded by thin walled sinusoids

- Number of vasovasorum increase in arteries crossing osteotomy site

Stability
- Increased wire diameter
- Increased wire tension
- Orthogonal pins
- Decreased ring to bone distance
- Multiple wires
- Olive wires
- Near apposition of ring and fracture site
- Adequate centering of the bone in the ring

Distraction Osteogenesis
- Latency 3–10 days following the procedure in some protocols
- Distraction is then initiated at 1 mm/day (0.25 mm four times a day)
- Consolidation: Once the desired length is achieved, patients must wait approximately 1 mo/cm for consolidation of the regenerate
- Different ideal distraction rates for different tissue types
- Nerve palsies and joint contractures can occur in patients who are distracted too quickly
- Following completion of distraction and removal of frame, contracture releases can be performed if necessary

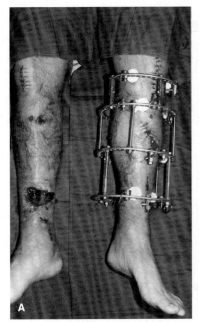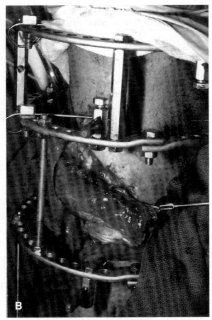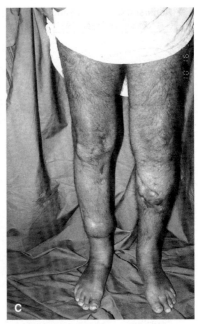

A: Patient with bilateral injuries. On the right leg, the distal third required free muscle transfer in the form of latissimus dorsi muscle flap covered with a split-thickness skin graft. The patient's left leg was stabilized with an Ilizarov fixator. The middle-third lesion required a hemisoleus transfer. **B:** The arc of rotation is seen. **C:** Patient standing at 9 months follow-up with both legs healed. (From Bucholz RW, Heckman JD, eds. Rockwood and Green's Fractures in Adults, 5th ed. Philadelphia, PA: Lippincott Williams & Wilkins; 2001.)

- Bone transport has become another means of distraction osteogenesis
- The procedure can be combined with an intramedullary nail to decrease the weight-bearing limitations during the consolidation phase of treatment
- Ring fixators represent a valuable tool which can be applied in a variety of manners to improve fracture management

Recommended Readings

Cierny G 3rd, Zorn KE. Segmental tibial defects: comparing conventional and Ilizarov methodologies. Clin Orthop Relat Res 1994;301:118–123.
Fleming B, et al. A biomechanical analysis of the Ilizarov external fixator. Clin Orthop Relat Res 1989;(278):95–105.
Ilizarov GA. The tension-stress effect on the genesis and growth of tissues. I. The influence of stability of fixation and soft tissue preservation. Clin Orthop Relat Res 1989;238:249–281.
Ilizarov GA. The tension-stress effect on the genesis and growth of tissues. II. The influence of the rate and frequency of distraction. Clin Orthop Relat Res 1989;239:263–285.

Upper Extremity

CLAVICLE FRACTURE

- Common injury in young populations
- Increasing frequency with increased sports, and high-risk activity participation
- 2.6% of all fractures
- Previously treated almost exclusively nonoperatively unless open, skin tenting
- Operative treatment now increasing in frequency
- Injuries are commonly the result of a fall directly onto the shoulder
- Must evaluate for other associated injuries in cases of high-speed trauma

Classification

- Middle third (80%)
- Distal third (15%)
  - I—Interligamentous (stable)
  - II—Displaced due to fracture medial to coracoclavicular (CC) ligaments or fracture with disruption of all or part of CC ligaments → **high nonunion** with superiorly displaced medial clavicle
  - III—Intra-articular AC joint
  - IV—Ligaments attached to periosteum, proximal fragment displaced
  - V—Comminuted
- Medial third (5%)
  - I—Minimal displacement (sternoclavicular [SC] ligament intact)

Robinson Cortical Alignment Fracture (Type 2A)

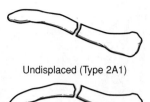

Undisplaced (Type 2A1)

Angulated (Type 2A2)

Robinson Displaced Fractures (Type 2B)

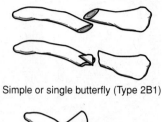

Simple or single butterfly (Type 2B1)

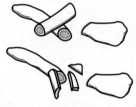

Segmental or comminuted (Type 2B2)

Allman Group I
Craig Group I

Robinson Cortical Alignment Fracture (Type 3A)

Extra-articular (Type 3A1)
Neer Type I
Craig Type I

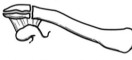

Intra-articular (Type 3A2)
Neer Type III
Craig Type III

Robinson Displaced Fractures (Type 3B)

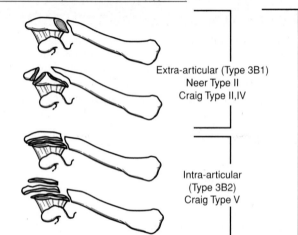

Extra-articular (Type 3B1)
Neer Type II
Craig Type II,IV

Intra-articular
(Type 3B2)
Craig Type V

Allman Group II
Craig Group II

Robinson Undisplaced Fractures (Type 1A)

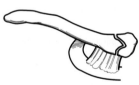

Extra-articular (Type 1A1)
Craig Type I

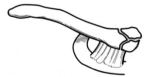

Intra-articular (Type 1A2)
Craig Type III

Robinson Displaced Fractures (Type 1B)

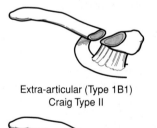

Extra-articular (Type 1B1)
Craig Type II

Extra-articular (Type 1B2)
Craig Type V

Allman Group III
Craig Group III

Clavicle fracture classification. (From Bucholz RW, Heckman JD, eds. Rockwood and Green's Fractures in Adults, 5th ed. Philadelphia, PA: Lippincott Williams & Wilkins; 2001, with permission.)

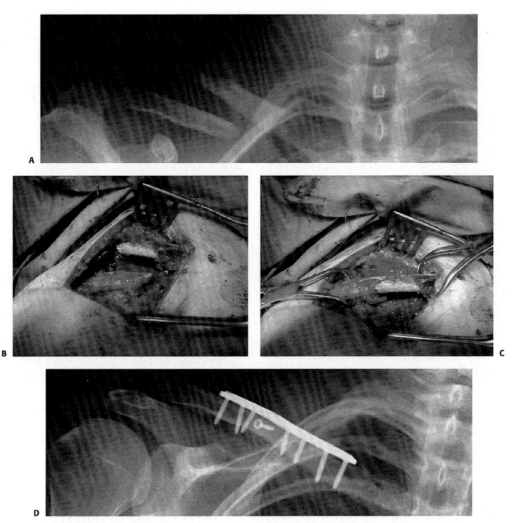

A: Anteroposterior radiograph of a displaced midshaft clavicle fracture. Note the difference in diameter of the proximal and distal fragments at the fracture site, suggesting that a significant degree of rotation has occurred. **B:** Intraoperative photograph of a displaced fracture, **(C)** reduced anatomically and held with a small fragment reduction forceps. **D:** Postoperative radiograph after open reduction and internal fixation with an anterior-to-posterior lag screw followed by fixation with an anatomic plate. (From Bucholz RW, Court-Brown CM, Heckman JD, Tornetta P. Rockwood & Green's Fractures in Adults, 7th ed. Philadelphia: Lippincott Williams & Wilkins; 2010.)

- II—displaced (SC ligament ruptured)
- III—intra-articular
- IV—Salter I
- V—Comminuted

Anatomy
- Bone with earliest ossification (5 wk in utero)
- Only long bone formed from intramembranous ossification without interval cartilage stage
- Medial growth plate closes last
- 80% growth occurs from the medial growth plate
- Flat when viewed anteroposterior (AP)
- S shaped when viewed from above
- Lacks a well-defined medullary cavity

- Stability maintained by ligamentous attachments to the shoulder girdle
- SC ligament maintains stability of the sternoclavicular ligament
- CC ligament is composed of the trapezoid and conoid ligaments
- CC ligaments are resist superior displacement of the clavicle

Radiographs
- AP of clavicle (angled 20 degrees superiorly)
- AP of chest can be utilized to evaluate shortening with the contralateral clavicle as a reference

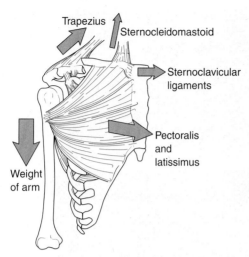

The displacing forces on a lateral clavicle fracture. (From Bucholz RW, Heckman JD, eds. Rockwood and Green's Fractures in Adults, 5th ed. Philadelphia, PA: Lippincott Williams & Wilkins; 2001, with permission.)

- Zanca view: Radiograph centered on AC joint with 15 degrees of cephalic tilt
- Consider CT scan for sternoclavicular dislocations or comminuted fractures

SC Dislocation
- Must differentiate physeal injury from SC dislocation
- 45-degree cephalic tilt view to see SC dislocation anterior vs. posterior
- Painful irreducible SC dislocation can be treated with distal clavicle resection if anterior/painful or posterior/unstable

- No more than 1.5 cm of clavicle can be resected to maintain the costoclavicular ligament attaches
- Nonunions most common in middle third, because most common fracture area
- Distal third: Most prone to nonunion

Functions
- Provides stability and power of upper extremity
- Forms the bony articulation which connects the axial skeleton to the upper limb
- Maintains appropriate lever arm for the upper extremity
- Protects the underlying neurovascular structures

Nonoperative Treatment vs. Operative Treatment
- Historically treatment has consisted of figure-of-eight sling and nonoperative management
- Neer (1960) showed a nonunion rate of 0.1% for nonoperative and 4.6% for operative fractures in a series of unstratified clavicle fractures
- Eskola (1986) a similar rate of union, but the clavicle fractures in the study had >15 mm of associated shortening
- Nordqvist (1998) evaluated patient outcomes in patients treated nonoperatively at 17 yr of follow and showed
  - Undisplaced fractures → 100% good/excellent outcomes
  - Fractures with no cortical contact → 83% good/excellent outcomes

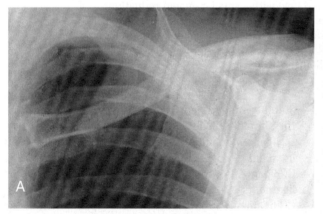
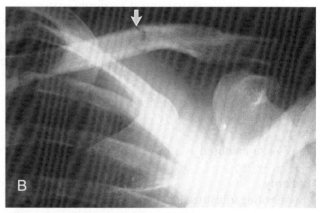

Clavicle fracture evaluation: angulated vs. nonangulated projections. **A:** Nonangulated anteroposterior clavicle. Note that no fracture line is visible on this view. **B:** Angulated clavicle. Observe that with 15-degree cephalad tube angulation, the fracture line is clearly evident (arrow). COMMENT: In evaluation of clavicular trauma, specific clavicle projections must be obtained to demonstrate fractures, particularly through the midportion of the clavicle. (Courtesy of Kenneth E. Yochum, D.C., St. Louis, Missouri.)

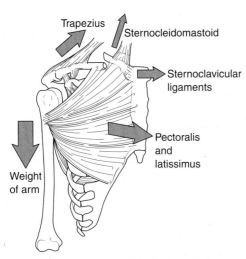

The displacing forces on a midshaft clavicle fracture. (From Bucholz RW, Heckman JD, eds. Rockwood and Green's Fractures in Adults, 5th ed. Philadelphia, PA: Lippincott Williams & Wilkins; 2001, with permission.)

- Fractures with an intermediary fragment → 73% good/excellent outcomes
- Treatment is now shifting toward operative management for specific indications
  - > 2 cm of shortening
  - > 2 cm of displacement
  - Significant comminution
  - Segmental fractures
  - Open fractures or fractures with tenting skin
- McKee (2006) showed that nonoperative treatment of displaced midshaft clavicle fractures were associated with significant disability:
  - Reduction in maximal abduction
  - Reduction in maximal internal rotation,
  - Worse Disabilities of the Arm, Shoulder, and Hand (DASH) score
  - Worse internal rotation and abduction endurance
- In a multicentered prospective randomized clinical trial, the Canadian Orthopaedic Trauma Society showed that patients who underwent operative fixation of displaced midshaft fractures had better DASH scores, faster time to union, decreased rate of symptomatic nonunions, and improved shoulder aesthetics

Or Tips and Tricks—Clavicle
- Incision along Langer's lines
- Incise platysma
- Supraclavicular nerves should be avoided to limit incisional parasthesias/numbness
- Fracture hematoma should be cleared with care taken not to completely strip the periosteum

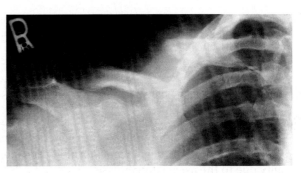

This x-ray shows the significant displacement that can occur particularly in the adult's fractured clavicle when the weight of the arm pulls the lateral fragment downward. (Modified from Connolly J. Fractures and Dislocations: Closed Management. Philadelphia, PA: WB Saunders; 1995, with permission.)

- Fix segmental piece to either medial or lateral fragments with 2.0- or 2.4-mm lag screw
- Small pointed reduction clamps applied to the fragments can be utilized for reduction of the fracture
- 2.4-mm locking compression plate can be placed anteriorly to act as a washer for fracture reduction.
- Apply 2.7 reconstruction plate superiorly to improve rotational control and fracture stability.
- 90:90 plating can be applied for increased stability when utilizing mini-fragment plates
- Precontoured 3.5 plates can be utilized, but due to the high variability of clavicle anatomy, the plate may not be appropriately contoured
- Six cortices should be completed on each side of the fracture
- Dimeneralized bone matrix may be included in extremely comminuted fractures to improve fracture healing rates

Recommended Readings
Canadian Orthopaedic Trauma Society. Nonoperative treatment compared with plate fixation of displaced midshaft clavicular fractures. A multicenter, randomized clavicular fractures. JBJS 2007;89-A(1);1–10.

Eskola, A et al. Surgery for ununited clavicular fracture. Acta Orthop Scand 1986;57:366–367.

Eskola A. Outcome of clavicular fractures in 89 patients. AOTS 1986;105(6):337–338.

McKee MD, et al. Deficits following nonoperative treatment of displaced midshaft clavicular fractures. JBJS 2006; 88-A(1): 35–40.

McKee MD, et al. Deficits following nonoperative treatment of displaced midshaft clavicular fractures. J Bone Joint Surg Am 2006;88(1):35–40.

Neer CS. Nonunion of the clavicle. JAMA 1960;172:1006–1011

Nordqvist A, Redlund-Johnell I. Mid-clavicle fractures in adults: ed result study after conservative treatment. J ORTHOP TRAUMA1998;12(8):572–576.

Zlowodzki M, et al. Treatment of acute midshaft clavicle fractures: systematic review of 2144 fractures. J Orthop Trauma 2005;19(7):504–507.

SCAPULAR FRACTURES

Background
- These fractures result from high-energy mechanisms and are associated with significant morbidity and mortality due to the associated injuries
- Patients presenting with these injuries often require ATLS protocols for stabilization and management of associated injuries
- The prevalence of scapular fractures is 1%
- These fractures most commonly result from high-energy blunt trauma but may also occur as a result of traction injury
- Rib fractures are the most common associated injury followed by head and chest/pulmonary injuries

History and Physical
- ATLS should utilized for first evaluation of these patients
- A detailed neurovascular exam should be performed, as 5%–13% of patients with scapular fractures may present with an associated brachial plexus injury
- 11% of patients report arterial injuries, so pulses should be documented carefully

Imaging
- AP chest radiograph, true AP scapula, and lateral of the scapula should be performed
- Additionally patients should undergo an axillary view of the shoulder or valpeau if the patient cannot tolerate an axillary
- The stryker notch view can be utilized to visualize the corocoid
  - Performed with the patient supine and the elbow flexed with the hand placed over the patient's head
  - The beam is directed caudally 10 degrees and centered over the coracoid process
- A West Point lateral or apical oblique allows visualization of glenoid rim fractures
  - Performed with the patient positioned prone with the injured shoulder abducted 90 degrees with the hand and forearm resting over the edge of the table.
  - The beam is aimed 25 degrees from horizontal to the table and 25 degrees medial to the patient's midline

- CT scan with 3D reconstructions provide the best visualization of these fractures and provide valuable templates for preoperative planning

Classification
- See "Classification section (anatomic)"
- Glenoid fractures
- Ideberg Classification
  - I. Fractures that may cause glenohumeral instability and often result from glenohumeral dislocation
    - A. Anterior margin of the glenoid (>25% leads to instability)
    - B. Posterior Margin of the glenoid (>33% leads to instability)
    - Instability increased if fragment displaced greater than 1 cm
  - II. Fracture line extends from the glenoid fossa to the lateral boarder of the scapular body
    - ORIF indicated in fractures with > 5 mm of displacement
  - III. Fracture involving the superior third of the glenoid fossa, including the coracoid and extending through the superior scapular body to the scapular notch
    - ORIF indicated if >5 mm displacement present
  - IV. Fracture line divides the glenoid fossa in two parts
    - ORIF indicated if >5 mm displacement present
  - V. Highest injury classification
    - A. Combination of types II and IV
    - B. Combination of types III and IV
    - C. Combination of types II, III, and IV
- VI. Highest-energy fracture with two articular fragments present with either combined fracture type

Associated Injuries
- 96% had associated injury
- Upper thoracic rib fracture most common
- Pulmonary injury
- Hemopneumothorax
- Pulmonary contusion
- Head injury
- Skull fracture
- Ipsilateral clavicle fracture (floating shoulder)
- C-spine 12%
- Permanent cord injuries
- Brachial plexus injury

Treatment
- The majority of scapular fractures are treated nonoperatively

BONE: SCAPULA (14)

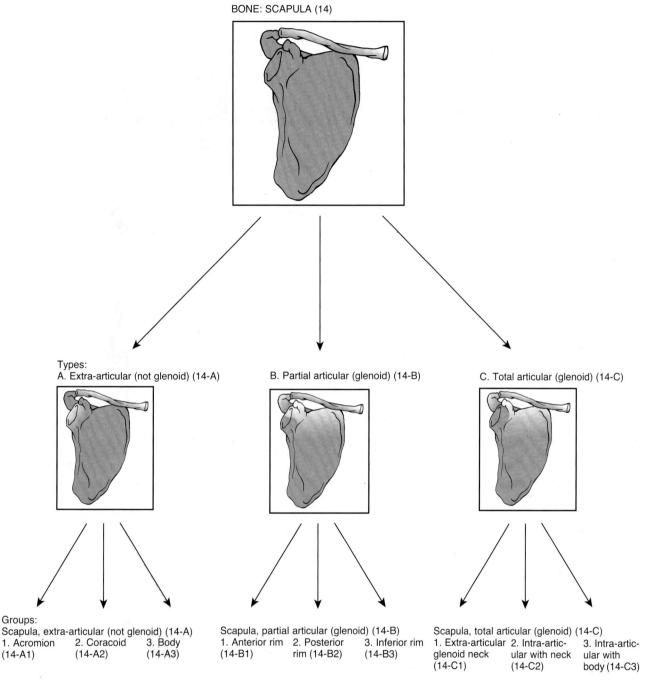

Types:
A. Extra-articular (not glenoid) (14-A)

B. Partial articular (glenoid) (14-B)

C. Total articular (glenoid) (14-C)

Groups:

Scapula, extra-articular (not glenoid) (14-A)
| 1. Acromion (14-A1) | 2. Coracoid (14-A2) | 3. Body (14-A3) |

Scapula, partial articular (glenoid) (14-B)
| 1. Anterior rim (14-B1) | 2. Posterior rim (14-B2) | 3. Inferior rim (14-B3) |

Scapula, total articular (glenoid) (14-C)
| 1. Extra-articular glenoid neck (14-C1) | 2. Intra-articular with neck (14-C2) | 3. Intra-articular with body (14-C3) |

The OTA classification of Scapular fractures. (From Bucholz RW, Court- Brown CM, Heckman JD, et al. *Rockwood & Green's Fractures in Adults*, 7th ed. Philadelphia: Lippincott, Williams & Wilkins, 2010.)

– Short-term immobilization is performed for most fractures followed by early range of motion (ROM) to improve return to function
– Due to the significant soft tissue attachments and blood supply, most fractures heal by 6 wk, alleviating the need for supportive slings

– Two reasons for high frequency of nonoperative treatment
  – Limited bone stock for hardware/fixation
  – Most fractures heal without intervention or loss of function

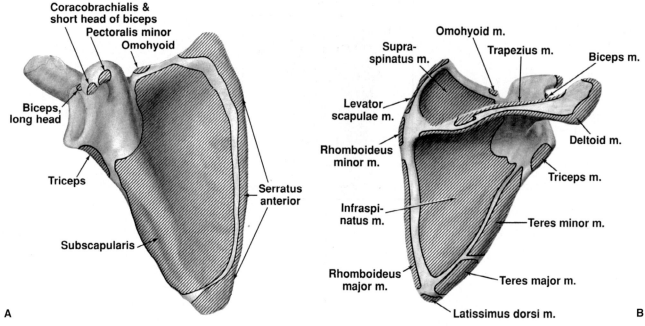

Muscle insertions onto the scapula. Anterior (**A**) and posterior (**B**) views. (From Bucholz RW, Court-Brown CM, Heckman JD, et al. *Rockwood & Green's Fractures in Adults*, 7th ed. Philadelphia: Lippincott, Williams & Wilkins, 2010.)

Surgical Indications
- >25% of glenoid involved with humeral subluxation
- Intra-articular step-off >5 mm
- >40-degree angulation or 1-cm translation of neck fracture with excessive medialization of glenoid
- Double disruption of the superior shoulder suspensory complex

Open Reduction Internal Fixation
- The goals of operative intervention are the reestablish the articular surface of the glenoid and its relationship with the scapula to maintain adequate glenohumeral mechanics
- By restoring the glenoid fossa, glenohumeral instability should be improved

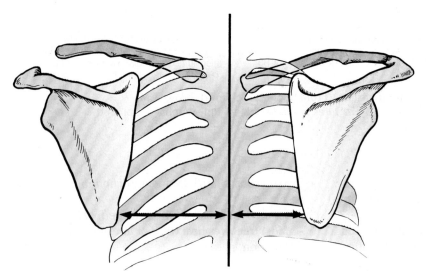

The diagnosis of scapulothoracic dissociation can be made on an AP radiograph by comparing the distance from the medial border of the scapula with the spinous processes between the affected (long arrow) and unaffected (short arrow) sides. Kelbel et al. 86 created the scapula index and reported a normal value to be a ratio of 1.07. (From Bucholz RW, Court-Brown CM, Heckman JD, et al. *Rockwood & Green's Fractures in Adults*, 7th ed. Philadelphia: Lippincott, Williams & Wilkins, 2010.)

- The primary regions where bone stock is strong enough to maintain internal fixation are
  - The glenoid neck
  - The scapular spine
  - The scapular border
  - The coracoid process
- A combination of appropriately contoured 3.5, 2.7, and 2.4 mm reconstruction plates provide excellent fixation

Scapulothoracic Dissociation

- Complete lateral displacement of the scapula and upper extremity from the axial skeleton with intact skin
- Results from high-energy rotational or traction force of the shoulder girdle
- Injury associated with a high incidence of neurologic injury (up to 94% with brachial plexus injury)
- 88%–100% of patients have an associated vascular injury
- Mortality rate with this injury is 10%
- Advance trauma life support (ATLS) protocols should be utilized in the evaluation of these patients to maintain hemodynamic stability
- AP chest radiograph shows scapular edge laterally displaced on nonrotated chest radiograph
- May have multiple associated musculoskeletal injuries including clavicle fractures, sternoclavicular dislocation, acromioclavicular separation, deltoid tear, pectoralis tear, or other muscles of the shoulder girdle
- Angiography may be required in those patients with vascular injuries once stabilized
- Goals of treatment are the re-establish the vascularity, stabilized the bone framework to improve functionality, protect the brachial plexus, and prevent nonunion/malunion

Outcomes/Complications

- The majority of scapular fractures are treated nonoperatively, with good to excellent results regarding return to function
- Displaced or malunited glenoid fractures may lead to glenohumeral arthritis or glenohumeral instability
- The most common complication of operative intervention is the need for removal of hardware secondary to pain
- Physical therapy is crucial for return to function in these patients
- Due to the infrequency of operative treatment of these injuries, most complication rates are based on small case series

BRACHIAL PLEXUS INJURY

Background

- Approximately 70% of traumatic injuries are due to motor vehicle accidents
- Can be the result of traction injuries, direct trauma, ore fracture
- Injury leads to significant physical disability and emotional distress
- Limitations following injury can be devastating
- Most injuries are treated closed initially and followed for progressive recovery
- GSW is not an indication for exploration because most are neurapraxia (vibration injury)
- Primary exploration indicated for
  - Sharp penetrating trauma
  - Open bony injury
  - Progressive neurologic deficit
  - Expanding hematoma
  - Vascular injury
- Better functional outcome with upper injury because the hand is preserved

Pre- vs. Postganglionic Injury

- Preganglionic
  - Cell body of distal root ganglion still attached to axon, thus sensory conduction intact
  - Flail arm, Horner's, scapular winging, weak rhomboids, diaphragm paralysis
  - Traumatic meningoceles
  - Nerves to paraspinals come off just distal to ganglion, thus atrophy in preganglionic injury
- Postganglionic
  - Only flail arm
  - Normal myelography
  - Motor and sensory conduction absent
  - Normal cervical paraspinal muscles

Surgical Management

- Surgical intervention is dependent on three factors
  1. Patient population
  2. Timing
     - Early intervention for high root injuries at 3–6 wk
     - Routine exploration at 3–6 mo postinjury
  3. Reconstructive priorities
- Elbow flexion
- Shoulder abduction
- Hand sensation
- Wrist extension, finger flexion
- Wrist flexion, finger extension
- Intrinsics

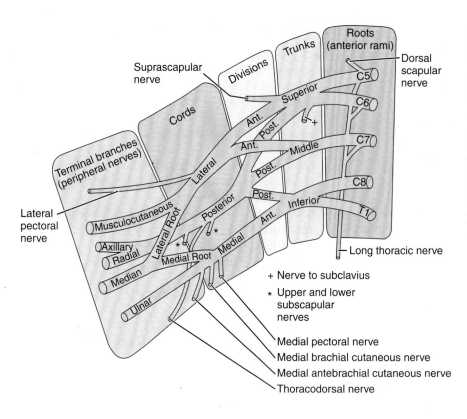

Schematic design of the brachial plexus. The many named components of this intricate plexus all serve the muscles of the upper extremity. The division of each trunk into anterior and posterior halves matches the opposition of the muscles of flexion (all served by anterior-division nerves) and the muscles of extension (all served by posterior-division nerves). (From Moore KL, Dalley AF, eds. Clinically Oriented Anatomy, 5th ed. Baltimore, MD: Lippincott Williams & Wilkins; 2006, with permission.)

+ Nerve to subclavius
* Upper and lower subscapular nerves

Reconstructive Options
- Nerve repair in acute sharp injury
- Nerve graft—sural, ipsilateral cutaneous, ipsilateral vascularized ulnar
- Neurotization (intact nerve sewn into stump of intact distal nerve)—cranial nerve XI, phrenic, intercostals, contralateral C7
- Gracilis free muscle transfer

Recommended Readings

Chuang DC, et al. Cross-chest C7 nerve grafting followed by free muscle transplantation for the treatment of avulsed brachial plexus injuries. Plast Reconstr Surg 1993;92:717.

Millesi H, et al. Further experience with interfascicular grafting of the median, ulnar and radial nerves. J Bone Joint Surg Am 1976;58:209.

Sturm JT, Perry JF Jr. Brachial plexus injuries from blunt trauma—a harbinger of vascular and thoracic injury. Ann Emerg Med 1987;16(4):404–406.

PROXIMAL HUMERUS FRACTURES

Background
- Common injury that is currently increasing in frequency with the country's aging population
- A large portion of these injuries are treated nonoperatively, but those which require fixation can lead to significant debilitation if not treated appropriately

- Annual incidence of injury is between 63 and 105 per 100,000 people
- These injuries most commonly occur in elderly patients as a result of a low-energy fall
- >75% occur as the result of a low-energy osteoporotic patient fall
- The remaining injuries are the result of higher-energy mechanisms in younger patients, including motor vehicle accidents, sports, or other mechanisms

Anatomy
- The proximal humerus is composed of four major fragments
- The **greater tuberosity** is the insertion point for the supraspinatus and infraspinatus
- The **lesser tuberosity** is the insertion point for the subscapularis
- The **long head of the biceps** runs in the bicipital groove between the greater and lesser tuberosity and provides a valuable landmark during fracture fixation
- The **anatomic neck** represents division between the articular portion of the proximal humerus and the nonarticular portion
- The **surgical neck** is located just below the lesser and greater tuberosity

Blood Supply

- Historically, humeral head blood supply was thought to be from the artery of Laing (a terminal branch from anterior humeral circumflex artery), which runs in bicipital groove
- Recent data has shown that the posterior humeral circumflex provides 64% of the blood supply to the humeral head (Hettrich et al. 2010).
- Posterior blood flow supports the low probability of avascular necrosis (AVN) with proximal humerus fractures
- Most common sign of axillary artery injury is paresthesias rather than pulselessness

- Be aware of axillary artery injuries masquerading as axillary nerve injuries

Nerve Supply

- The axillary nerve is the primary structure at risk during operative fixation and proximal humerus fracture
- The nerve is located 6 cm distal to the acromion and travels along the anterior aspect of the surgical neck of the proximal humerus along with the anterior humeral circumflex artery
- Patients may present with inferior subluxation of the glenohumeral joint as a result of axillary nerve insult
- This subluxation resolves over time after return of axillary nerve function

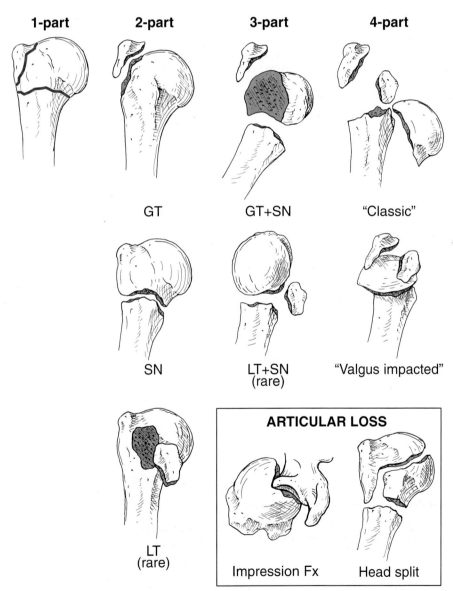

The Neer classification of proximal humerus fractures. (Reprinted with permission from Neer CS. Displaced proximal humeral fractures: I. Classification and evaluation. J Bone Joint Surg Am 1970;52:1077–1089.)

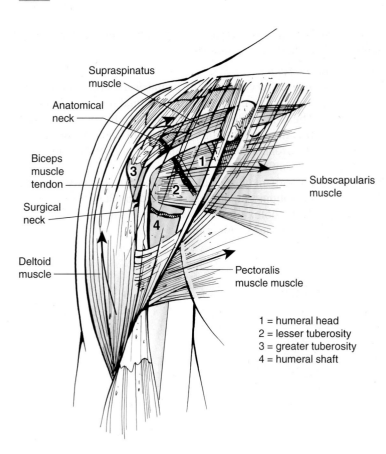

Supraspinatus muscle

Anatomical neck

Biceps muscle tendon

Surgical neck

Deltoid muscle

Subscapularis muscle

Pectoralis muscle muscle

1 = humeral head
2 = lesser tuberosity
3 = greater tuberosity
4 = humeral shaft

Displacement of the fracture fragments depends on the pull of the muscles of the rotator cuff and the pectoralis major. (From Bucholz RW, et al., eds. Rockwood and Green's Fractures in Adults, 6th ed. Philadelphia, PA: Lippincott Williams & Wilkins; 2006.)

Radiographs
- AP internal rotation, AP external, scapular Y, and axillary views should be performed
- AP films are Grashey views that are taken with 30-degree lateral oblique orientation tangential to the glenohumeral joint
- CT scan with 3D reconstructions allow detailed visualization for operative planning

Classifications
- Neer classification system based on a retrospective evaluation a series of proximal humerus fractures
- Fracture fragments are described as parts based on displacement and/or angulation
  - Greater tuberosity
  - Lesser tuberosity
  - Anatomic head
  - Surgical head
- A fracture part is defined as a one of the above fragments with >1 cm of displacement (0.5 cm in greater tuberosity fractures) or >45 degrees of angulation

Two Part

Surgical Neck
- Shaft pulled anteromedially by pectoralis
- Posterior angulation better tolerated than varus or anterior displacement

- Closed reduction and nonoperative treatment is the treatment of choice
- Early motion should be initiated at 4 wk
- If displaced, reduction/sling if stable
- If unstable/irreducible, ORIF should be performed
- If unstable, closed reduction and percutaneous pinning can be considered in some patients

Anatomic Neck
- Rarely occur in isolation

Greater Tuberosity
- Supraspinatus, infraspinatus, teres minor pull fragment posterosuperiorly leading to displacement in most injuries
- ORIF should be performed if >5-mm displacement
- Subacromial impingement may occur in displaced fragments leading to a block of external rotation and abduction.

Lesser Tuberosity
- Rarely occur in isolation, but when present, likely the result of a posterior dislocation

Three Part
- In surgical neck/greater tuberosity, subscapularis internally rotates head to face posteriorly

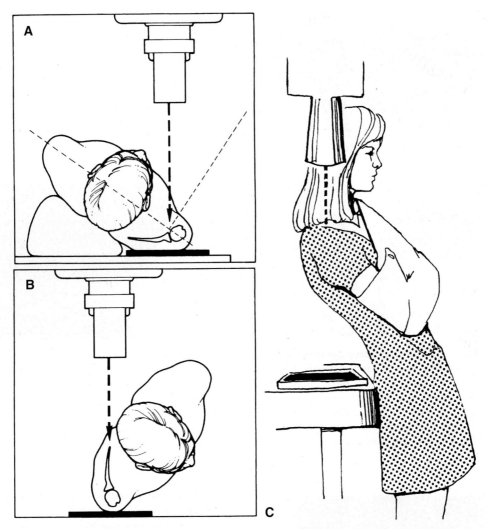

Trauma series. The trauma series consists of anteroposterior and lateral x-rays in the scapular plane as well as an axillary view. These views may be done with the patient sitting, standing, or prone. The lateral is called the tangential or Y-view of the scapula. This series allows evaluation of the fracture in three perpendicular planes so fracture displacement can be accurately assessed. The scapula sits obliquely on the chest wall, and the glenoid surface is tilted 35 to 40 degrees anteriorly. Therefore, the glenohumeral joint is not in the sagittal or the coronal plane. **A:** For the anteroposterior x-ray in the scapular plane, the posterior aspect of the affected shoulder is placed against the x-ray plate, and the opposite shoulder is tilted forward approximately 40 degrees. **B:** For the lateral x-ray in the scapular plane, the anterior aspect of the affected shoulder is placed against the x-ray plate, and the other shoulder is tilted forward approximately 40 degrees. The x-ray tube is then placed posteriorly along the scapular spine. **C:** The Velpeau axillary view is preferred after trauma when the patient can be positioned for this view, because it allows the shoulder to remain immobilized and avoids further displacement of the fracture fragments. (From Bucholz RW, Heckman JD, eds. Rockwood and Green's Fractures in Adults, 5th ed. Philadelphia, PA: Lippincott Williams & Wilkins; 2001.)

– In surgical neck/lesser tuberosity, cuff externally rotates head to face anteriorly
– In younger patients, fracture should undergo ORIF
– If displaced in older patient with limited functionality, hemiarthroplasty should be considered

Four Part
– Usually occur in elderly osteopenic
– ORIF can be performed with the assistance of a structural graft to provide increased stability (fibular allograft, endosteal plate) in addition to

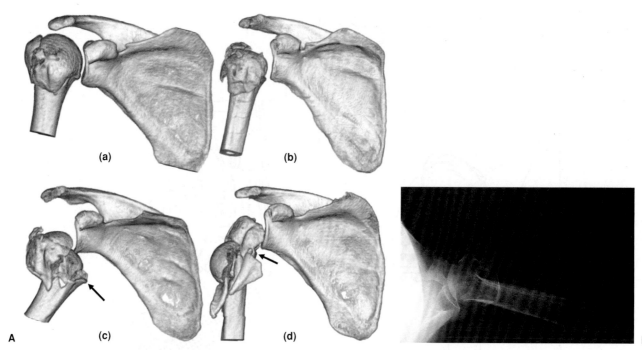

Three- and four-part varus fractures are less common than valgus injuries, and radiographically give rise to inferior subluxation of the humeral head on conventional radiography **(A)** and on three-dimensional reconstructions of computerised tomograms **(B)**. (A from Bucholz RW, et al., eds. Rockwood and Green's Fractures 97 in Adults, 7th ed. Philadelphia, PA: Lippincott Williams & Wilkins; 2010, B from From Koval KJ, Zuckerman JD. Atlas of Orthopaedic Surgery: A Multimedia Reference. Philadelphia, PA: Lippincott Williams & Wilkins; 2004 with permission.)

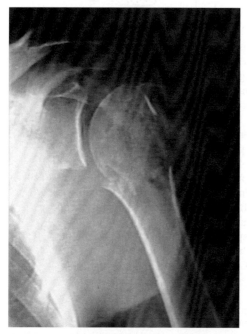

Hemiarthroplasty of the proximal humerus. Anteroposterior view. (From Koval KJ, Zuckerman JD. Atlas of Orthopaedic Surgery: A Multimedia Reference. Philadelphia, PA: Lippincott Williams & Wilkins; 2004.)

the proximal humeral locking plate (angular stable device)
- Hemiarthroplasty can be considered in patients with low functionality

Recommended Readings

Brooks CH, et al. Vascularity of the humeral head after proximal humeral fractures: an anatomical cadaver study. J Bone Joint Surg Br 1993;75:132–136.

Flatow EL, Bigliani LU. Open reduction and internal fixation of two-part displaced fractures of the greater tuberosity of the proximal part of the humerus. J Bone Joint Surg Am. 1991;73(8):1213–1218.

Hettrich CM, et al. Quantitative assessment of the vascularity of the proximal part of the humerus. J Bone Joint Surg 2010;92(4):943–948.

Neer CS. Displaced proximal humeral fractures. I. Classification and evaluation. J Bone Joint Surg Am 1970;52:1077–1089.

Treatment
Options
- Closed reduction, sling
- Closed reduction, percutaneous pins
- IM nail
- Tension band
  - Suture or wire

- Blade plate
- Cloverleaf plate
- Locking proximal humerus plate

Closed Reduction and Percutaneous Pinning
- Less commonly performed
- 2.5-mm threaded wires can be utilized in patients with contraindications to formal ORIF
- Should be reserved for simple surgical neck fractures
- Jaberg and Warner (1992) showed good to excellent results in 56% of patients

Locked Intramedullary Nail
- Provides additional less invasive method of treatment for surgical neck fractures
- Allows for early ROM
- Care should be taken to avoid radial nerve injury with insertion of distal interlocks

Blade Plate
- Utilized for revision fixation in addition to primary fracture treatment of proximal humerus fractures
- A blade plate is a technically demanding implant, which is highly successful when utilized appropriately
- Hinterman et al. (2000) evaluated 42 patients after treatment of displaced three- and four-part proximal humerus fractures
  - All fractures healed, and 30/41 patients had good or excellent results
  - The rate of AVN was 5% in the study

Proximal Humeral Locking Plate
- Now the most common method of fixation
- Locking plate technology provides an angular stable construct to combat the osteoporotic bone located in the humeral head
  - Augment with allograft fibula, which can be used as both a reduction device and structural strut

Recommended Readings
Hawkins RJ. The three-part fracture of the proximal part of the humerus. Operative treatment. J Bone Joint Surg Am. 1986;68(9):1410–1414.
Jaberg H, Warner JJ, Jakop RP. Percutaneous stabilization of unstable fractures of the humerus. J Bone Joint Surg 1992;74(4):508–515.
Lin J, et al. Locked nailing for displaced surgical neck fractures of the humerus. J Trauma 1998;45(6):1051–1057.
Rowles DJ, McGrory JE. Percutaneous pinning of the proximal part of the humerus. An anatomic study. J Bone Joint Surg 2001;83-A(11):1695–1699.

Hemiarthroplasty
- Utilized for patients with significant comminuition, articular extension or failed fixation

- Should also be considered in patients with limited functional requirements or inability to aggressively perform postoperative occupational therapy
- Goldman et al. (1995) showed a 75% rate of minor or no pain at 3 yr post hemiarthroplasty for 3/4 part proximal humerus fractures
- Despite improved pain control, functional recovery was somewhat unpredictable
- Activities requiring lifting, carrying weight or using the hand at or above the shoulder were limiting activities for many patients
- Norris and Green (1995) showed that late shoulder arthroplasty for malunion, or nonunion or proximal humerus fractures was more technically challenging and resulted in worse results
- Prosthetic arthroplasty reduced the shoulder pain in 95% of the patients.
  - Despite the improvement in pain and improved ROM, the final results were worse than those achieved by Goldman et al. in 1995

Or Tips and Tricks—Proximal Humerus
Deltopectoral
- C-arm can be positioned with the intensifier behind the humerus while the patient is placed in the beach chair position
- A bump can be placed under the elbow to abduct shoulder
- Incision is made from the coracoid to the deltoid insertion
- Locate the cephalic vein
- In trauma cases, cephalic vein often brought medially because the vein runs medial at distal aspect of extended exposure.
- Locate the deltoid insertion and detach 3 cm of it from bone from medial to lateral (leave small cuff for repair)
- Retract the deltoid
- The clavicopectoral fascia is continuous with corocoacromial ligament
- Incise the rotator interval, then elevate the head
- Tag and mobilize the lesser and greater tuberosities around the head
- Collagraft, allograft fibula, plexur or other bone graft substitute can be utilized to improve fixation in the humeral head
- The plate should be placed lateral, which can be difficult through this interval
- Following plating, repair the rotator interval and deltoid insertion

Anterolateral
- The palpable landmarks include the anterolateral aspect of the acromion and the lateral epicondyle

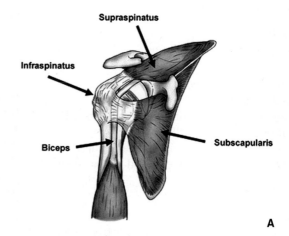

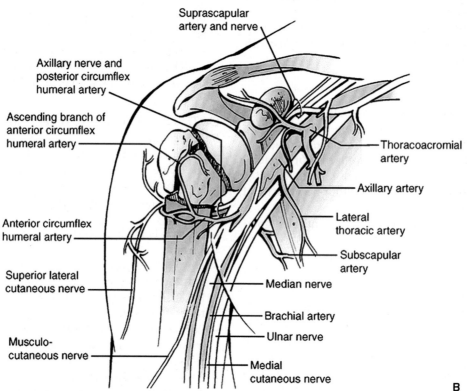

Soft-tissue anatomy of shoulder showing the rotator cuff musculature **(A)** and the neurovascular structures **(B)**. (From Bucholz RW, Court-Brown CM, Heckman JD, Tornetta P. Rockwood & Green's Fractures in Adults, 7th ed. Philadelphia, PA: Lippincott Williams & Wilkins, 2010.)

- A 10-cm incision should be made and taken down to the deltoid
- Dissection should be taken through the raphe separating the anterior and middle heads of the deltoid down to the level of the overlying bursa
- The axillary nerve should be maintained in a cuff of deltoid rather than fully dissecting the nerve from the surrounding soft tissues to provide additional protection

- Homan retractors can be placed anteriorly and posterior to exposure the humeral head
- Modified Mason-Allen sutures should be placed in the subscapularis, infraspinatus, and supraspinatus to allow for mobilization of the humeral head
- An appropriately sized fibula allograft can be contoured to provide structural support as well as assist with reduction

Incision is made from the coracoid to the deltoid insertion.

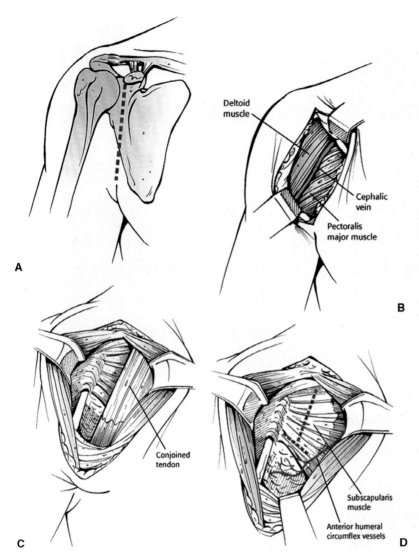

- Fibula should be potted medially and proximally utilizing a bone tamp
- Fibula should be oriented vertically in valgus fractures to maintain position and more angular in varus fractures to prevent failure into valgus orientation
- Following adequate positioning the proximal humeral locking plate can be fixed (oblong hole first) to the shaft
- Following shaft fixation, a second shaft screw can be placed to maintain rotation and fibular strut positioning
- Proximally, locking screws can be placed with care taken to capture the fibular strut to provide additional cortical fixation strength
- A cortical screw should be placed in the calcar screw position if the fibula is captured to enhance strength and ability to reduce the fracture

- Cuff sutures should be tied to the plate followed by layered closure
- ROM is initiated postoperative day 1 with a continuous passive motion machine for unlimited forward flexion

Or Tips and Tricks—Shoulder Hemiarthroplasty
- Release subdeltoid adhesions
- Define fracture with elevator
- Locate the biceps tendon. The lesser tuberosity is media and the greater tuberosity if lateral
- Tag the tuberosities at the bone-tendon junction with #5 Ethibond
- Take down the rotator interval as needed to allow for removal of the head

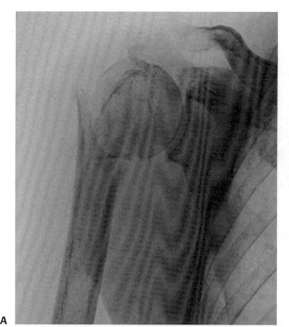

A

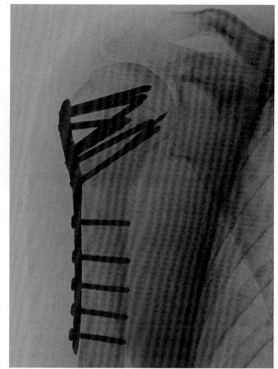

B

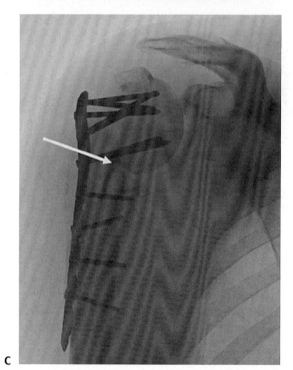

C

The defect produced after reduction of a varus displaced fracture **(A)** is larger on the side of the medial calcar (medially based triangular defect). These fractures require support from structural bone graft and low calcar screws as show in this case **(B)**. In another case, failure to provide adequate calcar support (arrow) resulted in early failure of the locking plate with the head falling back into varus **(C)**. (From Bucholz RW, Court-Brown CM, Heckman JD, Tornetta P. Rockwood & Green's Fractures in Adults, 7th ed. Philadelphia, PA: Lippincott Williams & Wilkins, 2010.)

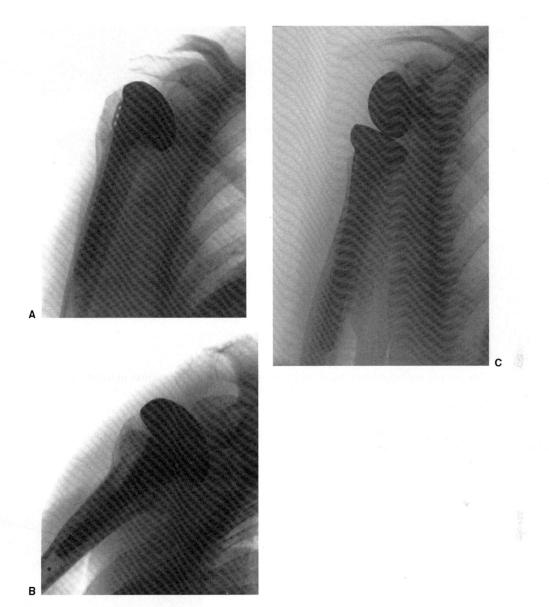

Nonreconstructable fractures may be treated with a humeral head arthroplasty. A conventional hemiarthroplasty may be associated with satisfactory shoulder function if the tuberosities heal, as shown in this case on anteroposterior and modified axial views **(A,B)**. Reverse shoulder arthroplasty joint is a newer technique, which does not rely on the integrity of the rotator cuff for function. The results of the use of this technique for acute fractures are largely unknown at present **(C)**. (From Bucholz RW, Court-Brown CM, Heckman JD, Tornetta P. Rockwood & Green's Fractures in Adults, 7th ed. Philadelphia, PA: Lippincott Williams & Wilkins, 2010.)

- Present the humerus shaft for reaming and broaching
- Place two drill holes in the shaft for suture placement
- Use biceps tension to set length
- Externally rotate the forearm 30 degrees, then place head to allow for 30 degrees of retroversion
- The implant keel should be 8 mm posterior to tuberosity
- Dial in the head with the majority of the head posterior
- There should be about 50% translation in A to P plane with trial head placed
- Fill the proximal stem with bone graft
- Attach the tuberosities to each other, to the stem, and to shaft through the previously drilled holes

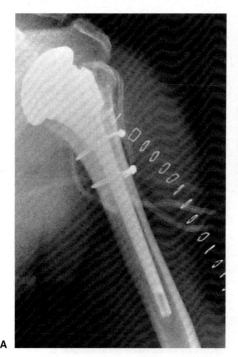

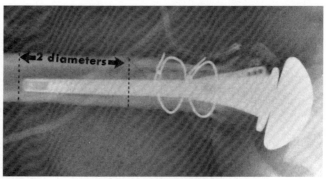

A: This patient sustained a comminuted three-part fracture dislocation of the proximal humerus that extended distally for several centimeters. Treatment consisted of a cemented hemiarthroplasty augmented with cerclage wires. **B:** Note that the humeral stem bypasses the distal extent of the fracture by about two cortical diameters. (From Bucholz RW, Heckman JD, eds. Rockwood and Green's Fractures in Adults, 5th ed. Philadelphia, PA: Lippincott Williams & Wilkins; 2001.)

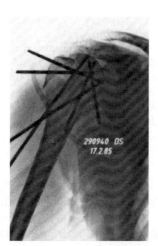

Closed reduction and percutaneous pinning of valgus-impacted fracture using multiple 2.5-mm AO pins. The head has been elevated and the tuberosities reduced. (Courtesy of Jon J. P. Warner, M.D, and Roland P. Jakob, M.D.)

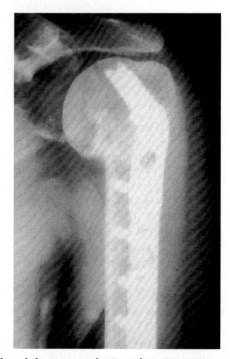

Surgical neck fracture malunion after osteotomy and repair with a blade plate. (From Bucholz RW, Heckman JD, eds. Rockwood and Green's Fractures in Adults, 5th ed. Philadelphia, PA: Lippincott Williams & Wilkins; 2001.)

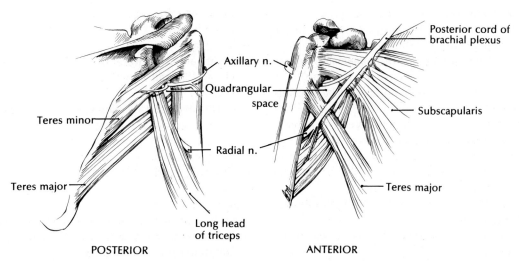

Relations of the axillary nerve to the subscapularis muscle, the quadrangular space, and the neck of the humerus. With anterior dislocations the subscapularis is displaced forward, which creates a traction injury to the axillary nerve. The nerve can't move out of the way because it is held above by the brachial plexus and below where it wraps around behind the neck of the humerus. (From Bucholz RW, Heckman JD, eds. Rockwood and Green's Fractures in Adults, 5th ed. Philadelphia, PA: Lippincott Williams & Wilkins; 2001.)

Recommended Readings

Gerber C, Werner CM, Vienne P. Internal fixation of complex fractures of the proximal humerus. J Bone Joint Surg Br 2004;86(6):848–855.

Goldman RT, et al. Functional outcome after humeral head replacement for acute three- and four-part proximal humeral fractures. J Shoulder Elbow Surg 1995;4(2): 81–86.

Hawkins RJ, Bell RH, Gurr K. et al. The three-part fracture of the proximal part of the humerus. Operative treatment. J Bone Joint Surg Am 1986;68(9):1410–1414.

Hawkins RJ, Switlyk P. Acute prosthetic replacement for severe fractures of the proximal humerus. Clin Orthop Relat Res 1993;289:156–160.

Hinterman B, et al. Rigid internal fixation of fractures of the proximal humerus in older patients. J Bone Joint Surg Br 2000;82:1107–1112.

Jaberg H, et al. Percutaneous stabilization of unstable fractures of the humerus. J Bone Joint Surg Am 1992;74: 508–515.

Lin J, et al. Locked nailing for displaced surgical neck fractures of the humerus. J Trauma 1998;45(6):105–1057.

Neer CS. I. Displaced proximal humeral fractures. II. Treatment of three-part and four-part displacement. J Bone Joint Surg Am 1970;52:1090–1103.

Norris TR, et al. Late prosthetic shoulder arthroplasty for displaced proximal humerus fractures. J Shoulder Elbow Surg 1995;4(4):271–280.

Resch H, et al. Minimally invasive reduction and osteosynthesis of articular fractures of the humeral head. Injury 2001;32(Suppl 1):25–32.

Rowles DJ, McGrory JE. Percutaneous pinning of the proximal part of the humerus. An anatomic study. J Bone Joint Surg 2001;83A:1695–1699.

HUMERUS—SHAFT

Background
- 1% of all presenting fractures
- Nonoperative/conservative treatment has been the primary treatment modality in most injuries
- Like most orthopaedic injuries, there is a bimodal distribution with a peak in young adolescent males and elderly osteoporotic females
- High-energy mechanisms common in young patients
- Low-energy mechanisms in young patients require evaluation for possible malignancy

Physical Examination
- The anatomy of the neurovascular structures surrounding the humeral shaft increase the risk of neurovascular compromise in association with this injury
- Radial nerve function should be evaluated closely following this injury as the radial nerve passes posteriorly around the midshaft region of the humerus increasing the risk of injury
- The radial nerve crosses the humerus at the spiral groove 14–20 cm proximal to the elbow
- The ulnar nerve exits the arcade of struthers 8–10 cm proximal to the medial epicondyle

Radial Nerve Palsy
- Radial nerve palsy most commonly associated with middle to distal third fracture

- High risk with transverse fracture
- Distal third spiral associated with lacerations or entrapment of nerve (Holstein-Lewis)
- Palsy has excellent prognosis with observation alone without exploration (>70% recovery over 3 mo)
- However, open fracture associated with lacerations and entrapments
- Electromyelogram/nerve conduction velocity at 6 wk, explore if fibrillations or sharp waves (polyphasic motor units, signs of denervation), and continue to observe if fasiculations/polyphasics (sign of renervation, predates clinical return by 2 mo)
- Consider external fixation in grade III open injuries, especially grade IIIB/C
- Distal pin should be placed with care to avoid the radial nerve

Radiographs
- AP and lateral humerus radiographs should be performed
- Elbow and shoulder films should be considered in the appropriate clinical context

Classification
- The AO/OTA classification is commonly used
- Fractures are classified according to
  - A: Simple
  - B: Wedge
  - C: Complex
- Fractures are then further classified in subgroups of each of these categories as shown in this figure

Treatment
Functional Bracing
- The majority of isolated humeral shaft fractures can be treated nonoperatively
- Patients are initially placed in coaptation splints for 1–2 wk
- Radiographs should be taken to confirm alignment
- At 2 wk, the coaptation splint is exchanged for a Sarmiento cast brace as the primary treatment modality
- Acceptable alignment includes <3 cm of shortening, <30 degrees of rotational malreduction, and <20 degrees of angulation in the sagittal or coronal plane
  - Average time to union is 10–12 wk in most patients

Contraindications to Bracing
- Brachial plexus palsy
- Soft tissue injury
- Unreliable patient
- Unable to maintain reduction (segmental)

Indications for Open Reduction with Internal Fixation
- Radial nerve palsy postreduction (relative)
- Nonunion

- Pathologic fracture (IM nail)
- Open fracture
- Vascular injury
- Multitrauma, bilateral upper extremity fracture, float elbow (IM nail allows early weight bearing in polytrauma)
  - However, plating allows better union rates and better function in floating elbows
- Ipsilateral plexus injury, Parkinson's (muscle tone needed for functional brace to work)
- Unstable/irreducible fracture

Intramedullary Nail
- Less invasive treatment for humeral shaft fractures
- Requires insertion of distal and proximal interlocks to maintain rotational alignment
  - Antegrade insertion is associated with increased shoulder pain
  - Fracture site is not opened/visualized during nailing → risk of radial nerve palsy with reaming, fracture reduction, and distal interlock insertion
  - Transverse fractures may result in nonunion due to distraction of the fracture site with nail insertion
  - Humerus is non–weight bearing → poorer results with nailing

Plating
- Primary treatment modality for ORIF of humeral shaft fractures
- Multiple surgical approaches exist as described below
- Standard AO principles should be utilized including overbending of the plate and standard compression plating
- Minifragment plates can be utilized in a 90/90 fashion as a provisional reduction device to maintain rotational control prior to placement of the primary plate
- Prasarn et al. (2010) described the use of a posterolateral 3.5 periarticular plate in conjuction with a 3.5 reconstruction plate placed primarily along the lateral aspect of the shaft to maintain length and rotation provisionally
  - Zagorski et al. (1988) showed good results in a study of 233 patients with prefabricated braces for humeral shaft fracture.
    - The patients averaged 10.6 wk to union
    - Average varus/valgus angulation was 5 degrees (usually varus).
    - Average AP angulation 3 degrees
    - Average radiographic (x-ray) shortening 4 mm
    - There were three nonunions
- Sarmiento et al. (1997) showed similar results in their study of 377 patients
  - There was a 2.6 % nonunion rate in the study with lower union rates in patients with distracted transverse fractures

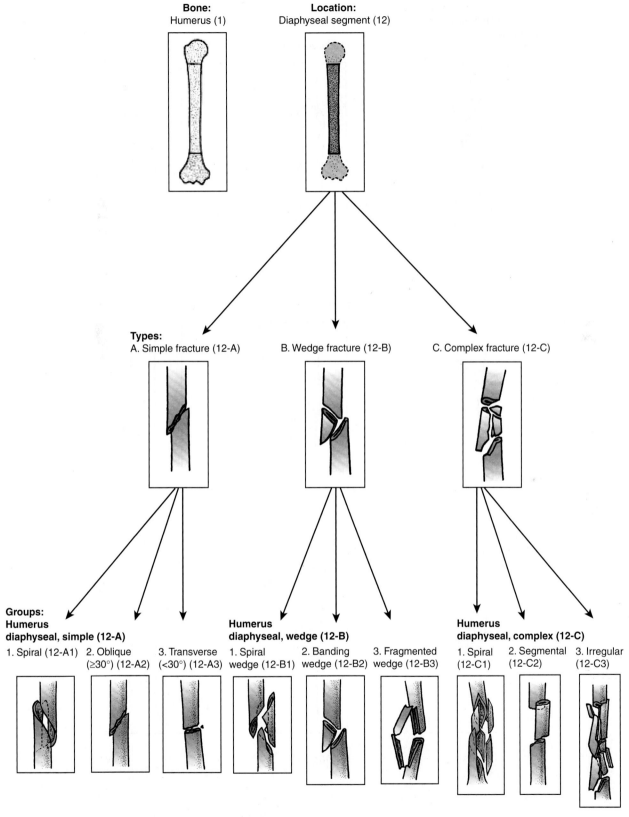

The OTA classification of humeral shaft fractures. (From Marsh JL, Slongo TF, Agel J, et al. Fracture and dislocation classification compendium—2007: Orthopaedic Trauma Association Classification, Database, and Outcomes committee. J Orthop Trauma 2007; 21(10 Suppl), with permission.)

**Subgroups and qualifications:
Humerus diaphyseal, simple,
spiral (12-A1)**
1. Proximal zone (12-A1.1) 2. Middle zone (12-A1.2) 3. Distal zone (12-A1.3)

A1

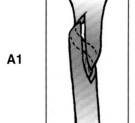 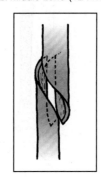 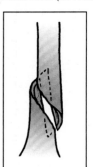

**Humerus diaphyseal, simple,
oblique (≥30°) (12-A2.2)**
1. Proximal zone (12-A2.1) 2. Middle zone (12-A2.2) 3. Distal zone (12-A2.3)

A2

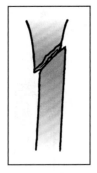 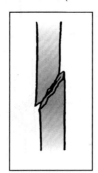 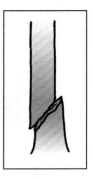

**Humerus diaphyseal, simple,
transverse (<30°) (12-A3)**
1. Proximal zone (12-A3.1) 2. Middle zone (12-A3.2) 3. Distal zone (12-A3.3)

A3

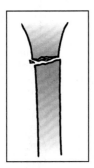 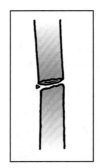 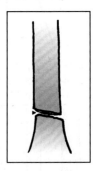

(Continued)

Humerus diaphyseal,
wedge, spiral (12-B1)
1. Proximal zone (12-B1.1)   2. Middle zone (12-B1.2)   3. Distal zone (12-B1.3)

B1

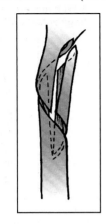 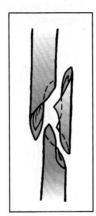 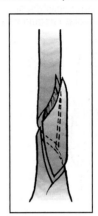

Humerus diaphyseal,
wedge, bending (12-B2)
1. Proximal zone (12-B2.1)   2. Middle zone (12-B2.2)   3. Distal zone (12-B2.3)

B2

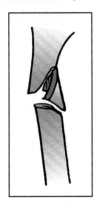 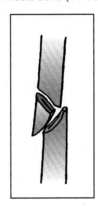 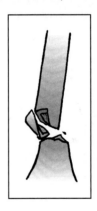

**Humerus diaphyseal,
wedge, fragmented (12-B3)**
1. Proximal zone (12-B3.1)   2. Middle zone (12-B3.2)   3. Distal zone (12-B3.3)

B3

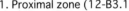

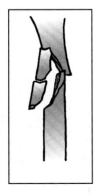 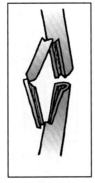 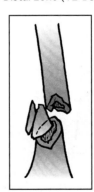

(Continued)

Humerus diaphyseal, complex, spiral (12-C1)
(1) Pure diaphyseal
(2) Proximal diaphylo-metaphyseal
(3) Distal diaphyslo-metaphyseal
1. With 2 intermediate fragments (12 -C1.1)

2. With 3 intermediate fragments (12-C1.2)

3. With more than 3 intermediate fragments (12-C1.3)

C1

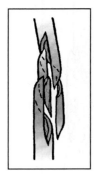
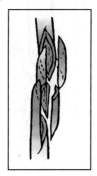
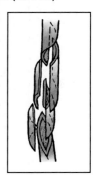

Humerus, diaphyseal, complex segmental (12-C2)
1. With 1 intermediate segmental fragment (12-C2.1)
(1) Pure diaphyseal
(2) Proximal diaphyslo-metaphyseal
(3) Distal diaphyslo-metaphyseal
(4) Oblique lines
(5) Transverse and oblique lines

2. With 1 intermediate segmental and additional wedge fragments (12-C2.2)
(1) Pure diaphyseal
(2) Proximal diaphyslo-metaphyseal
(3) Distal diaphyslo-metaphyseal
(4) Distal wedge
(5) Two wedges, proximal and distal

3. With 2 intermediate segmental fragments (12-C2.3)
(1) Pure diaphyseal
(2) Proximal diaphyslo-metaphyseal
(3) Distal diaphyslo-metaphyseal

C2

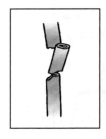
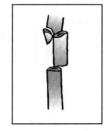
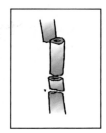

Humerus, diaphyseal, complex irregular (12-C3)
1. With 2 or 3 intermediate fragments (12-C3.1)
(1) 2 main intermediate fragments
(2) 3 main intermediate fragments

2. With limited shattering (<4 cm) (12-C3.2)
(1) Proximal zone
(2) Middle zone
(3) Distal zone

3. With extensive shattering (>4 cm) (12-C3.3)
(1) Pure diaphyseal
(2) Proximal diaphyslo-metaphyseal
(3) Distal diaphyslo-metaphyseal

C3

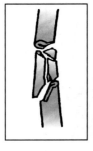
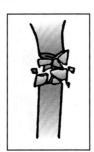
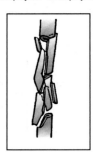

(Continued)

Surgical Exposures to the Humerus

Approaches
- Anterolateral: proximal 2/3
- Posterior: distal 1/2
- Straight lateral: distal 2/3 that requires radial nerve repair. Can be extended to anterolateral humeral shaft approach
- Six cortices above and below fracture
- Prebend plate to avoid gap opposite to plate
- Broad 4.5-mm dynamic compression plate with offset holes to avoid splitting the humerus

Gerwin (1996)
- Radial nerve 21 cm from medial epicondyle and 14 cm from lateral epicondyle; pierces IM septum 10 cm from lateral epicondyle
- Posterior triceps splitting approach visualizes up to 15 cm from the lateral epicondyle
- If radial nerve mobilized with this approach, an additional 6 cm proximally can be seen

Modified Posterior Approach
- Entire triceps retracted medially
- Lower lateral brachial cutaneous nerve found near posterior aspect of lateral IM septum and traced proximally to find main trunk of radial nerve as it passes through septum
- IM septum divided 3 cm distally over radial nerve to allow nerve mobilization
- Medial and lateral heads elevated subperiosteally and retracted medially
- Able to do this because along the posterior humeral diaphysis, there are many branches of radial nerve to lateral head and no branches to medial head
- Branch to medial (deep) head comes off distally lateral to bone at trifurcation of nerve (branch to medial head, lower lateral brachial cutaneous, and main trunk of radial nerve)
- Allows visualization of 26 cm from lateral epicondyle proximally

Or Tips and Tricks—Humerus and Humerus Nonunions
Anterolateral
- Start the incision 2 cm distal to coracoid, along deltopect groove, 1 cm lateral to lateral border of biceps, to 6 cm proximal to lateral epicondyle
- Retract biceps medially
- Deep dissection longitudinally through the brachialis, lateral to its midline, aiming for bone
- The radial nerve is lateral to brachialis and is protected
- Innervation to lateral brachialis from radial nerve is also protected

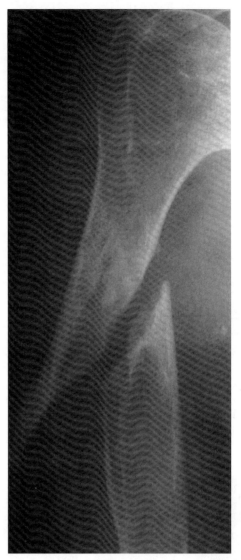

Atrophic nonunion of a humeral shaft fracture 18 months after fracture. Note the absence of callus. (From Bucholz RW, Court-Brown CM, Heckman JD, Tornetta P. Rockwood & Green's Fractures in Adults, 7th ed. Philadelphia, PA: Lippincott Williams & Wilkins, 2010.)

- Flexion of elbow and partial detachment of the deltoid insertion aid visualization

Posterior Triceps Splitting
- Lateral decubitus positioning with a triangle under arm
- Incision from the posterolateral acromion, along lateral edge of lateral head triceps, to the olecranon tip
- Proximally, the interval is between the long and lateral heads
- Distally, the triceps tendon is divided longitudinally
- Careful dissection should be performed to find the radial nerve and deep head of the triceps

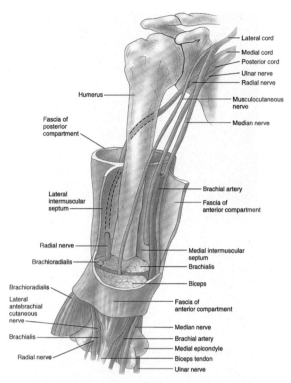

The neurovascular anatomy of the upper arm. (From Bucholz RW, Court-Brown CM, Heckman JD, Tornetta P. Rockwood & Green's Fractures in Adults, 7th ed. Philadelphia, PA: Lippincott Williams & Wilkins, 2010.)

- There is usually no defined plane between the deep and long/lateral heads. The radial nerve should be present 14 cm from lateral epicondyle
- Place a vessel loop or penrose around nerve/deep brachial artery
- Divide the lateral intermuscular septum.
- The deep triceps should be split centrally after localization of the radial nerve.
- In nonunions, all callous should be removed
- An eight-hole 3.5 or 4.5 locking compression plate can be utilized with six cortices above and below fracture
- Screws close to fracture sites should be placed for compression followed by those at the end of the plate
- Fix the plate with a compression screw initially to still allow rotation, then place a second screw to lock in position
- Provisional fixation may be performed utilized small pointed reduction clamps or K-wires
- The most distal hole can be used for the articulated tensioning device for improved compression
- Tension until red line (100 lb). Green line is 75 lb of pressure
- Fix the distal fragment to the plate through the screw closest to the fracture site using a standard compression screw

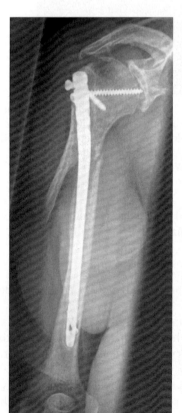
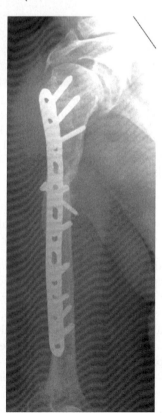

A

B

A. Aseptic nonunion in a 74-year-old healthy women 12 months following fixation with a locked nail. The fracture was never adequately reduced and one screw penetrated the joint. There were no signs of bone healing with instability in rotation and severe pain. **B.** Three months after reoperation with fixation with a compression screw and a locked plate and BMP for biologic stimulation. The fracture went on to uneventful healing. (From Bucholz RW, Court-Brown CM, Heckman JD, Tornetta P. Rockwood & Green's Fractures in Adults, 7th ed. Philadelphia, PA: Lippincott Williams & Wilkins, 2010.)

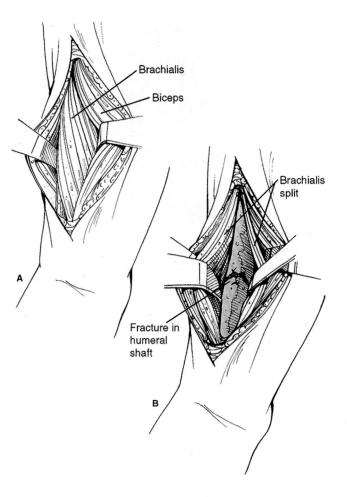

The anterolateral surgical approach to the humeral shaft. After skin and subcutaneous tissue dissection, the interval between the biceps anteriorly and the triceps posteriorly is developed. The shaft is identified distally by splitting the brachialis muscle in line with its fibers. The dissection can be extended into the delto-pectoral interval to gain access to the proximal humeral shaft and, if necessary, the humeral head. (From Bucholz RW, Heckman JD, eds. Rockwood and Green's Fractures in Adults, 5th ed. Philadelphia, PA: Lippincott Williams & Wilkins; 2001.)

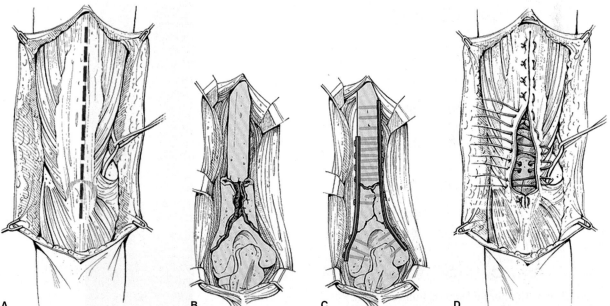

A–D. The posterior surgical approach to the humeral shaft. If necessary, the approach can be extended distally by reflecting the triceps from the olecranon, providing exposure of both medial and lateral columns. The triceps is then reattached through drill holes in the olecranon. (From Bucholz RW, Heckman JD, eds. Rockwood and Green's Fractures in Adults, 5th ed. Philadelphia, PA: Lippincott Williams & Wilkins; 2001.)

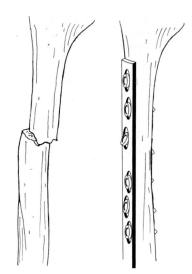

Ideal configuration of compression plate and screws for fixation of a short oblique fracture. Six points of cortical fixation are used proximally and distally with a lag screw placed across the fracture. (From Bucholz RW, Heckman JD, eds. Rockwood and Green's Fractures in Adults, 5th ed. Philadelphia, PA: Lippincott Williams & Wilkins; 2001.)

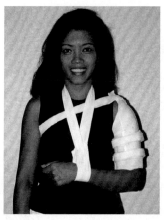

A functional orthosis consists of rigid plastic anterior and posterior pieces connected by Velcro straps. The anterior shell has a distal cutout to accommodate the biceps tendon and allow elbow flexion. The straps are tightened as swelling decreases. The proximal flare over the deltoid is optional. (From Bucholz RW, Heckman JD, eds. Rockwood and Green's Fractures in Adults, 5th ed. Philadelphia, PA: Lippincott Williams & Wilkins; 2001.)

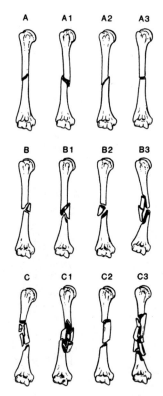

Open reduction with internal fixation: humeral shaft fracture. The AO/ASIF classification of humeral shaft fractures. (From Zuckerman JD, Koval KJ. Fractures of the shaft of the humerus. In: Rockwood CA, et al., eds. Rockwood and Green's Fractures in Adults, 4th ed., Vol. 1. Philadelphia, PA: Lippincott Williams & Wilkins; 1996:1025–1053, with permission.)

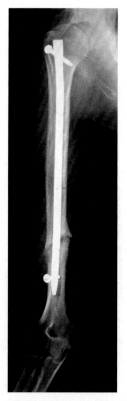

Nonunion of humeral shaft fracture in polytrauma patient 12 months after fixation with an unreamed, interlocked humeral nail. (From Bucholz RW, Heckman JD, eds. Rockwood and Green's Fractures in Adults, 5th ed. Philadelphia, PA: Lippincott Williams & Wilkins; 2001.)

- The fragment that is fixed to plate first is determined by obliquity at the fracture site to form an axilla for compression of the second fragment

Lateral
- Incision made from deltoid insertion to the lateral epicondyle
- The distal interval is between the brachialis and brachioradialis and can be developed using gentle blunt dissection to localize the radial nerve
- Retract the nerve laterally and develop the interval between the brachialis and triceps proximally
- May need to incise the intramuscular septum as the nerve courses proximally and posteriorly
- At the most distal aspect of the approach, the interval between the triceps and brachioradialis is found. The brachioradialis is then retracted anteriorly to protect the radial nerve

Recommended Readings

Amillo S, et al. Surgical treatment of the radial nerve lesions associated with fractures of the humerus. J Orthop Trauma 1993;7(3):211–215.

Bell MJ, et al. The results of plating humeral shaft fractures in patients with multiple injuries: the Sunnybrook experience. J Bone Joint Surg Br 1985;67(2):293–296.

Brumback RJ, et al. Intramedullary stabilization of humeral shaft fractures in patients with multiple trauma. J Bone Joint Surg Am 1986;68(7):960–670.

Gerwin M, et al.. Alternative operative exposures of the posterior aspect of the humeral diaphysis with reference to the radial nerve JBJS 1996;78A(11):1690–1706.

Ingman AM, Waters DA. Locked intramedullary nailing of humeral shaft fractures: implant design, surgical technique, and clinical results. J Bone Joint Surg Br 1994;76(1):23–29.

Mast JW, et al. Fracture of the humeral shaft: a retrospective study of 240 adult fractures. Clin Orthop Relat Res 1975;(112):254–262.

Prasarn ML, Ahn J, Paul O, Morris EM, Kalandiak SP, Helfet DL, Lorich DG. Dual plating for fractures of the distal third of the humeral shaft. J Orthop Trauma. 2011;25(1):57–63.

Sarmiento A, et al. Functional bracing of fractures of the shaft of the humerus. Orthop Trans 1997;21:1166.

Sarmiento A, et al. Functional bracing of fractures of the shaft of the humerus. J Bone Joint Surg Am 1977;59(5):596–601.

Zagorski JB, et al. Diaphyseal fractures of the humerus. Treatment with prefabricated braces. J Bone Joint Surg Am 1988; 70(4):607–610.

DISTAL HUMERUS FRACTURES

Background
- Complex fracture
- Bimodal presentation of injury, which includes osteoporotic low-energy injuries and high-energy mechanisms
- Pain-free motion, mobility, and early return to function require precise/stable fixation, which will allow early and excellent rehabilitation participation
- Represent 2% of all fractures
- High-energy injuries are more common in young active males, whereas low-energy injuries commonly occur in elderly female patients
- Despite the bimodal presentation, elderly patients represent the majority of distal humerus fractures
- Treatment and management is highly dependent on both fracture and patient factors

History and Physical Examination
- Determination of the mechanism of injury usually directs your physical examination
- Be cognizant of any associated injuries
- Evaluate for any signs of skin penetration or joint instability
- A detailed neurovascular exam should be performed immediately
- As many as 26% of patients may present with incomplete ulnar nerve neuropathy
- Confirm adequate perfusion
- History should examine the patient's current functionality and social situation to evaluate for treatment options

Radiographs
- AP, lateral, and oblique elbow radiographs should be performed for all patients
- Consider traction AP or lateral radiographs if there is significant shortening of the fragments
- Computed tomography (CT) scan with 3D reconstructions should be performed to better delineate articular injury and provide a guide for treatment

Anatomy
- The distal humerus is described as two columns with a spool in between
- The trochlea is in 94 degrees of valgus, 3–4 degrees of external rotation, and is more distal than the capitellum
- Overall the elbow is in 10–17 degrees of valgus when fully extended
- In general, the distal humerus is angulated 35–40 degrees anterior to the humeral shaft and is aligned in 4–8 degrees of valgus
- Radial fossa part of lateral column and vulnerable to screw penetration

Classification
Posada's Fracture
- Transcondylar fracture with displacement of distal fragment anteriorly and dislocation of radius and ulna from displaced fragment, usually in osteoporotic bone

Muller/AO Classification
- The most comprehensive classification system

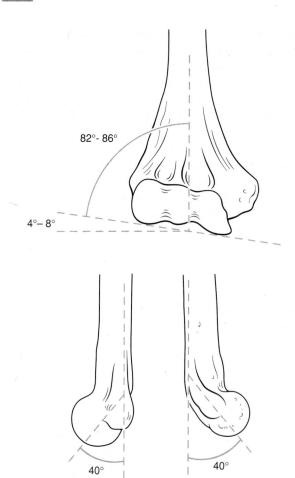

The joint surface to shaft axis is 4 to 8 degrees of valgus—the A-carrying angle **(A)**. The articular segment juts forward from the line of the shaft at 40 degrees and functions architecturally as the tie arch at the point of maximum column divergence distally. It is important to note that the medial epicondyle is on the projected axis of the shaft, whereas the lateral epicondyle is projected slightly forward from the axis **(B, C)**. (From Bucholz RW, Heckman JD, eds. Rockwood and Green's Fractures in Adults, 5th ed. Philadelphia, PA: Lippincott Williams & Wilkins; 2001.)

- Fractures of the distal humerus are designated as 13
- They are then separated into their appropriate type based on location in the distal humerus
  - A: Extra-articular
  - B: Partial articular
  - C: Complete articular
- They are further defined as shown in the chart on the following pages.

Jupiter Classification
- Classification is based on geometry of fracture lines
  - High T: Transverse fracture proximal to or at the olecranon fossa
  - Low T: Transverse fracture proximal to the trochlea
  - Y: Oblique fracture line through both columns with a distal vertical fracture line
  - H: Trochlea is a free fragment
  - Medial lambda: Proximal fracture exists medially
  - Lateral lambda: Laterally exiting proximal fragment line
  - Multiplane T: T Type with an associated fracture in the coronal
  Reference Skeletal Trauma: Chapter 42, pg 1552–1553

Treatment/Approach
Olecranon Osteotomy
- Chevron osteotomy of the olecranon allows visualization of both columns without threatening the triceps insertion stability
- Following completion of the procedure, the olecranon can be repaired utilizing tension band wiring, tension band plating, or utilization of a 6.5 cancellous screw in association with a tension band construct

Triceps Sparing Approach
- Utilize a standard posterior approach followed by ulnar nerve decompression and transposition
- Exposure of both the lateral and medial columns can be performed by following the intramuscular septum to the medial and lateral condyles to expose the fracture

Triceps Splitting
- May provide better visualization for extra-articular fragments
- Care should be taken when extending the incision proximally to avoid the radial nerve posteriorly

Triceps Reflecting
- Following ulnar nerve decompression, the triceps can reflected from ulnarly to radially subperiosteally to expose the distal humerus articulation

Fixation
- The goals of fixation are to reestablish the columnar anatomy while restoring the articular surface
- Reduce articular surface by utilizing the olecranon fossa as one of many fixation landmarks
- K-wires can be utilized to provisionally fix the articular surface so that it can then be restored to the shaft
- 90/90 dual plating provides a stable construct as demonstrated by Helfet and Hotchkiss (1990)
- A posterior plate to lateral column, medial plate to medial column for 90/90 construct
- Mini-fragment plating can be performed after appropriate plate contouring
- Most companies have now developed contoured periarticular plates, which can also be utilized in a bicolumnar or 90/90 plating orientation

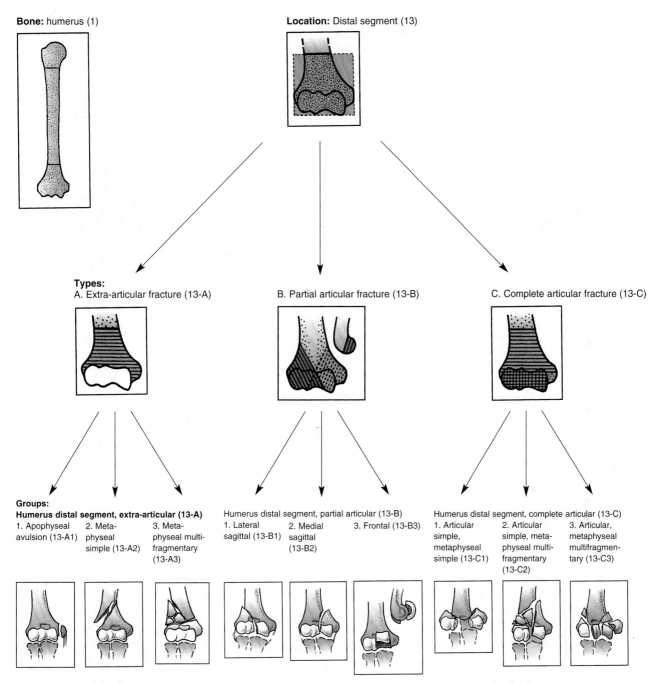

Bone: humerus (1)

Location: Distal segment (13)

Types:
A. Extra-articular fracture (13-A)

B. Partial articular fracture (13-B)

C. Complete articular fracture (13-C)

Groups:

Humerus distal segment, extra-articular (13-A)

1. Apophyseal avulsion (13-A1)
2. Meta-physeal simple (13-A2)
3. Meta-physeal multi-fragmentary (13-A3)

Humerus distal segment, partial articular (13-B)

1. Lateral sagittal (13-B1)
2. Medial sagittal (13-B2)
3. Frontal (13-B3)

Humerus distal segment, complete articular (13-C)

1. Articular simple, metaphyseal simple (13-C1)
2. Articular simple, meta-physeal multi-fragmentary (13-C2)
3. Articular, metaphyseal multifragmen-tary (13-C3)

The AO/OTA Classification of Distal Humerus Fractures. (Redrawn from Marsh JL, Slongo TF, Agel J, et al. Fracture and dislocation classification compendium—2007: Orthopaedic Trauma Association classification, database, and outcomes committee. J Orthop Trauma 2007;21(10 Suppl):S1–133, with permission.)

- Early ORIF and early ROM/physical therapy (postoperative days 3–5) are keys to restoring function
- Helfet and Schmeling (1993) showed 75% good/excellent results, 2% nonunion, 5% each of fixation failure, heterotopic ossification, infection, ulnar palsy in their series described in 1992

Total Elbow Arthroplasty
- Nonoperative treatment often leads to poor results in patients due to limited motion, pain, and risk of nonunion
- Despite the desire for ORIF for nearly all distal humerus fractures, feasibility should be determined before proceeding

Subgroups and Qualifications:
Humerus, distal, extra-articular apophyseal avulsion (13-A1)

1. Lateral epicondyle (13-A1.1)

2. Medial epicondyle, nonincarcerated (13-A1.2)
(1) nondisplaced
(2) displaced
(3) fragmented

3. Medial epicondyle, incarcerated (13-A1.3)

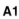

A1

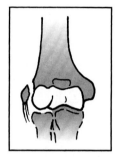

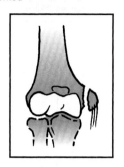

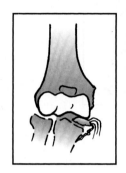

Humerus, distal, extra-articular metaphyseal simple (13-A2)

1. Oblique downward and inward (13-A2.1)

2. Oblique downward and outward (13-A2.2)

3. Transverse (13-A2.3)
(1) transmetaphyseal

(2) juxtaepiphyseal with posterior displacement (Kocher I)

(3) juxtaepiphyseal with anterior displacement (Kocher II)

A2

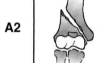

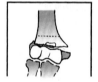

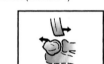

Humerus, distal, extra-articular metaphyseal multifragmentary (13-A3)

1. With intact wedge (13-A3.1)
(1) lateral
(2) medial

2. With fragmented wedge (13-A3.2)
(1) lateral
(2) medial

3. Complex (13-A3.3)

A3

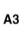

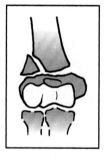

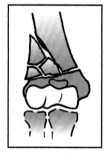

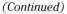

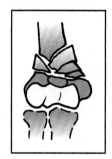

(Continued)

– Osteoporotic bone provides an additional challenge to fixation, especially in patients with preinjury arthritis, loss of motion, or low functional requirements
– Acute total elbow arthroplasty should be considered in these patients
– Contraindications include poor soft tissue coverage and infection

– Patients should be informed of the functional limitations of a total elbow replacement prior to consideration of these treatment modality

Complications

– Olecranon osteotomy → nonunion (higher with transverse cuts)

Humerus, distal, partial articular, lateral sagittal (13-B1)

1. Capitellum (13-B1.1)
(1) through the capitellum (Milch I)
(2) between capitellum and trochlea

2. Transtrochlear simple(13-B1.2)
(1) medial collateral ligament intact
(2) medial collateral ligament ruptured
(3) metaphyseal simple (classic Milch II)
lateral condyle
(4) metaphyseal wedge
(5) metaphysio-diaphyseal

3. Transtrochlear
multifragmentary (13-B1.3)
(1) epiphysio-metaphyseal
(2) epiphysio-meta-
physeal-diaphyseal

B1

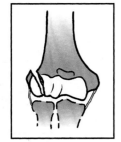
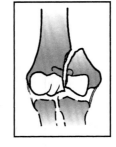
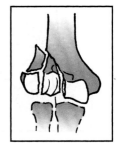

Humerus, distal, partial articular, medial sagittal (13-B2)

1. Transtrochlear simple, through
medial side (Milch I) (13-B2.1)

2. Transtrochlear simple, through
the groove (13-B2.2)

3. Transtrochlear multifragmentary
(13-B2.3)
(1) epiphysio-metaphyseal
(2) epiphysio-metaphyseal-diaphyseal

B2

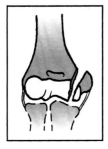
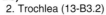
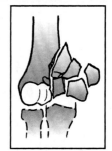

Humerus, distal, partial articular, frontal (13-B3)

1. Capitellum (13-B3.1)
(1) incomplete (Kocher-Lorenz)
(2) complete (Hahn-Steinthal 1)
(3) with trochlear component
(Hahn-Steinthal 2)
(4) fragmented

2. Trochlea (13-B3.2)
(1) simple
(2) fragmented

3. Capitellum and trochlea (13-B3.3)

B3

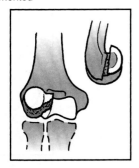
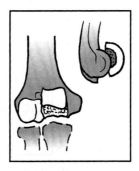
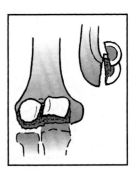

(Continued)

Humerus, distal complete, articular simple, metaphyseal simple (13-C1)

1. With slight displacement (13-C1.1)
(1) Y-shaped
(2) T-shaped
(3) V-shaped

2. With marked displacement
(13-C1.2)
(1) Y-shaped
(2) T-shaped
(3) V-shaped

3. T-shaped epiphyseal (13-C1.3)

C1

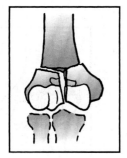

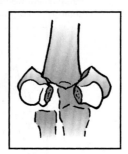

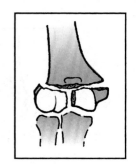

Humerus, distal, complete articular simple metaphyseal multifragmentary (13-C2)

1. With intact wedge (13-C2.1)
(1) metaphyseal lateral
(2) metaphyseal medial
(3) metaphysio-diaphyseal-lateral
(4) metaphysio-diaphyseal-medial

2. With a fragmented wedge (13-C2.2)
(1) metaphyseal lateral
(2) metaphyseal medial
(3) metaphysio-diaphyseal-lateral
(4) metaphysio-diaphyseal-medial

3. Complex (13-C2.3)

C2

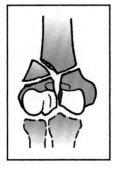

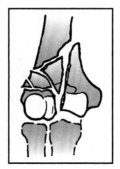

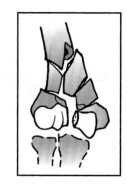

Humerus, distal, complete multifragmentary (13-C3)

1. Metaphyseal simple (13-C3.1)

2. Metaphyseal wedge (13-C3.2)
(1) intact
(2) fragmented

3. Metaphyseal complex (13-C3.3)
(1) localized
(2) extending into diaphysis

C3

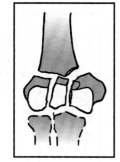

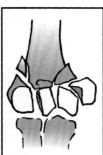

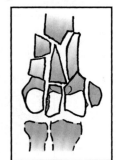

(Continued)

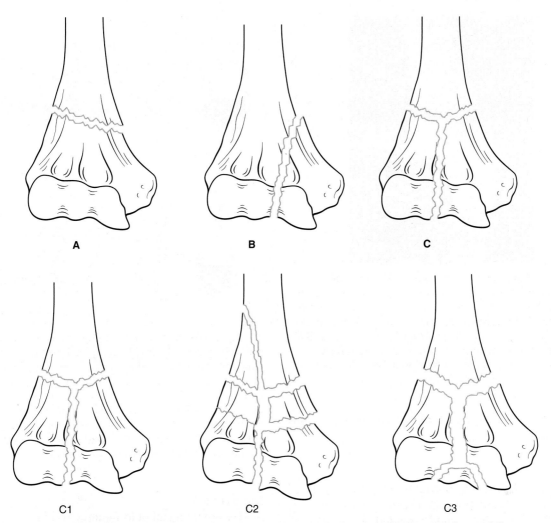

A: The fractures are divided into three types: A, nonarticular; B, partially articular; and C, no articular fracture fragments remain in continuity with the shaft fragment. Each of these types is further subdivided into three groups. **B:** The three groups for C-type fractures: C1, simple T or Y fractures; C2, those in which the articular fracture is simple but the nonarticular supracondylar area is segmental or comminuted; and C3, those in which the articular segment is segmental or comminuted. (From Bucholz RW, Heckman JD, eds. Rockwood and Green's Fractures in Adults, 5th ed. Philadelphia, PA: Lippincott Williams & Wilkins; 2001.)

- Heterotopic ossification
- Elbow stiffness requiring contracture release
- Nonunion (6%)
- Ulnar nerve neuropathy
- Infection
- Failure/infection of total elbow arthroplasty

Recommended Readings

Helfet DL, Hotchkiss RN. Internal fixation of the distal humerus: a biomechanical comparison of methods. J Orthop Trauma 1990;4(3):260–264.

Helfet DL, Schmeling GJ. Bicondylar intraarticular fractures of the distal humerus in adults. Clin Orthop Relat Res 1993;(292):26-36.

Jupiter JB, et al. Intercondylar fractures of the humerus. An operative approach. J Bone Joint Surg Am 1985;67:226–239.

Schildhauer TA, et al. Extensor mechanism-sparing paratricipital posterior approach to the distal humerus. J Orthop Trauma 2003;17:374–378.

CAPITELLAR FRACTURE

Background

- Very rare injury
- Compose 0.5%–1% of all elbow fractures
- More common in females than males secondary to osteoporosis

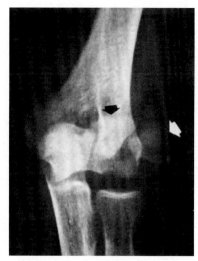

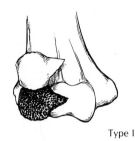 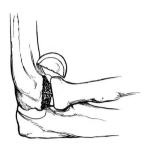

Type I

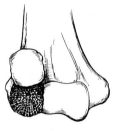 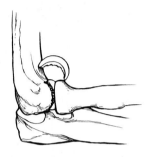

Type II

The type I (Hahn-Steinthal) capitellar fracture. The anteroposterior x-ray is often useful in demonstrating the degree of trochlear involvement. The arrows point to two fragments off the capitellotrochlear surface. This may be difficult to recognize on a lateral view. (From Bucholz RW, Heckman JD, eds. Rockwood and Green's Fractures in Adults, 5th ed. Philadelphia, PA: Lippincott Williams & Wilkins; 2001, with permission.)

The type I (Hahn-Steinthal) capitellar fracture. A portion of the trochlea may be involved in this fracture. In the type II (Kocher-Lorenz) capitellar fracture, very little subchondral bone is attached to the capitellar fragment. There is no fracture through the lateral condyle in the sagittal plane in either the type I or II capitellar fracture. (From Bucholz RW, Heckman JD, eds. Rockwood and Green's Fractures in Adults, 5th ed. Philadelphia, PA: Lippincott Williams & Wilkins; 2001, with permission.)

– May occur in association with radial head fractures and elbow dislocations.

Anatomy
– Capitellum has an anterior/inferior articular surface
    – Anterior articulates when flexed
    – Inferior articulates when extended
– Radial fossa: Depression in anterior humerus just above capitellum accommodates radial head in flexion

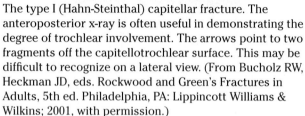

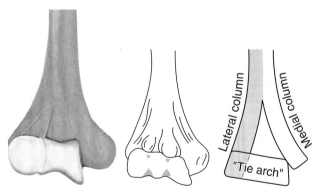

The distal-most part of the lateral column is the capitellum, and the distal-most part of the medial column is the nonarticular medial epicondyle. The trochlea is the medial-most part of the articular segment and is intermediate in position between the medial epicondyle and capitellum. The articular segment functions architecturally as a "tie arch."

Mechanism
– May be the result of low-energy trauma
– Axial directed force from the radial head with the elbow flexed may lead to shearing of the capitellum
– May have an associated radial head or neck fracture

Classification
– I: Hahn-Steinthal
    – Large part of osseous capitellum
    – May contain part of trochlea
    – More common
– II: Kocher-Lorenz
    – Anterior cartilage shell with little bone
    – Rare
– III (Bryan and Morrey): comminuted capitellar fracture
– IV (McKee): Type I fracture with medial extension into the lateral ridge of trochlea
– Johannson reported that medial collateral ligament (MCL) was commonly ruptures in capitellar fractures

Treatment
– Complete recovery possible but reduction must be anatomic

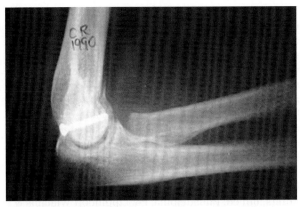

Progressive arthritis following radial head excision. A post-operative lateral radiograph following capitellar open reduction and internal fixation and radial head excision. The elbow joint is congruent, with no evidence of arthrosis. (From Koopman WJ, Moreland LW, eds. Arthritis and Allied Conditions: A Textbook of Rheumatology, 15th ed. Philadelphia, PA: Lippincott Williams & Wilkins; 2005, with permission.)

- ORIF is required, but if fragment severely comminuted, consider excision.
- Kocher (posterolateral) approach to the elbow can be considered for fixation
- Anterior to posterior buried headless lag screws, or 2.4-mm countersunk screws are utilized for fixation
- Small antiglide anterolateral mini fragment L plate or distal radius plate can be considered as well

Recommended Readings

Clough TM, et al. Fractures of the capitellum: A new fixation method using a maxillofacial plate. Clin Orthop Relat Res 2001;384:232–236.
Mehdian H, McKee MD. Fractures of capitellum and trochlea. Orthop Clin North Am 2000;31:115–127.
Oppenheim W, et al. Concomitant fractures of the capitellum and trochlea. J Orthop Trauma 1989;3(3):260–262.
Ward WG, Nunley JA. Concomitant fractures of the capitellum and radial head. J Orthop Trauma 1988;2:110–116.

ELBOW DISLOCATION

Anatomy
- Elbow articulation is dependent on inherent bony stability and ligamentous connections to prevent dislocation
- Ulnohumeral articulation provides 50% resistance to varus stress at extension, 75% with flexion to 90 degrees
- Radiocapitate articulation provides 30% of resistance to valgus stress; MCL provides other 70%
- Anterior medial collateral ligament (AMCL) inserts into medial base of coronoid (sublime tubercle)

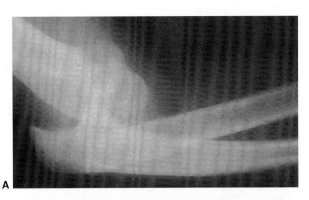

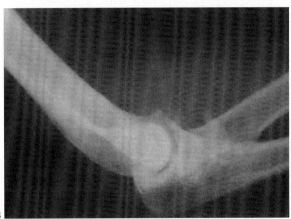

A: A fracture-dislocation with displaced fracture of the radial head. **B:** Reduction of elbow dislocation. (From Bucholz RW, MD and Heckman JD, MD. Rockwood & Green's Fractures in Adults, 5th ed. Lippincott, Williams & Wilkins, 2001)

- Lateral collateral ligament inserts into annular ligament and just lateral to semilunar notch
- Ulnar portion of lateral collateral ligament prevents posterolateral rotatory instability as detected by pivot shift test

Posterolateral Rotatory Instability
- Flexed forearm is supinated/externally rotated with axial and valgus load with patient supine

Evaluation
- Median age 30 yr
- 90% of dislocations are posterior or posterolateral
- 10% associated radial head fracture
  - Rule out Essex-Lopresti if radial head fracture and tender distal radioulnar joint (DRUJ)
- 18% of dislocations have an associated coronoid fracture
  - Instability increased with > 50% of the coronoid surface fractured
- Results of dislocation are worse in the setting of an associated fracture
- 5%–13% brachial artery injury

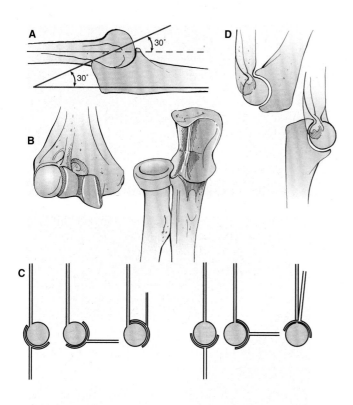

The elbow is an inherently stable joint. **A:** The trochlear notch of the ulna provides a nearly 180-degree capture of the trochlea, which tilts posteriorly ~30 degrees. **B:** The ridge in the center of the trochlear notch interdigitates with a groove on the trochlea, further enhancing stability. **C:** Flexion of the elbow is enhanced by the anterior translation of the trochlea with respect to the humeral shaft as well as the coronoid and radial fossae on the anterior surface of the humerus that accept the coronoid process and radial head, respectively. **D:** Posteriorly, the olecranon fossa enhances extension by accommodating the olecranon process. (From Bucholz RW, et al., eds. Rockwood and Green's Fractures in Adults, 6th ed. Philadelphia, PA: Lippincott Williams & Wilkins; 2006, with permission.)

- 90% incidence of osteochondral fracture upon operative exploration

Reduction

- Consider conscious sedation or intra-articular injection
- Maneuver should be performed in supination to allow the trochlea to clear the coronoid
- Place thumb on olecranon to palpate reduction
- ROM should be evaluated after reduction
- Care should be taken when extending the elbow, as redislocation is more common in extension
- Test valgus stability in pronation to tighten lateral structures; if stable and anterior aspect of the medial collateral is intact, the elbow can be taken though an arc of motion
- Pronation isolates the MCL
- Instability in supination can be attributed to lateral ulnar collateral ligament or MCL
- If reduction incongruent, operative intervention is necessary to either clear entrapped tissue or intra-articular fracture
- Simple elbow dislocations stable beyond 45 degrees of flexion can be splinted in 90 degrees of flexion
- Active range of motion (AROM) with patient supine on days 5–10 to prevent stiffness and maintain reduction
- If unstable in extension, consider a Bledsoe
- The ulnar nerve and medial nerve are uncommonly injured due to traction or entrapment, but an appropriate neurovascular exam should be performed both before and after reduction
- 70% of patient radiographs may have evidence of heterotopic ossification, but <5% will actually limit ROM or functionality motion

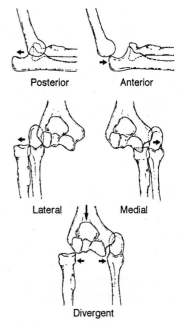

Elbow dislocations. (From Browner BD et al., eds. Skeletal Trauma: Fractures, Dislocations, and Ligamentous Injuries. Philadelphia, PA: WB Saunders; 1992:1142, with permission.)

Natural History
- 1%–2% will present with recurrent instability following simple dislocations
- Loss of 15 degrees of terminal extension is a common complication
    - Aggressive occupational therapy program should be initiated to prevent stiffness
- Surgical intervention is rare following simple dislocations

Associated Ligamentous Injuries
- Potential for instability is higher in elderly patients and younger patients following a high-energy injury
- Ligamentous injury is commonly the culprit of unstable elbow dislocations
- Josefsson (1987) showed that dislocations with associated MCL, LCL ruptures are at risk for redislocation
- Additionally, associated tears of the flexor/pronator mass and extensor mass can contribute to elbow instability during exam under anesthesia
- In those cases, LCL and MCL reconstruction/repair should be performed
    - O'Driscoll and Morrey (1992) performed a biomechanical study and was able to show that posterior elbow dislocations occur in a posterolateral rotatory circle from lateral to medial
- Based on the mechanism, the AMCL was commonly intact as evidenced by valgus stability in pronation
- AMCL is major valgus stabilizer
- The mechanics of the injured elbow are reproduced by the pivot shift test
- Post reduction, test for valgus stability in pronation (to tighten lateral structures that prevent external rotator subluxation); if stable, AMCL must be intact and safe to start ROM with elbow in pronation

Classification
Posterolateral Instability Classification
Stage I
- LCL rupture with persistent snapping due to posterolateral rotatory instability
- Positive pivot shift

Stage II
- Subluxation despite attempts at reduction
- LCL, anterior and posterior capsule torn
- Varus instability
- Coronoid is "perched" under trochlea
- Stable to valgus stress because AMCL intact
- Positive pivot shift
- Recurrent dislocations recover with lateral repair alone

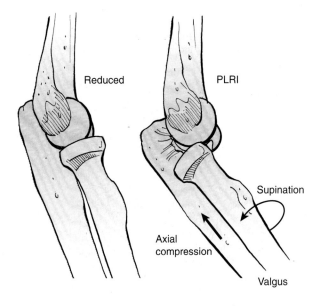

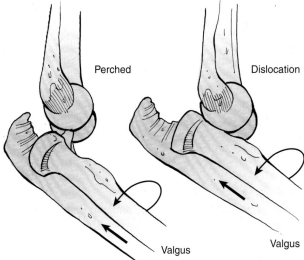

Posterolateral rotatory instability (PLRI) occurs in several stages. Elbow dislocation is the final stage. (From Bucholz RW, et al., eds. Rockwood and Green's Fractures in Adults, 6th ed. Philadelphia, PA: Lippincott Williams & Wilkins; 2006, with permission.)

Stage IIIA
- Coronoid clears trochlea; complete dislocation
- LCL, anterior and posterior capsule, and posterior MCL disrupted
- Stable to valgus because AMCL intact

Stage IIIB
- Complete dislocation with AMCL torn
- Grossly unstable
- Relies on muscle tension and articular congruity for stability
- Maintain reduction by keeping the elbow at 30–45 degrees of flexion

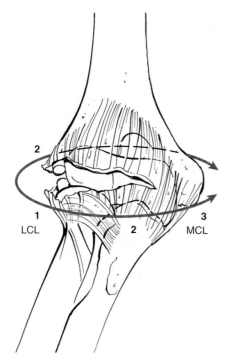

The capsuloligamentous structures of the elbow are injured in a lateral to medial progression during dislocation of the elbow. The elbow can dislocate with the anterior band of the medial collateral ligament (MCL) remaining intact. LCL, lateral collateral ligament. (From Bucholz RW, et al., eds. Rockwood and Green's Fractures in Adults, 6th ed. Philadelphia, PA: Lippincott Williams & Wilkins; 2006, with permission.)

Stage IIIC
– Complete soft tissue disruption from distal humerus
– Stability maintained at 90 degrees of flexion

Treatment
– Indicated in patients with symptomatic elbow instability

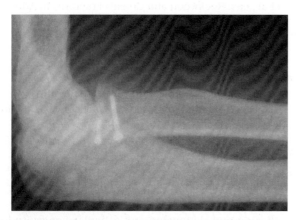

Appearance after internal fixation using minifragment screws in the safe zone. (From Bucholz RW, Heckman JD, eds. Rockwood and Green's Fractures in Adults, 5th ed. Philadelphia, PA: Lippincott Williams & Wilkins; 2001.)

– Isolated posterolateral instability: LCL complex reconstruction
– Posterolateral instability with increased medial joint space: MCL and LCL reconstruction
– Posterolateral instability with elbow arthritis: individualize treatment based on patient preference and functional requirements

Recommended Readings
Josefsson PO. Ligamentous injuries in dislocations of the elbow joint. Clin Orthop Relat Res 1987;221:221–225.

Josefsson PO, et al. Surgical versus nonsurgical treatment of ligamentous injuries following dislocation of the elbow joint: a prospective randomized study. J Bone Joint Surg 1987;69(4):605–608.

Josefsson PO, et al. Long-term sequelae of simple dislocation of the elbow. J Bone Joint Surg 1984;66(6):927–930.

Melhoff TL, et al. Simple dislocation of the elbow in the adult: results after closed treatment. J Bone Joint Surg 1988;70(2):244–249.

Morrey BF, An KN. Functional anatomy of the ligaments of the elbow. Clin Orthop Relat Res 1985;(201):84–90.

O'Driscoll SW, Morrey BF. Elbow subluxation and dislocation. A spectrum of instability. Clin Orthop Relat Res 1992;280:186–197.

MONTEGGIA FRACTURE

Background
– Proximal ulna fracture with an associated radial head dislocation
– Patients often present with both pain and loss of motion secondary to the radial head dislocation
– Radial head dislocation may be subtle, and should be evaluated closely in all proximal ulna fractures
– Wrist and elbow should be evaluated closely in these patients

Radiographs
– AP, lateral, and oblique radiographs of the elbow should be performed in addition to AP and lateral forearms films

Classification
Bado Classification
– I: apex anterior (ulna diaphysis fracture) and anterior dislocation—most common
– II: apex posterior (ulna diaphysis fracture) and posterolateral dislocation
– III: ulnar metaphyseal fracture and lateral or anterolateral dislocation of radial head
    – PIN palsy from radial head pressure
– IV: anterior dislocation with both-bone fracture

Jupiter Classification
– IIA: ulnar fracture involves coronoid and olecranon
– IIB: ulnar fracture at metaphyseal–diaphyseal junction
– IIC: ulnar fracture diaphyseal

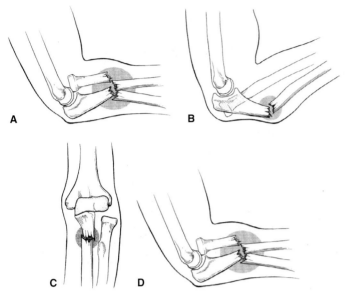

The Bado classification of Monteggia fractures. **A:** Type I. An anterior dislocation of the radial head with associated anteriorly angulated fracture of the ulnar shaft. **B:** Type II. Posterior dislocation of the radial head with a posteriorly angulated fracture of the ulna. **C:** Type III. A lateral or anterolateral dislocation of the radial head with a fracture of the ulnar metaphysic. **D:** Type IV. Anterior dislocation of the radial head with a fracture of the radius and ulna. (From Bado JL. The Monteggia lesion. Clin Orthop Relat Res 1967;50:70–86.)

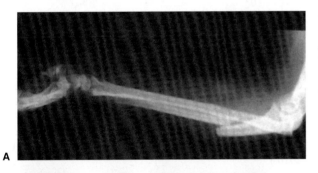

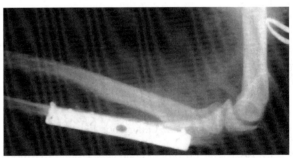

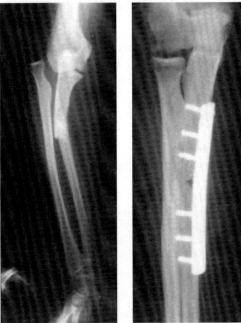

A, B: Type II Bado fracture with a posterolateral dislocation of the radial head in a 26-year-old woman. **C, D:** The ulna was fixed with a seven-hole dynamic compression plate, and the radial head was closed and reduced with satisfactory stability to permit early motion at 7 days. (From Bucholz RW, Heckman JD, eds. Rockwood and Green's Fractures in Adults, 5th ed. Philadelphia, PA: Lippincott Williams & Wilkins; 2001.)

- IID: ulnar fracture involves proximal third ulna
- Closed reduction (CR) in children
  - Reduce ulna first
  - Then reduce radial head
  - Ulnar bow deformation with radial head dislocation challenges idea of isolated radial head dislocation
- ORIF ulna, CR radial head in adults
  - Posterior plate (3.5 LC-DCP) on tension side
  - If radial head malreduced after ulna ORIF, take down the fixation and reassess

Late Diagnosis
- Closed or open reduction and reconstruct annular ligament if within 3 mo
- Restoration of ulnar length and alignment allows radial head reduction
- Assess for convex radial head
  - Indicates congenital dislocation and is irreducible (head is normally concave)
- Options are
- Annular ligament reconstruction alone
- Annular ligament reconstruction with ulnar corrective osteotomy
- Overcorrection lengthening ulnar osteotomy without annular ligament reconstruction
- Radial head excision contraindicated in the skeletally immature
- 20% PIN injury

Recommended Readings

Bado JL. The Monteggia lesion. Clin Orthop Relat Res 1967;50: 71–76.
Jupiter JB, et al. The posterior Monteggia lesion. J Orthop Trauma 1991;5:395–402.
Morrey BF. Current concepts in the treatment of fractures of the radial head, the olecranon, and the coronoid. J Bone Joint Surg 1995;77A:316–327.
Ring D, et al. Monteggia fractures in adults. J Bone Joint Surg 1998;80A:1733–1744.

OLECRANON FRACTURE

Background
- Isolated olecranon fractures require special attention
- These intra-articular fractures requires adequate fixation and evaluation of the proximal radioulnar and radiocapitellum articulation to confirm reduction
- The prevalence of proximal ulna fractures is about 5%
- The predominant mechanism is fall from standing, but there is also a cohort of patients who present falling high-energy trauma

Imaging
- AP, lateral, and oblique views of the elbow should be performed
- Consider CT scan to evaluate any articular depression in communited injuries

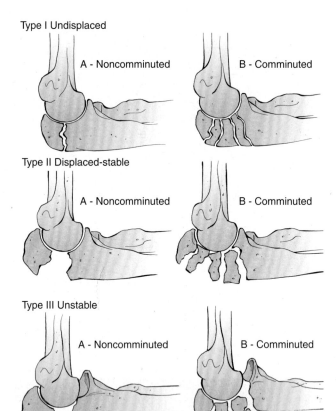

Type I Undisplaced
A - Noncomminuted   B - Comminuted

Type II Displaced-stable
A - Noncomminuted   B - Comminuted

Type III Unstable
A - Noncomminuted   B - Comminuted

The Mayo classification of olecranon fractures divides fractures according to displacement, comminution, and subluxation/dislocation. (From Bucholz RW, Court- Brown CM, Heckman JD, et al. *Rockwood & Green's Fractures in Adults*, 7th ed. Philadelphia: Lippincott, Williams & Wilkins, 2010.)

Physical Examination
- Close evaluation of the skin is necessary due to the subcutaneous position of the olecranon
- Elbow stability should be evaluated as well

Classification
Schatzker
- A: transverse
- B: transverse, central impaction
- C: oblique
- D: comminuted
- E: oblique distal (barely articular)
- F: fracture dislocation

Mayo
- Type I: Undisplaced
- Type 2: Displaced Stable
- Type 3: Displaced unstable
- Each category is divided into A (noncomminuted) and B (comminuted)

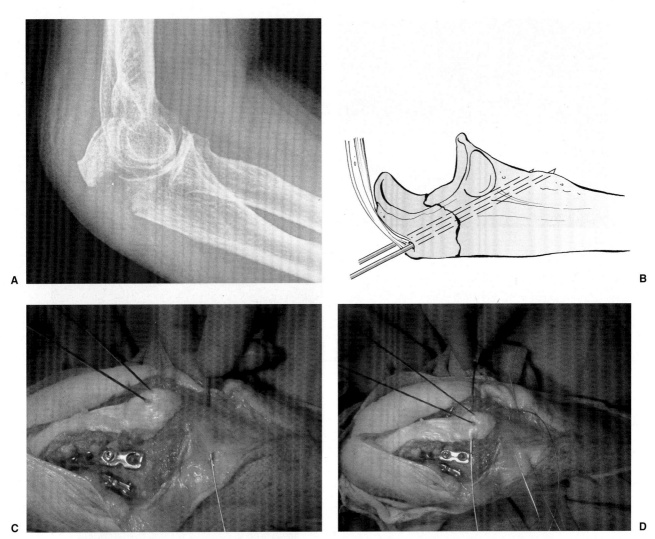

Tension band wiring is useful for simple isolated fractures of the olecranon. **A.** Lateral radiograph demonstrates a transverse fracture of the olecranon. **B.** The fracture is realigned and secured with two 0.045-inch Kirschner wires drilled obliquely so that they engage the anterior ulnar cortex distal to the coronoid. **C.** Two 22-gauge stainless steel wires are passed through drill holes in the ulna distal to the fracture. **D.** The wires are passed underneath the triceps insertion adjacent to the Kirschner wires. *(continued)*

Treatment
- The goals of treatment are restoration of trochlear notch of the ulna to maintain the ROM of that articulation

Nonoperative Treatment
- Can be considered in nondisplaced fractures or poorly functioning patients with an intact extensor mechanism
- Triceps function has a high likelihood of displacing the fracture with extension, so nonoperative treatment is rarely indicated

Operative Treatment
- Restoration of the cortical surfaces is important, but care must be taken to adequately evaluate and restore the articular surface
- Die punch lesion or articular depression may require autograft to restore joint height
- Multiple treatment modalities exist

Figure-of-8 Tension band
- Utilized in simple transverse fractures with or without impaction
- Method utilizes triceps tension to compress the fracture at the articular surface

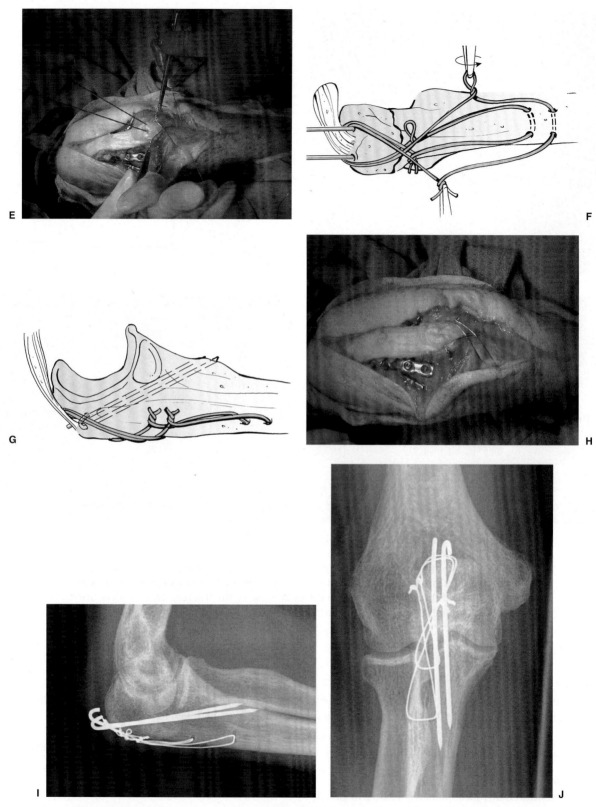

(Continued) **E, F.** The wires are then tensioned both medially and laterally. **G.** The Kirschner wires are then bent 180 degrees and impacted into the olecranon beneath the triceps insertion. **H.** The wires are bent into the adjacent soft tissues so that the entire construct has a very low profile. **I.** Postoperative lateral radiograph. **J.** Postoperative anteroposterior radiograph (From Bucholz RW, Court- Brown CM, Heckman JD, et al. *Rockwood & Green's Fractures in Adults*, 7th ed. Philadelphia: Lippincott, Williams & Wilkins, 2010.)

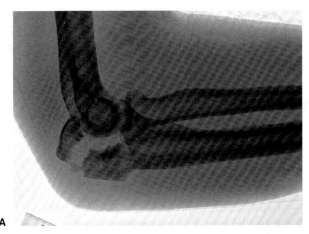 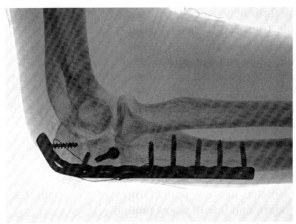

Comminuted olecranon fractures require plate and screw fixation. **A.** This injury created a small olecranon fragment. **B.** In addition to the plate and screws used to maintain alignment of the trochlear notch, a tension band wire is used to gain hold of the small proximal fragment. (From Bucholz RW, Court- Brown CM, Heckman JD, et al. *Rockwood & Green's Fractures in Adults*, 7th ed. Philadelphia: Lippincott, Williams & Wilkins, 2010.)

- Allows early motion to prevent stiffness and loss of function
- Following clearing of the fracture site a large tenaculum can be utilized to reduce the fracture fragments
- If necessary, a unicortical drill hole distal to fracture can be used to assist with tenaculum placement
- Bicortical 1.6-mm K-wires are placed from the tip of the olecranon just distal to the coronoid
- A bicortical 2.5-mm drill hole is made distal to the fracture fragment
- Two 18-gauge wires are passed in a figure-of-8 fashion and two knots are tensioned simultaneously to compress the fracture
- Tension band must be dorsal to midaxis of ulna
- Split the distal portion of the triceps and bend the K-wires deep to tendon

Cancellous Screw Tension Band
- Following reduction of the fracture
- 3.2 drill in drilled intramedullary in the proximal ulna (at least 80–100 mm)
- 6.5 tap is inserted with the fracture reduction maintained
- 6.5 partially threaded cancellous screw with washer is inserted while fracture reduction is maintained
- Triceps is splint to provide coverage of screw and fully seating of the screw
- 18-gauge wire passed through triceps and proximal ulna in figure-of-8 fashion and tensioned simultaneously

Plate Fixation (2.7 or 2.4 reconstruction plates)
- Utilized in cases with severe communcation to avoid tension band mediated collapse of the articular surface

- Also recommended in distal fractures involving the coronoid, oblique fractures distal to the trochlea, nonuninos and monteggia fracture/dislocations
- May require augmentation by 2.0 or DCP or 2.4 reconstruction plate along the radial or ulnar border of the olecranon if wall if distorted

Excision of Fragment and Triceps Advancement
- Consider in osteoporotic bone
- <50% of joint involved
- Attach triceps right at articular surface to create sling for trochlea
- Used as salvage procedure

Complications
- Hardware prominence commonly leads to the need for future removal
- Patients commonly report a loss of 15 degrees of terminal extension following the procedure
  - Rehab should be focused on early ROM to improve return to function
- Ulnar neuritis occurs in 2%–12% of patients but it usually resolves without intervention
- High likelihood of resolution

RADIAL HEAD FRACTURES

Background
- Radial head fractures represent 1.5%–4% of all fractures and 33% of presenting elbow fractures
- Most common mechanism is fall from standing onto an outstretched hand
- The axial force of the radial head on the capitellum leads to the resultant fracture

- Fractures may occur in isolation or as part of the terrible triad (radial head fracture, coronoid fracture, ulnohumeral dislocation)
- The radial head is important in resisting external joint forces and preventing valgus instability of the elbow
- Additionally, wrist and forearm forces are transferred proximally to the radiocapitellar articulation

History and Physical Examination
- In isolated injuries, patients present with pain, discomfort, and loss of elbow motion
- Even with nondisplaced fractures, patients may have a large palpable joint effusion that limits activity
- Care should be taken to examine the wrist for any instability or pain in the DRUJ
- In minimally displaced fractures, hematoma aspiration and lidocaine injection can be utilized to determine whether there is a block to elbow motion, which may require operative intervention
  *Please see section on terrible triad regarding further evaluation of ligamentous injury and elbow instability

Imaging
- AP, lateral, and oblique views of the elbow should be performed
- CT scan can be considered in minimally displaced cases or cases where 3D imaging is necessary to further evaluate the injury

Classification
Mason Classification as Modified by Hotchkiss
- Type 1: Nondisplaced with <2-mm intra-articular displacement
  - No block to supination/pronation
  - Treatment: sling and early ROM/supination/pronation (48 hr)
- Type 2: Displaced >2 mm displaced or angulated
  - With or without mechanical blocks to motion, these patients are treated with ORIF
- Type 3: Comminuted fractures which are irreparable
  - Excision if medial elbow stable, no IO membrane injury or no DRUJ injury
  - Radial head arthroplasty is becoming the most common method of treatment in these patients due to wrist of elbow and wrist instability with radial head excision
- Type 4 (Johnston et al. 1962)
  - Radial head fracture with associated elbow dislocation

- Treat radial head according to the modified Mason classification and treat ulnohumeral dislocation according to treatment algorithm discussed in elbow dislocation section

Treatment
- Treatment algorithm was discussed in the previous section
- Goals of treatment are re-establishing the articular surface of the radial head and stabilizing the radiocapitellar joint
- Two common approaches to the radial head are taken for radial head fixation or arthroplasty
  - **Kocher:** Posterolateral approach between the extensor carpi ulnaris (PIN innervation) and the anconeus (radial nerve)
    - Incision: From the lateral epicondyle distally along the proximal ulna
    - The PIN is protected with pronation of the wrist
  - **Kaplan:** More anterior based interval between the extensor carpi radialis brevis (radial nerve) and the extensor digitorum communis (PIN)
    - Allows better protection of the LCL complex, but anterior positioning places the PIN at increased danger
    - Wrist should be maintained in pronation to protect the PIN
- Both approaches can be utilized from a directly posterior approach with the elevation of a large lateral flap and cases, which may require olecranon fixation or MCL reconstruction in the setting of terrible triad fractures
- In cases of comminuted olecranon or proximal ulna fractures, the radial head may exposed through the fracture site through a direct posterior approach
- The safe zone (nonarticulating zone) for placement of hardware is lateral 110 degrees with forearm in neutral
- Coronoid fixation and LUCL reconstruction or repair should be performed as well if necessary
- Late contractures may result, leading to significant postoperative stiffness and loss of function in patients who fail to undergo adequate occupational therapy
  - These contractures are best treated with release after intra-articular causes ruled out
- Fracture fixation is performed utilizing mini-fragment screws or plate fixation (1.5–2.0 headless screws or minifragment plating)
- Fractures that extend into the radial neck may require plating of the neck with the assistance of T-plates, which can be contoured to fit appropriately and avoid articular surfaces

Or Tips and Tricks

- Kocher posterolateral approach between ECU (PIN) and anconeus (radial nerve)
- Pronate to protect PIN
- The safe zone is lateral 110 degrees with forearm in neutral
- Safe zone is the zone nonarticulating and can accept hardware
- Fix coronoid and LCL injury as well if necessary
- Late contractures best treated with release after intra-articular causes ruled out; manipulation under anesthesia makes stiffness worse from hematoma, progressive fibrosis

Or Tips and Tricks—Radial Head Arthroplasty

- Kaplan approach may provide better exposure to the radial head
- Pronate to protect the PIN
- All radial head fragments should be removed and utilized to reconstruct the radial head for appropriate sizing of the implant
- If the joint is incongruent, consider three factors
  - Is the joint overstuffed?
    - Too large causes point loading at the sigmoid notch
    - Can also lead to inappropriate loading of the radiocapitellar joint
    - Capitellar erosion
    - Early-onset arthritis
    - Loss of flexion
  - Is there a coronoid fracture?
    - Can lead to resultant instability, which precludes adequate fitting and persistent elbow instability
  - Is there a loose body in joint?
- All factors must be evaluated closely to determine the appropriate implant

Outcomes/Results

- Ring et al. (2002) evaluated 56 patients with radial head fractures
  - 13/14 patients with Mason type 3 fractures with more than three articular fragments had poor results compared to type 2 fractures that underwent fixation
- Early complications are most commonly secondary to inadequate fixation, stiffness, and PIN injury
- Early ROM should be initiated to decrease the risk of persistent stiffness and loss of motion

Recommended Readings

Johnston Gw, et al. A follow-up of one hundred cases of fracture of the head of the radius with a review of the literature. Ulster Med J. 1962;31:51–56

Ring D, Quintero J, Jupiter JB. Open reduction and internal fixation of fractures of the radial head. J Bone Joint Surg Am 2002;84:1811–1815.

GALEAZZI FRACTURE

- Fractures of the distal third of the radius should be evaluated for associated dislocation of the DRUJ
- Injury is associated with instability, which can limit function if not treated appropriately
- Force is transmitted through the DRUJ down the IO membrane and can propagate to the triangular fibrocartilage complex (TFCC) leading to further instability

Radiographic Evaluation

- AP, and lateral radiographs of the forearm, and AP, lateral, and oblique radiographs of the wrist

Treatment

- Surgical fixation is essential in adults
- Rigid fixation of the radius should be performed followed by reduction of the DRUJ
- Stability of the DRUJ should be evaluated through a full arc of motion
- If instability remains, two K-wires should be placed from the radius to the ulna with the arm in supination

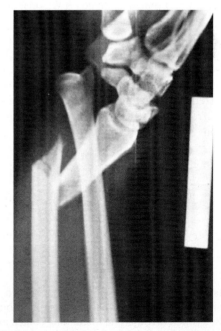

Galeazzi's fracture. A lateral projection shows the dorsally angulated distal radial fracture and the obvious disruption of the distal radioulnar joint. The ulna is intact. (From Eisenberg RL. An Atlas of Differential Diagnosis, 4th ed. Philadelphia, PA: Lippincott Williams & Wilkins; 2003, with permission.)

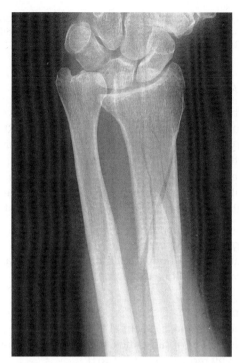

Galeazzi's fracture. Note that a comminuted fracture of the radius is present at the junction of the middle and distal thirds, with an associated dislocation of the distal radioulnar joint. There has been an overall shortening of the distal radius, which is a common finding in this fracture-dislocation. (From Yochum TR, Rowe LJ. Yochum and Rowe's Essentials of Skeletal Radiology, 3rd ed. Philadelphia, PA: Lippincott Williams & Wilkins; 2004.)

- Immobilization postoperatively should limit pronation and supination of the wrist
- Intermittently, the extensor carpe ulnaris tendon may lead to irreducible DRUJ, which requires further exploration

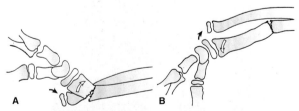

Walsh classification. **A:** The most common pattern, in which there is dorsal displacement with supination of the distal radius (open arrow). The distal ulna (black arrow) lies volar to the dorsally displaced distal radius. **B:** The least common pronation pattern. There is volar or anterior displacement of the distal radius (open arrow), and the distal ulna lies dorsal (black arrow). (From Walsh HPJ, McLaren CANP. Galeazzi fractures in children. J Bone Joint Surg Br 1987;69:730–733.)

Recommended Reading
Bruckner JD, et al. Complex dislocations of the distal radioulnar joint. Recognition and management. Clin Orthop Relat Res 1992;(275):90–103.

FOREARM FRACTURES

Background
- Fractures of the radius/ulna result from multiple mechanisms
- Dependent on precise radial and ulnar relationship to maintain rotation and motion of the forearm
- Considered intra-articular due to the importance of the radius/ulna rotational relationship
- Can lead to instability in both the DRUJ and the proximal radioulnar joint
- Care should be taken to restore anatomic alignment
- Incidence: 11.7/100,000 per yr

Physical Examination
- Motor and sensory function should be evaluated closely
- Any signs or symptoms of compartment syndrome should be investigated fully by measuring CPs
- Evaluation of the wrist and elbow should be included to prevent missing radioulnar joint injuries

Imaging
- AP and lateral radiographs of the forearm should be performed
- Elbow and wrist films to evaluate for Galeazzi or Monteggia fractures
- Widening at DRUJ should be further investigated in the setting of isolated radius fractures
- The radial head should be in line with the capitellum in all radiographic views

Classification:
- The AO classification is the most common and comprehensive classification available
  - Please see figure

Treatment
- Indications for surgical treatment
  - Displaced fractures of both radius and ulna
  - Open fractures
  - Patients should be stabilized initially and monitored for signs and symptoms of compartment syndrome
  - Nonoperative treatment should be limited to isolated minimally displaced ulnar fractures (nightstick fracture)

APPROACHES

Surgical Approaches

– Separate approaches to the ulna and radius should be performed to limit to risk of synostosis
– The radial exposure is often more difficult and should be performed first unless there is comminuition or bone loss with may limit the ability to reestablish the physiologic bow
– Consider ulnar fixation in simple fractures

– Consider provisional fixation of both fractures prior to closing the wounds to confirm adequate reduction

Volar Approach of Henry (Radius)

– Proximal: Interval between the brachioradialis and pronator teres
– Distal: Interval is between the brachioradialis/radial artery and the flexor carpi radialis

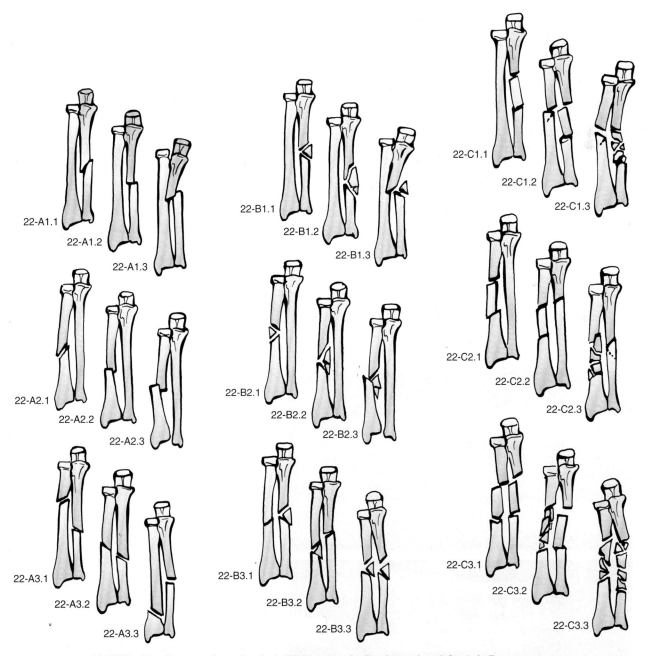

AO/OTA classification (from Bucholz RW, et al., eds. Rockwood and Green's Fractures in Adults, 7th ed. Philadelphia, PA: Lippincott Williams & Wilkins; 2010 with permission)

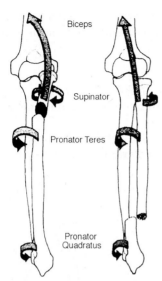

Deforming muscle forces in both-bone forearm fractures.
(From Cruess RL. Importance of soft tissue evaluation in
both hand and wrist trauma: statistical evaluation. Orthop
Clin North Am 1973;4:969.)

Dorsal Thompson Approach
- Proximal: Interval between the extensor carpi radialis
  brevis and the extensor digitorum communis
- Distal: Interval between extensor carpi radialis brevis
  and extensor pollicis longus (EPL)
- Allows for improved soft tissue coverage of the
  ulna

- Approach puts radial sensory nerve at risk, so care
  should be taken at the proximal dissection

Direct Approach to Ulna
- Along the subcutaneous boarder of the ulna between
  the extensor carpi ulnaris (ECU) and the flexor carpe
  ulnaris (FCU)
- The ulnar plate should be placed under either the
  ECU or the FCU to prevent pain at the subcutaneous
  boarder of the ulna
- Both bone forearm fractures should be plated in compression with absolute stability in stable fractures to
  allow for primary healing
- Comminuted fractures should be bride plated
- Locking compression plates have become the plate
  of choice, as they provide adequate compression and
  are sturdy enough to permit early motion without fracture displacement

Open Fractures
- External fixation should be considered in open frac-
  tures with significant contamination or bone loss
- Care should be taken to maintain appropriate length in
  polytrauma patients that cannot undergo immediate
  ORIF
- Ulnar pins can be placed easily due to the subcuta-
  neous nature of the bone
- In general, open fractures should be treated with
  immediate internal fixation, irrigation, and debride-
  ment
  - Redebridement should be performed at 24–48 hr

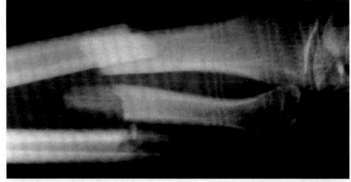

Displaced fractures of both bones of the forearm
in a 34-year-old woman as a result of a motor
vehicle accident. The radial fracture was
segmental. All fractures have been fixed with
plates and screws. Two separate plates were
required for fixation of the radial fractures. (From
Bucholz RW, Heckman JD, eds. Rockwood and
Green's Fractures in Adults, 5th ed. Philadelphia,
PA: Lippincott Williams & Wilkins; 2001, with
permission.)

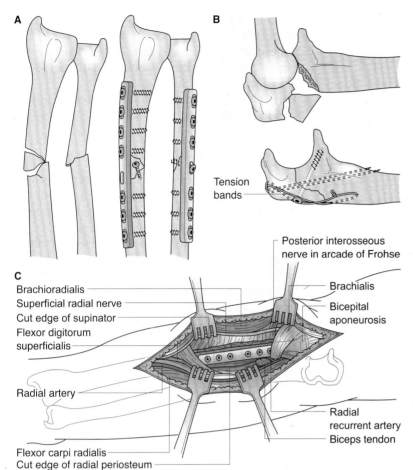

A: Both-bone fractures of the radius and ulna in adults are best treated by anatomic open reduction and internal fixation. **B:** Displaced fractures of the olecranon require open reduction and internal fixation. Tension band technique and interfragmentary fixation are illustrated. **C:** Open reduction and internal fixation of a proximal radius fracture. This fracture may be associated with a dislocation of the radial head (Monteggia fracture). An anterior approach is illustrated, although a posterior approach is more commonly used. The posterior interosseous branch of the radial nerve is at risk because it lies in the supinator muscle. It must be carefully identified and protected. (From Mulholland MW, et al., eds. Greenfield's Surgery Scientific Principles and Practice, 4th ed. Philadelphia, PA: Lippincott Williams & Wilkins; 2006.)

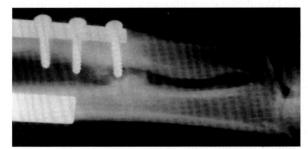

Radiograph before resection of heterotopic ossification arising due to impingement of screws used to fix one forearm bone against the opposite forearm bone. With rotation of the forearm, the internal fixation mechanically irritates the intervening soft tissues and heterotopic ossification can occur. This patient was treated by plate removal and resection of the heterotopic ossification. (From Bucholz RW, Heckman JD, eds. Rockwood and Green's Fractures in Adults, 5th ed. Philadelphia, PA: Lippincott Williams & Wilkins; 2001.)

Complications

Nonunion
- Results from inadequate fixation due to fracture gap or instability
- May result from soft tissue stripping and bone devitalization
- May require revision fixation with bone graft
- Rate of nonunion is <2% with plate fixation

Malunion
- Common complication that results in significant loss of rotational ROM of the forearm
- If functional limitation present, osteotomy should be performed in addition to revision fixation

Synostosis
- More common in patients who undergo
  - ORIF at >2 wk from injury
  - Use of single incision
  - Screws that protrude into the IO membrane
- Progressive synostosis can limit forearm rotation and limit functional improvement
- Consider excision of the syntostosis to improve outcomes
- 30% recur

Refracture
- 4%–20% refracture following plate removal
- Refracture usually occurs through old fracture site or previous screw holes
- Bone mineral density at fracture site does not normalize until 21 mo post fixation
- Patients should avoid contact sports for apptoximately 2 yr after removal of the plates to contact sports

Recommended Readings

Chapman MW, et al. Compression-plate fixation of acute fractures of the diaphyses of the radius and ulna. J Bone Joint Surg 1989;71(2):159–169.

Duncan R. Immediate internal fixation of open fractures of the diaphysis of the forearm. J Orthop Trauma 1992;6(1):25–31.

Moed BR, Kellam JF. Immediate internal fixation of open fractures of the diaphysis of the forearm. JBJS Am 1986;68(7):1008–1017.

Stern PJ, Drury WJ. Complications of the plate fixation of forearm fractures. Clin Orthop Relat Res 1983;(175):25–29.

Schemitsch EH, Richards RR. The effect of malunion on functional outcomes after plate fixation of fractures of both bones of the forearm in adults. J Bone Joint Surg 1992;74(7):1068–1078.

Wright RR, Schmeling GJ. The necessity of acute bone grafting in diaphyseal forearm fractures: a retrospective review. J Orthop Trauma 1997;11(4):288–294.

ULNAR SHAFT FRACTURES

Background
- Uncommon injury
- Occurs as a result from a direct blow to the forearm over the subcutaneous border of the olecranon
- Commonly treated nonoperatively
- Monteggia fracture should be ruled out in more proximal injuries
- DRUJ should be evaluated for any signs of instability

Imaging
- AP and lateral forearm films should be performed
- Elbow and wrist films should be considered in patients

Classification
- Isolated ulna fractures are classified as AO/OTA 22A1 or B1 injuries

Treatment
- Nonoperative treatment
  - Distal two-thirds ulna fractures with
  - <10 degrees of angulation
  - <50% displacement of the shaft
- Evaluate the DRUJ for stability with distal fractures.

- Nonunion can lead to stress fracture of radius and gradual radial head subluxation
- Functional short arm brace, early ROM as treatment
  - Operative intervention is performed through compression plating of the ulna if unstable
  - Percutaneous nail fixation is associated with high nonunion rates

DISTAL RADIUS FRACTURE

- 16% of all fractures treated by orthopaedic surgeons
- Trimodal distribution of injury which begins in childhood, extends to active adolescent/middle-aged males, and finally to females older than age 40
- Represents an insufficiency fractures in women older than age 40
  - Frequency in elderly female patients increases significantly
- Elderly patients and women older than age 40 more commonly the result of a fall from standing onto an outstretched hand
- May be the result of high-energy sports, or polytrauma in young active males

Anatomy
- Articulates with scaphoid and lunate distally (biconcave surface), three facets
- 80% of axial load is radius, 20% ulna and triangular fibrocartilage complex
- Volar ligaments are stronger

Classification
Fernandez Classification
- Mechanism based classification to assist in treatment recommendations
  - Type I: Bending extra-articular (Colle's or Smith's)
  - Type II: Shearing intra-articular (Barton's and radial styloid fractures)
  - Type III: Compression fractures of the joint surface (Die punch injuries)
  - Type IV: Avulsion fractures or radiocarpal fracture-dislocations
  - Type V: Combined fractures from high-velocity injuries

Frykman Classification
- Classification based on involvement of wrist joint, DRUJ, and ulnar styloid

Imaging
- PA, lateral, and oblique radiographs should be performed
- Important radiographic anatomical findings:
  - Radial inclination: 23 degrees (13–30 degrees)
  - Radial length: 13 mm (8–18 mm)

- Volar tilt: 11 degrees (1–21 degrees)
- Carpal alignment should be evaluated to avoid missing concomitant scaphoid fractures, scapholunate instability, or carpal ligament injury
- CT scan to evaluate intra-articular injury and articular congruity

Fracture Patterns

- **Colles:** Both extra- and intra-articular fracture demonstrating dorsal angulation, dorsal displacement, radial shift, and shortening
  - >90% of distal radius fractures
  - Intra-articular fracture more common in younger patient with higher-energy fracture
- **Smith's:** Describes fracture that collapses into volar flexion
  - Unstable fracture pattern—usually requires ORIF
- **Barton's:** Results in subluxation of the wrist
  - Volar Barton's is more common
  - Most stable in volar flexion and supination
  - Most are unstable and require ORIF with buttress plate
  - External fixation and ligamentotaxis is insufficient for adequate fixation of this fracture type
- Radial styloid fracture (Hutchinson's fracture, Chauffeur's fracture)
  - Mechanism: avulsion fracture 2 degrees to scaphoid compressing radial styloid

Radial Styloid

- Mechanism: Occurs secondary to scaphoid compression of the radial styloid with forced dorsiflexion
- Associated with intercarpal ligamentous injuries
- Scapholunate dissociation, perilunate dislocation should be evaluated
- Fixation of the radial styloid enhances fixation of associated distal radius fracture and maintenance of radial length to prevent carpal shift
- Ulnar impaction syndrome can result from failure to restore radial height

Stable Fracture

- For nondisplaced or acceptably reduced fractures (near anatomic volar tilt, radial height, radial inclination) and stable fracture pattern
- Radiographs should be performed every week for the first 2–3 wk
- Cast application at 2 wk once swelling has subsided
- 6–8 wk of cast wear followed by volar resting splint for protection

Acceptable Reduction

- Change in volar tilt <10 degrees
- Radial shortening <2 mm
- Change in inclination <5 degrees
- Articular step-off <2 mm

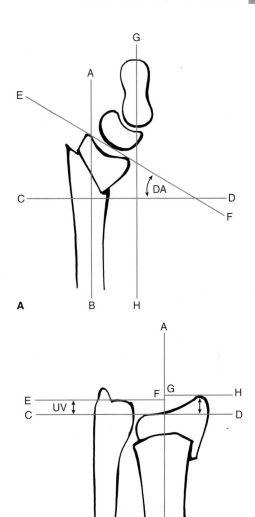

A. The dorsal angle (DA) is measured by finding the angle between a line (CD) perpendicular to the long axis of the radius (AB) and a line joining the dorsal and volar extremities of the radiocarpal joint (EF). Carpal alignment is assessed by the point of intersection of the line parallel to the long axis of the radius (AB) and a line parallel to the long axis of the capitate (GH). If these intersect outwith the carpus or do no intersect as in this illustration, then the carpus is malaligned. **B.** Ulnar variance (UV) is the distance between two lines perpendicular to the long axis of the radius (AB). The first is tangential to the ulnar corner of the radius (CD) and the second tangential to the ulnar head (EF). Radial length is the distance between line EF and a line tangential to the radial styloid (GH). (From Court-Brown C, McQueen M, Tornetta P. Orthopaedic Surgery Essentials: Trauma. Philadelphia: Lippincott Williams & Wilkins, 2006, with permission.)

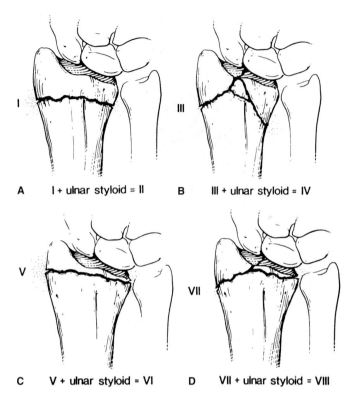

A   I + ulnar styloid = II   B   III + ulnar styloid = IV

C   V + ulnar styloid = VI   D   VII + ulnar styloid = VIII

Frykman classification of distal radius fractures. **A:** Frykman types I and II, extra-articular. **B:** Frykman types III and IV, intra-articular radiocarpal joint. **C:** Frykman types V and VI, intra-articular distal radioulnar joint. **D:** Frykman types VII and VIII, intra-articular radiocarpal and distal radioulnar joints. (From Rockwood CA, et al., eds. Rockwood and Green's Fractures in Adults, 4th ed., Vol. 1. Philadelphia, PA: Lippincott Williams & Wilkins; 1996, with permission.)

- If not achieved, one attempt at rereduction can be performed
- If rereduction not inadequate, then consider ORIF

La Fontaine Criteria, Injury (1989) (Belgium)
- Evaluated factors that are correlated with risk of failure of closed treatment of distal radius fractures post reduction
- Fractures are considered unstable if
  - Prereduction radiograph with >20 degrees dorsal angulation
  - Marked dorsal comminution
  - Intra-articular radiocarpal fractures
  - Associated ulnar or ulnar styloid fractures
  - Occur in patients >60 yr
  - >5–10-mm loss of radial length
- Other instability associated factors—Barton's, Chauffeur's, and Smith's fractures
  - High-energy fractures with significant articular comminution
- Rule of 2's for stability
  - Radial shortening >2 mm
  - Translation in AP plane >2 mm
  - Intra-articular displacement >2 mm
  - >5-mm displacement
  - Dorsal impaction or comminution past midaxial plane

ORIF should be considered in these cases

Treatment—Unstable Fracture
Percutaneous Pinning
- Can be used for extra- articular fracture and two-part intra-articular fracture in which volar cortex is intact
- Does not maintain length in volar or bicortical fractures comminution
- Styloid ± dorsal pin (See OR Tips and Tricks)
- Pins removed at 6–8 wk
- Must splint or externally fix postoperative
- Pin tract infections are common complications

External Fixation
- Success rates have been reported as high as 80%–90% success
- Consider in unstable extra-articular fractures with both column involvement
- In cases of severe comminuted intra-articular fracture, may be applied for ligamentotaxis
- Open fracture, multiple injuries
- As augmentation to fixation or percutaneous pinning
- Low complication rates
- Can restore radial length and inclination, but volar tilt is difficult to control due to the imbalance of volar and dorsal ligaments
- The radiocarpal joint should not be distracted for >5 mm
- Fixator should be maintained for approximately 8 wk

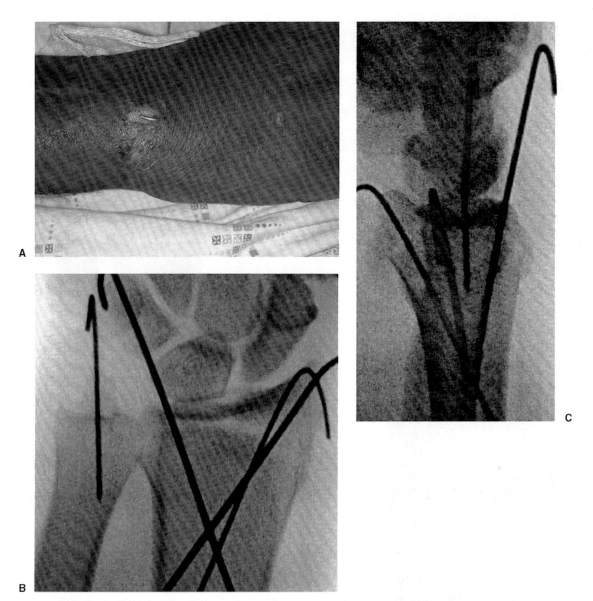

A–C. Comminuted radius fracture in a poly trauma patient treated with percutaneous pinning technique. (From Bucholz RW, Heckman JD, eds. Rockwood and Green's Fractures in Adults, 5th ed. Philadelphia, PA: Lippincott Williams & Wilkins; 2001, with permission.)

- Complications include reflex sympathetic dystrophy, stiffness, fracture through pin sites, radial sensory neuritis, and pin tract infection

Open Reduction Internal Fixation
- Frequency of volar plating has increased significantly
- Allows from accurate articular reduction of fractures as well as earlier ROM postoperatively
- Required in certain fracture types as mentioned above (Barton's and unstable Smith's)
- Comminuted, intra-articular fractures
- See OR Tips and Tricks for detailed explanation

Complications
Median Nerve Dysfunction
- If lesion occurs after reduction, splint should be taken down and wrist placed in the neutral position
- Complete median nerve lesion with no improvement following reduction requires surgical exploration

Posttraumatic Arthritis
- EPL rupture can occur following ORIF
  - Extensor indicis proprius can be utilized for transfer to EPL
- Midcarpal instability with increased dorsal tilt of the lunate secondary to the injury

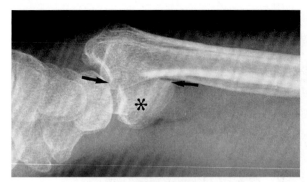

Classic volar Barton fracture. The oblique intraarticular fracture (arrows) involves the volar aspect of the distal radius. The separate fragment (asterisk) and the bones of the wrist and hand are volarly and proximally displaced. (From Harris JH Jr, Harris WH. The Radiology of Emergency Medicine, 3rd ed. Philadelphia: Lippincott-Raven, 2000:388, with permission.)

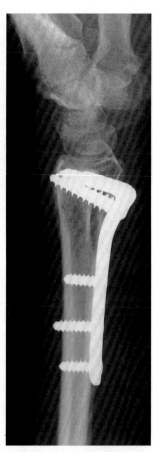

A fossa lateral radiograph in neutral position. (From Bucholz RW, Heckman JD, eds. Rockwood and Green's Fractures in Adults, 5th ed. Philadelphia, PA: Lippincott Williams & Wilkins; 2001, with permission.)

- Infection
- Volkmann's contracture secondary to compartment syndrome is also a concern

Recommended Readings

LaFontaine M. Instability of fractures of the lower end of the radius: apropos of a series of 167 cases. Acta Orthop Belg 1989;55(2):203–216.
LaFontaine M, Hardy D. Stability assessment of distal radius fractures. Injury 1989;20(4):208–210.

Or Tips and Tricks—Distal Radius

Volar Buttress Plate

- Incision along flexor carpi radialis to the palmar wrist crease
- Retract flexor carpi radialis ulnarly to improve exposure of radial aspect to the radius for elevation of the pronator quadratus
- Entering the posterior sheath of flexor carpi radialis reveals the flexor pollicis longus
- Flexor pollicis longus, radial artery and vein are retracted radially

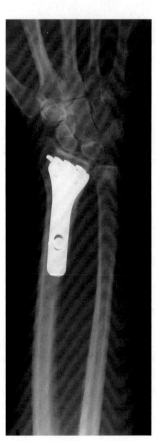

PA radiograph showing full supination and pronation of the DRUJ 6 months postsurgery. (From Bucholz RW, MD and Heckman JD, MD. Rockwood & Green's Fractures in Adults, 5th ed. Philadelphia: Lippincott Williams & Wilkins; 2001, with permission.)

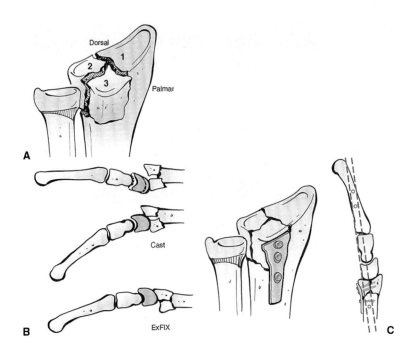

A: Typical three-part intra-articular fracture of the distal radius. **B:** Depression of the lunate facet palmarly is difficult to reduce by closed methods. **C:** A plate applied palmarly to the lunate facet reduces and mortars both the DRUJ and the radiocarpal joint. (From Bucholz RW, Heckman JD, eds. Rockwood and Green's Fractures in Adults, 5th ed. Philadelphia, PA: Lippincott Williams & Wilkins; 2001, with permission.)

- Everything else should retracted ulnarly to fully expose the pronator quadratus
- The pronator quadratus is elevated off the radial aspect of the radius
- Elevate the ulnar 1/4 of brachioradialis tendon with pronator to allow easier closure
- Provisional fixation with K-wire from the subchondral bone just proximal to the articular surface
- Plates are often placed too proximal
  - Insert initial screw in distal aspect of the oblong hole to allow movement of the plate and appropriate positioning.

Dorsal Buttress Plate
- Incision should be on the dorsoradial aspect of the radius, lateral to Lister's tubercle
- The third compartment (EPL) should be incised just distal to the extensor retinaculum and extended proximally

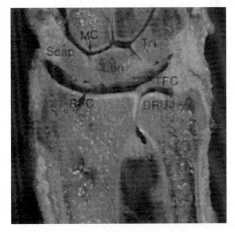

Cross-section anatomy (coronal view) demonstrates the intraosseous ligaments (small arrows) that imperceptibly blend the scaphoid (Scap), lunate (Lun), and triquetrum (Tri) to each other and separate the radiocarpal joint (RC) from the midcarpal joint (MC). The triangular fibrocartilage (TFC) is an ulnar extension of the articular surface of the distal radius and separates the radiocarpal from the distal radioulnar joint (DRUJ). It is the main stabilizer of the distal radioulnar joint. (From Bucholz RW, Heckman JD, eds. Rockwood and Green's Fractures in Adults, 5th ed. Philadelphia, PA: Lippincott Williams & Wilkins; 2001, with permission.)

The cross-sectional anatomy of the radius with comminution dorsally and radially. Note the tendency to dorsal collapse is the result of dorsal comminution and the collapse at the midcarpal joint. (From Bucholz RW, Heckman JD, eds. Rockwood and Green's Fractures in Adults, 5th ed. Philadelphia, PA: Lippincott Williams & Wilkins; 2001, with permission.)

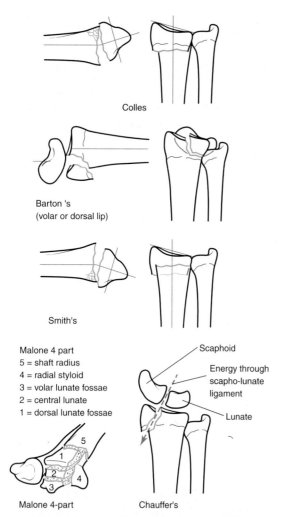

Colles

Barton 's
(volar or dorsal lip)

Smith's

Malone 4 part
5 = shaft radius
4 = radial styloid
3 = volar lunate fossae
2 = central lunate
1 = dorsal lunate fossae

Malone 4-part

Scaphoid

Energy through
scapho-lunate
ligament

Lunate

Chauffer's

Eponymic classification of five basic types of distal radius fractures: four classic (Colles, Barton, Smith, and Chauffeur's) fracture descriptions, and the Malone four-part fracture, which was described more recently and represents an increasing understanding of the importance of the distal radioulnar joint and the ulnar column of the radius.

- The EPL is retracted radially to allow entry into the floor of the third compartment
- The soft tissues should be elevated over the second and fourth compartments. They should be retracted radially and ulnarly, respectively
- Small Hohman retractor placed around the distal radius allow for adequate visualization
- Following reduction and plating, the dorsal retinaculum should be repaired
- The EPL can be left radially displaced out of compartment during closure

Closed Reduction Percutaneous Pinning
- Indicated for extra-articular fractures with intact volar cortex or polytrauma patients who may not be able to tolerate ORIF

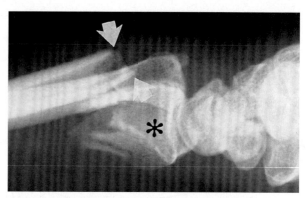

Smith fracture characterized by a transverse fracture (arrows) of the distal radius, with volar and proximal displacement of the distal radial fragment (asterisk). (From Harris JH Jr., Harris WH. The Radiology of Emergency Medicine, 3rd ed. Philadelphia, PA: Lippincott-Raven; 2000:386, with permission.)

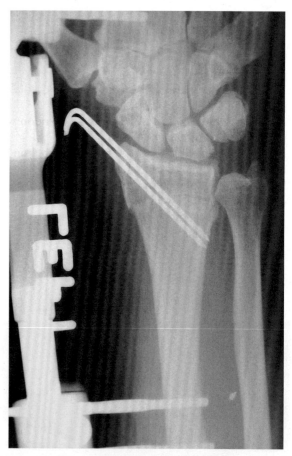

Distal radius fractures: external fixation and supplemental K-wires. Anteroposterior radiograph of distal radius fracture after closed reduction and external fixation with supplemental Kirschner wire. Radiocarpal and midcarpal articulations are seen without overdistraction. (From Koval KJ, Zuckerman JD. Atlas of Orthopaedic Surgery: A Multimedia Reference. Philadelphia, PA: Lippincott Williams & Wilkins; 2004 with permission.)

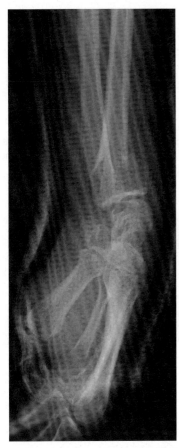

An extra-articular distal radius fracture poorly stabilized by adequate cast support with early loss of reduction and longitudinal collapse apparent. (From Bucholz RW, Heckman JD, eds. Rockwood and Green's Fractures in Adults, 5th ed. Philadelphia, PA: Lippincott Williams & Wilkins; 2001, with permission.)

- For most procedures, two pins may be utilized
- Reduce by traction, palmar translation of the distal fragment
- First pin is placed dorsal to volar. The entry site is ulnar to Lister's (in middle of wrist) on AP view
- The pin should be driven into the volar cortex
- Traction and ulnar deviation should be applied again for placement of the styloid pin
- Styloid pin starting point is at very distal tip of styloid on AP, at midwrist on lateral view.
- They should be aimed slightly dorsal to utilize the dorsal cortex

Recommended Readings

Abbaszadegan H, et al. Prediction of instability of Colles' fractures. Acta Orthop Scand 1989;60(6):646–650.

Bradway JK, et al. Open reduction and internal fixation of displaced, comminuted intra-articular fractures of the distal end of the radius. J Bone Joint Surg 1989;71(6):839–847.

Cooney WP III, et al. Complications of Colles' fractures. J Bone Joint Surg 1980:613–619

Fernandez DL. Distal radius fracture: the rationale of a classification. Chir Main. 2001;20(96):411–425.

Fernandez DL, Jupiter JB. Fractures of the Distal Radius. New York: Springer; 1995.

Howard PW, et al. External fixation or plaster for severely displaced comminuted Colles' fractures? A prospective study of anatomical and functional results. J Bone Joint Surg 1989;71(1):68–73.

Knirk JL, Jupiter JB. Intra-articular fractures of the distal end of the radius in young adults. J Bone Joint Surg 1986:232–233

Seitz WH Jr., et al. Limited open surgical approach for external fixation of distal radius fractures. J Hand Surg 1990;15(2):288–293.

Lower Extremity

PELVIC FRACTURES

- Commonly result from high-energy mechanisms (MVCs, motorcycles, falls from height) and are associated with significant morbidity and mortality
- May result from low-energy mechanisms in geriatric, osteoporotic patients
- These injuries require thorough evaluation of the patient and the associated injuries to allow for adequate treatment and stabilization of these patients

Evaluation

- ATLS protocols should be followed closely during the initial evaluation
- The patient's hemodynamic status should be monitored closely to avoid falling behind in fluid and blood resuscitation
- Hypothermia, acidosis, hypocalcemia should all be avoided as they can lead to coagulopathy and increased blood loss
- Patients should be evaluated for limb length equality and rotation

Stability

- Push/Pull examination of the pelvis should be performed as part of the initial assessment to determine stability of the pelvis
  - Unstable type C can usually be diagnosed by physical exam
  - The hemipelvis will rotate with compression and may also translate vertically and posteriorly with no endpoint when push–pull force applied

Radiographic signs of instability

- >1 cm of posterior or vertical displacement of iliac wings
- >5-mm posterior sacroiliac (SI) opening
- Pubic symphysis widening >2.5 cm
- Posterior fracture gap in open book–type injuries
- L5 transverse process avulsion/fractures (represent lumbosacral ligamentous instability)

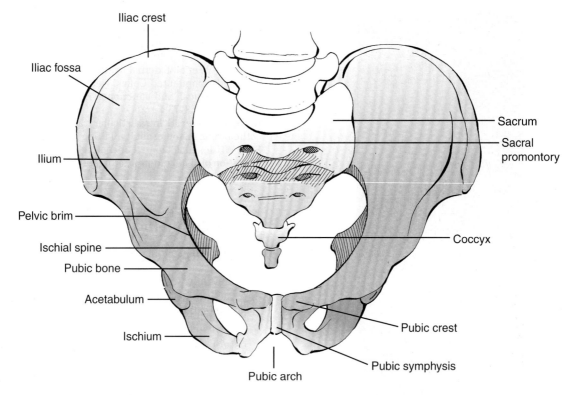

Iliac crest

Iliac fossa

Ilium

Pelvic brim

Ischial spine

Pubic bone

Acetabulum

Ischium

Sacrum

Sacral promontory

Coccyx

Pubic crest

Pubic symphysis

Pubic arch

A

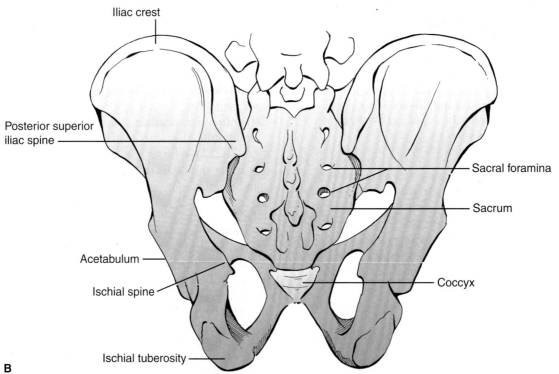

Iliac crest

Posterior superior iliac spine

Acetabulum

Ischial spine

Ischial tuberosity

Sacral foramina

Sacrum

Coccyx

B

Schematic showing bony architecture of the pelvic ring (**A**) from anterior and (**B**) from posterior. (From Bucholz RW, Court-Brown CM, Heckman JD, et al. *Rockwood & Green's Fractures in Adults*, 7th ed. Philadelphia: Lippincott, Williams & Wilkins, 2010.)

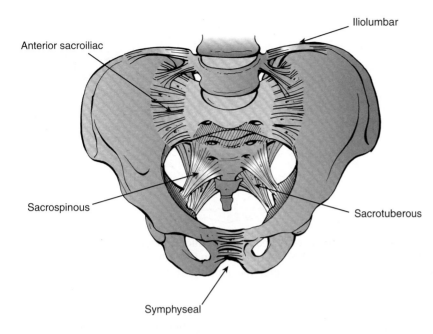

Iliolumbar

Anterior sacroiliac

Sacrospinous

Sacrotuberous

Symphyseal

Schematic drawing demonstrating the supporting ligamentous structures of the pelvic ring. (From Bucholz RW, Court-Brown CM, Heckman JD, et al. *Rockwood & Green's Fractures in Adults*, 7th ed. Philadelphia: Lippincott, Williams & Wilkins, 2010.)

– Sacral spine or Ischial tuberosity avulsions (represent sacrospinus or sacrotuberous ligamentous instability)

Open Fractures
– Any wounds or laceration in the pelvic region should be explored to rule out open fractures
  – 50% mortality in open pelvic fractures
  – Rectal (sigmoidoscopy) and vaginal (digital) examination may be necessary to rule out
  – Diverting colostomy may be necessary in patients with rectal lacerations

Shock and Mortality
– Overall 15%–25% mortality with high-energy pelvic fracture; leading cause of death is blood loss
– 20% of patients presenting are hemodynamically unstable
– Retroperitoneum can hold up to 4 L of blood
– Superior gluteal artery is most commonly injured vessel in posterior ring disruptions
– Internal pudendal artery bleeds are complicated by their location and the volume of blood lost from that region
– Shock and hypovolemia are associated with highest mortality rates in these patients

Genitourinary
– Watnik et al. (1996) showed that 12% of patients have genitourinary injuries in high-energy pelvic fracture (most commonly at bulbous urethra)
– Urethrogram indicated in severely displaced anterior fractures, patients with a high-riding prostate, or any meatus bleeding

– Be aware that urethrogram dye can interfere with angiography if necessary in hemodynamically unstable patients

Neurologic
– The lumbosacral plexus should be evaluated closely
  – 50% of patients with type C injuries were noted to have lumbosacral plexus injuries, while 8% of all patients suffering from pelvic fractures exhibit these injuries

Venous Thromboembolism
– 30%–50% of patients will develop a deep vein thrombosis (DVT)
– 2% pulmonary embolus rate in polytrauma patients with pelvic fractures compared with patients without an associated pelvic fracture
– Inferior vena cava filters should be considered in these patients as they may also have a head injury or other contraindication to pharmacologic anticoagulation
– 0.5%–2% fatal pulmonary embolism

Imaging
Radiographs
– Three views of the pelvis are utilized

AP Pelvis
– Provides an overall assessment of pelvic alignment
– True AP pelvis shows the pubic symphysis collinear with the sacral spinous processes
– The intersection of the iliopectineal line and the sacral ala should be at the superior margin of S2

Inlet
– Taken with the x-ray beam directly caudally 45 degrees to the radiographic film

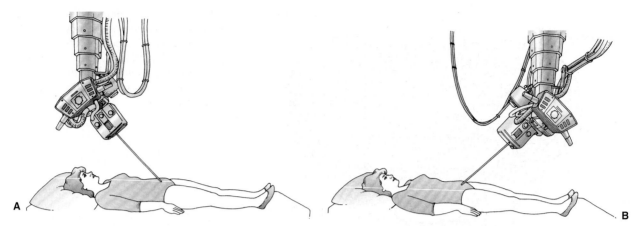

Schematic representing the direction of the incident x-ray beam for (**A**) inlet projection and (**B**) outlet projection of the pelvic ring. (From Bucholz RW, Court- Brown CM, Heckman JD, et al. *Rockwood & Green's Fractures in Adults*, 7th ed. Philadelphia: Lippincott, Williams & Wilkins, 2010.)

- Allows direct view into the pelvis to evaluate the rotation of the hemipelvis, widening of the pubic symphysis, and AP translation of the sacrum

Outlet
- Taken 45 degrees cephalad to the pelvis and radiographic film
- The sacrum is seen en face
- Allows visualization of vertical component of pelvis fractures

CT Scan
- Provides valuable 3D evaluation of the pelvis
- Subtle posterior injuries are missed in patients who appear to have an isolated injury
- The ring structure of the pelvis makes isolated fractures impossible
- 2-mm CT cuts should be performed to further evaluate and characterize those injuries

Anatomy/Biomechanics
- The pelvis is composed of two innominate bones and the sacrum
- Stability of the pelvis is dependent on the surrounding ligamentous structures
- Three primary components to pelvic stability
  1. Anterior symphysis and rami contributes 40% of stiffness of pelvis
  2. SI complex with SI IO ligament
     - The posterior structures provide approximately 60% of the strength of the pelvis
  3. Pelvic floor with sacrospinal and sacrotuberous ligaments
     Ability of pelvic ring to withstand physiologic forces without abnormal deformation is dependent on ligamentous attachments

- Vertically placed ligaments resist vertical shear or migration
  - Long posterior SI
  - Sacrotuberous
  - Lateral lumbosacral
- Transversely placed ligaments resist rotational forces
  - Short posterior SI
  - Sacrospinous
  - Iliolumbar

External Rotation Force
- Rotational forces (anterior posterior compression [APC]) disrupt the pubic symphysis leading to tears in the pelvic floor followed by the anterior SI ligaments tear until the ilium impinges on sacrum
- These injuries are partially stable if injury stops at the ilium and is not translated posteriorly or vertically
- Tearing of pelvic floor leads to associated visceral injuries and significant blood loss as seen in high-grade injuries

Internal Rotation Force
- Rotational forces (lateral compression [LC]) break anterior rami, but the pelvic floor is maintained
- Anterior sacrum is compressed if posterior SI ligaments remain intact, making the pelvis partially stable and preventing posterior or vertical translation
- There is a lower risk of visceral injury, but up to 50% of patients may have closed head injury or traumatic with these injuries

Classifications
Tile Classification

Tile Type A—Stable
- A1—Avulsion fracture

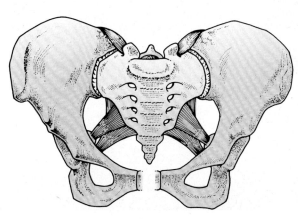
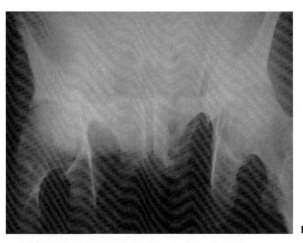

(**A**) Schematic and (**B**) outlet radiograph of a typical APC I injury. (From Bucholz RW, Court-Brown CM, Heckman JD, et al. *Rockwood & Green's Fractures in Adults*, 7th ed. Philadelphia: Lippincott, Williams & Wilkins, 2010.)

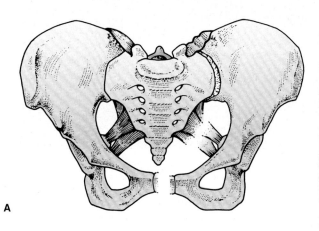
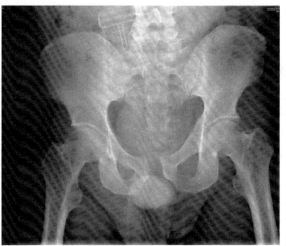
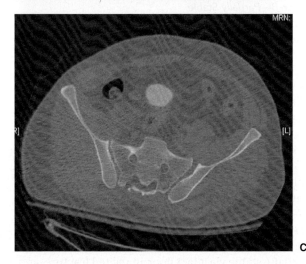

(**A**) Schematic and (**B**) AP radiograph with (**C**) CT scan of a typical APC II injury. (From Bucholz RW, Court-Brown CM, Heckman JD, et al. *Rockwood & Green's Fractures in Adults*, 7th ed. Philadelphia: Lippincott, Williams & Wilkins, 2010.)

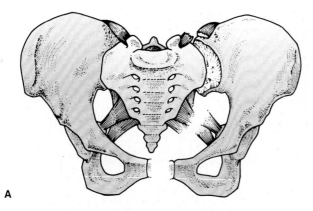

A

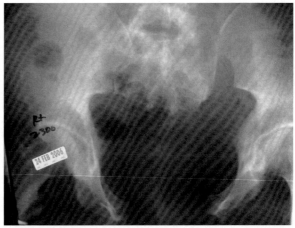

B

C

(**A**) Schematic and (**B**) AP radiograph with (**C**) CT scan of a typical APC III injury. (From Bucholz RW, Court-Brown CM, Heckman JD, et al. *Rockwood & Green's Fractures in Adults*, 7th ed. Philadelphia: Lippincott, Williams & Wilkins, 2010.)

- A2—Nondisplaced pelvic ring fracture (ramus fracture)
- A3—Transverse fracture coccyx/sacrum

Tile Type B—Partially Stable
- May be rotationally unstable
- The pelvis usually has an endpoint on physical exam
- Rami may be stuck in a displaced position
- Incomplete posterior ligamentous or SI injury is present
- The pelvis is stable to posterior and vertical stress
- B1—Open-book pelvic injury (external rotation force)
- Stage 1—diastasis <2.5 cm
  - Pelvic floor and SI joint intact
- Stage 2—diastasis >2.5 cm
- Pelvic floor disrupted
- Anterior SI ligaments disrupted
- B2—Internal rotation
- May be unstable to internal rotation
- May be stuck, impacted, internally rotated
- Partially stable via intact floor, impacted fracture, and remaining posterior ligaments
- B2-1—ipsilateral internal rotation injury

- Anterior inferior and superior rami fracture or
- Anterior overlapped locked pubis symphysis
- Posterior impaction of sacrum or ilium
- B2-2—contralateral internal rotation injury
- "Bucket handle"
- Hemipelvis rotates anteriorly and superiorly
- Anterior lesion is contralateral to posterior injury
- Affected hip is elevated with a shortened limb
- B3—bilateral, partially stable
- B3-1—bilateral open book
- B3-2—bilateral LC

Tile Type C—Rotationally and Vertically Unstable
- Complete posterior disruption
- Translates posteriorly and vertically
  - Grossly unstable, no endpoint on physical examination
- C1—ipsilateral anterior and posterior pelvic injury
- C1-1—disruption through the ilium
- C1-2—disruption through SI joint fracture-dislocation
- C1-3—through sacrum
- C2—unstable one side, partially stable on other side
- C3—bilateral hemipelvis unstable

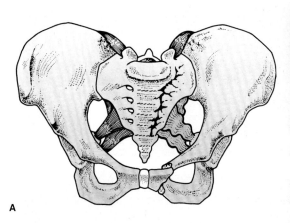

A

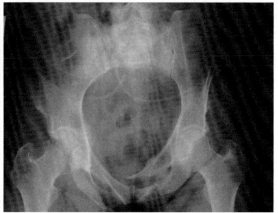

B

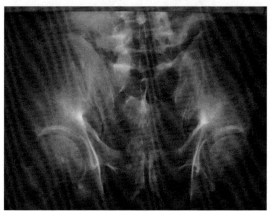

C

(**A**) Schematic and (**B**) inlet radiograph with (**C**) CT scan demonstrating a typical LCI injury with a sacral impaction fracture posteriorly and rami fractures anteriorly. (From Bucholz RW, Court-Brown CM, Heckman JD, et al. *Rockwood & Green's Fractures in Adults*, 7th ed. Philadelphia: Lippincott, Williams & Wilkins, 2010.)

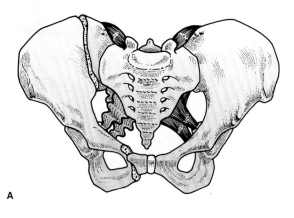

A

B

C

(**A**) Schematic and (**B**) AP radiograph with (**C**) CT scan of a typical LCII injury associated with an iliac wing fracture. (From Bucholz RW, Court- Brown CM, Heckman JD, et al. *Rockwood & Green's Fractures in Adults*, 7th ed. Philadelphia: Lippincott, Williams & Wilkins, 2010.)

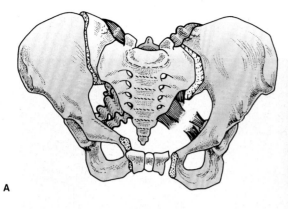

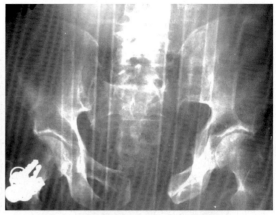

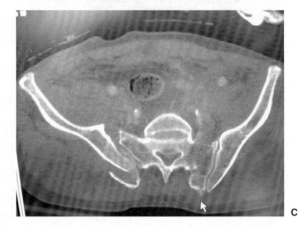

(**A**) Schematic and (**B**) AP radiograph with (**C**) CT scan of a typical LCIII injury. (From Bucholz RW, Court- Brown CM, Heckman JD, et al. *Rockwood & Green's Fractures in Adults*, 7th ed. Philadelphia: Lippincott, Williams & Wilkins, 2010.)

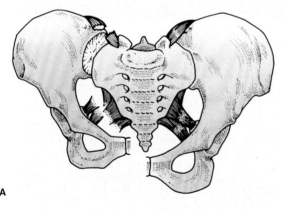

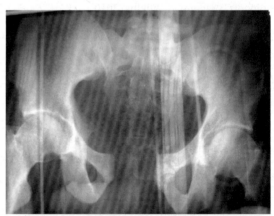

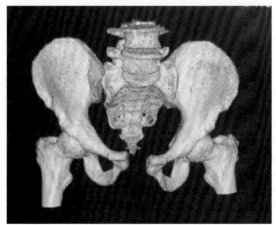

(**A**) Schematic and (**B**) AP radiograph with (**C**) CT scan of a typical VS injury. (From Bucholz RW, Court- Brown CM, Heckman JD, et al. *Rockwood & Green's Fractures in Adults*, 7th ed. Philadelphia: Lippincott, Williams & Wilkins, 2010.)

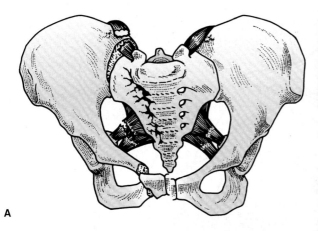

A

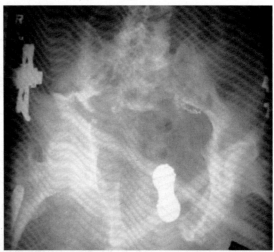

B

C

Schematic and (**B**) AP radiograph with (**C**) CT scan of a typical CM injury. (From Bucholz RW, Court-Brown CM, Heckman JD, et al. *Rockwood & Green's Fractures in Adults*, 7th ed. Philadelphia: Lippincott, Williams & Wilkins, 2010.)

Young and Burgess Classification
- Classification is based on the mechanism of injury/ direction of force
- 50% of presenting patients have LC fractures while 21% are APC fractures.

Anterior Posterior Compression I—Vertical Ramus Fracture
- Diastasis 1–2 cm
- SI ligaments intact

Anterior Posterior Compression II
- Diastasis >2 cm
- Anterior SI ligaments disrupted
- Sacrotuberous ligament disrupted
- Posterior SI ligaments intact

Anterior Posterior Compression III
- Complete hemipelvic separation
- No vertical displacement
- High risk of hemorrhage
- Diastasis >5 cm to open completely posteriorly

Lateral Compression I—Oblique Anterior Fracture
- Anterior pelvic ring injury
- Ipsilateral sacrum impaction

Lateral Compression II
- Anterior pelvic ring injury
- Crescent fracture of iliac wing or near SI joint

Lateral Compression III
- LC I or II plus open-book SI injury on contralateral side
  - Hemipelvic internal rotation on one side, external rotation on the contralateral side
- High incidence of head injury, which can also lead to hypotension
- High mortality from associated injuries

Vertical Shear
- Usually SI rupture but may also occur via fracture of ilium or sacrum
- High incidence hemorrhage and hemodynamic instability

Combined Mechanism
- Any combination of LC or APC injuries

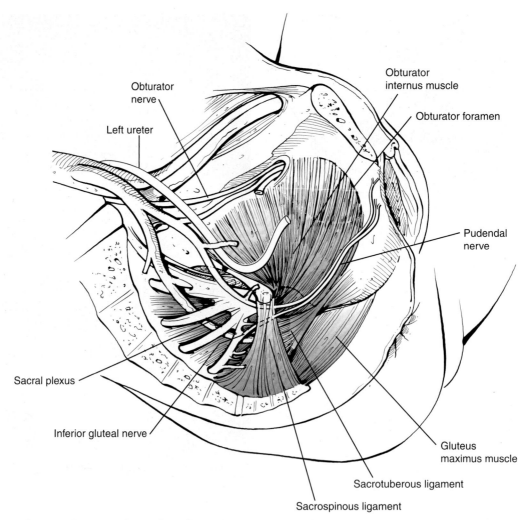

Picture showing relationship of vascular structures to ligamentous structures within pelvic cavity. (From Bucholz RW, Court- Brown CM, Heckman JD, et al. *Rockwood & Green's Fractures in Adults*, 7th ed. Philadelphia: Lippincott, Williams & Wilkins, 2010.)

Treatment

External Fixation

- External fixation is part of resuscitation process in hemodynamically unstable patients
- Vertically unstable patients benefit from early placement of a tibial/femoral traction pin to stabilize the fracture
- External fixation is indicated in lesions that increase pelvic volume such as Tile B1, B3-1, and all Tile C's, with ongoing bleed or signs of hemodynamic instability
- Posterior ligamentous injury without pelvic widening are generally not life threatening

Iliac Wing External Fixation

- Position: Supine on radiolucent table
- Incision: Palpate the iliac wing and make a small 2–4-cm incision proximal to the AIS perpendicular to the iliac wing

- Technique:
  1. Place a guidewire along the inner table to provide orientation of the pelvic slope
  2. Palpate the Iliac wing and position drill along the inner third of the iliac wing
     Too Lateral can violate the inner table.
  3. Insert the 5-mm schanz pin between the two tables aiming toward the hip joint
  4. The second pin should be placed anteriorly or posteriorly in a converging fashion
  5. Following compression of the pelvis and application of the frame, hemodynamic stability may be maintained

Supracetabular Pins

- Considered more biomechanically stable
- Additionally, patients able to sit up more comfortably with the fixator in place when placed as definitive treatment

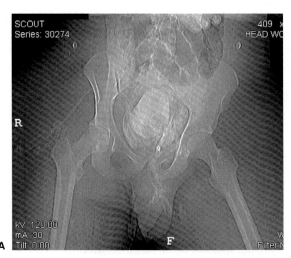 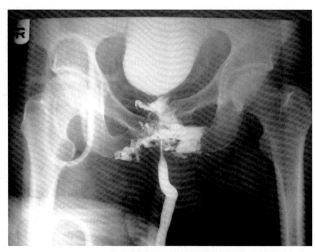

Radiographic appearance of (**A**) bladder rupture and (**B**) urethral disruption. (From Bucholz RW, Court-Brown CM, Heckman JD, et al. *Rockwood & Green's Fractures in Adults*, 7th ed. Philadelphia: Lippincott, Williams & Wilkins, 2010.)

Incision: Palpate the ASIS and locate an area 2–3 cm distal directly in line. Make a small 2–3-cm incision

Technique
1. Spread the soft tissues aiming 20–30 degrees internally
2. Confirm the anterior inferior iliac crest starting point
3. The pin should be in the apex of the AIIS on the iliac oblique view
4. Place the pin and advance in the direction of the sciatic notch
5. Confirm with iliac/obturator oblique views
6. Connect the pins to crossbar and reduce as necessary

7. Supracetabular and iliac wing pinc can be placed for improved rqtational stability.

Dangers
– Lesion of the **LFCN:** occurs in 1%–13% of cases.
– Joint perforation
– Pin site infection
– External fixation alone does not stabilize posterior ring disruption
– 80% failure rate in definitive treatment of unstable type C pelvis with external fixation

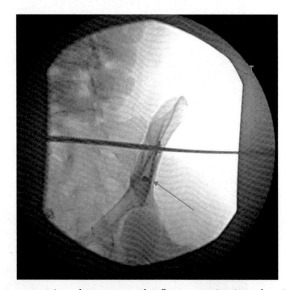

Clinical photograph showing an anterior external fixator placed low enough to provide access to the abdomen for laparotomy. (From Bucholz RW, Court-Brown CM, Heckman JD, et al. *Rockwood & Green's Fractures in Adults*, 7th ed. Philadelphia: Lippincott, Williams & Wilkins, 2010.)

Intraoperative obturator outlet fluoroscopic view showing teardrop for supra-acetabular pin placement. (From Bucholz RW, Court-Brown CM, Heckman JD, et al. *Rockwood & Green's Fractures in Adults*, 7th ed. Philadelphia: Lippincott, Williams & Wilkins, 2010.)

Nonoperative
- Tile A
- Most Tile B1-1, B2-1
- May require external fixation in multitrauma if no obvious signs of the cause of hemodynamic stability
- May require SI screw fixation for posterior injuries to maintain stability
- B1-1 = APC with <2.5-cm diastasis
- B2-1 = LC with sacral impaction

Indications for Operative Fixation
- Early internal fixation may lead to increased complications but may be indicated in posterior injuries with pubic symphysis (PS) diastasis/medial ramus fractures in patients undergoing exploratory laparoscopy
- Single plating of the PS if >2.5-cm displacement in type B injuries
- SI screw placement is crucial to fixation in fractures with anterior and posterior injuries
- Insertion may lead to L5 root
- Transsacral screws are not applicable in patients with a dysmorphic pelvis
- Pre- and postoperative neurovascular exams are crucial for evaluation of possible neurologic injury

- Posterior extra-articular ORIF of crescent fractures (SI fracture-dislocation) may be necessary
- Tilt fractures: superior pubic ramus fracture with pubic symphysis widening, disruption, and overlap
  - Lead to dyspareunia
- Most type Cs should undergo ORIF of the front and back after temporizing with external fixation and traction

Indications for Surgery for Lateral Compression Fractures
- Limb length discrepancy >1.5 cm
- Severe internal or external rotation deformity
- Bony impingement of vagina or perineum
- SI involvement → instability
- External fixation or SI screw fixation is performed in patients with severe pain from ambulation

Or Tips and Tricks—SI Screw
- The sacrum is angulated 45 degrees from the axis of the spine and pelvis
- The patient is positioned supine and should be prepped as posteriorly as possible
- Lines should be drawn on the abdomen to visualize the wire positioning

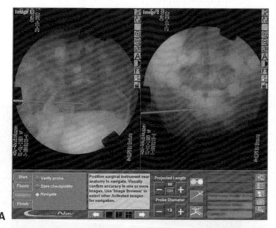
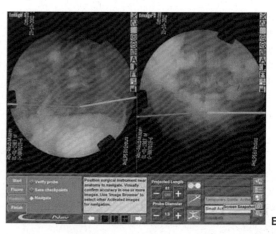
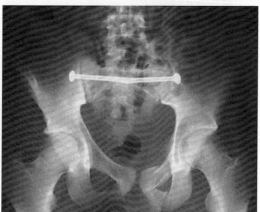

Bilateral sacroiliac screws. **A, B.** Typical intraoperative display of computer screen during bilateral insertion of two sacroiliac screws. The live spatial position of the drill guide is simultaneously presented on two views (inlet and outlet) with a virtual continuation representing the track of the guidewire. **C.** Postoperative verification radiograph showing the accurate real position of the two sacroiliac screws after the navigation process. (Images property of Drs. Meir Liebergall, Rami Mosheff, Leo Joskewicz.)

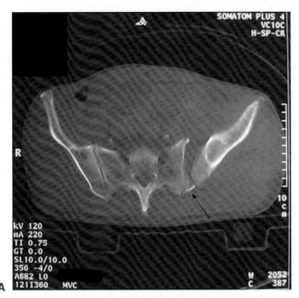 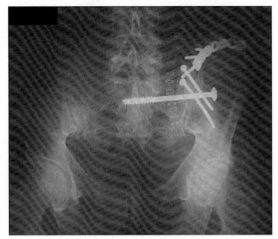

(A) Axial CT scan and **(B)** postoperative radiograph demonstrating a small crescent fragment with significant involvement of the SI joint treated with ORIF and a supplemental SI screw. (From Bucholz RW, MD. Court-Brown CM, Heckman JD, Tornetta P. Rockwood & Green's Fractures in Adults, 7th ed: Philadelphia: Lippincott Williams & Wilkins, 2010.)

- The wires should be shown in the proper location on the inlet and outlet
- The entry line is the intersection of two planes created by the two views showing proper positioning of the wire
- Draw lines depicting x-ray beams in outlet and inlet views
- On the inlet view, move anterior or posterior on sacrum by moving perpendicular to inlet beam
- On the outlet view, move proximal or distal on the sacrum by moving perpendicular to outlet beam
- The screws should be placed perpendicular to the fracture lines if a sacral fracture is present.
- Do not compress across sacral fracture if the fracture transverses the foramen (Denis II)
- Place the SI screw perpendicular to the SI joint if there is no fracture present.

Recommended Readings
Dujardin FH. Long-term functional prognosis of posterior injuries in high-energy pelvic disruption. J Orthop Trauma 1998;12(3):145–151
Watnik NF, Goldberger M. Urologic injuries in pelvic ring disruptions. Clin Orthop Relat Res 1996;329:37–45.

ACETABULAR FRACTURE

Anatomy
- The acetabulum is composed of two columns in the shape of an inverted "Y"

- Anterior column: Anterior half of the iliac wing to the superior pubic ramus
- Posterior column: Superior aspect of greater sciatic notch to the ischial tuberosity

Mechanism of Injury
- Acetabular fractures are caused by force generated through the femoral head into the acetabulum.
- Patients may present with low- or high-energy mechanism of injury
- Mechanism of injury dictates the patient evaluation

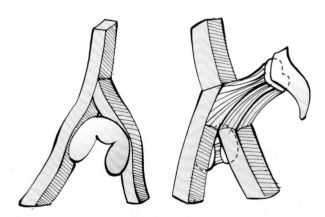

The acetabulum is supported by two columns in the shape on an inverted "Y." These are in turn linked to the sacrum by the sciatic buttress. From Bucholz RW, Court-Brown CM, Heckman JD, et al. *Rockwood & Green's Fractures in Adults*, 7th ed. Philadelphia: Lippincott, Williams & Wilkins, 2010.)

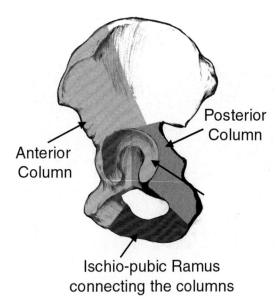

Columns of the acetabulum as described by Letournel and Judet. 76 (Copyright Berton R. Moed, MD.)

High Energy
– Young population
– Motor vehicle injuries most common
– Polytrauma or high-energy blunt trauma
– ATLS principles with care taken during the secondary survey for associated injuries
– Associated injuries include extremity, CNS, nerve palsy, genitourinary injury, and spine injury
– Thorough evaluation is essential to missing additional injuries

Low Energy
– Older population
– Osteoporotic patients
– Result from fall onto lateral side

– Often isolated injury
– Despite low energy may be comminuted and displaced due to poor bone quality

Radiographs
– Obturator oblique
  – Best view for visualizing hip dislocation
  – Visualizes the anterior column, posterior wall
  – Obturator foramen is seen en face
– Iliac oblique
  – Visualizes the posterior column, anterior wall
  – Iliac wing is seen en face

Letournel's Elementary Fracture
(Direct reduction of only one column needed)
– Posterior wall (most common)
– Posterior column
– Anterior wall
– Anterior column
– Transverse (involves both columns)

Letournel's Associated Fracture
(Multiple fragments and multiplanar injury)
– Posterior wall, posterior column
– Posterior wall, transverse
– Anterior column, posterior hemitransverse
– T shaped (worst prognosis)
– Both columns (floating acetabulum)

Six Lines
– 1—iliopectineal: anterior column
– 2—ilioischial: posterior column
– 3—teardrop: quadrilateral plate
– 4—roof
– 5—anterior rim
– 6—posterior rim (more lateral)

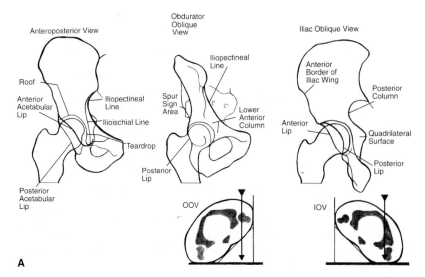

Radiographic assessment of acetabular fractures. **A:** The anteroposterior, obturator oblique, and iliac views are essential for the definition of the fracture. (From Hansen ST, Swiontkowski MF. Orthopaedic trauma protocols. New York, NY: Raven; 1993:249.)

A

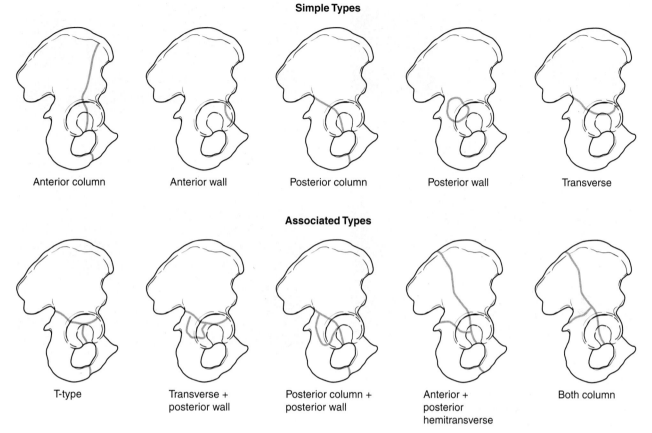

Simple Types

Anterior column   Anterior wall   Posterior column   Posterior wall   Transverse

Associated Types

T-type   Transverse + posterior wall   Posterior column + posterior wall   Anterior + posterior hemitransverse   Both column

Letournel classification of acetabular fractures. (From Bucholz RW, Heckman JD, eds. Rockwood and Green's Fractures in Adults, 5th ed. Philadelphia, PA: Lippincott Williams & Wilkins; 2001.)

Posterior Wall Fractures
- Ilioischial line intact
- Gull sign
- Most common simple fracture
- Poor results associated with articular comminution
- Associated with posterior hip dislocation

Posterior Column Fractures
- Only involve ischium
- Exits out greater sciatic notch and obturator foramen
- Ilioischial line disrupted

Anterior Wall Fractures
- Central portion of anterior column is most often injured
- Iliopectineal line involved
- Inferior pubic ramus and obturator foramen intact

Anterior Column Fractures
- Iliopectineal line disrupted
- Roof usually displaces medially
- Inferior pubic ramus and obturator foramen disrupted

Transverse Fractures
- Horizontal/oblique fracture across acetabulum
- Both iliopectineal and ilioischial disrupted
- Infratectal (through fossa acetabuli) vs. transtectal (through acetabular dome) vs. juxtatectal (through junction between dome and fossa acetabuli)

T-Type
- Transverse with vertical component that exits out obturator foramen
- Associated with heterotopic ossification (HO)

Anterior Column, Posterior Hemitransverse
- May be difficult to distinguish from T-type fractures
- Anterior column (AC) fracture with fracture line that involves posterior column (PC)

Both Columns
- Acetabular roof (with an associated part of the anterior ilium) is separated from pelvis
- The posterior ilium is free floating
- Can be misdiagnosed as a T-type fracture.

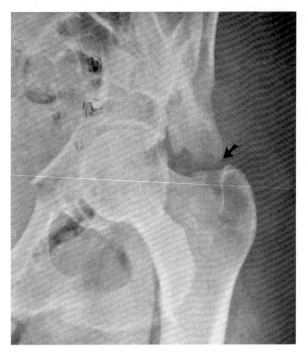

The classic spur sign of this fracture (arrow) is seen on the obturator oblique view showing the division on both columns above the acetabulum. Note the further fracture line through the anterior column with a T fracture dividing the obturator foramen. (From Tile M, ed. Fractures of the Pelvis and Acetabulum, 2nd ed. Baltimore, MD: Williams & Wilkins; 1995.)

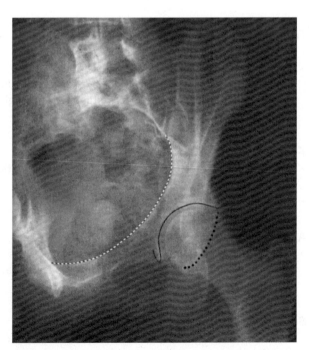

Obturator oblique x-ray of the left hemipelvis. (From Tile M, ed. Fractures of the Pelvis and Acetabulum. Baltimore, MD: Williams & Wilkins; 1984.)

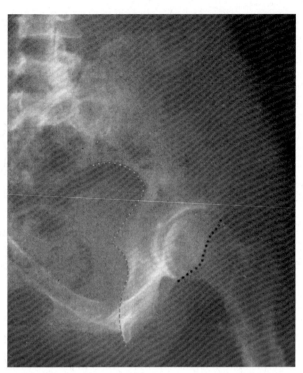

Iliac oblique radiographic view of the left hemipelvis. (From Tile M, ed. Fractures of the Pelvis and Acetabulum, 2nd ed. Baltimore, MD: Williams & Wilkins; 1995.)

- Can be distinguished by additional fracture line that separates posterior ilium from roof
- "Spur" sign = Visualized on obturator oblique. Posterior iliac wing is lateral to the displaced acetabular roof
- Acetabulum and lower extremity are dissociated from axial skeleton

CT Scan
- Horizontal line = fracture of one or both columns
- Vertical line = transverse fracture
- Provides visualization of the extent of articular involvement
- Allows visualization of loose bodies
- Marginal impaction (in 25% of posterior walls)
- Posterior wall size

Treatment
- Skeletal traction if hip unstable or head impacted into pelvis (protrusio)

Nonoperative Criteria
(Matta, 1993)
- 10-mm CT subchondral arc without fracture line
- >45-degree medial roof arc angle (vertical line from center head vs. line from center head to fracture) without fracture on all views
- >50%–80% posterior wall intact

- Femoral head congruent on three views
- Negative fluoroscopic stress views with flexion to 90 degrees showing no subluxation or dislocation of the hip
- Secondary congruence on both-column fracture (especially in elderly)
- Touch-toe weight bearing for 10–12 wk
- Close radiographic follow-up

Contraindications to Surgery
- Morbid obesity
- Open contaminated wound
- DVT unless inferior vena cava filter placed and patient stable from pulmonary standpoint

Indications
- Dome displacement >2 mm
- Posterior wall fracture >40%, unstable
  - Intra-articular loose body
- Irreducible fracture—dislocation
- Morel-Lavalle closed degloving
  - Requires incision and drainage due to high risk of infection
  - May require serial debridements followed by wound vacuum application
  - 12% have a risk of infection despite incision and drainage

Approaches
- Most common reason for suboptimal fixation and intra-articular hardware is inappropriate surgical approach

Kocher-Langenbeck (K-L) Approach
- Posterior wall
- Posterior column
- Most transverse (displacement usually greatest posteriorly)
  - T-type
  - Flex knee 90 degrees to relax sciatic nerve
- 2%–10% sciatic nerve iatrogenic injury
- Damage to femoral head blood supply
- Approach is associated with a high incidence of HO

Ilioinguinal Incision
- Anterior column, anterior wall
- Anterior column, posterior hemitransverse
- Both column; ± T type
- Allows one to visualize medial acetabulum
- Lateral femoral cutaneous nerve (LFCN) injury more common than femoral nerve
- Femoral vessel thrombosis
- Laceration of corona mortis
- Lowest incidence of HO

Extended Iliofemoral Approach
- Highest incidence of HO
- Stripping of gluteal muscle from the iliac crest increases risk of gluteal artery injury and gluteal muscle necrosis

Fixation
- Most common fixation with lag screws in combination with reconstruction plate placement
- "Spring plate": One-third tubular plate, which is cut and bent to allow for fixation of small posterior wall fragments that do not tolerate screw fixation

Poor Prognosis
- Old age
- Cartilage damage/impaction to femoral head
- Malreduction on postoperative radiograph

Complications
- 7% HO as defined by loss of 20% of hip ROM; associated with iliofemoral approach, T type
- Sciatic nerve palsy
  - 31% incidence preoperative
  - 2%–16% iatrogenic
- 1.5% deep infection with K-L approach
- 5% significant HO with K-L
- 34% DVT, 2% pulmonary embolism with surgery
- 6%–7% AVN with all acetabular fractures, 18% of posterior fracture patterns
- Postfixation total hip replacement requires increased operative time, increased blood loss, and higher requirement for bone grafting.

Operative Anatomy
Anatomy of Kocher-Langenbeck
- Split gluteus maximus, tensor fascia latae, section external rotations
- Identify greater and lesser sciatic notch
- Superior gluteal nerve and artery exit superior/deep to piriformis
- Exiting inferior/deep to piriformis
  - Inferior gluteal nerve and artery
  - Pudendal nerve and artery
  - Nerve to obturator internus
  - Nerve to quadratus femoris
  - Sciatic nerve
  - Posterior femoral cutaneous nerve

Sciatic and Piriformis Variations
- 84%—sciatic nerve runs deep to piriformis and superficial to other short external rotators, thus taking off and peeling back piriformis only does not protect sciatic nerve
- 12%—peroneal division passes through muscle and tibial division passes deep to it

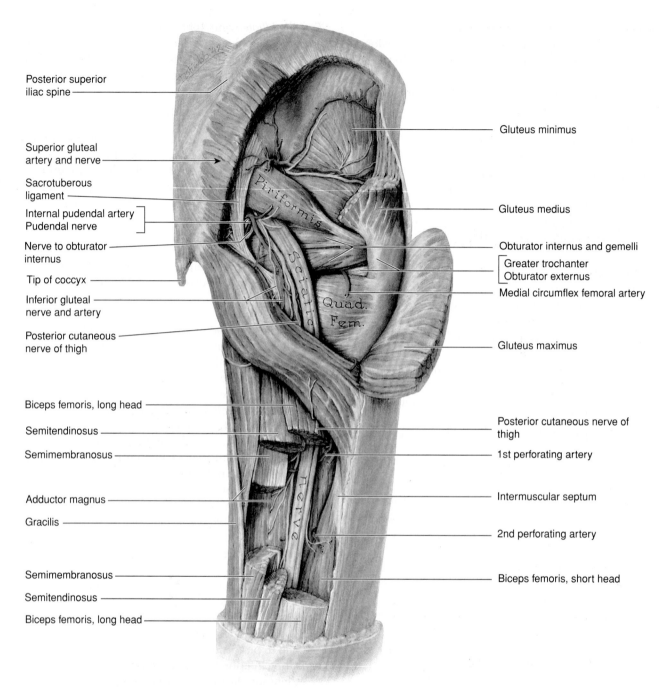

Posterior superior iliac spine

Superior gluteal artery and nerve

Sacrotuberous ligament

Internal pudendal artery
Pudendal nerve

Nerve to obturator internus

Tip of coccyx

Inferior gluteal nerve and artery

Posterior cutaneous nerve of thigh

Biceps femoris, long head

Semitendinosus

Semimembranosus

Adductor magnus

Gracilis

Semimembranosus

Semitendinosus

Biceps femoris, long head

Gluteus minimus

Gluteus medius

Obturator internus and gemelli

Greater trochanter
Obturator externus

Medial circumflex femoral artery

Gluteus maximus

Posterior cutaneous nerve of thigh

1st perforating artery

Intermuscular septum

2nd perforating artery

Biceps femoris, short head

Deep dissection of the gluteal region and the posterior aspect of thigh. Most of the gluteus maximus and medius are removed, and segments of the hamstrings are excised. Note that the superior gluteal artery and nerve emerge from the pelvis superior to the piriformis to lie between the gluteus medius and minimus. The inferior gluteal artery and nerve, the sciatic nerve, and the posterior cutaneous nerve of the thigh typically emerge inferior to the piriformis; however, exceptions occur. (From Moore KL, Dalley AF II, eds. Clinical Oriented Anatomy, 4th ed. Baltimore, MD: Lippincott Williams & Wilkins; 1999.)

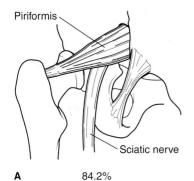

Piriformis

Sciatic nerve

A   84.2%

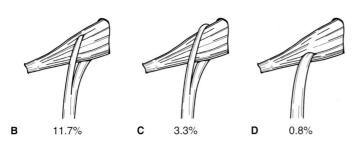

B   11.7%   **C**   3.3%   **D**   0.8%

A–D: The sciatic nerve is a single structure that emerges from the greater sciatic notch anterior to the piriformis in 84% of cases. In 16%, a portion of the nerve passes through the piriformis or posterior to it, placing it at greater risk. (From Bucholz RW, Heckman JD, eds. Rockwood and Green's Fractures in Adults, 5th ed. Philadelphia, PA: Lippincott Williams & Wilkins; 2001.)

– 3%—peroneal passes superficial to piriformis, tibial passes deep
– 1%—entire sciatic nerve passes through piriformis

Gluteus Maximus
– Superior gluteal artery supplies upper one-third
– Inferior gluteal artery supplies lower two-thirds
– Fat plane exists in this intervascular interval > split there
– Entire innervation from inferior gluteal nerve, thus stop split when first branch to upper part of muscle seen
– Safest way to find sciatic nerve is to follow quadratus femoris on its posterior surface
– Following obturator internus proximally leads to ischial tubercle and lesser sciatic notch
– Obturator internus comes from inner surface of obturator foramen, takes 90-degree turn through lesser sciatic notch, then to hip
– Gemelli come from near ischial spine and insert into oburator internus tendon

Or Tips and Tricks—Ilioinguinal Approach
– Position the patient supine on a Jackson table
– The incision is midline 3 cm above pubis, lateral to anterior superior iliac spine, along anterior two-thirds of crest
– The iliacus is elevated off the inner wall posteriorly to SI joint and medially to brim
– Expose the aponeuorosis of external oblique to further visualize the rectus abdominis. The incision should be extended 1 cm proximal to external inguinal ring

– The external oblique is then reflected distally to unroof inguinal canal
– Place a penrose around the round ligament/spermatic cord and ilioinguinal nerve in the medial aspect of canal
– Incise the inguinal ligament sharply to leave a 2-mm cuff with common origins of internal oblique, transversus abdominis, and transversalis fascia. (The neurovascular structures are underneath.)
– The LFCN exits into thigh under inguinal ligament 2 to 3 cm medial to ASIS
– The external iliac vessels are just below the incised ligament
– Cut the insertion of the conjoined tendon into pubis medial to the vessels
– The rectus abdominis may need to be elevated from the pubis
– Pack retropubic space of Retzius
– The anterior aspects of femoral vessels and lymphatics within lacuna vasorum are located in the middle of the wound
– The lacuna musculorum, the iliopsoas, the femoral nerve, and the LFCN are located laterally
– The iliopsoas sheath or iliopectineal fascia separates these two lacunas
– Separate penrose drains are placed around the contents of vasorum and musculorum
– The iliopectineal fascia is then developed and incised to the pectineal eminence and detached from pelvic brim
– Detaching the iliopectineal fascia allows access to the true pelvis, quadrilateral surface, and posterior column

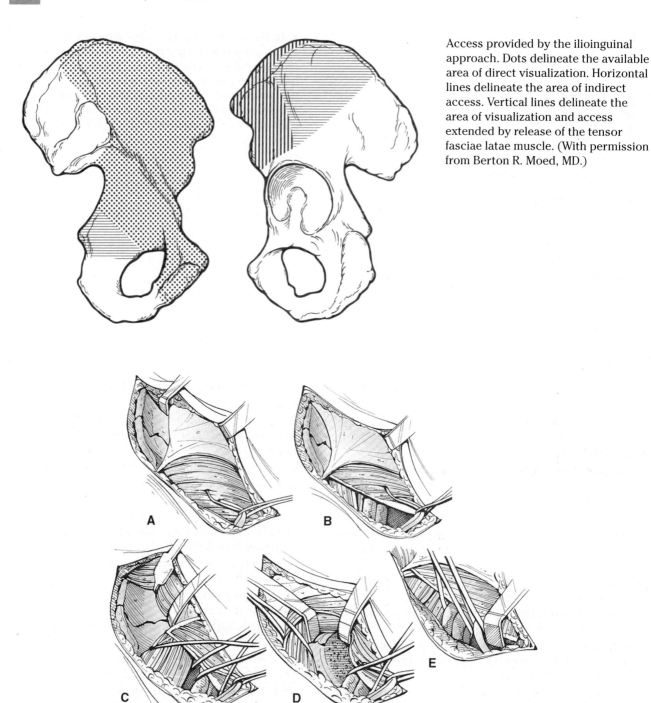

Access provided by the ilioinguinal approach. Dots delineate the available area of direct visualization. Horizontal lines delineate the area of indirect access. Vertical lines delineate the area of visualization and access extended by release of the tensor fasciae latae muscle. (With permission from Berton R. Moed, MD.)

The ilioinguinal approach. **A.** The skin incision extends from just posterior to the gluteus medius tubercle, paralleling the iliac crest to the anterior superior iliac spine and then coursing medially to the midline ending two finger-breaths above the pubic symphysis. **B.** The iliacus muscle has been dissected subperiosteally from the internal iliac fossa, and the external oblique aponeurosis has been incised from the anterior superior iliac spine to the midline, passing at least 1 cm superior to the superficial inguinal ring, and reflected distally. The spermatic cord in the male or the round ligament in the female is bluntly isolated along with the ilioinguinal nerve and retracted using a rubber sling. The now-exposed inguinal ligament is split through its entire length and the iliopectineal fascia is seen to be separating the femoral nerve and iliopsoas from the external iliac vessels. **C.** The iliopectineal fascia has been released and the exposure is complete. The lateral window exposes the internal iliac fossa to the sacroiliac joint and pelvic brim. **D.** The middle window exposes the pelvic brim to the pectineal eminence, the quadrilateral surface, and the anterior wall. **E.** The medial window is shown here with retraction of the spermatic cord laterally. The rectus abdominis tendon has been transected. The space of Retzius, superior ramus, and symphysis pubis are visualized. (From Bucholz RW, Court-Brown CM, Heckman JD, Tornetta P. Rockwood & Green's Fractures in Adults, 7th ed. Philadelphia: Lippincott Williams & Wilkins, 2010.)

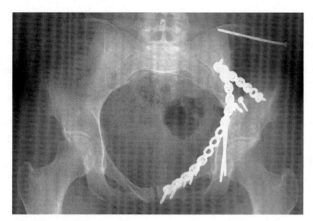

Radiographic appearance at 2 years. This patient was treated through the Ilioinguinal approach. Obliquely oriented screws were placed from just lateral to the pelvic brim and directed posteriorly toward the superior iliac extension of the posterior wall fragment. (With permission from Berton R. Moed, MD.)

- Prior to retracting the external iliac vessels, locate the obturator artery and nerve posteromedially
- Locate the obturator artery and nerve prior to retracting the external iliac vessels

First (Lateral) Window
- Medial retraction of iliopsoas and the femoral nerve. This allows access to internal iliac fossa, SI joint, and pelvic brim

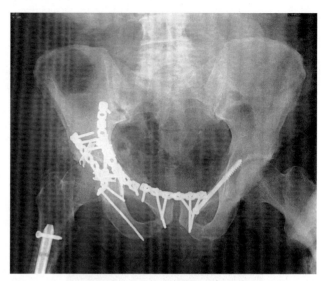

The same patient, 6 weeks after staged open reduction and internal fixation of right acetabular fracture and pubic diastasis with pelvic reconstruction plates, retrograde left superior ramus lag screw, and retrograde interlocked intramedullary rod for associated right femoral fracture. (From Mulholland MW, et al., eds. Greenfield's Surgery Scientific Principles and Practice, 4th ed. Philadelphia, PA: Lippincott Williams & Wilkins; 2006.)

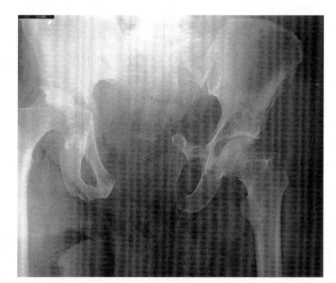

Polytrauma victim. Grade III open pelvic disruption with associated urogenital injury. Orthopedic injuries include pubic diastasis, left sacroiliac dislocation, left superior and inferior pubic rami fractures, right acetabular fracture and hip dislocation, and right femoral fracture. (From Mulholland MW, et al., eds. Greenfield's Surgery Scientific Principles and Practice, 4th ed. Philadelphia, PA: Lippincott Williams & Wilkins; 2006.)

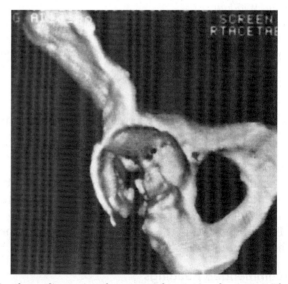

The three-dimensional computed tomography scan with the head subtracted shows the large posterior wall fragment that has the potential for instability and comminution, best seen from the posterior view. (From Bucholz RW, Heckman JD, eds. Rockwood and Green's Fractures in Adults, 5th ed. Philadelphia, PA: Lippincott Williams & Wilkins; 2001.)

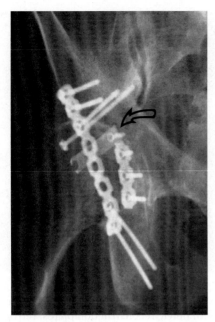

X-rays show excellent anatomic reduction, stabilization of the posterior wall fragment by a lag screw, and, in this case because of the marked comminution, a spring plate held under the main buttress plate (arrow). A second reconstruction plate was used to buttress the multiple fragments along the lesser notch. The long buttress plate is in the typical location, and no screws are placed in the danger zone centrally. (From Bucholz RW, Heckman JD, eds. Rockwood and Green's Fractures in Adults, 5th ed. Philadelphia, PA: Lippincott Williams & Wilkins; 2001.)

Second Window
- Lateral retraction of the iliopsoas and femoral nerve
- Medial retraction of the external iliac vessels shows the pelvic brim from the SI joint to the pectineal eminence and quadrilateral surface

Third (Medial) Window
- Lateral retraction of the external iliac vessels and medial or lateral retraction of the spermatic cord shows superior pubic ramus and symphysis
- Repair all layers
- The inguinal ligament remnant should be repaired to the transversalis fascia, conjoined tendon of the internal oblique, and the transversus abdominis
- The aponeurosis of the external oblique should then be repaired

Recommended Readings

Hoppenfeld S, Deboer P, Thomas HA, eds. Surgical Exposures in Orthopedics: The Anatomic Approach, 2nd ed. Philadelphia: JB Lippincott; 1994.

Judet R, et al. Fractures of the acetabulum: classification and surgical approaches for open reduction. Preliminary report. J Bone Joint Surg 1964;1615–1646.

Letournel E. Acetabulum fractures: classification and management. Clin Orthop Relat Res 1980;151:81–106.

Letournel E, Judet R, eds. Fractures of the Acetabulum, 2nd ed. New York: Springer-Verlag; 1993.

Letournel E. Acetabulum fractures: Classification and management. Clin Orthop 1980:81–107.

Letournel E. The treatment of acetabular fractures through the ilioinguinal approach. Clin Orthop 1993:62–76.

Letournel E, Judet R. Fractures of the Acetabulum, 2nd edition. New York: Springer-Verlag; 1993.

Matta JM. Operative treatment of acetabular fractures through the ilioinguinal approach: a 10-year perspective. Clin Orthop 1994:10–19.

Mayo KA. Open reduction and internal fixation of fractures of the acetabulum. Results in 163 fractures. Clin Orthop 1994:31–37.

HIP DISLOCATION

Background
- The hip joint is inherently stable
- Acute native hip dislocation requires urgent intervention
- Predominately results from high-speed/high-energy mechanism
- Posterior hip dislocations result from motor vehicle accidents due to the resultant dashboard injury → posterior-directed force on a flexed and adducted hip
- These are also associated meniscal and ligamentous injuries of the knee
- Patients must be evaluated according to ATLS protocol to avoid missing additional injuries

Mechanism
- Posterior: Flexed hip, adduction, and internal rotation
- Posterior fracture dislocation: Partial flexion, less adduction, internal rotation
- Anterior: Hyperabduction, extension, and external rotation

Imaging
- AP pelvis, AP, and lateral views of the ipsilateral hip and femur
- Consider Judet views, or inlet/outlet films in patients with associated pelvic or acetabular injuries (should be reserved for after reduction of the hip)
- Following reduction, CT scan should be performed to evaluate for associated
  - Acetabular fracture
  - Intra-articular retained fragment
  - Femoral head fracture
  - Symmetry of reduction

Classification
See figure OTA classification page 291
- Classification determined by location of dislocation
- Pipkin classification includes fracture dislocations of the femoral head
  - Type 1: Posterior dislocation with femoral head fracture caudad to the fovea

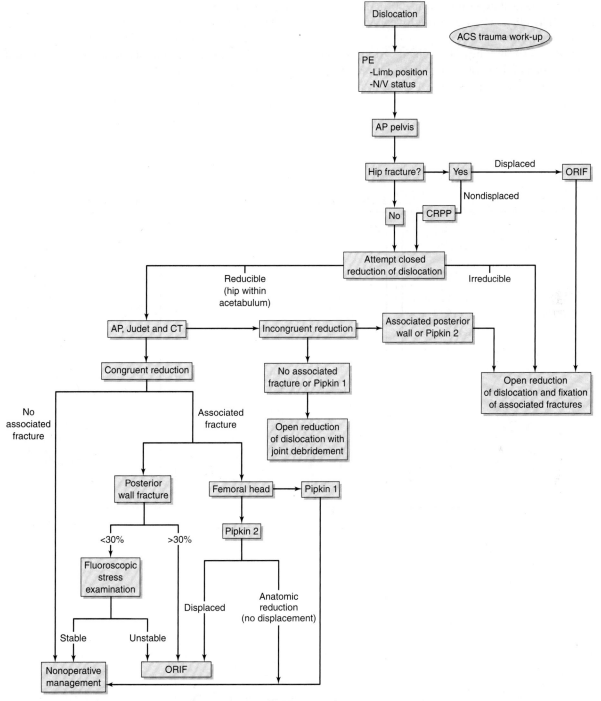

Algorithm for the management of hip dislocation and femoral head fractures (From Bucholz RW, Court-Brown CM, Heckman JD, et al. *Rockwood & Green's Fractures in Adults*, 7th ed. Philadelphia: Lippincott, Williams & Wilkins, 2010

- Type 2: Posterior dislocation with femoral head fracture cephalad to the fovea
- Type 3: Femoral head fracture with associated femoral neck fracture
- Type 4: Any of the three other categories with associated acetabular fracture

Femoral Head Vascular Anatomy
- The primary blood supply to the femoral head is from the medial femoral circumflex artery
- The superior and posterior vessels provide the majority of the femoral heads blood flow

- Additional blood flow comes from both the lateral femoral circumflex artery and the foveal artery (obturator artery branch)
- Dislocation of the hip can lead to blockage of the vessels supplying the head, making the femoral head more dependent on collateral circulation

Treatment
- The goal is to reduce the hip as soon as possible to limit insult to femoral head vascularity
- Continuous traction in line with deformity should be performed to reduce the joint
- Assess stability post reduction, especially in cases with associated acetabular fracture

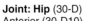

Joint: Hip (30-D)
Anterior (30-D10)   Posterior (30-D11)   Obturator (30-D30)

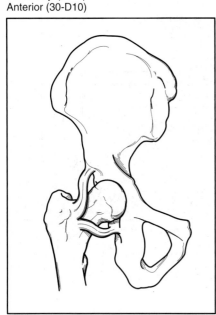 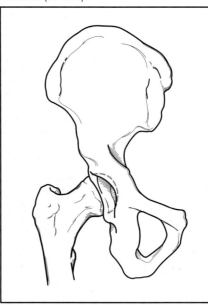 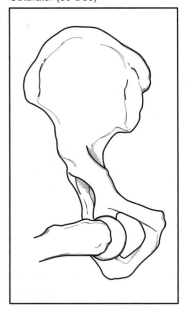

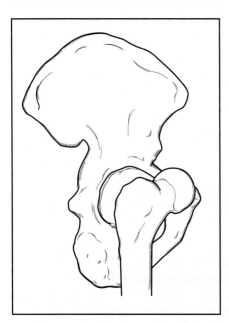 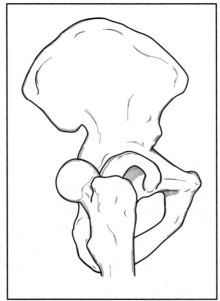

The Orthopaedic Trauma Association classification of hip dislocations. (From Bucholz RW, Heckman JD, eds. Rockwood and Green's Fractures in Adults, 5th ed. Philadelphia, PA: Lippincott Williams & Wilkins; 2001, with permission.)

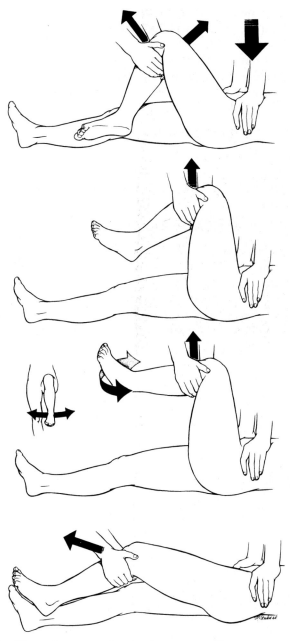

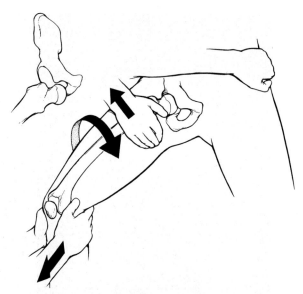

The Allis maneuver for anterior dislocations. (From Bucholz RW, Heckman JD, eds. Rockwood and Green's Fractures in Adults, 5th ed. Philadelphia, PA: Lippincott Williams & Wilkins; 2001, with permission.)

- Approach for fragment extraction is dependent on the direction of the dislocation and the location of the acetabular fracture
- ORIF femoral head or acetabular fracture if criteria apply

The Allis reduction technique for posterior hip dislocations. (From Bucholz RW, Heckman JD, eds. Rockwood and Green's Fractures in Adults, 5th ed. Philadelphia, PA: Lippincott Williams & Wilkins; 2001, with permission.)

- CT scan should be performed following reduction to confirm concentric reduction and evaluate for intra-articular fragments
- Small fragments in the fovea (avulsion off femoral head by ligamentum teres), which does not impinge need not be removed
- Any incarcerated fragments causing asymmetric reduction should be removed through open reduction of the hip

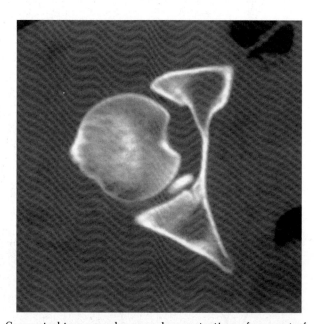

Computed tomography scan demonstrating a fragment of bone interposed between the femoral head and posterior articular surface that requires removal. (From Bucholz RW, Heckman JD, eds. Rockwood and Green's Fractures in Adults, 5th ed. Philadelphia, PA: Lippincott Williams & Wilkins; 2001, with permission.)

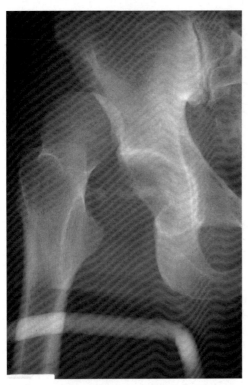

A 53-year-old woman with a posterior hip dislocation demonstrating fragments in the joint prior to hip reduction and an inferior femoral head fracture. (From Bucholz RW, Heckman JD, eds. Rockwood and Green's Fractures in Adults, 5th ed. Philadelphia, PA: Lippincott Williams & Wilkins; 2001, with permission.)

- In patients with a stable joint without associated injuries, **partial weight bearing (PWB)** for 2–4 wk should be initiated
- An irreducible hip dislocation is an orthopaedic emergency requiring emergent surgical intervention
- Surrounding soft tissue is often the cause of an irreducible hip dislocation

Recommended Readings

Dreinhofer KE, et al. Isolated traumatic dislocation of the hip. J Bone Joint Surg Br 1994;76:6–12.

Tornetta P III, Mostafavi HR. Hip dislocation: current treatment regimens. J Am Assoc Orthop Surg 1997;5:27–36.

FEMORAL HEAD FRACTURE

Background

- Femoral head fractures are uncommon isolated injuries
- Majority occur in conjunction with hip dislocations
- Can be a potentially debilitating injury
- 7% incidence in patients who suffer a posterior hip dislocation
- Usually result from high-energy mechanism
- 95% of patients with hip fracture or hip dislocation have an associated injury, which requires hospitalization
- Proper diagnosis is crucial to appropriate treatment and timing

Imaging

- AP pelvis
- AP and lateral hip radiographs

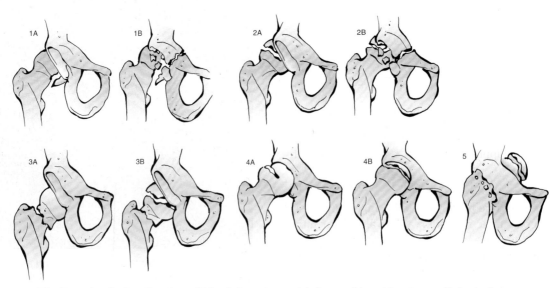

The Brumback classification of hip dislocations with femoral head fractures. (Adapted from Stannard JP, Harris HW, Volgas DA, et al. Functional outcome of patients with femoral head fractures associated with hip dislocations. Clin Orthop Rel Res 2000;377:44–56. From Bucholz RW, Court-Brown CM, Heckman JD, et al. *Rockwood & Green's Fractures in Adults*, 7th ed. Philadelphia: Lippincott, Williams & Wilkins, 2010 with permission.)

- CT scan to evaluate fracture fragments
- If associated with a dislocation, postreduction CT is essential to evaluate joint congruency and rule out retained fragments, which can lead to chondrolysis

Classification
- Schemes have been based on both the location of the fracture and the associated direction of dislocation
- Please see figures regarding the Brumback and Pipkin classifications

Immediate Treatment
- Immediate treatment should focus on ATLS principles
- Early reduction of any associated dislocation should be performed to decrease risk of avascular notice
- Reduction of the hip should not be performed in the setting of associated femoral neck fractures (Pipkin III or Brumback 3B)
- Prereduction neurovascular exam should be performed to evaluate the sciatic nerve and distal vascular status
- Postreduction should neurovascular exam should be carefully performed
- Irreducible fractures require operative intervention for both reduction of the dislocation and fracture fixation

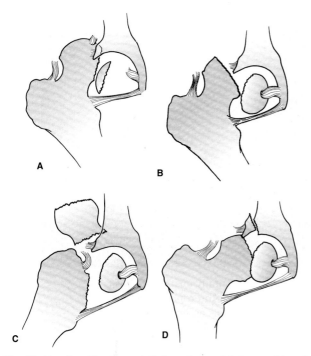

The Pipkin classification of dislocations with femoral head fractures. **A:** Type I. **B:** Type II. **C:** Type III. **D:** Type IV. (From Bucholz RW, et al., eds. Rockwood and Green's Fractures in Adults, 6th ed. Philadelphia, PA: Lippincott Williams & Wilkins; 2006, with permission.)

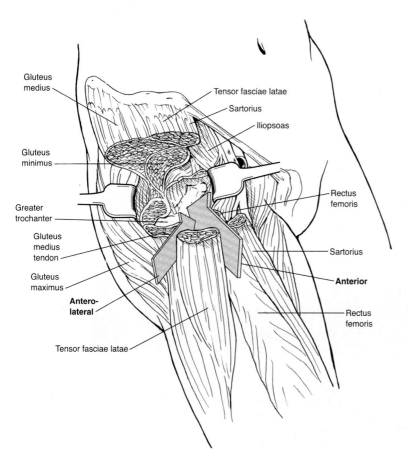

The Smith-Peterson (direct anterior) and the Watson-Jones (anterolateral) approaches to the hip take the same deep interval but pass on different sides of the tensor in their superficial dissections. The anterior approach is well suited for femoral head fractures, while the anterolateral approach is best for irreducible anterior dislocations. (From Bucholz RW, Heckman JD, eds. Rockwood and Green's Fractures in Adults, 5th ed. Philadelphia, PA: Lippincott Williams & Wilkins; 2001, with permission.)

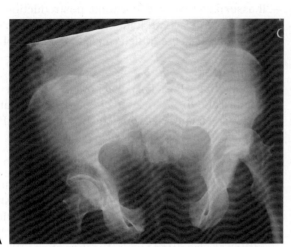
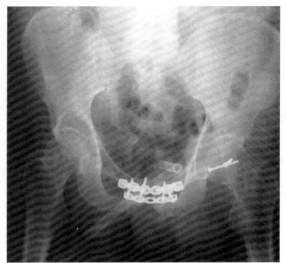

A: Wide pubic diastasis, characteristic of an "open book" horizontally unstable pelvis (type B), with associated femoral head fracture and hip dislocation. **B:** Anteroposterior radiograph after open reduction and dual plating of pubic diastasis and open reduction and internal fixation of femoral head fracture. The patient had associated bladder rupture requiring repair and suprapubic cystostomy. (From Mulholland MW, et al., eds. Greenfield's Surgery Scientific Principles and Practice, 4th ed. Philadelphia, PA: Lippincott Williams & Wilkins; 2006.)

Definitive Treatment

- I—Consider nonoperative approach if fragment stable
  - Consider fragment excision if small
  - ORIF of larger fragments and those above the fovea
- II—ORIF in incongruent or nonanatomic reductions
- III—Stabilize the femoral neck prior to femoral head fixation
- IV—Approach to fixation dictated by acetabular fracture. Most commonly associated with posterior wall

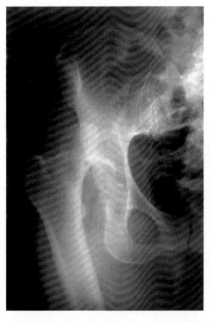
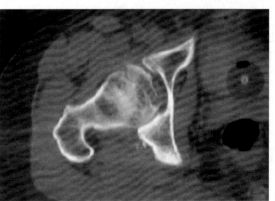

Anteroposterior view of a posterior hip dislocation with associated femoral head fracture **(A)**. Computed tomography scan after reduction of the hip demonstrates an anatomic reduction of the fragment at the level of the fovea and a congruent joint **(B)**. (From Bucholz RW, Heckman JD, eds. Rockwood and Green's Fractures in Adults, 5th ed. Philadelphia, PA: Lippincott Williams & Wilkins; 2001, with permission.)

fractures → Kocher-Langenbeck to allow for femoral head fixation and acetabulum reconstruction

Open Reduction Internal Fixation
- Malreduction (>1-mm displacement)
- Loose body
- Associated femoral neck or acetabular fracture
- Polytrauma patient
- Anterior (Smith-Petersen) preferred to avoid injury to femoral head vascularity and decrease risk of AVN
- Internervous plane superior gluteal nerve (tensor fascia latae) and femoral nerve (sartorius) superficially and direct head of the rectus and gluteus medius deep
- This allows visualization of the femoral head fragment, as it is commonly inferior and anterior
- HO prophylaxis should be considered
- Surgical hip dislocation is a valuable tool for fracture fixation
- Consider in most injuries to improve visualization, limit vascular compromise, and allow for fracture fixation

Recommended Readings
Brumback RJ, et al. Fractures of the femoral head. In: The Hip Society, ed. Proceedings of the Fourteenth Open Scientific Meeting of the Hip Society. St. Louis, MO: CV Mosby; 1987:181–206.

DeLee JC, et al. Anterior dislocation of the hip and associated femoral head fractures. J Bone Joint Surg Am 1980;62:960–964.

Epstein HC. Traumatic anterior and simple posterior dislocations of the hip in adults and children. Instr Course Lect 1973;22:115–145.

HIP FRACTURE—FEMORAL NECK

Background
- One of the most commonly treated orthopaedic injuries
- Commonly the result of a low-energy fall from standing in an elderly osteoporotic patient
- Incidence is increasing with the concurrent increasing age of the US population
- Sequelae of the injury are severe including loss of independence and mortality
- Femoral neck fractures in patients younger are commonly the result of high-energy trauma and carry their own associated risks, injuries, and sequelae
- Management for these two groups should be carefully distinguished

Physical Examination
Low Energy
- Patients present with shortened and externally rotated extremity
- Associated medical problems should be evaluated
- Patients who live independently should be evaluated for dehydration, anemia, and rhabdomyolysis as a

result from prolonged time down if extrication by paramedics necessary
- Medical evaluation should be performed to risk assess the patient prior to proceeding with surgery
- Early surgical intervention indicated in those healthy patients (ASA 2 and lower) following medical evaluation
- No advantage to early intervention in ASA 3/4 patients due to associated medical risks

High Energy
- ATLS protocol should be initiated
- Care should be taken to evaluate for associated injuries
- Early intervention is indicated to prevent further vascular insult to the femoral head
- There should be a high suspicion for ipsilateral femoral neck fractures in patients with femoral shaft fractures

Garden Classification
- I: Valgus impacted, incomplete
- II: Complete, nondisplaced
- III: Complete, displaced <50%
- IV: Completely displaced

Pauwels Classification
- Based on orientation of fracture line
- I: <30 degrees
- II: 30–50 degrees
- III: >50 degrees
- IV: Associated with higher nonunion, avascular necrosis, and is more common in young patients presenting with femoral neck fractures and AVN
- Higher shear forces lead to poorer outcomes when treated with cannulated screws

Imaging
- AP pelvis, AP, and cross-table lateral of the hip
- Frogleg lateral should be avoided to prevent displacement of nondisplaced fractures

Treatment
Determinants of Treatment Modality
- Age
- Displacement
- Medical comorbidities
- Associated injuries (high-energy mechanism)

Nondisplaced/Valgus Impacted (Elderly)
- Percutaneous screw placement
- Inverted triangle configuration with insertion of 6.5 or 7.3 cannulated partially threaded screws
- Entry point should be at or above to prevent a stress riser, which can lead to subtrochanteric hip fractures

Displaced Fractures (Elderly)
– Hemiarthroplasty vs. total hip arthroplasty
– Increased push toward total hip replacement in active individuals
– Care should be taken to avoid total hip replacement in patients with neuromuscular diseases including Alzheimer's, multiple sclerosis, and Parkinson's due to high risk of dislocation
– Risk of dislocation following total hip replacement in the setting of femoral neck fractures may be attributed to lack of capsular tension and increased flexibility in these patients
– No significant difference seen in bipolar vs. unipolar hemiarthroplasty

Displaced Femoral Neck Fractures (Young)
– Considered a surgical emergency due to risk of vascular status of the femoral head
– Three major sources of blood flow to the femoral head are in danger
    – Capsular vessels
    – Intramedullary vessels
    – Foveal artery
– Predominant blood flow comes from the medial femoral circumflex
– Patients require ORIF via the anterolateral Watson-Jones approach (internervous plane: gluteus medius and tensor fascia latae)
– Following reduction, fixation with cannulated screws or a sliding hip screw depending on surgeon preference

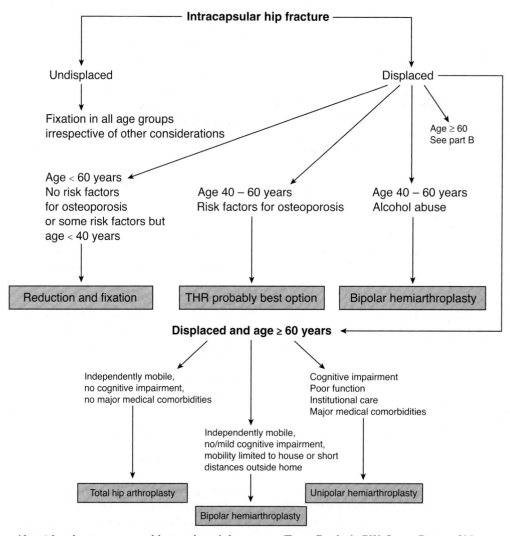

Algorithm for treatment of femoral neck fractures. (From Bucholz RW, Court-Brown CM, Heckman JD, et al. *Rockwood & Green's Fractures in Adults*, 7th ed. Philadelphia: Lippincott, Williams & Wilkins, 2010 with permission.)

Complications

Mortality

- 25% 1-yr mortality
- 15 times greater mortality in first month postoperative; associated with males, cardiopulmonary disease, dementia, pneumonia
- No difference in short- or long-term mortality with general vs. regional anesthesia
- Complications associated with preoperative cardiopulmonary and electrolyte abnormalities
- Cemented: 6-mo mortality 20%, 1-yr mortality 28%
- Albumin <3.0 associated with >3 times mortality
- Preoperative hemoglobin <12 for females, or hemoglobin <13 for males associated with increased hospital stay, increased 1-yr mortality (Koval 2002)
- Pillow under leg for IT and FN fracture more comfortable and less pain medications than 5 lb of skin traction (Koval 2001)

Associated Pathology

- Distal radial fracture
- Proximal humerus fracture

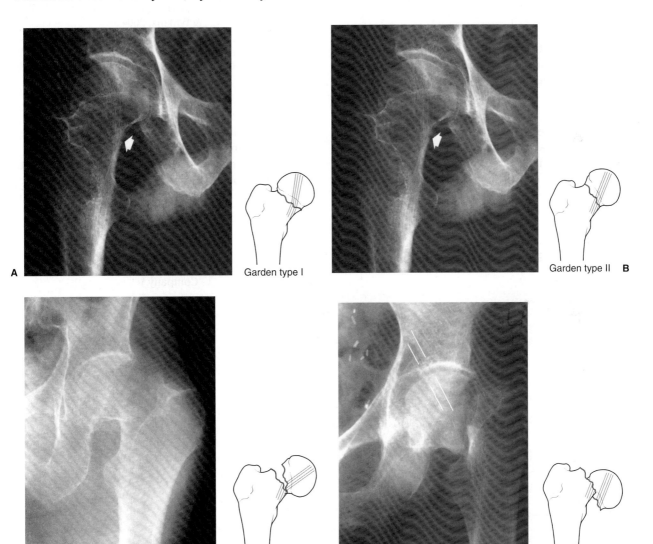

A   Garden type I

B   Garden type II

C   Garden type III

D   Garden type IV

The Garden classification of femoral neck fractures. Type I fractures can be incomplete but much more typically are impacted into valgus and retroversion **(A)**. Type II fractures are complete, but undisplaced. These rare fractures have a break in the trabeculations but no shift in alignment **(B)**. Type III fractures have marked angulation but usually minimal to no proximal translation of the shaft **(C)**. In the Garden type IV fracture, there is complete displacement between fragments and the shaft translates proximally **(D)**. The head is free to realign itself within the acetabulum, and the primary compressive trabeculae of the head and acetabulum realign (white lines). (From Bucholz RW, et al., eds. Rockwood and Green's Fractures in Adults, 6th ed. Philadelphia, PA: Lippincott Williams & Wilkins; 2006.)

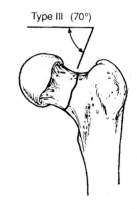

Type I (30°)   Type II (50°)   Type III (70°)

Femoral neck fracture: closed reduction and internal fixation. The classification system proposed by Pauwels is based on the angle of inclination of the fracture line: type I, fracture line 30 degrees from the horizontal; type II, fracture line 50 degrees from the horizontal; and type III, fracture line 70 degrees from the horizontal. (From Koval KJ, Zuckerman JD. Atlas of Orthopaedic Surgery: A Multimedia Reference. Philadelphia, PA: Lippincott Williams & Wilkins; 2004.)

- Subdural hematoma
- Myocardial infarction
- Cerebrovascular accident

Nonunion
- Defined as unhealed at 12 mo
- 5% in nondisplaced and valgus impacted fracture
- 10%–30% in displaced fracture
- In young patient with nonunion and viable femoral head by bone scan/MRI, treatment: valgus osteotomy, 80% chance of healing

- In young patient with acute fracture, 84% union with multiple screws vs. 64% with dynamic hip screw (DHS)

Avascular Necrosis
- 8% in nondisplaced and valgus impacted fracture
- 15%–30% in displaced fracture
- Increased risk with worse initial displacement, time to reduction, nonanatomic reduction
- Treatment: valgus IT osteotomy in young patient, if <50% femoral head necrosis

Cross-section of Hip Joint Area

Hip joint area cross section. (Asset provided by Anatomical Chart Company.)

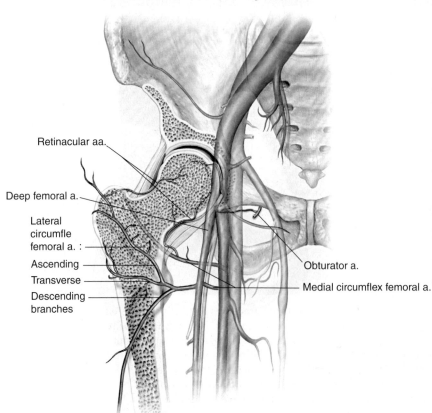

Retinacular aa.

Deep femoral a.

Lateral circumfle femoral a. :

Ascending

Transverse

Descending branches

Obturator a.

Medial circumflex femoral a.

- If >50% necrosis: free fibula or total hip arthroplasty (THA)
- If older patient, THA

Infection
- 25% of hip fractures and 40% of FN fractures get urinary tract infection during hospital stay; more risk if preoperative delay >48 hr

Transfusion
- 40% of hip hemiarthroplasty require transfusion
- 20% of DHS require transfusion
- 0% with screw fixation required transfusion
- Patients requiring transfusion twice as likely to get postoperative infection

Recommended Readings

Bout CA, et al. Percutaneous cannulated screw fixation of femoral neck fractures: the three point principle. Injury 1997;28:135–139.

Greenough CG, Jones JR. Primary total hip replacement for displaced subcapital fracture of the femur. J Bone Joint Surg Br 1988;70:639–643.

Orosz GM, Hannan EL, Magaziner J, Koval K, Gilbert M, Aufses A, et al. Hip fracture in the older patient: reasons for delay in hospitalization and timing of surgical repair. J Am Geriatr Soc 2002;50:1336–1340.

Rosen JE, Koval KJ. Efficacy of preoperative skin traction in hip fracture patients: a prospective, randomized study. J Orthop Trauma 2001;15(2):81–85.

Swiontkowski MF, et al. Laser Doppler flowmetry for bone blood flow measurement: correlation with microsphere estimates and evaluation of the effect of intracapsular pressure on femoral head blood flow. J Orthop Res 1986;4:362–371.

HIP FRACTURE—INTERTROCHANTERIC

Background
- Generally older than those patients presenting with femoral neck fractures
- Increased number of comorbidities → higher mortality rate than femoral neck fractures
- Result from fall from standing onto the GT → laterally directed force
- Patients will present with a shortened, externally rotated leg on presentation
- Care should be taken in those patients presenting with an isolated lesser trochanteric fracture as that injury is pathognomonic for pathologic lesion

Imaging
- AP and cross-table lateral hip and femur films should be performed
- AP pelvis should be performed as well
- Full-length femurs should be used to evaluate site of distal interlocking screws for cephalomedullary devices

Characteristics of Fracture
- Fractures can be divided into stable vs. unstable categories, which directs treatment modalities

Stable Fractures
- Resist medial compressive loads and are axially stable once reduction is performed
- Stable once reduced
- No extension of fracture line into lateral buttress
- Lesser trochanter (LT) intact

Unstable Fractures
- Posteromedial comminuition
- Reverse obliquity fractures
- Sliding hip screws should be avoided as the fracture lines are in line with the sliding hip screws → further displacement of the fracture
- Intertrochanteric fractures with subtrochanteric extension
- Unstable fractures have a tendency to fall into varus or develop medial displacement of the shaft
- Unstable if posteromedial buttress lost

Dynamic Hip Screw
- Commonly used implant for treatment of stable intertrochanteric hip fractures
- Cost-effective valuable implant in the right patient
- Sliding compression screw allows compression across fracture site with ambulation → fracture healing
- Avoid in unstable fractures as the mechanism of action allows medial displacement of shaft until stable impacted position reached (shortening is poorly tolerated due to limb-length discrepancy and alternation of joint reaction forces)

Essentials to DHS
- Standard lateral approach to the proximal femur is utilized
- After splitting iliotibial band, vastus can be elevated off the intermuscular septum or split pending surgeon preference
- Tip-apex distance (TAD) (tip of screw to apex of head based on line drawn along femoral nect) on AP added to TAD on lateral must be <25 mm to minimize risk of screw cut out (Baumgaertner 1995)
- Screw should be placed in the center–center (both AP and lateral)
- Second best positioning for the screw is posterior inferior in the femoral head
- Anterior superior position places the implant at highest risk for cutout
- Screw should be placed within 5–10 mm of subchondral bone

- 150-degree plate decreases varus moment and slides better but increases distal stress riser because entry point is more distal
- Most common complication is varus displacement with screw cut
  - Improper screw placement
  - Stable reduction not obtained
  - Excess collapse
  - Inadequate screw barrel engagement (jamming), which prevents sliding
  - Severe osteoporosis

Intramedullary Nail
- Resists fracture collapse and medialization of shaft (nail acts as a stop to proximal fragment sliding)
- Percutaneous, less blood loss
- IM hip screw risk femoral shaft fracture at distal interlock

95-Degree Fixed-Angle Device
- Can be utilized in reverse obliquity fractures where the DHS is contraindicated
- Can also be utilized in revision of intertrochanteric nonunions or femoral neck malunions to perform valgus osteotomies

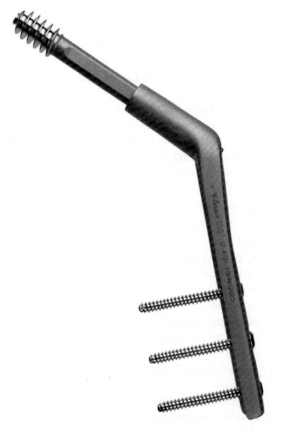

Compression hip screw components: lag screw, blunt tip, side-plate of fixed angle and cortical shaft screws. (From Bucholz RW, Court-Brown CM, Heckman JD, Tornetta P. Rockwood & Green's Fractures in Adults, 7th ed. Philadelphia, PA: Lippincott Williams & Wilkins, 2010.)

Or Tips and Tricks—DHS
- Patient should be placed on fracture table
- Goal is to achieve stable reduction by traction and internal rotation under fluoro before starting case
- Incise from gluteus flare proximally to length of marking pen, along femur looking from lateral
- If unable to palpate the flare, utilize fluoroscopy to find point of guide pin insertion
- This can be used as the proximal aspect of the incision
- In contrast, an incision can be made from the palpable aspect of the vastus ridge to just below the LT depending on the length of the side plate
- Fascia of the vastus lateralis can be incised posteriorly and the muscle swept anteriorly using a periosteal elevator to expose the lateral femoral cortex
- Submuscular dissection limits perforating bleeders.
- Electrocauterize any bleeders to improve visualization of the femoral perforators
- The best bone is located inferiorly and posteriorly in the femoral head
- Avoid wire placement in the anterosuperior head
- A wide Bennett can be used to retract the vastus lateralis superiorly.
- The guide pin should be placed with 135-degree guide (depending on the blade) to hit *center–center
- Tip of screw should be within 6 mm of subchondral bone for adequate purchase and to decrease risk of cut out.
- *Avoid anterosuperior head
- An antirotational guide pin can be inserted 2 cm proximal to the first pin under fluoroscopic guidance to prevent rotation of the head during lag screw insertion
- If another fracture line or lateral buttress thin/small, start hole more distally to avoid fracture line and use higher-degree side plate
- Indirect measuring device was used to determine the depth of the guide pin
- Set triple reamer 5 mm less than pin with Richards, 10 mm less with Synthes
- Utilize the DHS triple reamer to simultaneously drill for the lag screw into the femoral head, ream for the plate barrel, and countersink for the plate/barrel junction
- The lag screw pathway should be tapped in patients with stronger bone to prevent rotation of the proximal fragment
- The lag screw can then be inserted over the guide pin under fluoroscopic guidance
- Short barrel when lag screw <85
- The handle should be aligned with the femoral shaft to allow proper placement of the sideplate

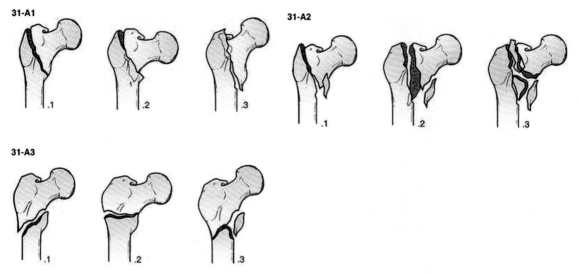

In the OTA alphanumeric fracture classification, intertrochanteric hip fractures comprise type 31A. These fractures are divided into three groups, and each group is further divided into subgroups based on obliquity of the fracture line and degree of comminution. Group 1 fractures are simple (two-part) fractures, with the typical oblique fracture line extending from the greater trochanter to the medial cortex. The lateral cortex of the greater trochanter remains intact. Group 2 fractures are comminuted with a posteromedial fragment. The lateral cortex of the greater trochanter, however, remains intact. Fractures in this group are generally unstable, depending on the size of the medial fragment. Group 3 fractures are those in which the fracture line extends across both the medial and lateral cortices. This group includes the reverse obliquity pattern. (From Bucholz RW, Court-Brown CM, Heckman JD, Tornetta P. Rockwood & Green's Fractures in Adults, 7th ed. Philadelphia, PA: Lippincott Williams & Wilkins, 2010.)

- After placement of the plate, the appropriate shaft screws should be inserted
- Release traction prior to inserting the lag screw
- Compression can be applied utilizing the lag screw

- The antirotational wire can be removed or a cannulated short thread 7.3 or 6.5 screw can be inserted after indirect measuring
- The hip should be rotated live on fluoroscopy following insertion of the lag screw to ensure that no penetration of the femoral head

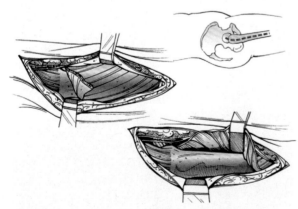

Lateral surgical approach to the hip. Slight curvature of proximal extent of incision to allow palpation of the anterior cortex. Vastus lateralis reflection distally as needed for length of plate. (From Bucholz RW, Court-Brown CM, Heckman JD, Tornetta P. Rockwood & Green's Fractures in Adults, 7th ed. Philadelphia, PA: Lippincott Williams & Wilkins, 2010.)

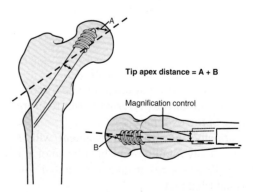

The tip-apex distance (TAD), expressed in millimeters, is the sum of the distances from the tip of the lag screw to the apex of the femoral head on both the AP and lateral radiographic views. (From Bucholz RW, Court-Brown CM, Heckman JD, Tornetta P. Rockwood & Green's Fractures in Adults, 7th ed. Philadelphia, PA: Lippincott Williams & Wilkins, 2010.)

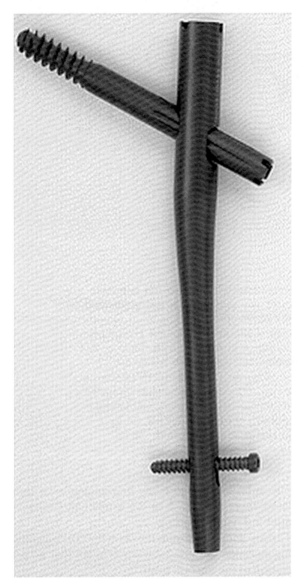

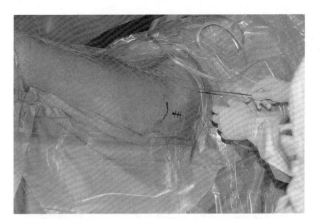

Intramedullary approach. Incision is placed center to slightly posterior to line of femoral shaft centered between the anterior superior and inferior iliac spines anteriorly. Incision length is 2 to 4 cm. (From Bucholz RW, Court-Brown CM, Heckman JD, Tornetta P. Rockwood & Green's Fractures in Adults, 7th ed. Philadelphia, PA: Lippincott Williams & Wilkins, 2010.)

Short gamma 3 intramedullary nail. (From Bucholz RW, Court-Brown CM, Heckman JD, Tornetta P. Rockwood & Green's Fractures in Adults, 7th ed. Philadelphia, PA: Lippincott Williams & Wilkins, 2010.)

Or Tips and Tricks—Gamma Nail
- The patient can be positioned on the fracture table
- Reduction should be performed prior to prepping and draping of the extremity
- Occasionally, the proximal fragment will be flexed and externally rotated requiring placed of a ball-spike pusher (Kugelspitze) at the inferomedial spike of the proximal fragment

Osteonics/Howmedica
- Reduce the fracture on the on fracture table prior to scrubbing if possible

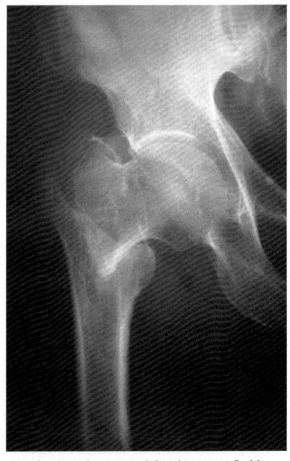

Intertrochanteric fractures: sliding hip screw. Stable fracture. Notice that the posteromedial cortex remains intact. (From Koval KJ, Zuckerman JD. Atlas of Orthopaedic Surgery: A Multimedia Reference. Philadelphia, PA: Lippincott Williams & Wilkins; 2004.)

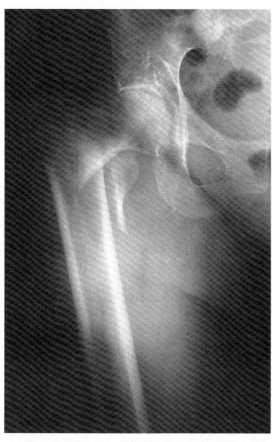

Intertrochanteric fractures: sliding hip screw. Unstable fracture. Notice the greater comminution of the posteromedial cortex. (From Koval KJ, Zuckerman JD. Atlas of Orthopaedic Surgery: A Multimedia Reference. Philadelphia, PA: Lippincott Williams & Wilkins; 2004.)

- Shoot lateral with beam approximately 15 degrees from floor to be parallel to neck
- Aim to neck should be referenced off center post
- 5-cm incision should be made from the tip of the GT extending proximally

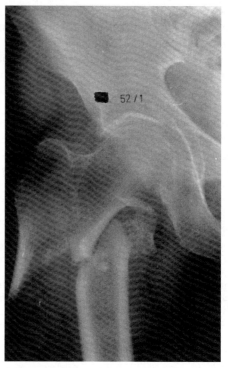

Anteroposterior radiograph demonstrating a reverse obliquity right intertrochanteric fracture. (From Bucholz RW, Heckman JD, eds. Rockwood and Green's Fractures in Adults, 5th ed. Philadelphia, PA: Lippincott Williams & Wilkins; 2001.)

- Start the awl insertion medially to prevent notching the medial calcar with the entry reamer
- The guide pin should be inserted to the level of the superior pole of the patella
- Ream proximally and medially with the entry reamer, taking care not to ream the medial calcar
- Remove inner sleeve to measure lag screw length. Remember, the measurement starts at end of threads, so add approximately 10 mm to measurement

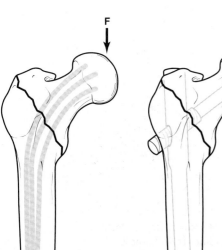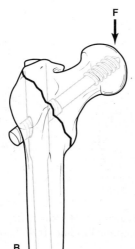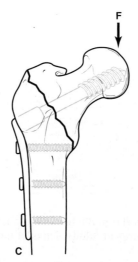

For stabilization of intertrochanteric fractures, intramedullary devices (A, B) are subjected to smaller bending moments than plate-and-screw devices (C) because they are positioned closer to the mechanical axis of the femur. (From Bucholz RW, Heckman JD, eds. Rockwood and Green's Fractures in Adults, 5th ed. Philadelphia, PA: Lippincott Williams & Wilkins; 2001.)

- Insert lag screw to the appropriate position
- Compression can be applied to the fracture after the extremity is taken off of traction
- Following insertion of the lag screw and application of compression, the set screw should be inserted through the proximal aspect of the guide to lock the lack screw in position
- Attention should then be turned distally to insert the distal interlocks utilizing perfect circles technique
- Place the distal interlocks with perfect circles

Recommended Readings

Baumgaertner MR. The value of the tip-apex distance in predicting failure of fixation of peritrochanteric fractures of the hip. J Bone Joint Surg Am 1995;77(7):1058–1064.

Bolhofner BR, et al. Results of intertrochanteric femur fractures treated with a 135-degree sliding screw with a two-hole side plate. J Orthop Trauma 1999;13(1):5–8.

Bridle SH, et al. Fixation of intertrochanteric fractures of the femur: a randomized prospective comparison of the gamma nail and the dynamic hip screw. J Bone Joint Surg 1991;73B: 330–334.

Koval KJ, et al. Effect of acute inpatient rehabilitation on outcome after fracture of the femoral neck or intertrochanteric fracture. J Bone Joint Surg Am 1998;80:357–364.

Koval KJ, Zuckerman JD. Postoperative weight-bearing after a fracture of the femoral neck or an intertrochanteric fracture. J Bone Joint Surg Am 1998;80(3):352–356.

Kyle RF, et al. Analysis of six hundred and twenty-two intertrochanteric hip fractures. J Bone Joint Surg Am 1979; 61(2):216–221.

FEMORAL SUBTROCHANTERIC FRACTURE

Background
- Between the lesser trochanter (LT) and the isthmus
- Within 5 cm of the LT distally

Anatomy
- High medial compressive and lateral tensile forces in subtrochanteric region
- Transition area from cancellous to cortical bone
- Strong deforming muscle forces
  - Proximal fragment is pulled into flexion, abduction, and external rotation by the iliopsoas, short external rotators, and hip abductors

Russell-Taylor Classification
- Based on fracture involving
  - Piriformis fossa
    - Evaluate lateral x-ray
  - LT
    - Assess for medial comminution
- Type I: Piriformis fossa intact—acceptable for IM nail
  - IA: LT intact
    - Can use conventional interlocking nail or reconstruction nail
  - IB: LT displaced
  - Reconstruction nail preferred
- Type II: Piriformis fossa fractured—may need blade plate or GT entry point nail
  - IIA: LT intact
    - No bone graft needed

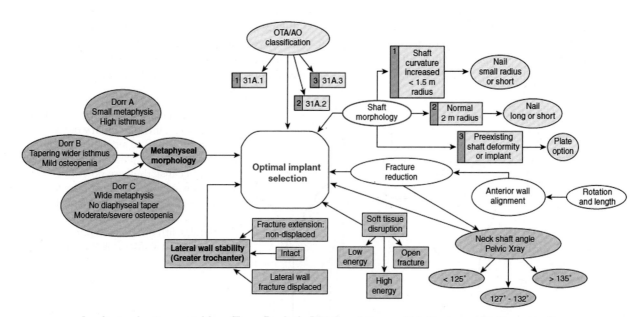

Implant selection variables. (From Bucholz RW, Court-Brown CM, Heckman JD, Tornetta P. Rockwood & Green's Fractures in Adults, 7th ed. Philadelphia: Lippincott Williams & Wilkins, 2010.)

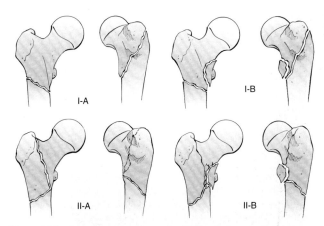

Russell-Taylor classification of subtrochanteric fractures. (From Bucholz RW, et al., eds. Rockwood and Green's Fractures in Adults, 6th ed. Philadelphia, PA: Lippincott Williams & Wilkins; 2006, with permission.)

- May use intramedullary hip screw/gamma/trochanter fixation nail or plate
- IIB: LT comminuted
  - May use plate: load-bearing device instead of load sharing
  - Indirect reduction techniques
  - GT entry nail

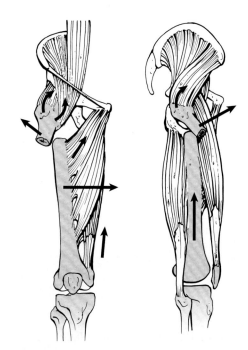

The deforming force by the unopposed pull of the iliopsoas causes the proximal femur in flexion and external rotation. (From Bucholz RW, et al., eds. Rockwood and Green's Fractures in Adults, 6th ed. Philadelphia, PA: Lippincott Williams & Wilkins; 2006, with permission.)

Seinsheimer Classification

- Considers higher rate of fixation failure with medial comminution
- I: Displaced <2 mm
- II: Two part
  - IIA: Transverse
  - IIB: Spiral, LT attached proximally
  - IIC: Spiral, LT attached distally
- III: Three part
  - IIIA: LT is part of third fragment
  - IIIB: Third part is lateral butterfly
- IV: Four parts or more, comminuted
- V: Subtrochanteric extension into GT
- High rate of implant failure before union
- Nonunion defined as 6 mo without bridging
- IM nail useful, but unlike shaft fracture, nail does not reduce fracture
  - Reduction critical prior to placing implant
- Varus malreduction is most common complication in piriformis entry nail for subtrochanteric fracture with displaced LT

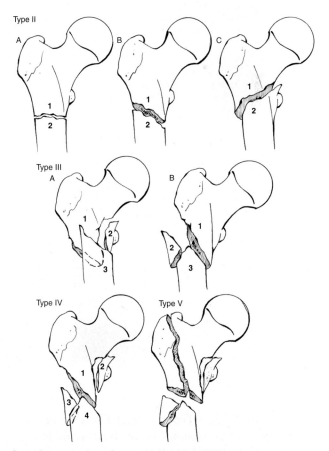

Seinsheimer classification of subtrochanteric fractures. (From Bucholz RW, et al., eds. Rockwood and Green's Fractures in Adults, 6th ed. Philadelphia, PA: Lippincott Williams & Wilkins; 2006, with permission.)

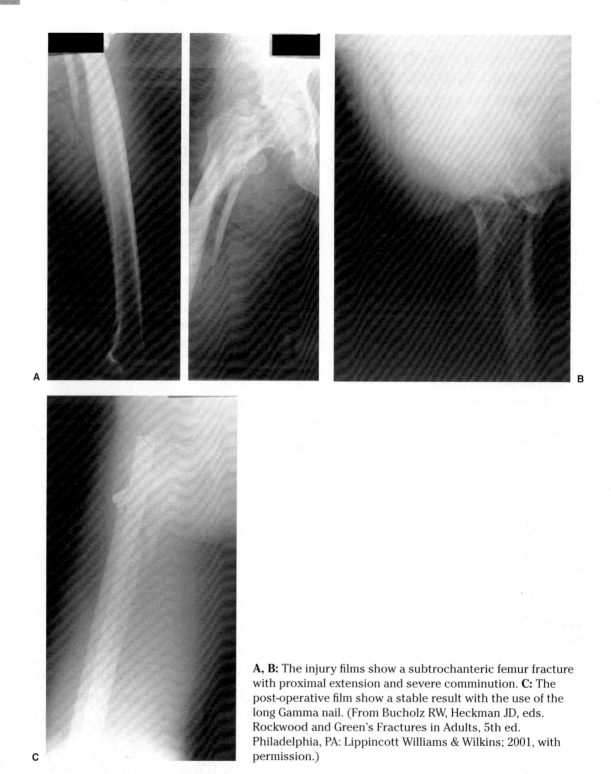

A, B: The injury films show a subtrochanteric femur fracture with proximal extension and severe comminution. **C:** The post-operative film show a stable result with the use of the long Gamma nail. (From Bucholz RW, Heckman JD, eds. Rockwood and Green's Fractures in Adults, 5th ed. Philadelphia, PA: Lippincott Williams & Wilkins; 2001, with permission.)

Or Tips and Tricks—Trochanteric Fixation Nail

- Patients can be positioned on the fracture table or in the lateral decubitus position
- Patient positioned on the fracture table
- Depending on the implant system, 10-, 11-, or 12-mm nails are available

- 125-, 130-, or 135-degree jigs for blade
- Two fluoroscopy machines can speed up the procedure but are not essential
- Insertion point for the guide pin is the intersection point of a line from the femoral shaft/GT with vertical line from ASIS.

Implant
- Percutaneously place guide pin in place at very tip of GT, then go in 15 cm
- Incision can be made prior to guidewire placement followed by incision of fascia
- Take incision three-quarters of an inch skin distal to pin and one quarter of an inch proximal to it
- Incise fascia in the same fashion
- Drill with 17-mm proximal opening reamer opener
- Ream medial to clear calcar bone
- Insert the ball-tipped guidewire to the superior aspect of the patella
- The F-tool, a crutch, or a ball-spike pusher can be utilized for the reduction.
- Ball-spike pusher can be placed on the inferomedial portion of the femoral neck/proximal fragment to counter the flexion/abduction force
- The crutch can be utilized to elevate the distal fragment to improve reduction
- The fracture reduction should be maintained throughout distal reaming
- Reaming should be performed to 1.5 mm larger than the expected nail
- Aiming guide should be applied following insertion of the nail
- Blade sleeve should be buttressed down to bone for adequate measurement. Reduction should be maintained throughout reaming and blade placement
- Guide wire should be placed within 5 mm of edge of head, center–center
- Place set screw as compression is not necessary in subtrochanteric fractures
- Distal interlocks can be placed using perfect circles or the Synthes "SureLock" aiming guide

Recommended Readings

Kinast C, et al. Subtrochanteric fractures of the femur: results of treatment with the 95 condylar blade-plate. Clin Orthop Relat Res 1989;28:122–130.

Russell TA, Taylor JC. Russell-Taylor classification of subtrochanteric fractures. In: Browner BD, et al., eds. Skeletal Trauma. Philadelphia: WB Saunders; 1998:1891–1897.

Seinsheimer F III. Subtrochanteric fractures of the femur. J Bone Joint Surg 1978;60A:300–306.

Wiss DA, Brien WW. Subtrochanteric fractures of the femur: results of treatment by interlocking nailing. Clin Orthop Relat Res 1992;283:231–236.

FEMORAL SHAFT FRACTURE

Background
- High energy, often in the setting of acute high-velocity trauma
- Frequency increasing in low-energy mechanisms in geriatric patients with a history of bisphosphonate use

- ABCs should be evaluated as with all trauma patient
- Associated injuries may include nondisplaced vertical shear femoral neck fractures
- Care must be taken for a complete evaluation of the patient and adequate evaluation of imaging to avoid missing associated injuries.
- Bilateral injuries are associated with an even higher risk of pulmonary insult

Classification
- Location
- Degree of comminution
- Winquist-Hansen
    - 0: No comminution
    - I: Minimal comminution
    - II Butterfly, >50% cortex intact
    - III: <50% cortex intact
    - IV: Segmental fracture

Traction
- One of the quickest methods of damage control orthopaedics
- Stabilization through traction decreases the risk of fat embolism, improves pain control, and prevents shortening secondary to muscular spasms
- In elderly, low-energy mechanism, consider skin traction up to 10 lbs or 2 kg.
- Skeletal traction should be performed in young patients of high-energy mechanism injuries. Consider 10% of body weight but can increase as needed to distract the fracture site
- Tibial pin is preferred to prevent tethering of quadriceps and avoid distal femoral interlocks
- Prior to placement, assess knee ligamentous stability
- Should be avoided in patients with any ligamentous instability
- 2 cm posterior to tibial tubercle, two to three fingerbreadths below joint line
- Pin should be inserted from lateral to medial to protect the superficial peroneal nerve
- Traction pin should be placed more distal in osteoporotic patients to avoid metaphyseal bone and pin pullout
- Main indication for distal femoral traction is ipsilateral knee instability
- Pin should be inserted medial to lateral to avoid the popliteal vessels
- Pin should be placed immediately superior to the condyles above the superior pole of the patella

Treatment
- Most common complication: Malrotation of the femur
- Care must be taken to adequately re-establish anatomic rotation and length

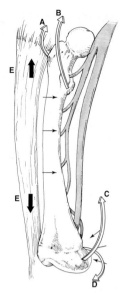

Deforming muscle forces on the femur; abductors (A), iliopsoas (B), adductors (C), and gastrocnemius origin (D). The medial angulating forces are resisted by the fascia lata (E). Potential sites of vascular injury after fracture are at the adductor hiatus and the perforating vessels of the profunda femoris. (From Bucholz RW, Heckman JD, eds. Rockwood and Green's Fractures in Adults, 5th ed. Philadelphia, PA: Lippincott Williams & Wilkins; 2001.)

- Increased risk of external rotation when the patient is supine, or internal rotation when patient placed in the lateral position

Intramedullary Nails
- First-generation nails involved interlocking screws primarily at the lesser trochanter
- Second-generation nails utilized an interlocking screw into the femoral head
- Third-generation nails utilized GT entry point with associated cephalomedullary device

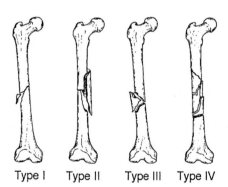

Winquist-Hansen classification of femoral shaft fractures. (From Browner BD et al., eds. Skeletal Trauma: Fractures, Dislocations, and Ligamentous Injuries. Philadelphia, PA: WB Saunders; 1992.)

- Interlocks: Only one distal interlock needed if fracture above distal third to maintain rotational control
- Wolinsky and Johnson (1995) evaluated 551 consecutive reamed IM nails in 1999 and showed a 94% primary healing rate following the first procedure and 99% healing rate overall
- 80 interlocking screws and 131 nails removed
- The most common complication of antegrade (GT entry) nail at >1 yr is Trendelenberg gait

Indications for Retrograde Nail
- Distal femur fracture
- Bilateral femur fractures
- Floating knee to save incision
- Ipsilateral neck, acetabular, pelvic fracture
- Obese, pregnant
- Unstable spine injury
- Contaminated hip wound
- Clean knee arthrotomy
- Technically easier but union rates lower, potential intra-articular infection, cruciate injury, cartilage damage

Temporary External Fixation
- Treatment of choice in hemodynamically unstable patient as part of damage control orthopaedics
- Temporizing measure in unstable patient, severe open injuries, or patients with vascular injury
- Minimizes blood loss and operating room time
- Can safely convert to nail within 2–3 wk without having to remove the pins
- Lateral to medial pins should be inserted at near-near far-far configuration

Plate
- Plating is usually reserved for special cases including:
  - Vascular injury after repair
  - Some open fractures
- Associated with higher rates of infection, nonunion, implant failure compared with nail
- Early stabilization (within 24 hr) associated with decreased pulmonary complications, DVT, cost due to elimination of intramedullary manipulation

Gunshot Wound (GSW)
- Low-velocity wound (<2,000 ft/sec): Immediate reamed nail; treat like closed fracture
- High-velocity wound (>2,000 ft/sec): Depends on soft tissue wound. If significant soft tissue injury or vascular injury, consider external fixation rather than immediate nailing

Union Rates
- Reamed antegrade nailing = 97%–99%
- Reamed retrograde nailing = 92%

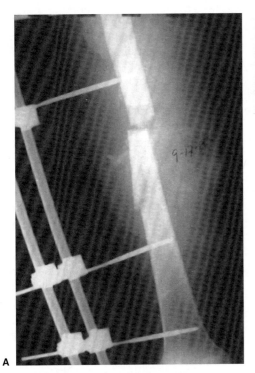

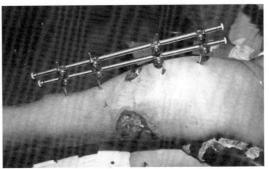

A, B: External fixation is an excellent way to temporarily stabilize femoral shaft fractures while avoiding the use of traction. In this 18-year-old woman with a Glasgow Coma Scale score of 6 and a subdural hematoma and frontal contusion requiring craniotomy, the external fixation was rapidly placed, after debridement of the open femoral shaft fracture, under the initial anesthesia after the neurosurgical procedure. (From Bucholz RW, Heckman JD, eds. Rockwood and Green's Fractures in Adults, 5th ed. Philadelphia, PA: Lippincott Williams & Wilkins; 2001, with permission.)

– Unreamed antegrade nailing = 96%
– Unreamed retrograde locked = 86%

Concomitant Shaft and Neck Fracture
(Wolinsky & Johnson, 1995)
– 1%–9% of femoral shaft fractures are associated with femoral necks
– Anywhere from 20%–50% of these injuries can be missed
– 95% of these injuries are midshaft
– Femoral neck fracture is usually high Pauwels angle, nondisplaced making it easy to list
– CT scan should be utilized to avoid missing the diagnosis due to the significant morbidity from a missed femoral neck fracture
– In high-energy injuries, close attention should be paid to the abdominal/pelvis ct performed by the primary trauma attention
– In 2007, Tornetta et al showed a reduction of delay of diagnosis of associated femoral neck fractures by 91% when utilizing a 15 % internal rotation ap radiograph and fine (2-mm) cut CT scan through the femoral neck, and an intraoperative fluoroscopic lateral radiograph prior to fixation followed by postoperative AP and lateral radiographs of the hip
– In patients age <50 yr, 20% of femoral neck fractures associated with femoral shaft fracture
– 30% of these are not diagnosed preoperatively
– If diagnosis after nail inserted, place lag screws anterior to nail
– Removing nail risks displacing neck fracture

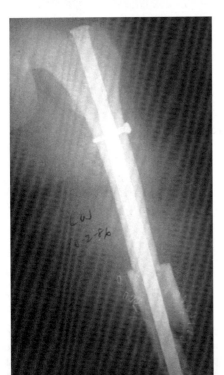

At day 7, after her condition had stabilized, the frame was removed and the fracture treated with standard interlocking nail, resulting in rapid union. Her functional recovery was excellent given the severity of her injury. (From Bucholz RW, Heckman JD, eds. Rockwood and Green's Fractures in Adults, 5th ed. Philadelphia, PA: Lippincott Williams & Wilkins; 2001, with permission.)

- 5% risk of head AVN, 5% risk of femoral neck nonunion in ipsilateral neck/shaft fractures
- **Treat femoral neck fracture first**
- If diagnosed preoperatively, options to consider:
  - Femoral neck screws, followed by standard nail
  - Reconstruction nail—may be hard to maintain reduction
- **Neck screws can be placed followed by retrograde nailing**

Or Tips and Tricks—Femoral Nail
- Rotation should be evaluated on contralateral extremity preoperatively
- Measure length, rotation, and canal diameter to determine appropriate nail

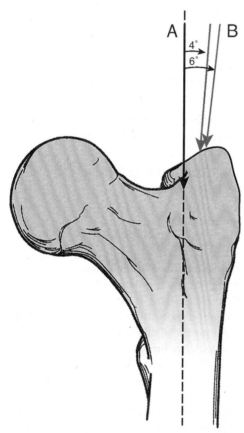

On the AP radiographic view, the entry location and direction for a piriformis nail is depicted with the black arrow and is parallel with the femoral shaft on both radiographic views. The entry angle and location for a trochanteric nail depends on the specific design parameters of the implant. Typically, a 4- to 6-degree entry angle is required (red and gray arrows) although some implants use a lateral entry on the proximal femur with a larger entry angle. (From Bucholz RW, Court-Brown CM, Heckman JD, Tornetta P MD, . Rockwood & Green's Fractures in Adults, 7th ed. Philadelphia: Lippincott, Williams & Wilkins, 2010.)

- The length is from tip of GT to adductor tubercle or superior aspect of the patella for diaphyseal fractures or the top of femoral notch for distal one third shaft fractures

Lateral Decubitus Position
- Allows for access to piriformis fossa especially in large patients or patients with decreased hip ROM
- Positioning can be utilized for trochanteric entry nail as well
- Disadvantages
  - Respiratory compromise due to positioning
  - Valgus angulation of the fracture may make reduction difficult
  - Rotational reduction is more difficult
  - Distal interlock placement may be more difficult
- Patient should be placed on a radiolucent table
  - Manual traction or femoral distractor may be utilized
  - Access to piriformis fossa improved with adduction of the hip

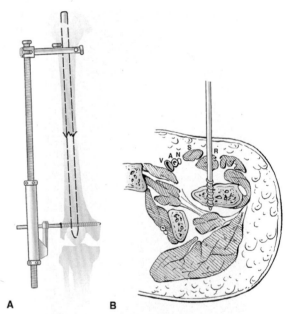

A: A femoral distractor can be placed to allow for restoration of femoral length and rotation. This requires strategic placement of the half pins to ensure that the path of the intramedullary nail is not violated. The distal pin can be placed transversely from lateral to medial in the metaphysis. The proximal pin can be placed from lateral to medial or from anterior to posterior as depicted. **B:** The location of the relevant soft tissue structures in the vicinity of a pin placed from anterior to posterior at the level of the lesser trochanter. (Redrawn after McFerran MA, Johnson KD. Intramedullary nailing of acute femoral shaft fractures without a fracture table: technique of using a femoral distractor. J Orthop Trauma 1992;6:271–278.)

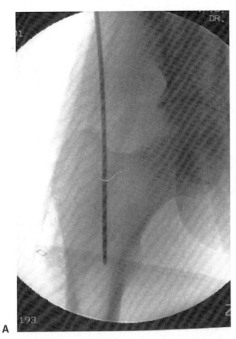
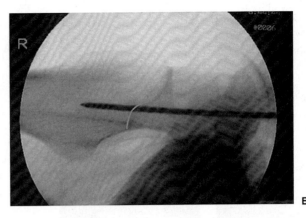

The starting point for a femoral nail is shown in the AP **(A)** and lateral **(B)** fluoroscopic images. The lateral image demonstrates the pin position relative to the femoral neck, greater trochanter, and calcar femorale. The outline of the piriformis (trochanteric) fossa should be apparent intraoperatively and is highlighted in red on the AP and lateral views. (From Bucholz RW, Court-Brown CM, Heckman JD, Tornetta P MD. Rockwood & Green's Fractures in Adults, 7th ed. Philadelphia: Lippincott Williams & Wilkins, 2010.)

- 5-cm incision just proximal to tip of GT in line with femur
- Starting awl tip should be in line with canal on AP and lateral
- On the lateral, the awl is at junction of the middle and posterior third of the neck
- Alternatively, a 5/32 Steinman or guide wire may be placed into the piriformis fossa followed by the 13-mm opening reamer
- Enlarge the canal with T-handle
- The guide wire must go into center of knee
- Eccentric guide wire placement can lead to excess reaming of one cortex
- Ream the canal in 1-mm increments until chatter of endosteal surface then advance by 0.5-mm increments
- Ream through isthmus until resistance lost, but refrain from reaming all the way down into the distal metaphysis to improve fixation in the cancellous bone
- The canal should be reamed 1.5 mm over size of nail
- The nail can be utilized over the guide wire to aid in reduction by joysticking the proximal fragment
- Impact the fracture once nail into distal fragment
- Two distal interlocks should be placed to maintain rotation.

Recommended Readings

Brumback RJ, et al. Intramedullary nailing of femoral shaft fractures. Part III: Long-term effects of static interlocking fixation. J Bone Joint Surg Am 1992;74(1):106–112.

Tornetta P. Diagnosis of femoral neck fractures in patients with a femoral shaft fracture. Improvement with a standard protocol. JBJS 2007;89(1):39–43.

Winquist RA, et al. Closed intramedullary nailing of femoral fractures. A report of five hundred and twenty cases. J Bone Joint Surg Am 1984;66(4):529–539.

Wolinsky PR, et al. Reamed intramedullary nailing of the femur: 551 cases. J Trauma 1999;46(3):392–399.

Wolinsky PR, Johnson KD. Ipsilateral femoral neck and shaft fractures. Clin Orthop Relat Res 1995;318:81–90.

FEMUR—SUPRACONDYLAR FRACTURE

Background

- Less common injury than femoral shaft, femoral neck, or intertrochanteric hip fractures
- Bimodal pattern of injury (high-energy vs. low-energy osteoporotic/osteopenic patients)
- Each group provides different fixation challenges, which must be addressed at the time of injury
- Injuries are commonly the result of axial loading in the setting of varus or valgus stress
- Like subtrochanteric fractures, associated muscular attachments lead to fracture fragment deformation

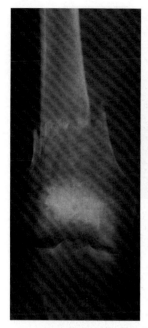
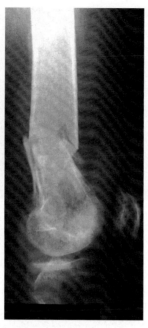

Type C2 distal femur fracture. (From Bucholz RW, Heckman JD, eds. Rockwood and Green's Fractures in Adults, 5th ed. Philadelphia, PA: Lippincott Williams & Wilkins; 2001.)

- – Gastrocnemius causes flexion of the distal fragment and this is complicated in the setting of intercondylar extension
- – In high-energy injuries, ABCs must be performed and detailed secondary survey is necessary to avoid missing additional injuries
- – 5%–10% of these injuries are open fractures necessitating irrigation and debridement
- – Although a small poke hole may be present, mechanism and associated soft tissue injury may further classify the fracture as a Gustilo Anderson IIIA fracture

Imaging
- – AP and lateral radiographs of the knee or distal femur should be performed
- – In cases with severe comminution, consider traction view or CT scan to evaluate articular extension

Classification
- – Arbeitsgemeinschaft Fur Osteosynthesefragen/ Association for the Study of Internal Fixation (AO/ASIF)
  - – A—extra-articular
    - – A1—condylar avulsion
    - – A2—transverse
    - – A3—comminuted
  - – B—partial articular
    - – B1—medial or lateral condylar split
    - – B2—intercondylar split
    - – B3—coronal split (Hoffa)

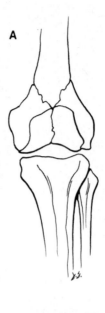
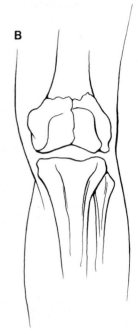

Distal femur fractures. **A:** Y-shaped intercondylar. **B:** T-shaped intercondylar. (From Harwood-Nuss A, et al. The Clinical Practice of Emergency Medicine, 3rd ed. Philadelphia, PA: Lippincott Williams & Wilkins; 2001.)

- – C—intra-articular, three or more parts
  - – C1—intercondylar split (Y)
  - – C2—intercondylar split (comminuted)
  - – C3—coronal split (comminuted articular surface)

Definition
- – Metadiaphyseal Junction
- – Distal 9 cm of femur
- – 5 cm above metaphyseal flare to articular surface

Deforming Forces
- – Adductors → varus deformity
- – Gastrocnemius → flexion of the distal fragment
- – Condylar attachment cause disjointed articular fragment deformation

Treatment
- – Before 1970, treatment was commonly nonoperative
- – Closed reduction, traction, and casting were initial treatment modalities

Treatment Difficulties
- – Closed reduction
  - – Incongruity
  - – Stiffness
  - – Delayed mobilization
- – ORIF
  - – Thin cortices may limit fixation strength

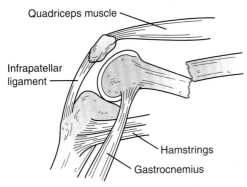

Lateral view showing muscle attachments and resulting deforming forces. These result in posterior displacement and angulation at the fracture site. (From Browner B, Jupiter J, Levine A, eds. Skeletal Trauma: Fractures, Dislocations, and Ligamentous Injuries, 2nd ed. Philadelphia, PA: WB Saunders; 1997.)

- Comminution may require bridging
- Wide canal may limit intramedullary fixation

Goals of Closed Treatment
- May accept up to:
  - 7 degrees varus/valgus
  - 7–10 degress flexion/extension
  - 1.5-cm shortening
  - 2-mm step-off

Indications for Nonoperative Treatment
- Nondisplaced, incomplete fracture
- Impacted, stable, elderly, osteoporotic
- Medically unstable
- Spinal cord injury

Associated Injuries
- Vascular: 2%–3% of patients will have an associated vascular injury
  - Consider angiography if no pulse present following reduction of fracture
- Ligamentous: uncommon
  - Anterior cruciate ligament (ACL) most common
  - Open repair may be performed for avulsions during fracture fixation
  - Midsubstance: Consider delayed reconstruction

Implants
Blade Plate 95 Degrees
- Technically difficult to implant due to precision necessary for insertion
- Most stable
- Three-plane alignment
- Consider nail with lateral comminution
- May displace occult intercondylar fracture

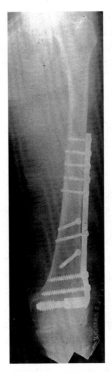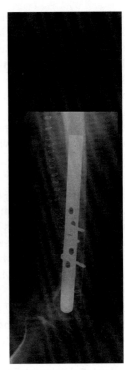

Direct open reduction and internal fixation with interfragmentary lag screws and a dynamic condylar screw. (From Bucholz RW, Heckman JD, eds. Rockwood and Green's Fractures in Adults, 5th ed. Philadelphia, PA: Lippincott Williams & Wilkins; 2001.)

- Need 2 cm of intact distal bone to adequately place the blade

Dynamic Compression Screw (DCS)
- Compression screw lags the condyles
- Provides better purchase in osteopenic patients
- Screw may be prominent distally
- Harder to maintain reduction in the sagittal
- May require an additional distal screw distally to improve fixation
- 4-cm intact distal bone necessary for compression screw placement

Condylar Buttress Plate
- Poor resistance to varus stress especially in patients with medial comminution
- May require screws outside of the plate for articular fixation
- Micromotion of the plate is essential for comminuted fractures treated with buttress plating. (Do not fill all the holes.)
- Locked compression plates provide the ability to utilize both compression plating techniques and locking screws as part of a fixed angle device

IM Nails: Retrograde Supracondylar Mail
- Load sharing device, which allows early motion
- Faster operative time and decreased blood loss
- Can be utilized in osteoporotic or periprosthetic fractures
- Despite ease of insertion, provides less axial and rotational stability
- Patients may develop postoperative knee pain due to violation of the knee joint with intra-articular insertion of the nail

Less Invasive Stabilization System (LISS) Plate
- Locked screw plate, which can be inserted percutaneously to limit blood loss
- Requires minimal bone distally
- Direct anatomic reduction of articular surface, indirect reduction of metaphysis, percutaneous plate insertion

Or Tips and Tricks—Retrograde Femoral Nail
- Preoperatively plan length, rotation, canal diameter to improve efficiency with implant choice
- A small medial parapatellar incision can be utilized
- Guide wire should be placed from the trochlear line to Blumensaat's line

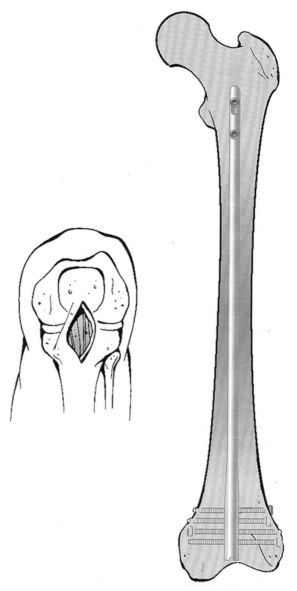

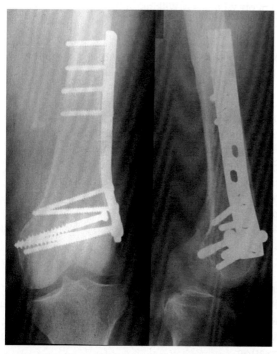

Post-operative films after open reduction and internal fixation using interfragmentary lag screws and a contoured 4.5-mm dynamic compression plate as a buttress plate. (From Bucholz RW, Heckman JD, eds. Rockwood and Green's Fractures in Adults, 5th ed. Philadelphia, PA: Lippincott Williams & Wilkins; 2001.)

Approach to the distal femur for retrograde femoral nailing. The knee is bent over a radiolucent triangle or bolster. The authors prefer a medial (or rarely lateral) approach to the patellar tendon. This can be extended into a formal parapatellar approach if necessary for articular reduction. (From Bucholz RW, Court-Brown CM, Heckman JD, Tornetta P. Rockwood & Green's Fractures in Adults, 7th ed. Philadelphia, PA: Lippincott Williams & Wilkins; 2010.)

- Confirm wire placement utilizing fluoroscopy
- Canting the AP image toward patient's head will allow a notch view of the distal femur
- Following placement of the guide wire, the 13-mm cannulated reamer can be utilized for placement of starting hole
- The knee should be flexed approximately 45 degrees to prevent reaming of the patella or the plateau

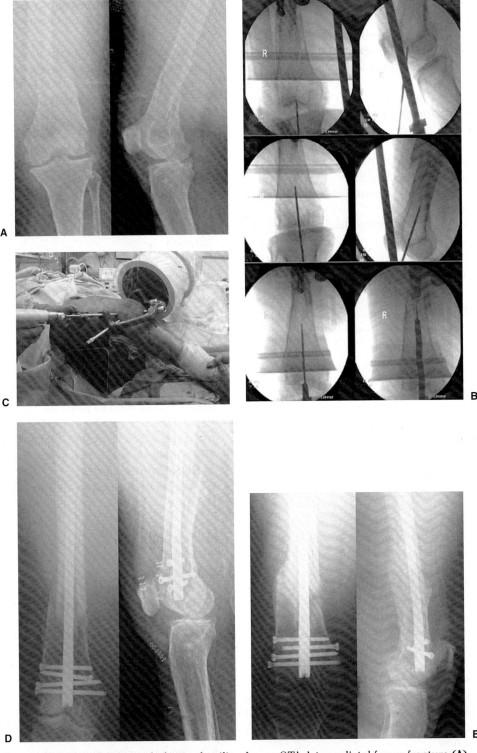

Illustrative case of retrograde femoral nailing for an OTA A-type distal femur fracture (A).
(B) Intraoperative fluoroscopy images showing the guide pin (or awl) is inserted in line
with the femoral canal in the intercondylar notch at the distal end of the Blumensaat line.
Indirect reduction methods are similar to those used for bridge plating. Protection of the
patella and soft tissues is mandatory. Intraoperative photograph during distal interlocking
(C). Postoperative (D) and 8-month follow-up (E) radiographs show stable fixation of
condyles using a modern nailing system that allows for maintenance of alignment. (From
Bucholz RW, Court-Brown CM, Heckman JD, Tornetta P MD. Rockwood & Green's Fractures
in Adults, 7th ed. Philadelphia, PA: Lippincott, Williams & Wilkins, 2010.)

- Reduce the fracture site and make note of the reduction maneuver
- Pass the long-tip guide wire with bend at tip through fracture site to the level of the lesser trochanter
- Ream with the fracture reduced to avoid eccentric reaming
- Overream nail by 1.5 mm
- Set up nail and confirm interlocks
- Following insertion of nail, rotation should be evaluated
- Compare cortical thickness at fracture site on AP view and lateral view to confirm rotation
- Be aware that the posterior cortex of femur thicker due to linea aspera
- Distal interlock or blade should be placed followed by compression of the fracture
- The two distal interlocks will control valgus/varus stress on the fracture site

Recommended Readings

Farouk O, et al. Effects of percutaneous and conventional plating techniques on the blood supply to the femur. Arch Trauma Surg 1998;117:438–441.

Kregor PJ. Distal femur fractures with complex articular involvement: management by articular exposure and submuscular fixation. Orthop Clin North Am 2002;33(1):153–175.

Krettek C, et al. Transarticular joint reconstruction and indirect plate osteosynthesis for distal supracondylar femoral fractures. Injury 1997;28:SA31–SA41.

KNEE DISLOCATIONS

Background
- Uncommon injury
- The majority of patients presenting with a knee dislocation present after spontaneous reduction of the injury
- Most commonly results from motor vehicle injuries
- Patients must be evaluated for other associated injuries, which may result from the high-energy trauma
- May also occur in low-energy situations
- ATLS protocol should be utilized in patient evaluation
- Three of the four major knee ligaments (cruciate/collateral) must be disrupted for dislocation to occur
- Evaluation of ACL, PCL, MCL, LCL, and PLC should be performed to determine ligamentous involvement.
- One-third of presenting patients may have an associated vascular injury
- Half of the vascular injuries occur with anterior posterior dislocations

Physical Examination
- Evaluation of the ligamentous structures should be performed to determine knee stability
- Neurovascular exam should be focused and detailed

- Due to the high frequency of vascular injury, ankle brachial index (ABI) should be performed
- Normal ABI is >0.9
- Angiography should be performed for ABI <0.9
- If hard signs of vascular injury present (absent pulse, bleeding, expanding hematoma, bruit, thrill), operative exploration/angiography, stabilization, or repair should be initiated early
- Angiogram should if soft signs present after reduction
- Usual repair is revascularization with saphenous vein graft
- Revascularize within 6 hr
- Green and Allen (1977) evaluated 245 knee dislocations showing 32% with popliteal artery injuries
- 86% of those not treated within 6–8 hr went on to amputation.
- Fasciotomy important with revascularization procedures
- 25% present with nerve (peroneal most common) injury
- Tibial nerve injuries are less common, but examiner should be aware of the possibility

Imaging/Radiographs
- AP, lateral, and oblique films of the knee should be performed as soon as possible
- Radiographs should be evaluated for subtle avulsion fractures, which represent ligamentous avulsions
- MRI should be performed in stable patients to evaluate ligamentous injuries
- CT can be performed as well to rule out associated fractures

Classification
Two Major Classifications
Directional
- Anterior: Most common
- Posterior: Commonly associated with extensor mechanism injury
- Posterolateral: Most commonly irreducible due to the femoral condyle buttonholing the capsule and thus preventing reduction

Anatomic
- Based on ligamentous injury (knee dislocation [KD] III most common)
- KD I: Single cruciate disruption
- KD II: Both cruciates disruption
- KDIIIM: Bicruciate with MCL tear
- KDIIIL: Bicruciate with lateral collateral ligament/posterolateral corner disruption
- KD IV: All four cruciates and collaterals disrupted
- KD V: Fracture dislocation (1–4 separated based on the number of ligamentous injuries)

Treatment

Nonoperative treatment
- Important to balance stability and stiffness with ROM and laxity
- Immobilization in extension for 6 wk can be considered, but these patients often require manipulation
- External fixation can be considered in patients with soft tissue injures that preclude operative fixation
- Closed treatment should be considered in sedentary patients or those too critically injured to undergo adequate operative treatment

Operative Treatment Indications
- Unsuccessful closed reductions
- Soft tissue interposition
- Open fractures
- Vascular injuries
- Timing of surgical repair for ligamentous injuries is dependent on the patient and limb
- KD IIIM injuries can be treated with ACL/PCL reconstruction at 6 wk after MCL healing
- KD IIIL injuries can undergo ACL/PCL/PLC reconstruction at 2–3 wk
- Goal of treatment is to identify and repair/reconstruct all pathology anatomically
- Consider external fixation in subluxing patient, multitrauma patient, or open fractures to temporize treatment
- Sisto and Warren (1985) evaluated 20 knee dislocations, 16 of which underwent operative fixation

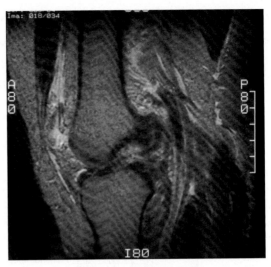

Mid-substance anterior cruciate ligament and posterior cruciate ligament tears on magnetic resonance imaging in a low-velocity knee dislocation. (From Bucholz RW, Heckman JD, eds. Rockwood and Green's Fractures in Adults, 5th ed. Philadelphia, PA: Lippincott Williams & Wilkins; 2001.)

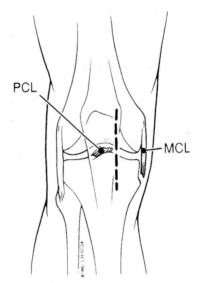

Medial exposure of the knee for reattachment of the posterior, anterior, and medial collateral ligaments. (From Bucholz RW, Heckman JD, eds. Rockwood and Green's Fractures in Adults, 5th ed. Philadelphia, PA: Lippincott Williams & Wilkins; 2001.)

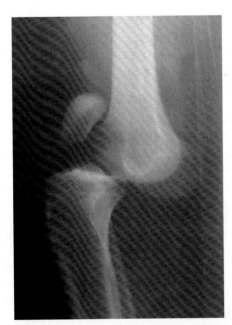

Lateral radiograph of a posterior cruciate ligament intact knee dislocation. (From Bucholz RW, Heckman JD, eds. Rockwood and Green's Fractures in Adults, 5th ed. Philadelphia, PA: Lippincott Williams & Wilkins; 2001.)

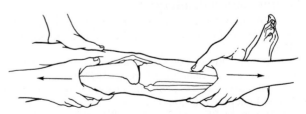

Technique for reduction of knee dislocation. (From Harwood-Nuss A, et al. The Clinical Practice of Emergency Medicine, 3rd ed. Philadelphia, PA: Lippincott Williams & Wilkins; 2001.)

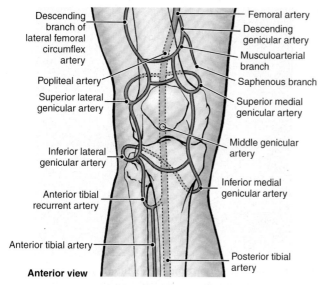

Descending branch of lateral femoral circumflex artery

Popliteal artery

Superior lateral genicular artery

Inferior lateral genicular artery

Anterior tibial recurrent artery

Anterior tibial artery

Anterior view

Femoral artery

Descending genicular artery

Musculoarterial branch

Saphenous branch

Superior medial genicular artery

Middle genicular artery

Inferior medial genicular artery

Posterior tibial artery

Arterial routes and the knee joint. The popliteal artery continuation of the femoral artery sends branches around the knee joint to support flow in any leg posture. The joint is well perfused by this thorough network. (Modified from LifeART image, copyright © 2007 Lippincott Williams & Wilkins. All rights reserved.)

- 16 of the operative cases had ACL and posterior cruciate ligament (PCL) ruptures.
- Bony avulsion was present in 14/16 PCLs, 10/16 ACLs.
- Acute repair was performed followed by manipulation at 3 mo
- In acutely repaired patients, there was no instability but stiffness was present
- 46% had chronic pain and 77% returned to vigorous sporting activities
- MCL was treated nonoperatively in this study
- Postoperative rehabilitation in these patients is crucial to improved patient outcomes
- ROM is usually initiated at 3 wk, with a goal of initiated full weight bearing by 6 wk
- Open-chain exercises are limited initially
- Most patients with lose approximately 10–15 degrees of terminal flexion

Recommended Readings

Dennis JW, et al. Reassessing the role of arteriograms in the management of posterior knee dislocations. J Trauma 1993; 35:692–697.

Green NE, Allen BL. Vascular injuries associated with dislocation of the knee. J Bone Joint Surg Am 1977;59A(2):236–239.

Meyers M, Harvey JP. Traumatic dislocation of the knee joint. J Bone Joint Surg Am 1971;53:16–29.

Sisto DJ, Warren RF. Complete knee dislocation: A follow-up study of operative treatment. Clin Orthop Relat Res 1985; 198:94–101.

Stannard JP, et al. Vascular injuries in knee dislocations following blunt trauma: Evaluating the role of physical examination to determine the need for arteriography. J Bone Joint Surg Am 2004;86:910–915.

Wascher DC, et al. Knee dislocation: Initial assessment and implications for treatment. J Orthop Trauma 1997;11:525–529.

FLOATING KNEE

Background

- Complex injury likely resultant from high-energy trauma
- May be associated with numerous injuries requiring comprehensive intervention
- ATLS principles should be applied to patients presenting with these injuries
- Incidence increasing with the concurrent motor vehicles and high-speed traffic
- Uncommon injury but should be evaluated closely
- Fraser and Waddell (1978) showed multiple associated injuries at high rates with patients presenting with floating knees
  - 27% intracranial trauma
  - 15% pelvic fracture
  - 10% chest injury
  - 1.4% compartment syndrome
  - 30% vascular injury, most common posterior tibial artery
  - 53% ligamentous injury
  - 18% ligament instability at 3.7-yr follow-up

Fraser-Wadell Classification

- I—extra-articular
- II—intra-articular and associated with worse prognosis
- IIA—femoral shaft with associated tibial plateau fracture
- IIB—distal femoral intra-articular and tibial shaft
- IIC—intra-articular tibial plateau fracture and distal femur fracture

Treatment

- All patients should be placed on a radiolucent table in the operating room, as the potential for nailing both fractures through one incision is present
- Femur should be stabilized initially because tibia can be splinted without traction if patient becomes unstable after femoral nailing
- Additionally, it is more manageable to stabilize tibia manually while nailing femur
- If tibia significantly unstable or femoral nailing appears challenging, consider external fixation of the tibia prior to femoral nailing to improve ability to perform fixation
- Retrograde femoral nail if fracture does not extend proximally to subtrochanteric region
- Subtrochanteric extension: Antegrade nailing of the femur should be performed

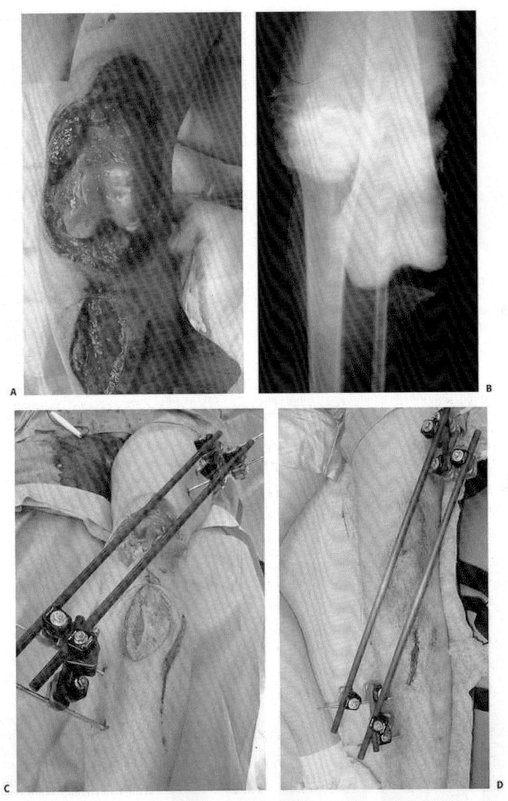

A, B: Severe open knee dislocation in conjunction with arterial disruption. **C, D:** Emergent knee-spanning fixator was applied at the time of initial surgical management, which included arterial repair and multiple débridements. The wound was eventually closed, and the patient underwent delayed ligamentous reconstruction at 10 weeks postinjury. (From Bucholz RW, Court-Brown CM, Heckman JD, Tornetta P MD. Rockwood & Green's Fractures in Adults, 7th ed. Philadelphia, PA: Lippincott, Williams & Wilkins, 2010.)

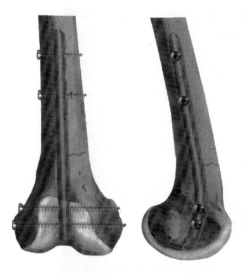

A: Type A distal femur fracture. **B:** Post-operative films after closed reduction and static locked reamed antegrade intramedullary nailing. (From Bucholz RW, Heckman JD, eds. Rockwood and Green's Fractures in Adults, 5th ed. Philadelphia, PA: Lippincott Williams & Wilkins; 2001.)

- Open knee wound: Debride the wound and nailing can be performed from the wound as long as an adequate debridement and irrigation is performed
- Grossly contaminated open knee wound: Antegrade nail femur and external fixation of the tibia should be performed
- Open tibia: I&D first and ex-fix before nailing femur, then nail tibia

- Proximal tibial fractures: Utilize distal femur traction pin if manual traction is too difficult
- Consider spanning external fixation for both fractures in intra-articular IIIC cases
- Ligamentous stability should be evaluated in all patients
- Patients should be braced for any MCL instability for at least 6 wk
- Meniscal tears, LCL, PLC injuries: Patients should undergo early repair to allow for early ROM and prevent stiffness
- ACL and PCL tear: Rehabilitation and delayed reconstruction

Or Tips and Tricks—External Fixation of the Knee

- Self-drilling and self-tapping 5-mm Schanz pins can be utilized, but care must be taken to prevent thermal necrosis and microfracture if placed unicortically
- Femur should be internally rotated so that patella in aligned appropriately
- Drill/pin guide should be used to appropriately position the pin
- Drill prior to insertion of the screw maintaining position with the triple sleeve
- Insert pin and advance just into the posterior cortex past the tapered edge
- Tibial pins are 5-mm Schanz pins that should be predrilled with a 3.5-mm drill bit just through the posterior cortex

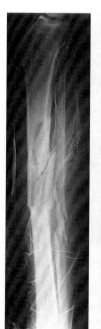
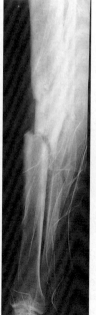
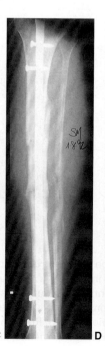
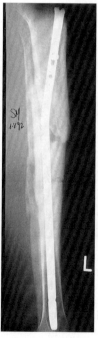

Displaced closed fractures of the tibia shaft, when shortened >1 cm or considered to be unstable, are best treated with interlocking nails. **A, B:** Preoperative radiographs of a shortened, unstable segmental fracture of the tibia shaft. **C, D:** The interlocking nail in place. The screws placed through the holes in the nail proximal and distal to the fracture provide length and rotational stability for the fracture. Nearly all fractures of the femoral shaft in skeletally mature individuals are treated with similar interlocking nails, allowing mobilization of the patient and early range of motion of adjacent joints. (From Swiontkowski MF. Manual of Orthopaedics, 6th ed. Philadelphia, PA: Lippincott Williams & Wilkins; 2006, with permission.)

- Stability is increased by bone-to-bone contact, large diameter pins, shorter distance from bar to bone and near/far near configuration of pins to fracture site
- Double stack rods when there is no bone-to-bone contact to increase stability
- Junction of the threads and nonthreaded portion of the pins may act as a stress riser and should be observed closely
- To improve pull out strength
  - Small diameter pins with lower pitch
- To improve pin strength
  - Increase pin diameter
- Consider box frame in femur and calcaneus to avoid pins in the tibia, which limit tibial nailing

Recommended Reading

Elmrini A, et al. Ipsilateral fractures of tibia and femur or floating knee. Int Orthop 2006;30(5):325–328.
Fraser RD, Waddwell JP. Ipsilateral fracture of the femur and tibia. J Bone Joint Surg Br 1978;60-B(4):510–515.

EXTENSOR MECHANISM INJURIES

- Injuries often occur as the result of a sudden forceful quadriceps contraction against full body weight (jumping, unexpected fall, or sudden hyperflexion of the knee)

History and Physical Examination

- Patients usually present with pain and may be unable to bear weight
- The major diagnostic sign in extensor mechanism injuries is the loss of active extension against gravity
- Patients also present with a large, effusion/hemarthrosis
- There is often a palpable defect in either the patellar or quadriceps tendon
- Patients with tendon ruptures often from undiagnosed tendon degeneration secondary to calcific tendonitis, repetitive microtrauma, mucoid degeneration, post dialysis chronic degeneration, chronic steroid use, diabetes, or other systemic diseases that may increase the propensity for suffering these injuries
- Healthy tendons should not rupture

Imaging

- AP and lateral knee radiographs should be performed to rule out patellar fracture as a cause of the loss of extensor mechanism function

- Lateral radiographs should be evaluated for signs of patella alta (patellar tendon ruptures) or patella baja (quadriceps tendon ruptures)
- Insall-Salvati ratio should be evaluated (30-degree flexion, lateral radiograph)
- The ratio of the patella length to patellar tendon length should be 1.0 (between 0.8 and 1.2)
  - <0.8 = patella alta
  - >1.2 = patella baja
- Ultrasound can be performed to evaluate the tendon void but is operator dependent for true diagnosis
- MRI can also be performed for more detailed evaluation in patients where the diagnosis is not completely consistent

Patellar Tendon Ruptures

- More common in patients <40 yr
- Patients may present with a prodromal patella tendonitis
- Insall-Salvati ratio is 0.8
- Most commonly the patellar tendon is avulsed off of the inferior pole of the patella

Treatment

- Direct repair can be performed utilizing two Krakow sutures in the remaining medial and lateral aspects of the patellar tendon splitting the tendon in thirds (#5 orthocord/#5 Fiberwire/#2 Ethibond)
- Three parallel drill holes should be placed in the patella and the sutures passed through the drill holes and tied in tension with the knee extended over the top of the patella
- The retinacular repair is essential to assist in return to function and patellar tendon repair strength
- The retinaculum is repaired utilizing #1 or 0 vicryl sutures closing down the retinaculum from deep to superficial
- 2.0 Ethibond can be considered to improve repair strength

Postoperative Management

- Repair should be evaluated intraoperatively
- Gentle passive ROM can be performed from 0 to 30 degrees if intraoperative evaluation is stable
- ROM is then advanced slowly over the course of 6 wk
- Patients are made weight bearing as tolerated with the knee locked in extension

Quadriceps Tendon Ruptures

- More common than patellar tendon ruptures
- More often seen in patients >40 yr
- These patients have a higher rate of comorbidities, which may contribute to tendon rupture

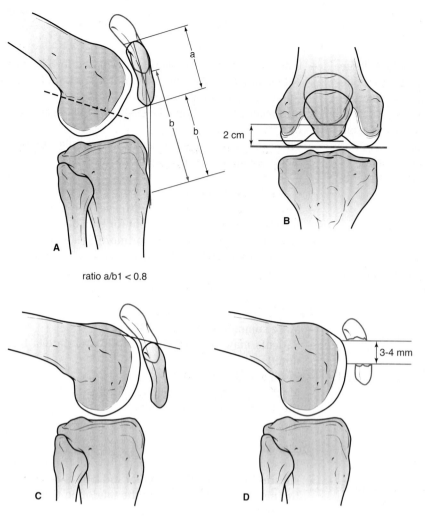

A. The length of the patellar tendon should approximate the midsagittal length of the patella and the inferior pole of the patella projects to the level of Blumenstaat line (dashed line). A ratio of <0.8 indicates possible injury to the patellar tendon (method of Insall). **B.** On the anteroposterior radiograph, the inferior pole of the patella should lie within 2 cm of a plane formed by the distal femoral condyles. **C.** At 90 degrees of flexion, the superior pole of the patella should lie inferior to the anterior surface of the femoral shaft. **D.** The lateral view gives the best view of the fracture pattern and of fragment separation. (From Bucholz RW, Court- Brown CM, Heckman JD, et al. *Rockwood & Green's Fractures in Adults*, 7th ed. Philadelphia: Lippincott, Williams & Wilkins, 2010.)

ratio a/b1 < 0.8

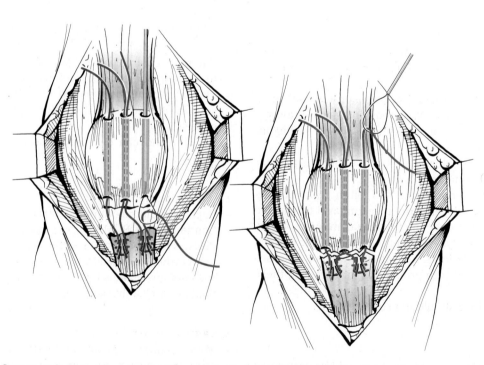

Suture technique of patellar tendon repair. **A.** A suture passer is used to guide the core sutures through the drill holes. **B.** The suture is retrieved and tied at the superior margin of the patella. (From Bucholz RW, Court- Brown CM, Heckman JD, et al. *Rockwood & Green's Fractures in Adults*, 7th ed. Philadelphia: Lippincott, Williams & Wilkins, 2010.)

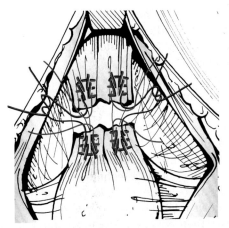

Acute repair using a Krackow suture technique. (From Bucholz RW, Court-Brown CM, Heckman JD, et al. *Rockwood & Green's Fractures in Adults*, 7th ed. Philadelphia: Lippincott, Williams & Wilkins, 2010.)

– One-third of patients with bilateral ruptures and one-fifth of unilateral rupture patients report an underlying systemic condition that weakens tendon
– Diagnosis may be more difficult and require the use of ultrasound or MRI
– Unfortunately, a large portion of these injuries are intrasubstance tears up to 2 cm above patella
– Direct primary surgical repair should be performed if patients are unable to actively extend the knee

Treatment
– Similar to patellar tendon ruptures, direct repair can be performed utilizing two Krackow sutures in the remaining medial and lateral aspects of the patellar tendon splitting the tendon in thirds (#5 orthocord/#5 Fiberwire/#2 Ethibond)

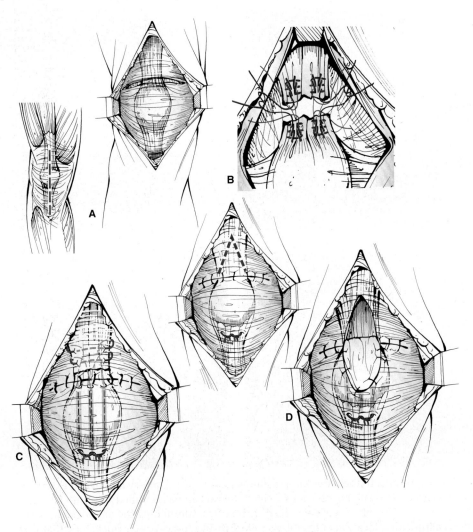

Acute quadriceps tendon repair. **A.** Approach is through a midline longitudinal incision. **B.** Acute repair using a Krackow suture technique. **C.** Repair through three parallel drill holes in the patella. **D.** Scuderi technique with a turndown flap reinforcement. (From Bucholz RW, Court-Brown CM, Heckman JD, et al. *Rockwood & Green's Fractures in Adults*, 7th ed. Philadelphia: Lippincott, Williams & Wilkins, 2010.)

- Three parallel drill holes should be placed in the patella and the sutures passed through the drill holes and tied in tension with the knee extended over the inferior pole of the patella
- These patients may also require a retinacular repair utilizing #1 or 0 vicryl suture

Scuderi Reinforcement
- A 2-inch triangle of partial thickness flap proximal to tear can be elevated to reinforce the repair

Postoperative Management
- Repair should be evaluated intraoperatively
- Gentle passive ROM can be performed from 0 to 30 degrees if intraoperative evaluation is stable

- ROM is then advanced slowly over the course of 6 wk
- Patients are made weight bearing as tolerated with the knee locked in extension with a Bledsoe or knee immobilizer

Chronic Quadriceps Tendon Rupture
- 10%–50% diagnostic failure rates
- Methods to close gap
- Elevate quadriceps from femur and release adhesion to improve muscle mobilization
- Consider the Codivilla technique
- Full-thickness inverted V flap proximal to tear.
- This allows tear to be approximated
- The flap then covers repair to reinforce it while the open triangle is sewed side to side

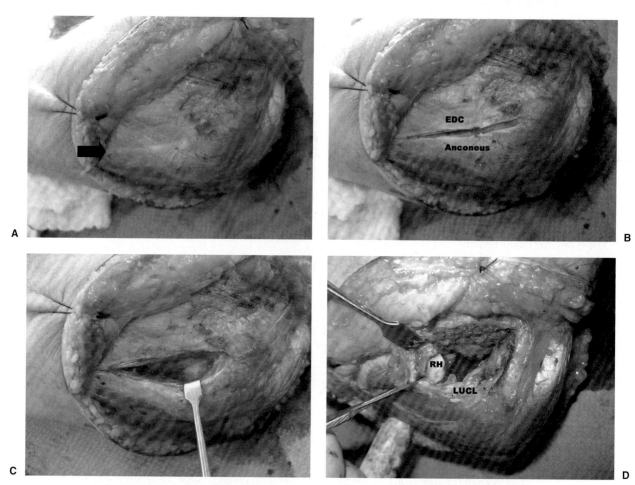

Kocher's approach to the anterolateral elbow joint uses the interval between extensor carpi ulnaris (ECU) and anconeus **(A).** This interval can be identified by a thin fat stripe (black arrow). The interval is developed by bluntly undermining the anconeus muscle, which allows identification of the elbow joint capsule and capsular thickening that is the lateral ulnar collateral ligament (LUCL) **(B, C).** The posterior portion of the common extensor tendon origin has to be elevated off the LUCL to allow an arthrotomy to be made anterior to the ligament **(D).** (RH, radial head.) (From Bucholz RW, Court-Brown CM, Heckman JD, et al. *Rockwood & Green's Fractures in Adults*, 7th ed. Philadelphia: Lippincott, Williams & Wilkins, 2010.)

Outcomes
- Most patients are able to return to function following the injury (most studies report good to excellent results in 70%–100% of patients)
- Persistent quadriceps weakness is common post repair complaint
- Adequate recovery regimen is necessary to prevent loss of motion and other functional limitations
- Early repair is associated with improved outcomes

PATELLAR FRACTURE

Background
- Represent approximately 1% of all presenting fractures
- Previous treatment has included nonoperative treatment and partial/complete patellectomy
- Further evaluation has shown the importance of the patella in maintenance of efficient extensor mechanism function
- Despite significant improvement in fixation methods, the injury continues to cause significant pain, discomfort, reoperation, and change in function
- Fracture treatment and union is dependent on a tenuous blood supply despite a vasculature
- The most common mechanism of injury is direct blow to anterior knee
- The majority of patients present with transverse fractures, but higher-energy injuries lead to stellate or more comminuted injuries, which provide additional challenges to fixation
- Elderly patients also provide a unique challenge to patella fracture fixation due to associated comorbidities and the high frequency of osteoporosis

History and Physical Examination
- Patients traditionally present with an inability to actively extend knee following a direct blow to the anterior knee
- Care must be taken to evaluate the skin for any signs of an open fractures, or abrasions that may preclude operative fixation
- Patients can be provisionally placed in a bulky jones dressing with knee immobilizer until decision made regarding surgical intervention

Radiographs
- AP, lateral, and oblique knee films
- Merchant views of the knee can be performed to evaluate vertical fracture lines
- Lazaro (2012)
  - CT alters treatment strategy when compared to plain radiographs

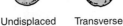

Descriptive classification of patellar fractures. (From Bucholz RW, Court- Brown CM, Heckman JD, et al. *Rockwood & Green's Fractures in Adults*, 7th ed. Philadelphia: Lippincott, Williams & Wilkins, 2010.)

- CT scan will show distal pole comminution in 88% of fractures which is often missed on plain radiographs

Treatment
Indications for Nonoperative Treatment
- Nondisplaced fractures with intact extensor mechanism
- Fractures with <2 mm of intra-articular step-off or displacement
- <3 mm of fragment separation
- Patients can be treated weight bearing as tolerated in a hinged knee brace

Operative Treatment
- Indicated in patients without extensor mechanism intact
- Open injury
- >2 mm of intra-articular step off or 2 mm of displacement
- >3 mm of fragment separation

Surgical Approach
- Traditionally, standard anterior approach to the knee is utilized for fixation
- Lateral parapatellar approach can be considered to avoid the major blood supply to the patella and allow for eversion of the patella to examine the articular surface (Gardner, Lorich 2005)
- **Anterior tension band**
  - 2 × 2 threaded K-wires parallel to the articular surface of the patella in the subchondral bone
  - 18-gauge wire placed in a figure 8 fashion deep to the exposed wires at the superior and inferior pole
  - A second cerclage wire can be threaded around the patella to improve fixation

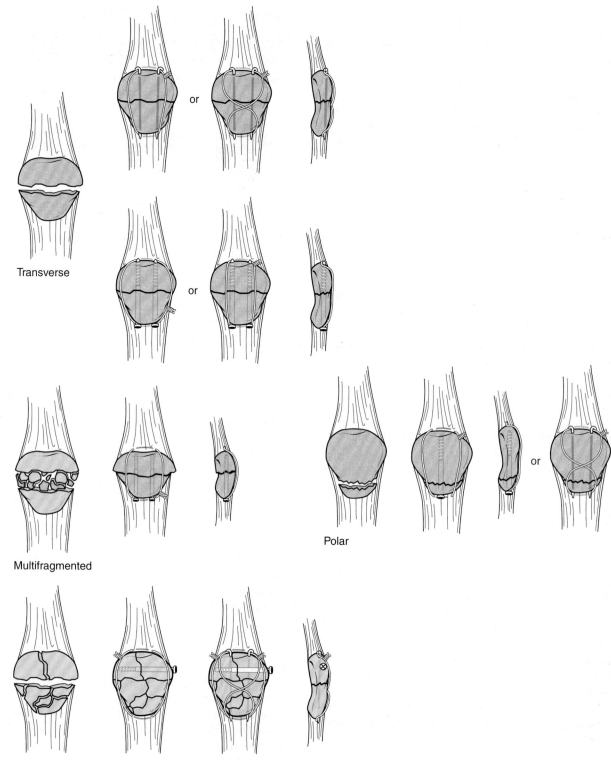

Transverse

Multifragmented

Polar

Fracture patterns and examples of internal fixation. (From Bucholz RW, Court- Brown CM, Heckman JD, et al. *Rockwood & Green's Fractures in Adults*, 7th ed. Philadelphia: Lippincott, Williams & Wilkins, 2010.)

- Avoid in fractures with significant comminution at the articular surface to avoid compression/shortening
- **Anterior tension band with cannulated screws**
  - 4.0 cannulated screws can be passed along the subchondral surface of the patella followed by passing of the 18-gauge wire in a figure 8 fashion
  - Wires are then tensioned symmetrically
  - 4.0 lag screws are utilized to improve interfragmentary compression
- Modifications to the tension band contructs are made based on the planes of the fractures
- Additional 2.0 threaded K-wires can be utilized for fixation of multiple fragments in comminuted fractures
- Additional support of the construct can be performed through augmentation of the patella tendon with krakow suture (#2 Ethibond) passed through the patellar tendon and passed through drill holes in the patella
- Distal pole extra-articular fractures are often better treated with patellar tendon augmentation as mentioned above if comminution prevents adequate fixation

Complications
- Anterior knee pain
- Painful hardware requiring removal
- 20% loss of reduction
- Technical error, patient noncompliance
- Nonunion <5%

Recommended Reading
Gardner MJ, Griffith MH, Lawrence BD, Lorich DG. Complete exposure of the articular surface for fixation of patellar fractures. J Orthop Trauma 2005;19(2):118–123.

Lazaro LE, Wellman DS, Pardee NC, Gardner MJ, Toro JB, Macintyre NR 3rd, Helfet DL, Lorich DG. Effect of computerized tomography on classification and treatment plan for patellar fractures. J Orthop Trauma 2012 Sep 4.

TIBIAL PLATEAU FRACTURES

Background
- Bimodal incidence (males in 40s, females in 70s)
- In younger patients, commonly result from higher-energy mechanisms, whereas older patient injuries result from low-energy falls from standing
- Intra-articular fracture, which requires accurate reconstruction of the articular surface
- May have multiple associated soft tissue injuries including:
  - 50% of patients with meniscal tears
  - 30% of patients with ligamentous injuries (MCL)
- Direction and type of force determine the fracture pattern
- Most common injuries result from a valgus load at the knee in combination with axial compression (lateral plateau injuries)
- Medial injuries result from varus stress with associated knee flexion and internal rotation

History and Physical Exam
- Patients with high-energy mechanisms should be evaluated closely for open injuries and should be managed utilizing ATLS protocols if necessary
- Adequate knee exam should be performed to evaluate for instability or associated ligamentous injury
- Neurovascular exam should be focused and detailed
- High-energy fractures are at highest risk for compartment syndrome and should be monitored closely
- Care must be taken to rule out compartment syndrome in all fractures, as approximately 10% of all tibial plateau fractures are diagnosed with compartment syndrome
- Open wounds should be examined closely as they may be communicate with the knee joint
- Swelling should be monitored closely, as fracture blisters may develop precluding operative intervention

Imaging
- Radiographs: AP, lateral, and two oblique views, 15-degree caudal view to visualize the plateau
- CT scan is essential for evaluating fracture fragments
- MRI may provide additional information regarding soft tissue injury, joint impaction, and cartilage damage

Schatzker Classification
- I—lateral split
  - Younger
  - Ligamentous injuries
  - Meniscus trapped in fracture
- II—lateral split/depression
- III—pure lateral central depression
  - Low energy
  - Elderly
  - Low risk of ligamentous injury
  - Stable due to intact rim
- IV—medial
  - High energy
    - Associated with peroneal nerve injury
- V—bicondylar splits of medial and lateral
  - No depressions
  - Combined anterolateral, posteromedial approaches with less infection
- VI—associated proximal shaft fracture
  - High energy
  - Associated with popliteal artery disruption due to high risk of dislocation

Treatment

Nonoperative

- Nonoperative treatment is reserved for minimally or nondisplaced fractures or patients with low functional demands or significant osteoarthritis
- Joint congruity and mechanical alignment should be evaluated prior to considering nonoperative intervention
- Consider hinged knee brace, non–weight bearing for 12 wk
- ROM can be initiated early to decrease the risk of stiffness, flexion contractures, and poor functional recovery
- No restriction at 4–6 mo

Operative Treatment

External Fixation

- Patients with severe soft tissue injury or swelling that precludes internal fixation should undergo early knee-spanning external fixation to expedite soft tissue recovery
- Goals of external fixation are the restore length and improve alignment prior to internal fixation

Internal Fixation

- Operative intervention is dependent on the fracture mechanism and pattern
- Indications for ORIF
    - >10-degree varus or valgus instability
    - Step-off >2 mm and all medial and bicondylar fractures
- Minimize soft tissue stripping in bicondylar fractures to maintain fragment vascularity
- Monitor skin bridges if two incisions considered

Splits—Schatzker I, IV, V

- Care must be taken to maintain vascularity of fragments during treatment of these fractures
- The articular surface should be palpated to confirm no palpable depression and adequate fracture alignment
- A large periarticular tenaculum clamp and the femoral distractor can be utilized to maintain reduction of the fractures
- Buttress plating is the standard of treatment to resist sheer forces across the fragment
- Anterolateral approach can be taken for lateral fragments while the posteromedial approach is utilized for large posteromedial fragments

Depressed—Schatzker III

- True Schatker III fractures are truly rare, as most fractures have an associated split, which is discovered upon intervention
- If articular surface is minimally depressed, a metaphyseal window may be made to elevate the depression.

- Elevate depressed bone en masse with tamp
- To prevent settling postoperatively, bone grafting should be performed in the void left by the depressed fragments
    - Consider allograft chips, fibular strut allograft, or calcium triphosphate cement
- Support graft with rafting screws in proximal aspect of the buttress plate or provisionally fix with K-wires, which can be left in place following definitive fixation

Split/Depressed—Schatker II

- ORIF is the treatment of choice
- Metaphyseal split should be booked open utilizing osteotomes or a laminar spreader to better visualize the depressed fragments
- Depressed articular segment should be elevated with the assistance of structural graft or osteotomes
- K-wires can be placed subchondrally to maintain elevation of the articular surface
- Allograft fibula, Plexur (Osteotech 2010) provides structural support, which can be cut and tamped into the void left by the depressed fragments
- Large periarticular clamp can then be placed followed by placement of buttress plate
- Split can be repaired using cortical screws to stabilize the split through both buttressing and lagging of the fragments

Schatzker VI

- Reconstruct articular surface using largest fragment as the constant fragment (commonly the medial fragment)
- Following reduction of the articular surface, attention can be turned to reducing the articular surface to the metaphyseal/shaft component
- Dual condylar plating may be performed as long as care is taken to avoid the small interincision flaps, which can lead to poor wound healing
- Solitary lateral locking plate fixation is considered in some cases but should be avoided in cases with large posteromedial coronal shear fractures that are not adequately captured by lateral locking plate
- Posteromedial buttress plating can be performed with an appropriately contoured 3.5-mm reconstruction plate
- Care should be taken with bicolumnar plating, as infection rates range from 8.4% to 18%

Or Tips and Tricks—Anterolateral Approach to the Tibial Plateau

- An oblique incision, from level at top of patella to four fingers below tibial tubercle can be used or the lazy S incision

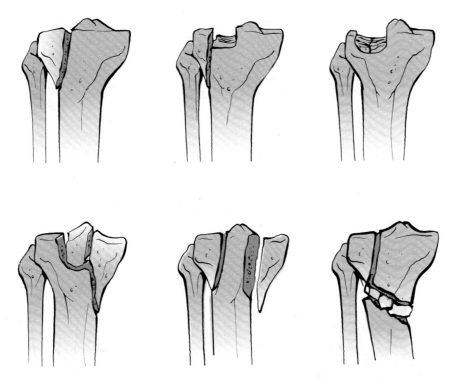

The Schatzker classification of tibial plateau fractures. (From Bucholz RW, Court-Brown CM, Heckman JD, et al. *Rockwood & Green's Fractures in Adults*, 7th ed. Philadelphia: Lippincott, Williams & Wilkins, 2010.)

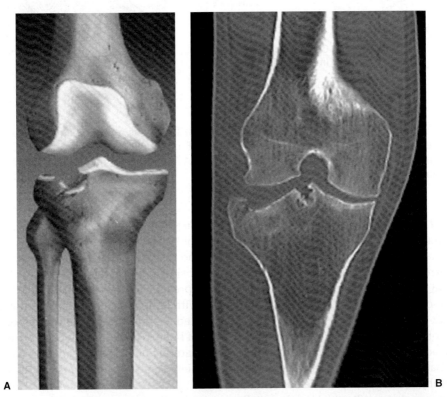

A local compression fracture (AO/OTA B-2, Schatzker 3) illustrated in (**A**) a drawing and (**B**) a coronal CT cut. There may be a subtle split fragment. (From Bucholz RW, Court-Brown CM, Heckman JD, et al. *Rockwood & Green's Fractures in Adults*, 7th ed. Philadelphia: Lippincott, Williams & Wilkins, 2010.)

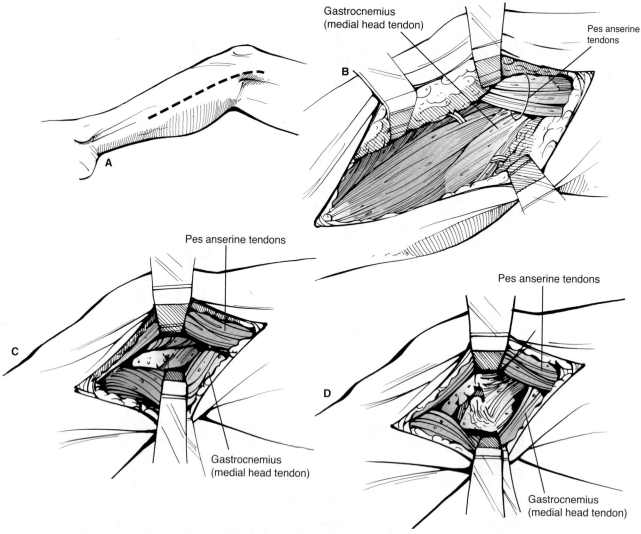

Posteromedial approach to the medial tibial plateau. The pes is retracted anteriorly and the medial gastrocnemius is retracted posteriorly. (From Bucholz RW, Court- Brown CM, Heckman JD, et al. *Rockwood & Green's Fractures in Adults*, 7th ed. Philadelphia: Lippincott, Williams & Wilkins, 2010.)

- Start from lateral epicondyle, passing through halfway point between Gerdy's tubercle and fibular head and ending 1 cm lateral to tibial spine
- Top of patella corresponds to metaphyseal flare where the distal femoral distractor pin can be placed
- Elevate anterior compartment off proximal tibia to Gerdy's, leaving 2-mm cuff for closure
- Take soft tissue off lateral plateau, posteriorly to the LCL or fibular head to allow for placement of the plate
- Incise iliotibial band in line with skin to Gerdy's and elevate flap laterally, leaving joint capsule underneath
- Bluntly separate capsule from iliotibial band medially as well
- Horizontal capsulotomy under meniscus, leaving cuff of coronary ligament for repair

- Polydioxanone sutures can be placed into anterior, middle, and posterior meniscus and retracted cephalad to expose the articular surface of the tibia
- If split depression, split the fracture with a laminar spreader to allow elevation of the articular surface with tamps or sequential osteotomes
- Reduce the surface and utilize bone graft to fill areas of bone loss or cancellous depression
- Lateral nonlocking 3.5-mm or 4.5 locking periarticular plate can be used to buttress the fragments

Outcomes/Complications

- Loss of reduction is one of the most common complications of tibial plateau fractures

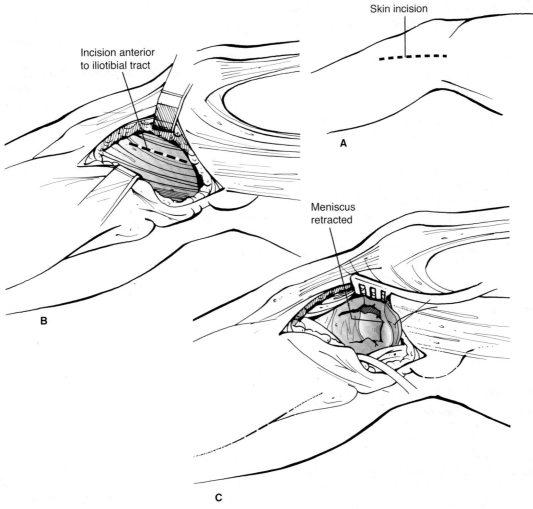

A. Anterolateral approach to the tibial plateau with alternate techniques to expose the lateral joint. **B.** A submeniscal arthrotomy through the coronary ligament. **C.** An anterior joint arthrotomy with detachment of the anterior horn of the meniscus. (From Bucholz RW, Court-Brown CM, Heckman JD, et al. *Rockwood & Green's Fractures in Adults*, 7th ed. Philadelphia: Lippincott, Williams & Wilkins, 2010.)

- 31%–79% of patients suffer loss of reduction of fractures
- Risk is high in elderly patients due to osteoporosis and inability to follow appropriate weight-bearing requirements
- Loss of reduction can lead to malalignment of the knee, which may require revision ORIF vs. possible arthroplasty to improve patient outcome
- Soft tissue management is crucial to outcomes in high-energy injuries
  - Inadequate management increases the risk of deep infection significantly leading to increased risk of nonunion, malunion, or the requirement for removal of hardware
  - These issues are compounded in patients requiring bicolumnar plating
- Loss of motion is another complication following operative treatment of tibial plateau fractures
  - Prior to hospital discharge, consider continuous passive motion and physical therapy instituted motion to 90 degrees to improve functional outcomes in patients
  - Patients requiring prolonged external fixation prior to definitive fixation are at the highest risk for postoperative stiffness
  - ROM may be improved with removal of lateral hardware, as the plate may cause pain and discomfort due to impinging on the iliotibial band
- Patients generally do well following tibial plateau fixation if mechanical alignment of the knee is maintained appropriately

- Patient outcomes have been shown to worsen in older patients in terms of functional outcomes and return to function

TIBIAL SHAFT FRACTURE

Background
- The most common presenting long bone fracture
- Majority of fractures occur in patients under the age of 40
- Wide spectrum of injury leads to variable treatment and patient outcomes
- Care should be taken in evaluation of these patients and their associated injuries

History and Physical Examination
- Patients may present following variety of energy mechanisms
- Mechanism of injury determines the injury pattern
- High-energy injuries may have associated injuries requiring ATLS for patient stabilization and evaluation
- Accurate and detailed neurovascular exam should be performed
- Due to the relatively thin soft tissue envelope surrounding the tibial shaft, approximately 20%–25% of these fractures are open
- Higher-energy mechanisms are at higher risk for soft tissue injury and open fractures
- Risk of compartment syndrome is highest in patients presenting with tibial shaft fractures – Prevalence from 1%–10% of tibial shaft fractures
  - Early fasciotomies should be considered in patients with impending compartment syndrome
  - Consider early evaluation of CPs (Delta pressure <30 or absolute pressure >30) to rule in or rule out compartment syndrome
  - Sequelae of missed compartment syndrome are significant and lead to poor functional outcomes

Low-Energy Injuries
- Result from torsional injury or indirect trauma
- Fibular fracture may be at a different level due to rotational injury

High-Energy Injuries
- Direct forces lead to significant comminution
- May have associated fibula fracture at same level
- Can be associated with severe soft tissue injury

Imaging
- AP and lateral tibia/fibula films on one plate should be performed to evaluate alignment and joint above and below the fracture

- Ankle films should be performed in distal third fractures to rule out components of rotational injuries (posterior malleolus fractures, oblique fibula fractures)
- CT scans should be performed for all distal third fractures to rule out nondisplaced posterior malleolus fractures, which may require additional intervention
- Boraiah et al. (2008) showed that 39% of patients presenting in a series of 62 patients had posterior malleolus fractures in spiral distal third tibial shaft fractures

Classification
AO/OTA Classification
A. Unifocal injury
B. Wedge fractures
C. Complex fractures

- Each grouping is further separated based on the fracture comminution

Treatment
Nonoperative Treatment
- Consider in low-energy injuries
- Patients are treated with a long leg cast for approximately 6 wk
- Can consider switching to non–weight-bearing short leg cast at 4 wk
- Care must be taken to adequately pad bony prominences to avoid pressure sores
- Closed treatment and casting is associated with an incidence of delayed union of 13% and a nonunion rate of 4%

Operative Treatment
Operative Indications
- Open, vascular injury, compartment syndrome, multiple injuries
- Significant shortening on injury
- Significant comminution
- Intact fibula—best predictor of varus if treated in brace
- Fibular fracture at same level as tibia

Intramedullary Nailing
- The standard of care and treatment of choice for most tibial fractures
- Goals of treatment are to restore length, alignment, and rotation of the tibial shaft
- Many factors should be considered in the treatment of tibial shaft fractures through IM nailing
- Fracture location should be considered as distal and proximal fractures have their own associated complications

Subgroups and Qualifications:

Tibia/fibula, diaphyseal, simple, spiral (42-A1)

(1) proximal zone
(2) middle zone
(3) distal zone

1. Fibula intact (42-A1.1)	2. Fibula fracture at different level (42-A1.2)	3. Fibula fracture at same level (42-A1.3)

A1

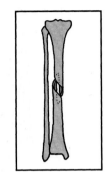 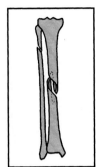 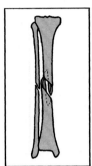

Tibia/fibula, diaphyseal, simple, oblique (>30˚) (42-A2)

(1) proximal zone
(2) middle zone
(3) distal zone

1. Fibula intact (42-A2.1)	2. Fibula fracture at different level (42-A2.2)	3. Fibula fracture at same level (42-A2.3)

A2

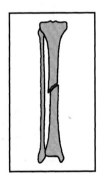 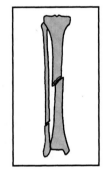 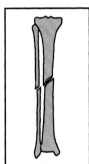

Tibia/fibula, diaphyseal, simple, transverse (<30°) (42-A3)

(1) proximal zone
(2) middle zone
(3) distal zone

1. Fibula intact (42-A3.1)	2. Fibula fracture at different level (42-A3.2)	3. Fibula fracture at same level (42-A3.3)

A3

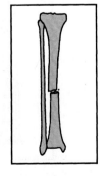 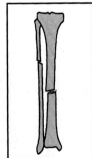 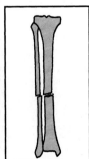

The Orthopaedic Trauma Association/AO classification of tibial diaphyseal fractures. (*continued*)

Tibia/fibula, diaphyseal, wedge, spiral (42-B1)
(1) proximal zone
(2) middle zone
(3) distal zone

1. Fibula intact (42-B1.1)

2. Fibula fracture at different level (42-B1.2)

3. Fibula fracture at same level (42-B1.3)

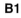 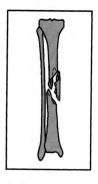 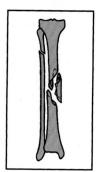 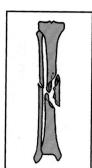

B1

Tibia/fibula, diaphyseal, wedge, bending (42-B2)
(1) proximal zone
(2) middle zone
(3) distal zone

1. Fibula intact (42-B2.1)

2. Fibula fracture at different level (42-B2.2)

3. Fibula fracture at same level (42-B2.3)

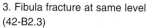 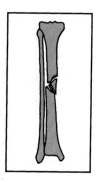 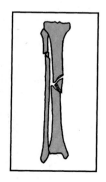 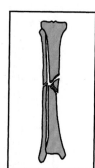

B2

Tibia/fibula, diaphyseal, wedge fragmented (42-B3)
(1) proximal zone
(2) middle zone
(3) distal zone

1. Fibula intact (42-B3.1)

2. Fibula fracture at different level (42-B3.2)

3. Fibula fracture at same level (42-B3.3)

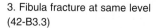 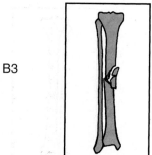 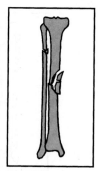 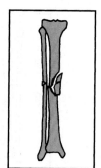

B3

(Continued)

Tibia/fibula, diaphyseal, complex, spiral (42-C1)
(1) pure diaphyseal
(2) proximal diaphysio-metaphysis
(3) distal diaphysio-metaphysis

| 1. With 2 intermediate fragments (42-C1.1) | 2. With 3 intermediate fragments (42-C1.2) | 3. With more than 3 intermediate fragments (42-C1.3) |

 C1

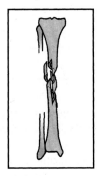 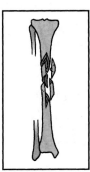 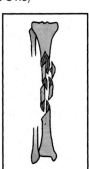

Tibia/fibula, diaphyseal, complex segmental (42-C2)

1. With an intermediate segmental fragment   (42-C2.1)
(1) pure diaphyseal
(2) proximal diaphysio-metaphyseal
(3) distal diaphysio-metaphyseal
(4) oblique lines
(5) transverse and oblique lines

2. With an intermediate segmental and additional wedge fragment(s) (42-C2.2)
(1) pure diaphyseal
(2) proximal diaphysio-metaphyseal
(3) distal diaphysio-metaphyseal
(4) distal wedge
(5) 3 wedges, proximal and distal

3. With 2 intermediate segmental fragments (42-C2.3)
(1) pure diaphyseal
(2) proximal diaphysio-metaphyseal
(3) distal diaphysio-metaphyseal

C2

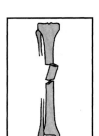 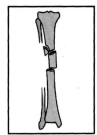 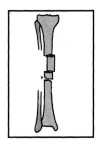

Tibia/fibula, diaphyseal, complex, irregular (42-C3)

1. With 2 or 3 intermediate fragments (42-C3.1)
(1) 2 intermediate fragments
(2) 3 intermediate fragments

2. Limited shattering (> 4cm) (42-C3.2)

3. Extensive shattering (> 4cm) (42-C3.3)
(1) pure diaphyseal
(2) proximal diaphysio-metaphyseal
(3) distal diaphysio-metaphyseal

C3

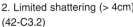

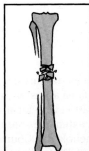 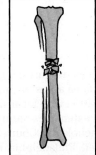 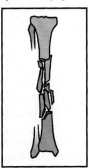

(Continued)

– The placement of medial and lateral femoral distractors through the posterior aspect of the tibia (physeal scar) and the calcaneus may improve maintenance of alignment during reduction and reaming minimizing the need for additional assistants to maintain traction

Proximal Third Fracture and Intramedullary Nail
– **Fractures tend to fall into valgus and procurvatum**
– Multiple techniques can be utilized to improve fracture reduction and prevent malreduction
  – More lateral starting point
  – Blocking screws placed laterally and posteriorly in the proximal fragment
  – Provisional reduction with unicortical screws through minifragment plates along the medial or anterior cortices
  – Tibial nailing in the semiextended position
  – Consider the suprapatellar nail

Distal Metaphyseal Fractures
– Shape of the distal metaphysis requires accurate reduction and reaming primary to nail placement
– Early use of large tenaculums for provisional reduction
– Wire should be centered directly in the tibial plafond
– It is essential to evaluate these fractures for associated posterior malleolus fracture which can displace with insertion of the nail
– Consider placement of an A-P screw prior to nail insertion
– ORIF of the fibula may be necessary in these rotational injuries, which may have associated ankle instability
– Two distal interlock screws should be available prior to the consideration of nailing distal third tibia fractures

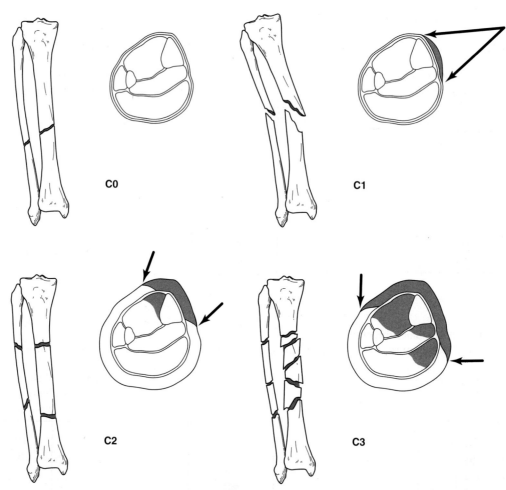

The Tscherne classification of closed fractures: C0, simple fracture configuration with little or no soft tissue injury; C1, superficial abrasion, mild to moderately severe fracture configuration; C2, deep contamination with local skin or muscle contusion, moderately severe fracture configuration; C3, extensive contusion or crushing of skin or destruction of muscle, severe fracture. (From Bucholz RW, Court-Brown CM, Heckman JD, et al. *Rockwood & Green's Fractures in Adults*, 7th ed. Philadelphia: Lippincott, Williams & Wilkins, 2010.)

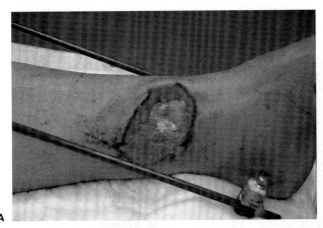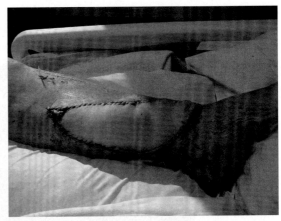

A. A patient was referred with exposed medial bone having had two previous irrigation and debridement procedures. **B.** After a further wound toilet and debridement of devitalized bone, we undertook definitive fixation, and an anterolateral thigh flap, which has healed. The patient awaits further bone grafting for a 2-cm bone defect. (From Bucholz RW, Court-Brown CM, Heckman JD, et al. *Rockwood & Green's Fractures in Adults*, 7th ed. Philadelphia: Lippincott, Williams & Wilkins, 2010.)

External Fixation
- Commonly utilized in high-energy severe fractures
- Primarily a temporizing method to allow for soft tissue management prior to definitive treatment
- Definitive treatment in external fixator associated with higher risk of malunion, superficial infection, poorer functional results, and increased time to union as compared to unreamed nails by Dervin (1996)
- Prolonged external fixation increases risk of deep infection when utilized as a temporizing measure (>2 wk)

Plating
- Usually limited to those fractures to proximal or distal to allow for adequate insertion of distal or proximal interlocking screws
- The use of compression plating and large invasive intervention are limited to those patients with simple fractures or nonunions requiring stiffer constructs
- Metaphyseal fractures or comminuted diaphyseal fractures are treated utilizing indirect reduction methods and less invasive plating with the assistant of locked plates to maintain alignment, rotation, and length

Open Tibia Fractures
- Infection is a common complication in tibia fractures with a rate ranging from 5%–50% in these cases
- Adequate debridement and irrigation must be performed in these patients prior to proceeding with definitive treatment
- Grading based on the Gustilo-Anderson classification
- Risk of deep infection is increased with increasing severity of soft tissue injury

- Most importantly, antibiotic treatment should be initiated immediately upon arrival to the emergency room (first-generation cephalosporin grade I and the addition of an aminoglycoside [Gentamicin] in grade II and III injuries)
- External fixation can be considered as part of damage control and to allow for soft tissue management and stabilization until definitive treatment is performed

Bone/Soft Tissue Defects and Flap Coverage
- Patients with sever soft tissue injury may require plastic surgery intervention to improve patient outcomes and decrease risk of infection and union
- Proximal third fractures with defects are treated with either medial or lateral gastrocnemius rotational flap
- Middle third defects require soleus rotational flap
- Distal third fractures benefit from gastrocnemius free flap or latissimus dorsi in patients with extensive soft tissue defects
- In patients with severe segmental defects, vascularized free fibula or bone transport with a ring fixator can be considered
- High-energy injury may require vascularized free flaps rather than local rotation flaps to improve outcomes due to associated muscle injury

Outcomes/Complications
- Court-Brown (1997)
  - Evaluated 169 reamed Grosse-Kempf nail for diaphyseal fracture
  - **56% knee pain (most common postoperative complaint)**

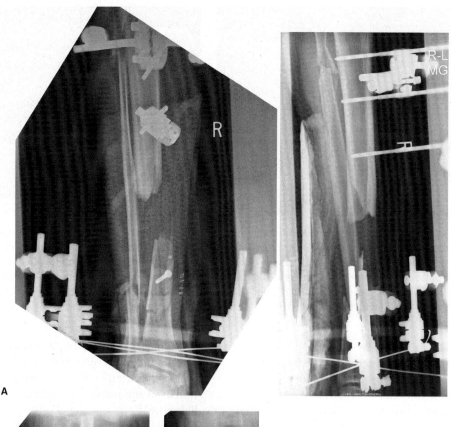

A

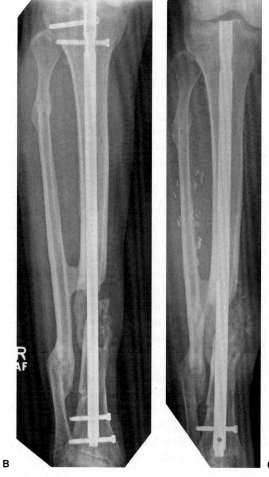

B

C

A. Anteroposterior and lateral radiographs of a Gustilo IIIB open distal tibial fracture with segmental bone loss. The fracture was initially treated with a hybrid external fixator. **B.** Intramedullary nailing was subsequently performed together with autogenous bone grafting. **C.** The patient required a second bone graft operation. A free anterolateral thigh flap was performed because of compromised soft tissues. The fracture united. (From Bucholz RW, Court-Brown CM, Heckman JD, et al. *Rockwood & Green's Fractures in Adults*, 7th ed. Philadelphia: Lippincott, Williams & Wilkins, 2010.)

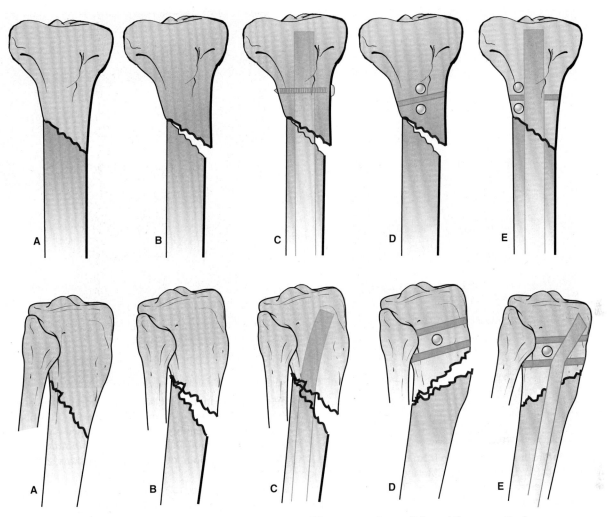

Diagram illustrating blocking screw technique. We commonly use 3.5- or 4.5-mm cortical screws. (From Bucholz RW, Court- Brown CM, Heckman JD, et al. *Rockwood & Green's Fractures in Adults*, 7th ed. Philadelphia: Lippincott, Williams & Wilkins, 2010.)

- Most common in younger patients
- 92% with kneeling, 37% at rest
- 1%–3% infection
- 2%–5% nonunion
- 0%–10% compartment syndrome
- The Lower Extremity Assessment Project (LEAP) was a multicentered evaluation of lower extremity injuries with severe soft tissue damage showed patient demographics and psychosocial factors were the most important determinants of outcomes in patients treated with amputation or limb salvage techniques

Healing Complications
- Delayed union—no progression of healing at 6–9 mo
- Nonunion—fracture not fully healed at >9 mo
- Dynamize nail if axially stable
- Exchange nail if not axially stable
- Posterolateral bone grafting if bone loss present
- Peroneal artery is at danger during revisions
- Consider electrical stimulation for fracture healing

Indications for Exchange Nailing
- <1 cm shortening
- No segmental defect
- Average time to union 4 mo

Recommended Readings

Boraiah S, et al. High association of posterior malleolus fractures with spiral distal tibial fractures. Clin Orthop 2008;466(7):1692–1628.

Bone LB, Stegemann P. Prospective study of union rate of open tibial fractures treated with locked undreamed intramedullary nails. J Orthop Trauma 1994;8(1):45–49.

Court-Brown CM, et al. Knee pain after intramedullary tibial nailing: its incidence, etiology and outcome. J Orthop Trauma 1997;11(2):103–105.

Dervin GF: Skeletal fixation of grade IIIB tibial fractures. The potential of metaanalysis. J Clin Orthop Relat Res 1996;332: 10–15.

Duwelius PJ, Green JM. Nonreamed interlocked intramedullary tibial nailing. One community's experience. Clin Orthop Relat Res 1995;315:104–113.

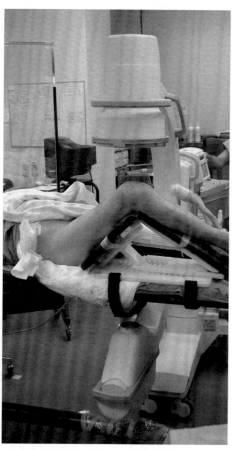

The image intensifier is brought in from the opposite side. (From Bucholz RW, Court- Brown CM, Heckman JD, et al. *Rockwood & Green's Fractures in Adults*, 7th ed. Philadelphia: Lippincott, Williams & Wilkins, 2010.)

Or Tips and Tricks-Tibial Nail
- A medial and lateral femoral distractors with Schanz pins can be placed into proximal and distal (or calcaneus) physeal scars may be utilized to improve reduction.
- Drill first with 3.2-mm drill bits to improve fixation of 5.0 Schanz pins
- Place long distractor rod posteriorly and sleeves anteriorly to allow for interlock placement
- Put proximal Schanz posteriorly and distal Schanz pin anteriorly to avoid rod

Lateral Parapatellar Approach
- Incision from level of oblique flat portion of plateau to lateral aspect of the midpoint of the patella
- Deep incision should made just lateral to the border of the patellar tendon
- A right angle can be placed under patellar tendon, retracting it medially, exposing fat pad
- A transverse incision through bursal layer behind fat pad to get to the starting point and avoid intrarticular nailing

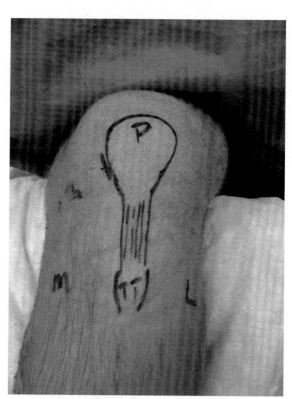

We use a high medial incision just medial to the edge of the patella. L, lateral; M, medial; P, patella; TT, tibial tubercle. (From Bucholz RW, Court- Brown CM, Heckman JD, et al. *Rockwood & Green's Fractures in Adults*, 7th ed. Philadelphia: Lippincott, Williams & Wilkins, 2010.)

- The Awl should be inserted in extension in line with tibial crest/tubercle and in line with the lateral tibial eminence
- External rotation of the tibia may be necessary to improve visualization with the distractor in place

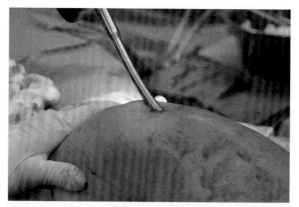

A curved awl is inserted behind the patellar tendon and is inserted into the tibia at the correct starting point as visualized on the image intensifier. As it is inserted, care is taken to keep the awl tip anterior in the tibia and in line with the canal. (From Bucholz RW, Court- Brown CM, Heckman JD, et al. *Rockwood & Green's Fractures in Adults*, 7th ed. Philadelphia: Lippincott, Williams & Wilkins, 2010.)

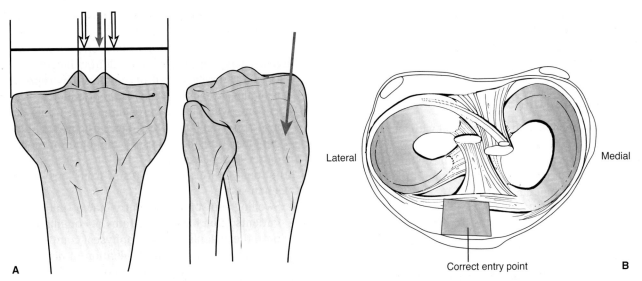

A. Diagram showing the high tibial extra-articular start point. **B.** Proper tibial nail start point. (From Bucholz RW, Court-Brown CM, Heckman JD, et al. *Rockwood & Green's Fractures in Adults*, 7th ed. Philadelphia: Lippincott, Williams & Wilkins, 2010.)

– General sagittal alignment can be performed with the distractor while finer points of reduction require manual manipulation or the use of large tenaculums to maintain reduction
– Care should be taken to avoid compression of the anterior compartment for prolonged periods of time during nailing
– Guidewire should be passed centrally in the distal plafond to adequate position the nail
– In sagittal plane, guidewire should be parallel to anterior tibial cortex
– Adequate fracture reduction must be performed before reaming to prevent malreduction of the fracture

– Goal is to improve stability with a 10-mm nail or greater by reaming
– Canal should be reamed at least 1–1.5 mm to accommodate nail insertion
– Depending on the type of nail, interlocking screws may increase in size with large diameter nails improving fixation
– Overream by 1–1.5 mm
– Perfect circles should be utilized for placing the interlocks
– When placing interlocks, start eccentric to hole to allow for interference fit with rod to improve rotational control

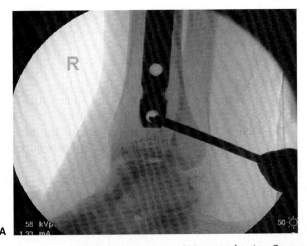

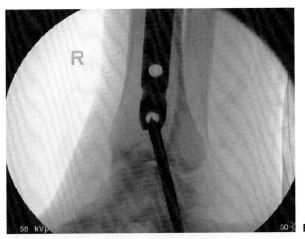

Distal cross screws are inserted using fluoroscopy and either a radiolucent or regular drill as shown in (**A**) or by first finding the hole and indenting the cortex with a Steinmann pin as shown in (**B**). (From Bucholz RW, Court-Brown CM, Heckman JD, et al. *Rockwood & Green's Fractures in Adults*, 7th ed. Philadelphia: Lippincott, Williams & Wilkins, 2010.)

- The first interlock should be placed at the end closer to the fracture. This allows reduction while interlocks are placed so that the other noninterlocked end is still free to move

PILON FRACTURES

- Technically difficult injury, fraught with multiple complicating factors affecting treatment
- Injury to the articular surface of the distal tibia carries high morbidity due to the significant force generated across the tibiotalar joint

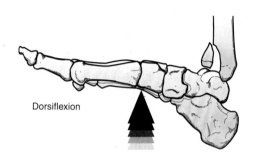

Dorsiflexion

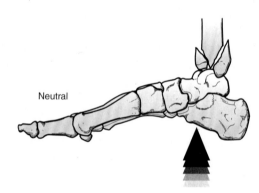

Neutral

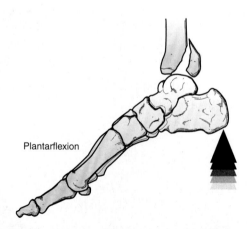

Plantarflexion

The position of the foot at the time of axial load determines which portion of the tibial plafond sustains the major impact of the talus. (From Bucholz RW, Court-Brown CM, Heckman JD, et al. *Rockwood & Green's Fractures in Adults*, 7th ed. Philadelphia: Lippincott, Williams & Wilkins, 2010.)

- Mechanism of energy may be high or low and result in differing patterns of injury
- Axial compression injuries most often result from higher-energy injuries such as fall from height
  - Proximal displacement of the talus may represent a significant factor in the resultant injury
  - Patients will often have resultant soft tissue damage or swelling that precludes early intervention
  - Articular and metaphyseal comminution complicate eventual fixation
- Rotational injuries usually result from lower-energy mechanisms
  - Swelling and soft tissue injury may be minimal
  - Patients often have lower rates of comminution in both the articular and metaphyseal component
- Care must be taken in the evaluation of high-energy mechanisms to rule out associated injuries (calcaneal fractures, lumbosacral injuries)
- ATLS protocol should be taken when necessary

History and Physical Examination

- Most important aspect of the history is evaluation of the mechanism of injury
- Physical examination should focus on neurovascular examination and the surrounding soft tissue envelope
- High-energy mechanisms increase the risk for compartment syndrome, abrasions, fracture blisters, or open wounds, which not only preclude early intervention but also represent factors that contribute to poor outcomes following operative intervention

Imaging

- AP, lateral, and mortise views of the ankle should be performed in addition to AP and lateral tibia/fibula films
- CT scan provides a valuable 3D evaluation of the injury and articular fragments

Classification

Ruedi-Algower Classification

- I—Cleavage fracture of the distal tibia without displacement of the articular surface
- II—Mild to moderate displacement of the articular surface but minimal comminution There is impaction of the metaphysis
- III—Comminution of the articular surface, metaphysis with significant impaction of the metaphysis

AO/OTA

- A—Extra-articular
  - A1—metaphyseal simple
  - A2—metaphyseal wedge
  - A3—metaphyseal complex

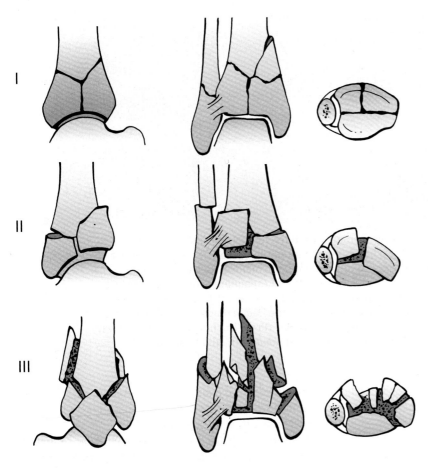

Ruedi-Allgower classification of tibial plafond fractures. Type I: cleavage fracture of the distal tibia without significant displacement of the articular surface. Type II: significant fracture displacement of the articular surface without comminution. Type III: Impaction and comminution of the distal tibial articular surface. (From Bucholz RW, Court- Brown CM, Heckman JD, et al. *Rockwood & Green's Fractures in Adults*, 7th ed. Philadelphia: Lippincott, Williams & Wilkins, 2010.)

- B—Partial articular (lateral plafond or large medial malleolus)
  - B1—pure split
  - B2—split depression
  - B3—multifragment depression
- C—Complete articular
  - C1—simple articular, simple metaphyseal
  - C2—simple articular, multifragment metaphysis
  - C3—articular multifragmentary

Fracture Fixation Considerations:
- Main fracture plane is coronal and intra-articular
- Secondary fracture plane is usually sagittal
- 75% of the patients have fibular fractures
- 33% of injuries are open
- Operative intervention should be delayed until the soft tissue permits
- Indirect reduction can be performed with a femoral distractor
- 7–10-cm skin bridge should be present between incisions in dual approach fixation
- Early plastics intervention should be performed for exposed bone, tendon, hardware
- If open, delay bone grafting until soft tissues are healed and uninfected

- Despite the morbidity, shortening can be considered in cases of severe comminution to decrease tension from soft tissue and decrease metaphyseal defect

Or Tips and Tricks—Pilon
Treatment
- Timing of operative intervention is crucial in limiting complications and improving patient outcomes
- Currently staged protocol of plating fibula and medial external fixation is one of the predominant methods of treatment
- Goal of primary fixation of the fibula is to help maintain length with the assistance of the external fixator
- Highly comminuted fibula fractures can lead to fibular shortening and complicate pilon fixation, so care should be taken with early fibula intervention
- Once soft tissues permit, definitive fixation can be considered
- Multiple approaches to the distal tibia exist
- Helfet and Grose (2007)
  - Extensile lateral approach to lateral tibia
  - Provides large soft tissue envelope for coverage of hardware
  - Incision made along the anterior border of the fibula

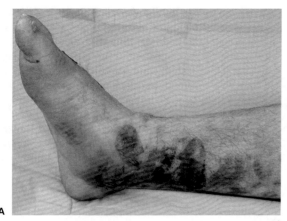
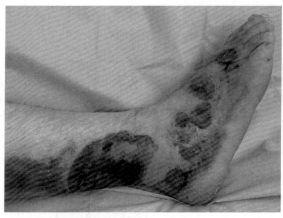

Clinical photographs of the right lower extremity from the medial (**A**), and lateral (**B**) perspectives 5 days after sustaining a highly comminuted tibial pilon fracture. A number of drained hemorrhagic fracture blisters can be identified, the majority of which are still covered by the overlying epidermal layer. Initial treatment (spanning external fixation) was delayed secondary to associated life-threatening injuries. The severity of soft tissue injury laterally, particularly the need for reepithelialization of the hemorrhagic fracture blister bed, precluded fibular fixation for approximately 3 weeks. (From Bucholz RW, Court-Brown CM, Heckman JD, et al. *Rockwood & Green's Fractures in Adults*, 7th ed. Philadelphia: Lippincott, Williams & Wilkins, 2010.)

- Taken subperiosteally over the fibula over the IO membrane elevating the anterior compartment

Anterolateral Approach
- Incision in line with the fourth ray up the anterolateral surface of the aspect of the fibula and as distal as the anterolateral talus
- Elevation of the anterior compartment exposes the distal tibia allowing for fixation of the chaput fragment and plate placement with soft tissue coverage

Posterolateral Approach to the Fibula/Tibia
- Utilized for fixation of Volkman's fragment
- Utilizes the interval between the peroneals and the flexor hallucis longus to allow exposure of the posterior surface of the fibula and the posterior tibia

Anteromedial Approach to the Tibia
- Historically the most common approach utilized, but limited soft tissue coverage increases the risk of painful hardware and wound complications
- The goals of fixation are restoration of the articular surface with care taken not to devitalize the articular fragments through extensive soft tissue dissection
- Additionally, length, rotation, and alignment of the distal tibia should be performed
- Skin bridges should be >7 cm to prevent risk for soft tissue breakdown
- Spanning external fixation with limited internal fixation to reduce articular surface
- Articulating external fixation maintains ROM

- Hybrid external fixation with limited internal fixation limits soft tissue devitalization
- Best indication to use external fixation as definitive treatment for pilon fractures with articular reduction
- Some feel hybrid fixation does not achieve adequate reduction and prefer minimally invasive fixation.

Outcomes
- Low-energy fractures have better outcomes secondary to improved soft tissue envelope and lower levels of articular comminution
- **Delay in surgery not proven to worsen outcomes**
- High energy associated with bone and soft tissue infection and poor results
- Posttraumatic arthritis is a serious complication of the procedure (arthrodesis rate ranged from 5% to 26% in most studies looking as patients for younger than 5 yr
- The chondral injuries associated with pilon fractures are often one area where treatment techniques are limited
- Patients are limited in the return to function including both wok and recreation due to stiffness, swelling, and pain postoperatively

Complications
- General soft tissue/wound sloughing and epidermolysis is seen in up to 10% of patients
- Deep infection rates range from 4% to 35%
- Pin site infection from prolonged external fixation is another common complication
- Care must be taken to avoid varus malunion

- The metaphyseal junction is the most common site of nonunion (rates from 0% to 16%)
- Teeny and Wiss (1993) evaluated 60 pilon fractures with 2.5-yr follow-up
  - 60% were high-energy injuries
  - Outcomes: 25% good/excellent, 25% fair, 50% poor
  - Complications
  - Wound dehiscence—17% in Ruedi II, 37% in Reudi III
  - Deep infection—none in Ruedi I and II, 37% in Ruedi III
  - Malunion—3% in I and II, 27% in III
- Sirkin and Sanders (1999) evaluated 56 type C fractures treated with fibular plate and medial external fixation within <24 hr followed by delayed ORIF average 12–14 days
  - For closed fractures, no dehiscence or full thickness skin necrosis; 17% partial thickness requiring local wound care; 3.4% late complications due to OM, draining sinus
  - For open fractures, 2/17 partial thickness and 10% with deep infection

Or Tips and Tricks—Pilon External Fixation
Medial Ankle Spanning External Fixation
- Two parallel pins should be placed in tibia, staying proximal to avoid plates for pilon fixation
- Predrilling of the tibia cortices should be performed to minimize the risk of thermal necrosis seen with self-drilling, self-tapping Schanz pins
- A long 3.5-mm drill bit is utilized by starting just medial to the tibial spine and aiming for posterolateral corner of the tibia
- Placing the Schanz pin by hand allows you to feel for resistance of opposite cortex followed by 5–6 half turns to engage the opposite cortex
- Medial oblique calcaneal incision should be placed in line with the calcaneal branch of the posterior tibial nerve 2–3 cm from posterior corner of heel
- A standard pin for medial external fixation can be used or a centrally threaded pin can be placed for a delta frame
- The calcaneal pin should be perpendicular to heel axis despite varus or valgus malalignment of the tibia to allow adequate provisional reduction
- Place a pin into the medial cuneiform, through the middle, then lateral cuneiform under fluoroscopic guidance
- Fix bar to tibial pins, followed by fixing calcaneal to cuneiform pins
- Spanning bar can then be applied allowing for reduction
- Ankle mortise or AP view allow one to judge varus/valgus orientation of the hindfoot by observing the calcaneal tuberosity

- In talonavicular dislocation, distraction, and manipulation through the cuneiforms can allow for adequate reduction

Recommended Readings
Grose A, Gardner MJ, Hettrich C, Fishman F, Lorich DG, Asprinio DE, Helfet DL. Open reduction and internal fixation of tibial pilon fractures using a lateral approach. J Orthop Trauma 2007;21(8):530–537.
Sirkin M, Sanders R. A staged protocol for soft tissue management in the treatment of complex pilon fractures. J Orthop Trauma 1999;13(2):78–84.
Teeny SM, Wiss DA. Open reduction and internal fixation of tibial plafond fractures. Variables contributing to poor results and complications. Clin Orthop Relat Res 1993;292:108–117.

ANKLE FRACTURE
Anatomy
- Talus wider anteriorly
- Axis of rotation of the ankle is in 20 degrees of external rotation
- Superficial deltoid
  - Origin: Anterior colliculus
  - Attachments: Talus, calcaneus, navicular
- Deep deltoid
  - Origin: posterior colliculus
  - Prevents anterolateral displacement of the talus
  - Main medial stabilizer
  - Prevents talus anterolateral displacement
- Syndesmosis (four parts)
  - IO membrane
  - Posterior inferior tibiofibular ligament (PITFL)
  - Anterior inferior tibiofibular ligament (AITFL)
  - IO ligament

Classification
Weber
- Based on location of fibula fracture
  A: Fibula fracture below the level of the Plafond
  B: Fibula fracture at the level of the plafond
  - Deltoid ligament integrity must be tested with the external rotation test to determine whether injury requires operative intervention. Medical clear space >4 mm indicative of deltoid ligament insufficiency and ankle instability.
  C: Above the level of the plafond
  - Syndesmotic membrane is torn and integrity of the syndesmosis should be tested
  - Operative intervention is indicated

Syndesmosis
- Tibiofibular syndesmosis is composed of four ligaments
  - AITFL
  - PITFL
  - IO ligament
  - IO membrane

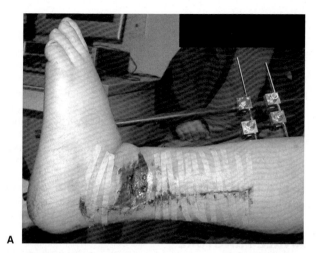

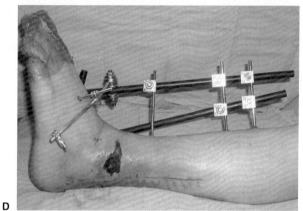

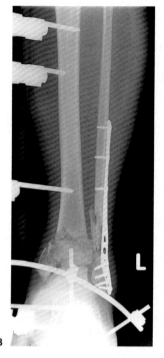

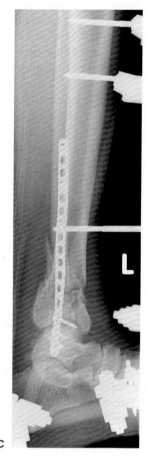

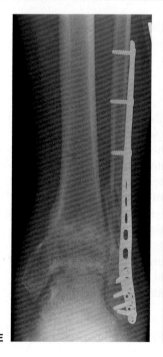

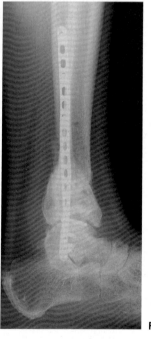

Two weeks after his injury, the severity of his soft tissue injury is still evident (**A**). Open treatment would likely have required soft tissue transfer or coverage but his nicotine use, hypertension, and age precluded this as a realistic option. He was definitively treated with tibiotalar spanning external fixation, modifying the external fixator to incorporate the lateral column of the foot, and to insert a tibial pin closer to the metaphyseal fracture (**B–D**). At 9 months, his fracture and soft tissue envelope have healed. Substantial articular incongruity remains and the prognosis for long-term satisfactory joint function is guarded (**E, F**). (From Bucholz RW, Court-Brown CM, Heckman JD, et al. *Rockwood & Green's Fractures in Adults*, 7th ed. Philadelphia: Lippincott, Williams & Wilkins, 2010.)

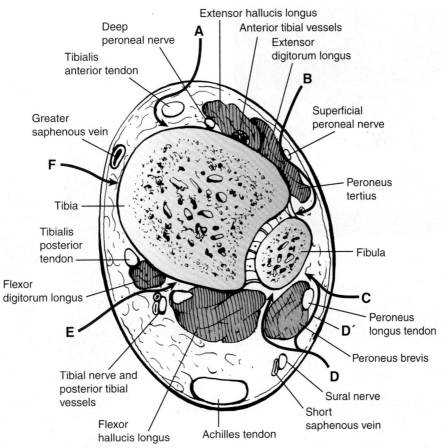

Axial view of the distal tibia just proximal to the distal tibiofibular syndesmosis demonstrating the relevant local surgical anatomy and surgical approaches for management of distal tibial plafond fractures. **A.** Anteromedial. **B.** Anterolateral. **C.** Posterolateral (fibula). **D.** Posterolateral (tibia). **D.** Posterolateral (fibula). **E.** Posteromedial. **F.** Medial. (From Bucholz RW, Court- Brown CM, Heckman JD, et al. *Rockwood & Green's Fractures in Adults*, 7th ed. Philadelphia: Lippincott, Williams & Wilkins, 2010.)

– Evaluation is syndesmosis is essential to ankle fracture treatment

    Radiographic signs of syndesmosis disruption: measure 1 cm proximal to the ankle joint.
    – Tibiofibular overlap
    AP: <10 mm
    Mortise <1 mm
    – Tibiofibular clear space
    AP >5 mm
– Must evaluate syndemosis case by case intraoperatively after fibula fixation performed

    Intraoperative Cotton test: Lateral traction applied to fibula with a pointed or serrated reduction clamp following fibular fixation. Radiographic measurements (tibiofibular overlap and tibiofibular clear space) should be evaluated.

    Treatment of syndesmotic injuries:
– Equivocal data regarding one vs. two screws and 3.5 vs 4.5 screw placement

– One-third of screws break once weight bearing is resumed
– Transsyndesmotic screws can be removed at 3 mo to prevent breakage and improve ROM (Miller 2010)
– Posterior malleolus fracture fixation has been shown to be equivalent to transsyndesmotic fixation without the need for hardware removal (Miller 2010)
– MRI may be useful to evaluate soft tissue integrity and fracture pattern.

Lauge Hansen Classification:
First name based on position of the foot, while second is based on the direction of force
– **Supination Adduction (20%)**
    1—lateral collateral ligament (LCL) or fibula avulsion below joint
    2—vertical shear of medial malleolus
    *Medial malleolus injury alone if laterally lax

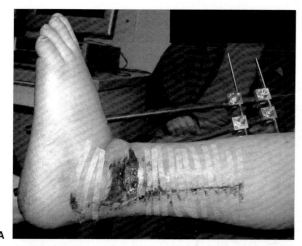

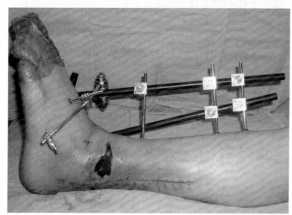

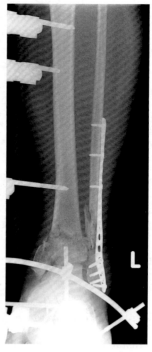

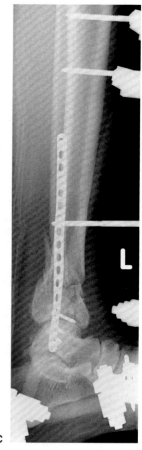

Two weeks after his injury, the severity of his soft tissue injury is still evident (**A**). Open treatment would likely have required soft tissue transfer or coverage but his nicotine use, hypertension, and age precluded this as a realistic option. He was definitively treated with tibiotalar spanning external fixation, modifying the external fixator to incorporate the lateral column of the foot, and to insert a tibial pin closer to the metaphyseal fracture (**B–D**). (From Bucholz RW, Court- Brown CM, Heckman JD, et al. *Rockwood & Green's Fractures in Adults*, 7th ed. Philadelphia: Lippincott, Williams & Wilkins, 2010.)

– **Supination-External Rotation (40%–75%)**
  1—AITFL ± bony avulsion - Tillaux-Chaput off tibia
  – Wagstaff-LeFort off fibula
  2—anterior distal, posterior proximal fibula spiral fracture
  3—PITFL ± Volkmann's posterior malleolus
  4—medial malleolus fracture or deltoid rupture
– **Pronation-Abduction (5%–21%)**
  1—medial malleolus fracture or deltoid rupture
  2—Chaput's tubercle or AITFL
  3—transverse fibular fracture, lateral comminution
  – ± lateral plafond impaction
– **Pronation-External Rotation (19%)**
  1—medial malleolus avulsion or deltoid rupture
  2—Chaput's tubercle or AITFL
  3—transverse fibular fracture above joint
  4—posterior malleolus fracture/PITFL rupture

– May be associated with maisonneuve fracture
– May have associated anterior colliculus fracture or deep deltoid rupture

Treatment
Weber A
– Nonoperative treatment if <3 mm of displacement
– Patient can be made weight bearing as tolerated and follow-up with regularly scheduled radiographs to confirm adequate healing

Weber B
– Deltoid competency should be evaluated with a stress view of the ankle
– Mortise view should be performed with the ankle slightly dorsiflexed and an external rotation force applied

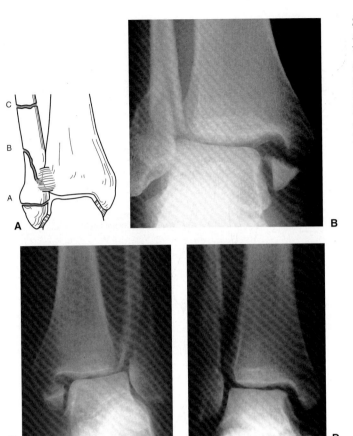

Schematic diagram of the Danis-Weber classification of ankle fractures. **A.** Comprehensive view of the Danis-Weber classification of ankle fractures. **B.** Supination external rotation type four ankle facture/Weber B lateral malleolus fracture. **C.** Supination external rotation type four ankle fracture/Weber B lateral malleolus fracture. **D.** Weber C ankle fracture. (From Bucholz RW, et al., eds. Rockwood and Green's Fractures in Adults, 6th ed. Philadelphia, PA: Lippincott Williams & Wilkins; 2006.)

– Medial clear space >4 mm is consistent with a deltoid ligament and an ankle fracture requiring operative fixation

Weber C
– Fibular fractures above the level of the plafond should undergo ORIF

Medial Malleolar Fractures
– ORIF is recommended for displaced fractures and fractures with associated fibular fracture

Special Considerations
Posterior Malleolus
– Posterior malleolus fixation is a controversial topic
– Historically, fractures composing >25% of the plafond undergo fixation
– Biomechanical studies have shown that posterior malleolous fixation regardless of the fragment size is associated with improved syndesmotic stability
– Fixation of the posterior malleolus may reestablish the PITFL fibular relationship allowing improved soft tissue healing

– PITFL is responsible for 40% of the syndesmotic strength
– Posterior malleolus fracture fixation has been shown to have equivalent functional outcomes to patients treated with transsyndesmotic fixation

Posttraumatic Arthritis
– The most common complication of fracture fixation
– The primary cause of ankle osteoarthritis (as many as 70% of patients with osteoarthritis)
– Fracture reduction is the primary factor
– Ramsey and Hamilton (1976) showed that 1 mm of fracture displacement leads to a 42% reduction in joint contact area and increased risk of posttraumatic arthritis
– Signs of fibular malunion
  – Medial joint widening
  – Shenton's line of ankle
  – Relation of medial fibula and lateral talus
  – Talocrural angle (angle of joint line with angle connecting ends of malleoli)
– 10% in anatomic reduced fractures
– 90% in malreduced fractures
– Seen by 18 mo postinjury

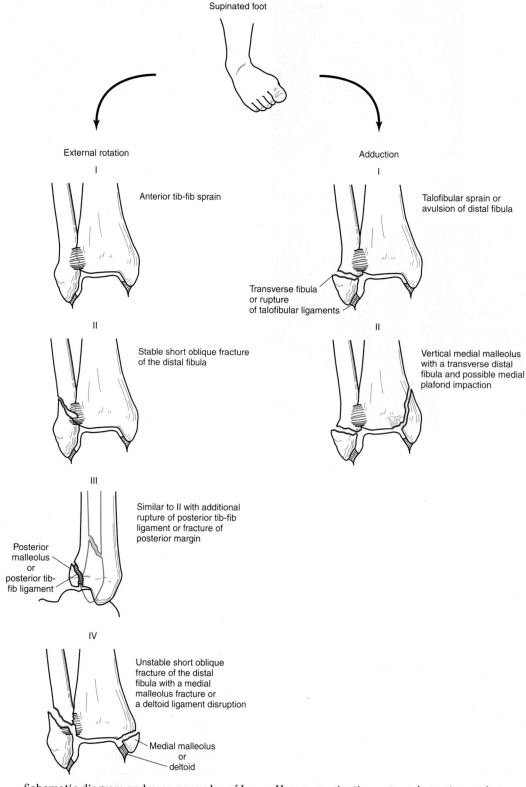

Supinated foot

External rotation

I

Anterior tib-fib sprain

II

Stable short oblique fracture of the distal fibula

III

Posterior malleolus or posterior tib-fib ligament

Similar to II with additional rupture of posterior tib-fib ligament or fracture of posterior margin

IV

Unstable short oblique fracture of the distal fibula with a medial malleolus fracture or a deltoid ligament disruption

Medial malleolus or deltoid

Adduction

I

Talofibular sprain or avulsion of distal fibula

Transverse fibula or rupture of talofibular ligaments

II

Vertical medial malleolus with a transverse distal fibula and possible medial plafond impaction

Schematic diagram and case examples of Lauge-Hansen supination-external rotation and supination-adduction ankle fractures. A supinated foot sustains either an external rotation or adduction force and creates the successive stages of injury shown in the diagram. The supination-external rotation mechanism has four stages of injury, and the supination-adduction mechanism has two stages. (From Bucholz RW, Heckman JD, eds. Rockwood and Green's Fractures in Adults, 5th ed. Philadelphia, PA: Lippincott Williams & Wilkins; 2001.)

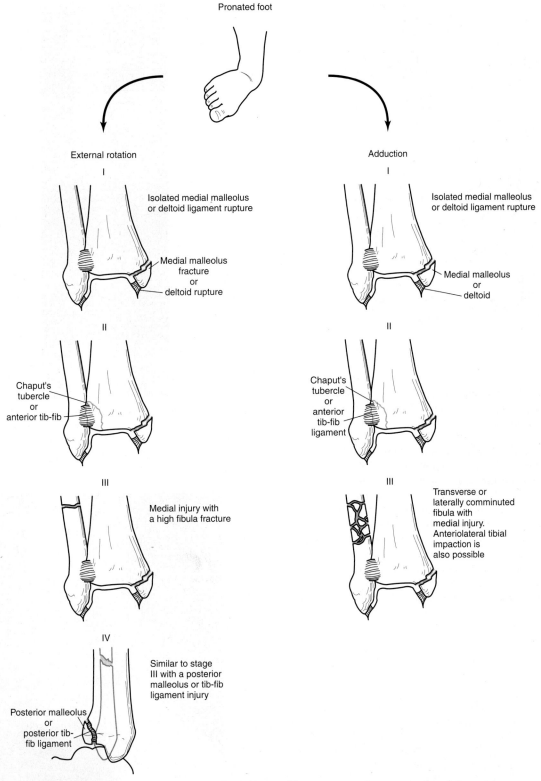

Schematic diagram and case examples of Lauge-Hansen pronation-external rotation and pronation-abduction ankle fractures. A pronated foot sustains either an external rotation or abduction force and creates the successive stages of injury shown in the diagram. The pronation-external rotation mechanism has four stages of injury, and the pronation-abduction mechanism has three stages. (From Bucholz RW, Heckman JD, eds. Rockwood and Green's Fractures in Adults, 5th ed. Philadelphia, PA: Lippincott Williams & Wilkins; 2001.)

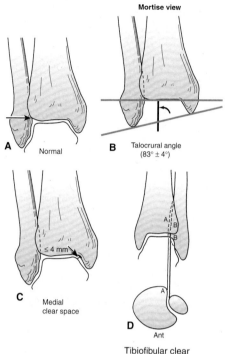

X-ray appearance of the normal ankle on mortise view. **A:** The condensed subchondral bone should form a continuous line around the talus. **B:** The talocrural angle should be approximately 83 degrees. When the opposite side can be used as a control, the talocrural angle of the injured side should be within a few degrees of the noninjured side. **C:** The medial clear space should be equal to the superior clear space between the talus and the distal tibia and ≤4 mm on standard x-rays. **D:** The distance between the medial wall of the fibula and the incisural surface of the tibia, the tibiofibular clear space, should be <6 mm. (Parts **A–C:** Adapted from Browner B, Jupiter J, Levine A, eds. Skeletal Trauma: Fractures, Dislocations, and Ligamentous Injuries, 2nd ed. Philadelphia, PA: WB Saunders; 1997; Part **D:** From Bucholz RW et al., eds. Rockwood and Green's Fractures in Adults, 6th ed. Philadelphia, PA: Lippincott Williams & Wilkins; 2006.)

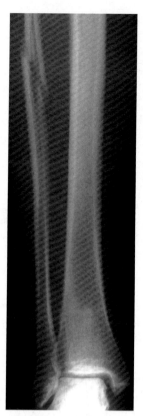

An anteroposterior radiograph of the ankle and tibia and fibula demonstrate a high fibula fracture. (From Bucholz RW, Heckman JD, eds. Rockwood and Green's Fractures in Adults, 5th ed. Philadelphia, PA: Lippincott Williams & Wilkins; 2001.)

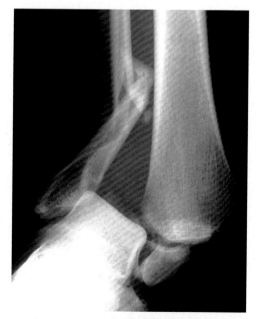

An anteroposterior radiograph of a typical pronation-abduction ankle fracture. The fibula is laterally comminuted. (From Bucholz RW, Heckman JD, eds. Rockwood and Green's Fractures in Adults, 5th ed. Philadelphia, PA: Lippincott Williams & Wilkins; 2001.)

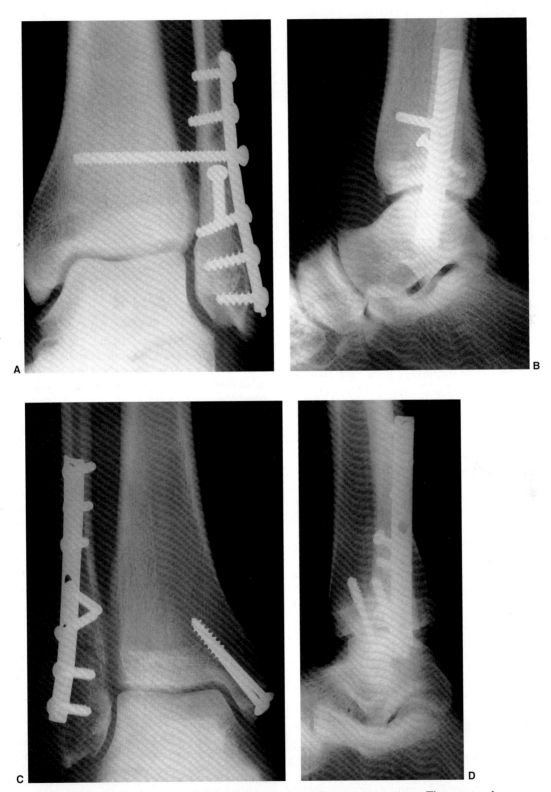

Distal fibular plates can be successfully applied in different orientations. Three sets of mortise and lateral radiographs illustrate straight lateral **(A, B)** and posterolateral **(C, D).** (From Bucholz RW, Heckman JD, eds. Rockwood and Green's Fractures in Adults, 5th ed. Philadelphia, PA: Lippincott Williams & Wilkins; 2001.)

Recommended Readings

Bauer M, Johnsson K. Ankle fractures. Foot Ankle 1987;8(1): 23–25.

Boden SD, et al. Mechanical considerations for the syndesmosis screw. A cadaver study. J Bone Joint Surg 1989;71(10):1548–1555.

Boden SD, Yamaguchi K. Operative treatment of syndesmotic disruptions without use of a syndesmotic screw: a prospective clinical study. Foot Ankle Int 1994;15(8):407–414.

Kannus P, Renstrom P. Treatment for acute tears of the lateral ligaments of the ankle: operation cast, or early controlled mobilization. J Bone Joint Surg 1991;73(2):305–312.

Lorich DG, Helfet HG. Radiographic measurements do not predict syndesmotic injury in ankle fractures: An MRI study. Clin Orthop Relat Res 2005;436:216–221.

Miller AN, Carroll EA, Parker RJ, Helfet DL, Lorich DG. Posterior malleolar stabilization of syndesmotic injuries is equivalent to screw fixation. Clin Orthop Relat Res 2010;468(4):1129–1135. doi: 10.1007/s11999-009-1111-4. Epub 2009 Oct 2.

Miller AN, Paul O, Boraiah S, Parker RJ, Helfet DL, Lorich DG. Functional outcomes after syndesmotic screw fixation and removal. J Orthop Trauma 2010;24(1):12–16.

Nielson JH, Sallis JG, Potter HG, Helfet DL, Lorich DG. Correlation of interosseous membrane tears to the level of the fibular fracture. J Orthop Trauma 2004;18(2):68–74.

Phillips WA, et al. A prospective, randomized study of the management of severe ankle fractures. J Bone Joint Surg Am 1985;67:67–78.

Ramsey PL, Hamilton W. Changes in tibiotalar area of contact caused by lateral talar shift. J Bone Joint Surg Am 1976; 58(3):356–357.

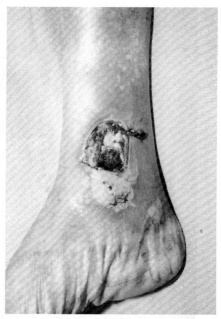

Example of surgical delay. Because of associated medical problems, the patient was not a candidate for microvascular tissue transfer. Lower-third tibial defect secondary to an open ankle fracture. Note exposed bone, which precludes use of a skin graft. (From Mulholland MW, et al., eds. Greenfield's Surgery Scientific Principles and Practice, 4th ed. Philadelphia, PA: Lippincott Williams & Wilkins; 2006.)

ANKLE FRACTURE—OPEN

Diabetic

- Diabetic patients are at increased risk of infection, wound breakdown, and poor fracture healing
- Those risks are magnified in the setting of open fractures
- White and Haidukeqwych (2003) evaluated 14 open fractures in diabetes mellitus patients
  - 19-mo follow-up
  - 64% wound healing problems
  - 42% below-knee amputation
  - Only three patients healed without complication

Immediate Open Reduction with Internal Fixation

- Open fracture management is dependent on soft tissue injury
- Irrigation and debridement of the wound should be performed in a timely fashion
- Most wounds will require 2–3 washouts prior to definitive treatment
- Fracture management consists of staged treatment with temporary delta frame external fixator and irrigation and debridement
- Definitive treatment is performed after wound declaration

- Large areas of soft tissue damage can be monitored with vacuum-assisted closure or wet to dry dressing
- Soft tissue coverage is essential to prevent wound breakdown, infection, and nonunion
- Staged treatment has been pre
- Wiss and Sarmiento (1988) evaluated 76 patients with open ankle fractures treated with immediate ORIF
  - Only 75% of the patients had satisfactory results
  - 8% of patients required ankle fusion
  - Infection related to
    - Energy of injury
    - Soft tissue damage
    - Level of wound contamination

Recommended Readings

Bray TJ, et al. Treatment of open ankle fractures. Immediate internal fixation versus closed immobilization and delayed fixation. Clin Orthop Relat Res 1989;(240):47–52.

Johnson EE, Davlin LB. Open ankle fractures. The indications for immediate open reduction and internal fixation. Clin Orthop Relat Res 1993;292:118–127.

Tho KS, et al. Grade III open ankle fractures—a review of the outcome of treatment. Singapore Med J 1994;35(1):57–58.

White CB, Haidukeqwych GJ. Open Ankle fractures in patients with diabetes mellitus. Clin Orthop Relat Res 2003;414:37–44.

Wiss DA, Sarmiento A. Immediate internal fixation of open ankle fractures. J Orthop Trauma 1988;2(4):265–271.

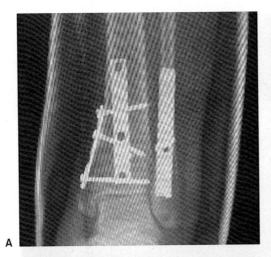

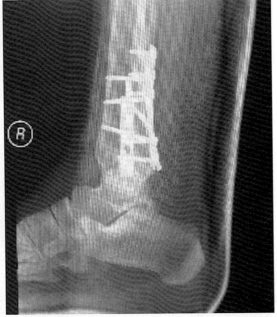

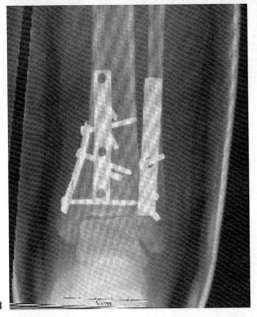

Posterior plating of the fibula, posterior malleolus, and antiglide fixation of medial malleolus. **A.** AP. **B.** Mortise. **C.** Lateral. (From Bucholz RW, Court-Brown CM, Heckman JD, Tornetta P. Rockwood & Green's Fractures in Adults, 7th ed. Philadelphia: Lippincott Williams & Wilkins, 2010).

Or Tips and Tricks—Ankle Fractures
Posterolateral Approach
- 12-cm curvilinear incision at the midpoint between the lateral aspect of the Achilles and the medial aspect of the fibula
- Incision taken down to the overlying fascia
- Fat strip/interval between the flexor hallucis longus (FHL) and peroneals should be visualized and dissected sharply
- Care should be taken to avoid exposure of muscle to improve visualization
- Short saphenous vein and sural nerve should be protected
- Elevate the peroneals off the posterior aspect of the fibula sharply, but avoid elevating the periosteum
- FHL should be elevated off the posterior aspect of the fibula

- Care should be taken with distal dissection to avoid injury to the PITFL
- A thin bent Hohman can be placed on the medial aspect of the posterior tibia to expose the posterior malleolus fractures or PITFL tears.
- Mini-fragment plating can be performed of both the fibula and the posterior malleolus
- 2.7 LCP/Reconstruction or 2.4 reconstruction plates can be placed posterolaterally on the fibula in an antiglide fashion
- 2.0 T-Plate or 2.0 DCP can be placed in an antiglide fashion over the posterior malleolus fracture following reduction with a large pointed reduction clamp
- PITFL tears can be repaired with an anteriorly 3.5 cortical screw and soft tissue washer
- Distal posterior malleolus and 3.5 cortical screw should be directed slightly posteroinferior to anterosuperior to avoid entry into the tibiotalar joint

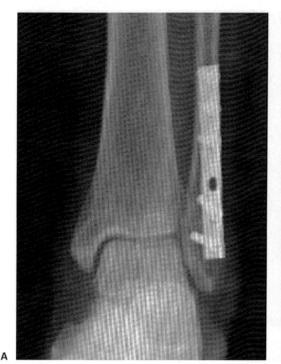

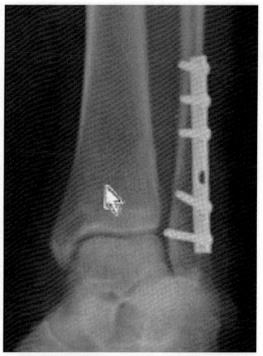

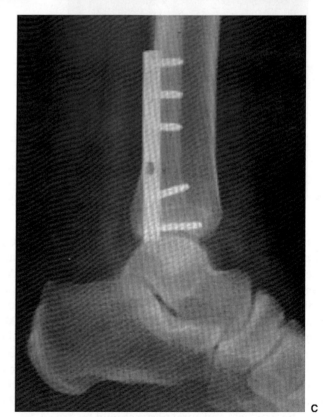

Posterior fibular plating. **A.** Antero-posterior. **B.** Mortise. **C.** Lateral. (From Bucholz RW, Court-Brown CM, Heckman JD, Tornetta P. Rockwood & Green's Fractures in Adults, 7th ed. Philadelphia: Lippincott Williams & Wilkins, 2010).

Advantages
- Posterior malleolus exposure
- Posterior plating of the fibula
- Increased soft tissue coverage of hardware
- Avoidance of superficial peroneal nerve

Lateral Approach
- Bump required for adequate positioning
- Straight incision on posterior half of fibula
- Superficial peroneal nerve pierces the crural fascia 10–12 cm from the lateral malleolus

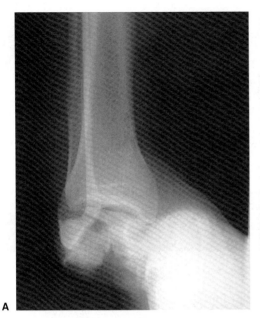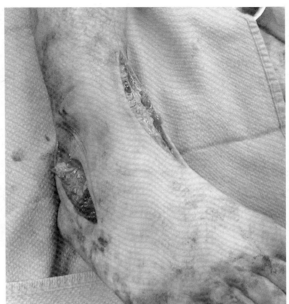

A   B

Talar body fracture with associated subtalar dislocation and comminution. **A.** Preoperative anteroposterior radiograph demonstrates dislocation and fracture comminution. **B.** Combined lateral and anteromedial surgical approaches were used. *(continued)*

- Two small cushions or a towel back can be placed under the ankle for positioning
- Utilize a bump for adequate positioning
- Straight incision on posterior half of fibula
- Find the superficial peroneal nerve for Weber C ankle fractures.
- Dissection can be taken down to bone to fully exposure the fibula and the fracture
- A surgeon should be alert when performing any proximal dissection
- Thin bent Hohman can be used to expose fibula along with sharp dissection
- Distally near posterior tip of lateral malleolus, the periosteum should become tougher signifying the peroneal retinaculum, which should be preserved
- Strip 2 mm of periosteum from the fracture site to allow reduction.
- Avoid dissection too far anterior to avoid AITFL
- Extract any fragments from the joint space
- Put bump under heel in supination external rotation (SERs) to help reduce then utilize small lion's jaw or thin bent reduction clamp to reduce the fracture
- Provisional fixation can be performed with a 1.6-mm K-wire from proximal anterior to distal posterior
- Plate can be placed directly lateral with or posterolateral (more biomechanically stable)
- If not lagging through plate, place K-wire away from where lag would go, pass wire to fracture site, reduce, then cross fracture site with K-wire
- Plan in advance for placing lag through plate

- Plate bending should be focused on twisting without bending proximally and providing a small lateral flare distally
- Fix posterolateral plate to proximal fragment first to use as antiglide
- If plating laterally, lag screw should be placed outside of the plate using standard AO technique
- Use proximal flare on most distal screw
- Lag screw through plate via 3.5-mm drill, then 2.5 mm
- If K-wire is the in way of the lag, put in a second K-wire to maintain reduction and move first one out of the way
- Distally, use long 22–26-mm-long posterior to anterior screw

Medial Approach (Colonna-Ralston)
- Straight incision about 3–4 cm over anterior half of medial malleolus
- Open to remove retained soft tissue in between fracture sites and the joint space
- Place two 1.6-mm K-wires for rotational control
- Drill over the K-wire and confirm that drills are not in joint space
- Place screws sequentially
- Be aware of pitfalls
  - Small bridge for lag, lag aimed too medially because soft tissue affects aiming, etc.

Immediate Postoperative Course
- Patients are placed in short leg splint. They are made non–weight bearing to protect the fixation

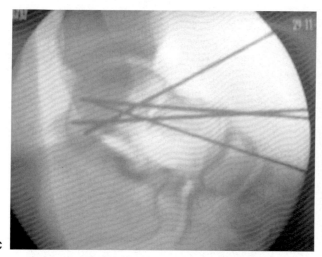

C

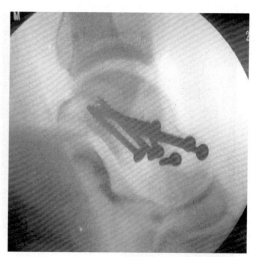

D

E

(Continued) Intraoperatively, Kirschner wires achieved provisional fixation (**C**) followed by definitive screw fixation (**D, E**). (From Bucholz RW, Court- Brown CM, Heckman JD, et al. *Rockwood & Green's Fractures in Adults*, 7th ed. Philadelphia: Lippincott, Williams & Wilkins, 2010.)

- Controlled active and passive ankle and subtalar joint motion is initiated 2 wk postoperatively
- Progressive weight bearing at 6–8 wk
- Expect full weight bearing at 10–12 wk

TALUS FRACTURES

Background
- Uncommon injury that requires appropriate evaluation, management and treatment to avoid the all too common poor outcomes, complications, and functional recovery
- Results from high-energy injury
- Result from hyperdorsiflexion of the foot or axial loading of the plantar surface of the foot
- The unique and tenous blood supply of the talus complicate fixation and postoperative outcomes
- High rates of nonunion, osteonecrosis should be considered and discussed with patients prior to intervention

History and Physical Exam
- Talus injuries represent <2% of extremity injuries
- Commonly present in young patients as the result of high-energy injuries
- Care must be taken to evaluate neurovascular status and soft tissue envelope
- High-energy injuries may have multiple associated injuries in trauma patients requiring ATLS protocols for evaluation
- Early reduction of talar dislocations should be performed to restore the blood supply and limit further soft tissue pressure
- Care must be taken to evaluate for other midfoot and ankle injuries

Imaging
- AP, lateral, and oblique views of the foot and ankle should be performed to evaluate the talus and associated joints

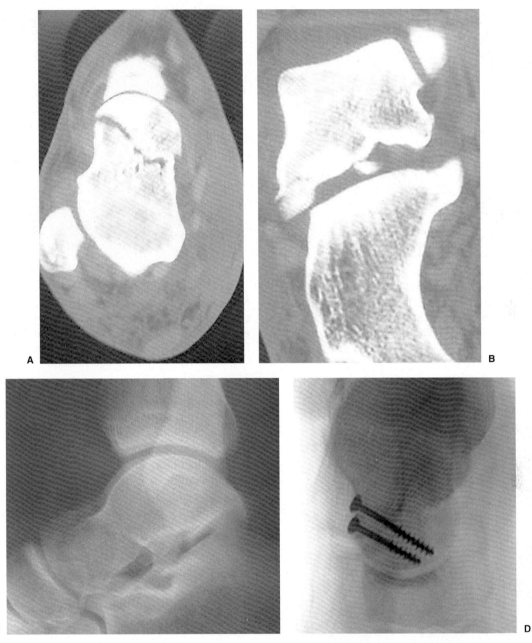

Talar head fracture treated with primary open reduction and internal fixation. Axial and coronal CT images demonstrate the fracture (**A**) and associated subtalar subluxation (**B**) better than plain radiographs (**C**). Open reduction and internal fixation was performed with compression screws (**D**). (From Bucholz RW, Court- Brown CM, Heckman JD, et al. *Rockwood & Green's Fractures in Adults*, 7th ed. Philadelphia: Lippincott, Williams & Wilkins, 2010.)

- Canale and Kelly view of the foot should be performed to better evaluate the talus should be performed
  - Beam should be directed 75 degrees to the perpendicular of a foot positioned 15 degrees oblique to the plate
- CT scan is essential for evaluation of low-energy injuries to rule out nondisplaced fractures
- CT also provides evaluation of the congruency of reductions

- MRI is crucial for evaluation of nondisplaced fractures in addition to being the best method of evaluating treated talus fractures for avascular necrosis

Talar Blood Supply
- Three primary vessels
  - Sinus tarsi artery: Can be a branch of the anterior tibial artery and peroneal artery supplies the talar head and neck

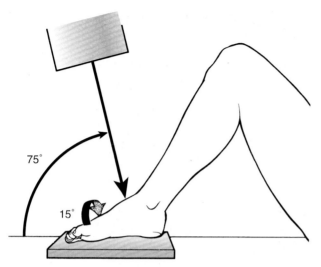

Canale and Kelly view of the foot. The correct position of the foot for x-ray evaluation of the talus is shown. (From Bucholz RW, Court- Brown CM, Heckman JD, et al. *Rockwood & Green's Fractures in Adults*, 7th ed. Philadelphia: Lippincott, Williams & Wilkins, 2010.)

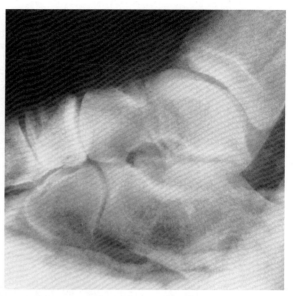

Nondisplaced vertical fracture of the talar neck, Hawkins' type I. (From Bucholz RW, Court- Brown CM, Heckman JD, et al. *Rockwood & Green's Fractures in Adults*, 7th ed. Philadelphia: Lippincott, Williams & Wilkins, 2010.)

- – Tarsal canal artery: Branch of the posterior tibial artery supplies the inferior neck and body
- – Deltoid artery: Branch of the posterior tibial artery that provides blood supply to the medial talar neck and the medial talar body
- – Tenuous blood supply → increased risk of AVN with increasing severity of injury
- – Prasarn and Lorich (2010) evaluated talar blood supply utilizing gadolinium and MRI to quantify major blood supply to the talus
  - – The anterior tibial artery supplied 36.3% of the total vasculature of the talus
  - – The peroneal artery supplied 16.9% of the vasculature
  - – The posterior tibial artery contributed 47%

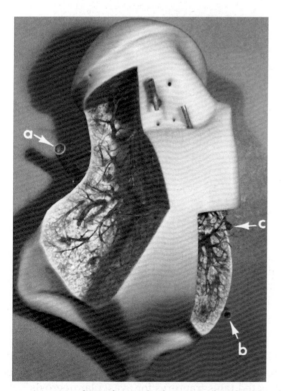

The anastomotic sling of vessels that provides the blood supply to the body of the talus. Laterally, the artery of the tarsal sinus (**A**); medially, the artery of the tarsal canal (**B**). Additional arteries enter dorsally through the neck and on the medial surface of the body (**C**). (From Kelly PJ, Sullivan CR. Blood supply of the talus. Clin Orthop 1963;30:38.)

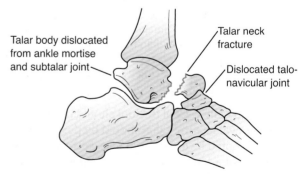

Hawkins type IV fracture of the talar neck with subluxation of the subtalar joint and dislocation of the talonavicular joint. (From Bucholz RW, Court- Brown CM, Heckman JD, et al. *Rockwood & Green's Fractures in Adults*, 7th ed. Philadelphia: Lippincott, Williams & Wilkins, 2010.)

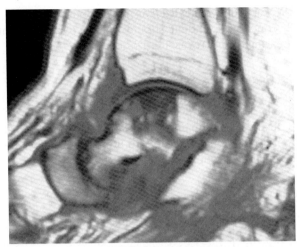

This T1-weighted MRI scan was obtained 6 mo after a talar fracture-dislocation and demonstrates osteonecrosis of the talar body. The region of osteonecrosis corresponds to the distribution of the artery of the tarsal canal. The scan also demonstrates arthritis of the talonavicular and subtalar joints, subluxation of the subtalar joint, and extensive fluid accumulation around the talus in keeping with a diagnosis of infection. (From Bucholz RW, Court-Brown CM, Heckman JD, et al. *Rockwood & Green's Fractures in Adults*, 7th ed. Philadelphia: Lippincott, Williams & Wilkins, 2010.)

- Additionally, when evaluating the vessels' contribution to each quadrant of the talus, the posterior tibial artery provided the major contribution to all regions except the anteromedial quadrant of the talus
- Through a variety of anastomosis with the anterior tibial artery the blood supply of the medial and superior surfaces received significant blood supply
- Additionally, the group showed antegrade blood flow to the talus through an anastomosis with the peroneal artery through the posterior tubercle of the talus

Classification:
AO/OTA Classification
- Separates fractures into categories based on location of the fracture
  - A: Avulsion, process, or head fracture
  - B: Talar neck fractures
  - C: Talar body fractures
- Talus fractures are classified are further classified according to location of fracture

Talar Neck Classification
Hawkins
- I—nondisplaced
  - Cast 6–8 wk
  - Osteonecrosis risk 0%–15%

- II—May or may not be associated with medial subtalar subluxation/dislocation
  - Reduce by plantarflexion
  - Higher risk of injury to the vasculature
  - Osteonecrosis risk 20%–50%
  - ORIF indicated
- III—May have associated displacement of body from ankle and subtalar joint (body travels posteromedial)
  - 50% of these fractures are open
- IV—Hawkins-Canale
  - 100% risk of osteonecrosis
  - Body dislocation from ankle and subtalar joints
    - Head dislocation from navicular

Talar Body Classification
Sneppen classification as modified by Delee
- I. Transchondral dome fracture
- II. Shear fracture
  - Coronal
  - Sagittal
  - Horizontal
- III. Posterior tubercle
- IV. Lateral Process
- V. Crush injury

Treatment
- Due to the blood supply, early intervention should be performed for displaced talar neck and body fractures
- Goal of treatment is anatomic reduction of the talar neck and body with congruent reduction of the joint
- Care should be taken when determining surgical approach to avoid further damage to the tenuous blood supply

Talar Neck Fractures
- Nonoperative management is limited to completely nondisplaced Hawkins I talus fractures
- Caused by forced dorsiflexion with axial load
- 20% associated with medial malleolus fracture
- 65% associated with other fractures
- Dorsomedial comminution in type II may lead to varus malunion with progressive arthritis and eventual need for triple fusion
- Varus deformity of the neck leads to short medial column, varus hindfoot, lateral foot overload, and decreased subtalar motion
- Posterior 4.0-mm screws are more rigid than anterior screws to better stabilize the fracture
- Consider combined anteromedial and anterolateral screws to prevent fracture gapping, which often occurs with unilateral anterior screws

- Consider medial malleolar osteotomy to reduce dislocated body if difficult or soft tissue interposition present
- Titanium screws can be utilized to allow for later MRI to evaluate postoperative avascular necrosis
- Following operative intervention 10–12-wk non–weight-bearing necessary to prevent hardware failure
- Hawkins sign: Subchondral lucency (Hawkins sign) seen at 6–8 wk on AP radiography confirming revascularization of the body

- AVN is usually visualized as a radiodensity
- If concerned, patient should remain partial weight-bearing during revascularization time

Talar Body Fractures
- Nonoperative treatment can be considered in minimally displaced fractures
- Calcaneal traction pins can be applied to patients with horizontal shear fractures to improve ability to perform closed reduction

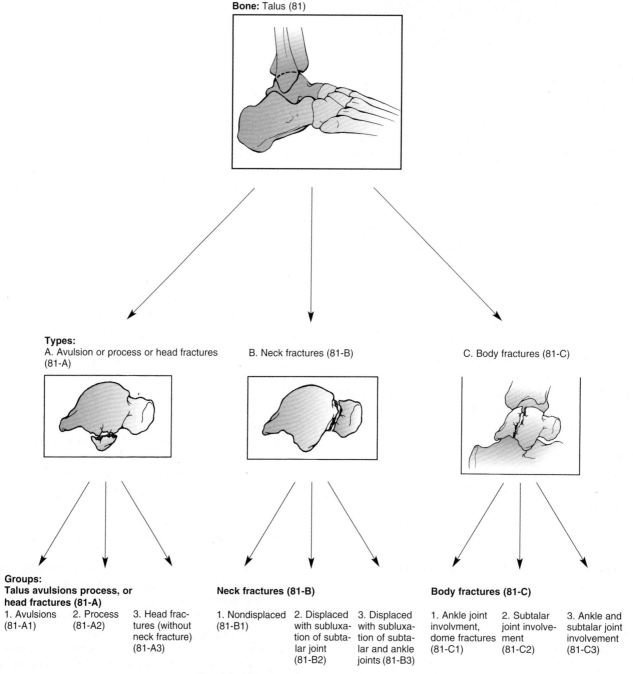

Bone: Talus (81)

Types:
A. Avulsion or process or head fractures (81-A)

B. Neck fractures (81-B)

C. Body fractures (81-C)

Groups:
Talus avulsions process, or head fractures (81-A)

1. Avulsions (81-A1)
2. Process (81-A2)
3. Head fractures (without neck fracture) (81-A3)

Neck fractures (81-B)

1. Nondisplaced (81-B1)
2. Displaced with subluxation of subtalar joint (81-B2)
3. Displaced with subluxation of subtalar and ankle joints (81-B3)

Body fractures (81-C)

1. Ankle joint involvment, dome fractures (81-C1)
2. Subtalar joint involvement (81-C2)
3. Ankle and subtalar joint involvement (81-C3)

The AO/OTA classification of talus fractures

Groups:

Talus avulsions, process or head fractures (81-A)

1. Avulsions (81-A1)

   1. Anterior (81-A1.1)

A

   2. Other (81-A1.2)

2. Process (81-A2)

   1. Lateral (81-A2.1)

   2. Posterior (81-A2.2)

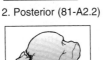

3. Head fractures (without neck fracture) (81-A3)

   1. Noncomminuted (81-A3.1)

   2. Comminuted (81-A3.2)

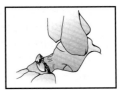

Groups:

Neck fractures (81-B)

1. Nondisplaced (81-B1)

B

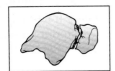

2. Displaced with subluxation of subtalar joint (81-B2)

   1. Noncomminuted (81-B2.1)

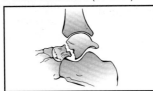

   2. Comminuted (81-B2.2)

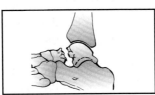

   3. Involves talar head (81-B2.3)

3. Displaced with subluxation of subtalar and ankle joints (81-B3)

   1. Noncomminuted (81-B3.1)

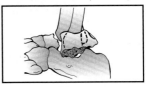

   2. Comminuted (81-B3.2)

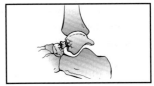

   3. Involves talar head (81-B3.3)

Groups:

Body fractures (81-C)

1. Ankle joint involvement, dome fractures (81-C1)

   1. Noncomminuted (81-C1.1)

C

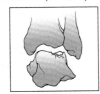

   2. Comminuted (81-C1.2)

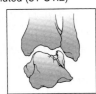

2. Subtalar joint involvement (81-C2)

   1. Noncomminuted (81-C2.1)

   2. Comminuted (81-C2.2)

3. Ankle and subtalar joint involvement (81-C3)

   1. Noncomminuted (81-C3.1)

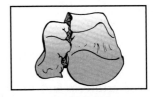

   2. Comminuted (81-C3.2)

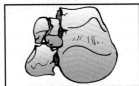

- Coronal shears are treated like talar neck fracture with A-P or P-A screws
- They are amenable to posterior screws if there is a large anterior fragment
- Sagittal shear fractures should be treated with open reduction fixation and anteromedial or anterolateral screw placement
- Posterior tubercle and lateral process fractures are usually treated nonoperatively with non–weight-bearing short leg cast for 6 wk
- Transchondral dome fractures usually treated with 6-wk short leg cast; ORIF only for acute lesion with more than one-third of dome involved

Talar Head Fractures
- Often missed due to associated injuries
- Shortens medial column
- Leads to talonavicular instability
- Main present with pain over talonavicular joint
- Nondisplaced, short leg cast for 6 wk
- Displaced, talonavicular unstable should be treated with ORIF
- Talonavicular fusion is salvage only because it makes calcaneal-cuboid and subtalar joints essential

Outcomes/Complications
- Risk of osteonecrosis, degenerative arthritis, and malunion increase with fracture severity
- Osteonecrosis
  - Hawkins I: 0%–13%
  - Hawkins II: 20%–50%
  - Hawkins III/IV: 80%–100%
- Degenerative joint disease
  - Hawkins I: 0%–30%
  - Hawkins II: 20%–90%
  - Hawkins III: 70%–100%

- Malunion
  - Hawkins I: 0%–10%
  - Hawkins II: 0%–25%
  - Hawkins III: 18%–27%
- Deep infection is more common in open fractures and extensive soft tissue injury
- Subtalar arthrosis and tibiotalar arthrosis are the most common complication of talus fractures
- Arthrosis may result in anywhere from 47% to 90% of patients
- Arthrodesis can be considered in patients with severe arthritis who fail conservative treatment

Recommended Reading
Prasarn ML, Miller AN, Dyke JP, Helfet DL, Lorich DG. Arterial anatomy of the talus: a cadaver and gadolinium-enhanced MRI study. Foot Ankle Int 2010;31(11):987–993. doi: 10.3113/FAI.2010.0987.

CALCANEUS FRACTURE
Background
- Approximately 2% of all fractures
- 60%–75% may be displaced intra-articular injuries
- Associated injuries should be ruled out
- Evaluation should include AP/lateral lumbosacral spine films (10% concomitant injury)
- Typically result from high-energy mechanism, including sporting trauma or falls from height
- Soft tissue injury should be monitored closely due to the complications of associated skin breakdown

Anatomy
- Surface anatomy composed of anterior, middle (sustentaculum), and posterior facets (main: major weight-bearing surface)
- Flexor hallucis longus runs on the undersurface of medial sustentaculum
- Lateral process of talus acts as a wedge, which dives into Gissane angle and posterior facet during trauma
- Letournel described the primary fracture line, which runs obliquely anterior to posterior through sinus tarsi or through posterior facet, behind the IO ligament
- The sustentaculum is called the constant fragment, which remains attached to talus by IO ligament
- There may be a secondary lateral to medial fracture line, creating anterolateral, superolateral, and superomedial fragments
- In tongue-type fractures, the fracture line enters the posterior facet and exits through the posterior tuberosity
- Soft tissue injury is commonly found on the medial aspect of the foot
- Fracture management should be delayed until blisters and swelling have resolved significantly

Imaging
Bohler's Angle (normal 25–50 degrees)
- Seen on lateral radiographs
- Measured from the highest part of anterior process to the highest part of posterior articular surface to most superior point on tuberosity
- Angle is smaller with depressed fractures

Crucial Angle of Gissane (normal 120–145 degrees)
- Seen on lateral radiographs
- Line parallel to posterior facet and line from sulcus to anterior process
- Increases with most fractures

Broden's View
- Patient supine, feet neutral, leg internally rotated 30 degrees

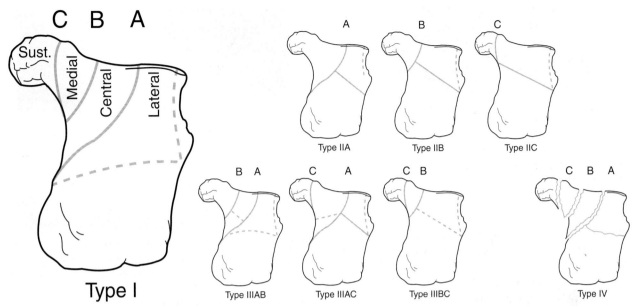

Schematic depiction of Sanders classification of intra-articular fractures of the calcaneus. Fracture lines A, B, and C describe the position of the primary fracture line in relation to the posterior facet and the subtalar joint. Types II and III have two or three fragments. Type IV represents severe comminution. (From Bucholz RW, Heckman JD, eds. Rockwood and Green's Fractures in Adults, 5th ed. Philadelphia, PA: Lippincott Williams & Wilkins; 2001, with permission.)

– Plate under ankle parallel to floor
– Beam shot anterior to posterior, angled caudally 10–40 degrees (as seen from side)
– 10-degree view shows posterior part of posterior facet
– 40-degree view shows anterior aspect

Harris Heel Axial View
– Allows visualization of calcaneocuboid joint
– Lateral wall blow out can be visualized
– Used intraoperatively to visualize fixation

Classification
Sanders et al. (1993)
– Number of displaced posterior facet fragments correlates best with postoperative outcome
– Based on coronal view on CT of widest view of posterior facet
– I—nondisplaced post facet
– II—single primary fracture line
– III—two fracture lines, three posterior facet fragments
– IV—three fracture lines, four fragments
– A—lateral joint fracture line
– B—midjoint fracture line
– C—medial fracture line through sustentaculum

Nonoperative Treatment
– Nondisplaced or minimally displaced extra-articular fractures

– Severe diabetes or peripheral vascular disease
– Minimally ambulatory elderly patients
– Sural neuritis
– Closed methods cannot reduce articular surface
– Care should be taken with smokers as fracture nonunion and wound complications are at a significantly higher risk

Or Tips and Tricks—Calcaneus
– Standard lateral L-shaped extensile incision is avoided to limit wound complications and infection
– Distal arm of extensile L-shaped incision utilized to expose the subtalar joint and calcaneocuboid
– Calcaneocuboid joint reduced initially utilizing K-wires

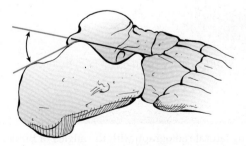

The Böhler angle. (From Bucholz RW, et al., eds. Rockwood and Green's Fractures in Adults, 6th ed. Philadelphia, PA: Lippincott Williams & Wilkins; 2006.)

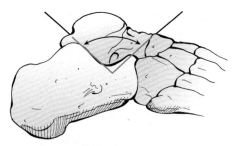

Angle of Gissane. (From Bucholz RW, et al., eds. Rockwood and Green's Fractures in Adults, 6th ed. Philadelphia, PA: Lippincott Williams & Wilkins; 2006.)

- K-wires into talus/fibula to retract
- If lateral wall blown out, then remove lateral wall removed to allow elevation of middle and posterior facet
- K-wires can be used to maintain reduction
- Consider IO structural bone graft to prevent collapse (allograft fibula or cancellous bone graft)
- Reduce sustentaculum to anterior process indirectly if possible
- Schanz pin can be placed in the tuber to assist reduction of tuberosity
- Primary goals are to restore height and correct heel varus
- Separate medial incision can be utilized at along the sustentaculum to expose the medial aspect of the calcaneus
- Medial plating can be considered under the neurovascular bundle to maintain reduction of the medial fragments
- Following medial and lateral plating, large fragment cannulated screws can be placed from proximal to distal and distal to proximal (into anterior process)
- Primary subtalar fusion for Sanders IV, highly comminuted fracture

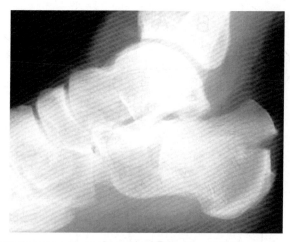

Percutaneous pin technique of Tornetta. Lateral radiograph showing tongue-type fracture. (From Bucholz RW, Heckman JD, eds. Rockwood and Green's Fractures in Adults, 5th ed. Philadelphia, PA: Lippincott Williams & Wilkins; 2001, with permission.)

Complications

- 20% if cases may have intra-articular hardware, which causes pain/discomfort
- Sural nerve injury is at risk with the extensile lateral approach
- Compartment syndrome should be monitored closely pre- and postoperatively
- Wound dehiscence and infection are some of the most common complications
- Up to 25% patients may have wound related complications
- 1%–2% of patients with wound infections require reoperation

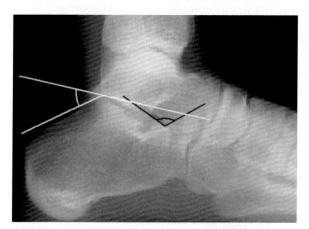

Standing lateral radiograph with the angles of Böhler and Gissane depicted. (From Bucholz RW, et al., eds. Rockwood and Green's Fractures in Adults, 6th ed. Philadelphia, PA: Lippincott Williams & Wilkins; 2006.)

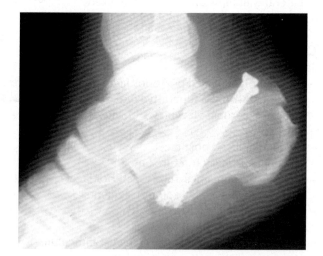

Percutaneous pin technique of Tornetta. Final lateral radiographic appearance. (From Bucholz RW, Heckman JD, eds. Rockwood and Green's Fractures in Adults, 5th ed. Philadelphia, PA: Lippincott Williams & Wilkins; 2001.)

- Soft tissue coverage with plastics assistance should be considered early to prevent deep wound infection
- Subtalar arthritis is common postoperatively due to the intra-articular nature of most fractures
- Peroneal tendinitis and stenosis can occur due to lateral impingement and compression
- Subtalar arthritis can lead to progressive tibiotalar arthritis and ankle pain
- Patient outcome is directly correlated with the rate of complications

Recommended Readings

Buckley RE, Meek RN. Comparison of open versus closed reduction of intraarticular calcaneal fractures: a matched cohort in workmen. J Orthop Trauma 1992;6(2):216–222.

Buckley RE, et al. Operative compared with nonoperative treatment of displaced intra-articular calcaneal fractures: a prospective, randomized, controlled multicenter trial. J Bone Joint Surg Am 2002;84:1733–1744.

Sanders R, et al. Operative treatment in 120 displaced intrarticular calcaneal fractures. Results using a prognostic computed tomography scan classification. Clin Orthop Relat Res 1993;290:87–95.

Tornetta P 3rd. Open reduction and internal fixation of the calcaneus using minifragment plates. J Orthop Trauma 1996; 10(1):63–67.

SUBTALAR DISLOCATION

Background
- Uncommon lower extremity dislocation of the talonavicular and talocalcaneal joint
- Most commonly occur in younger patients as the result of inversion or eversion of the foot
- May result from high-energy mechanisms with multiple associated foot injuries
- Other patients present following sports-related injuries (most commonly basketball), which are usually isolated

Physical Exam
- Patients present with significant midfoot deformity
- Up to 40% of patients may present with an open subtalar dislocation
- A detailed neurovascular exam should be performed to rule out any deficiencies prior to attempts at reduction

Imaging
- AP, lateral, and oblique views of the foot should be performed
- CT scan can be performed after reduction to rule out fracture or interposed fracture fragments
- MRI can be considered to rule of osteochondral lesions secondary to the injury or reduction

Classifications/Treatment
Medial
- 85% of subtalar dislocations are medial
- Calcaneus, navicular become medially displaced
- Foot appears plantarflexed, supinated
- Talar head may button hole extensor digitorum brevis
- 10% of patients will require open reduction
- Incision can be focused over the prominent talar head

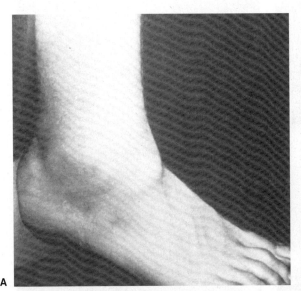
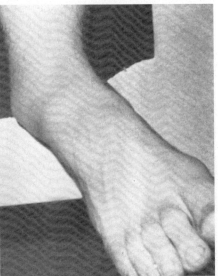

In this medial subtalar dislocation, the head of the talus (**A**) is palpable on the dorsum of the foot. The heel (**B**) is displaced medially. (From Buckingham WW Jr. Subtalar dislocation of the foot. J Trauma 1973;13:754.)

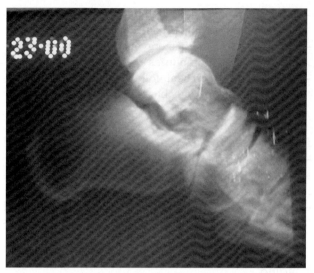

Medial subtalar dislocation. The head of the talus is directed inferior to the navicular. (From Bucholz RW, Court- Brown CM, Heckman JD, et al. *Rockwood & Green's Fractures in Adults*, 7th ed. Philadelphia: Lippincott, Williams & Wilkins, 2010.)

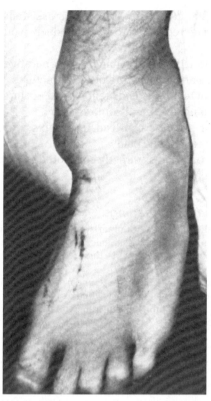

In this lateral subtalar dislocation, the head of the talus is prominent medially while the rest of the foot is dislocated laterally. (From Buckingham WW Jr. Subtalar dislocation of the foot. J Trauma 1973;13:757.)

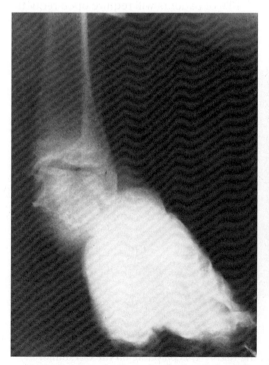
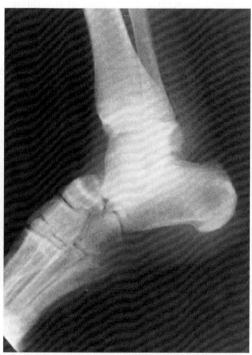

Radiographs of a lateral subtalar dislocation. (From Buckingham WW Jr. Subtalar dislocation of the foot. J Trauma 1973;13:758.)

Lateral
- 15% lateral
- Calcaneus and navicular are displaced laterally
- The foot appears pronated
- The talar head can be interposed on the posterior tibial tendon or flexor digitorum longus leading to difficulties with closed reduction
- 20% require open reduction
- The incision is placed over the sinus tarsi to allow for adequate removal of interposed soft tissue
- Knee flexion can help to help reduce the dislocation in both medial and lateral dislocations
- Following reduction, short leg splint can be applied initially if swollen followed by casting for 4 wk of immobilization total
- ROM should then be initiated following cast removal

LISFRANC—TARSOMETATARSAL FRACTURE/DISLOCATION

Background
- Common foot injury that results from multiple mechanisms
- The most common mechanisms are direct loading of the tarsometatarsal joint on the dorsal surface (crush injury) or indirect longitudinal loading of a plantar-flexed foot
- Physical exam is crucial for evaluation of the injury as radiographic findings may be subtle

Anatomy
- Joint stability from keystone effect of second metatarsal base recessed between the medial and lateral cuneiform
- Medial cuneiform joined to second metatarsal base by strong plantar Lisfranc ligament
- Tightens with pronation, abduction
- Common vascular injury to perforating dorsalis pedis artery

Classification
- A—homolateral
  - All metatarsals displaced in one direction
- B—isolated
  - One or two metatarsals displaced from others
- C—divergent
  - Metatarsal displaced in coronal and sagittal planes
  - Associated with navicular fracture

Imaging
- AP, lateral, and oblique radiographs should be performed
- 20% of injuries are missed on plain films

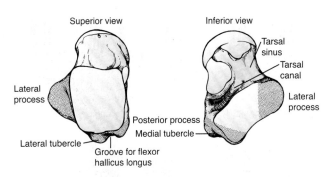

Superior and inferior views of the talus (stippling indicates the posterior and lateral processes). (From Bucholz RW, Court-Brown CM, Heckman JD, et al. *Rockwood & Green's Fractures in Adults*, 7th ed. Philadelphia: Lippincott, Williams & Wilkins, 2010.)

- Weight-bearing films provide a stress view to better evaluate ligamentous instability
- AP
  - The lateral border of the first cuneiform should be in line with the first metatarsal base
  - **The second metatarsal base should be in line with the middle cuneiform**
- Oblique
  - The medial border of the lateral cuneiform should line up with the third metatarsal base
  - **The medial border of the fourth metatarsal should be in line with the medial border of the cuboid**
  - **(Bold statements are the indicators of stability)**

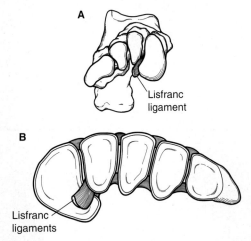

The anatomy of the tarsometatarsal joints of the foot. **A:** Proximal view of the cuneiform and cuboid articular surfaces. **B:** Distal view of the corresponding articular surfaces of the metatarsals. (From Bucholz RW, Heckman JD. Rockwood & Green's Fractures in Adults, 5th ed. Philadelphia, PA: Lippincott, Williams & Wilkins, 2001.)

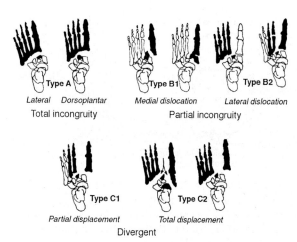

Myerson classification of Lisfranc fracture-dislocations. (From Myerson MS, et al. Fracture-dislocations of the tarsometatarsal joints: end results correlated with pathology and treatment. Foot Ankle 1986;6:225–242.)

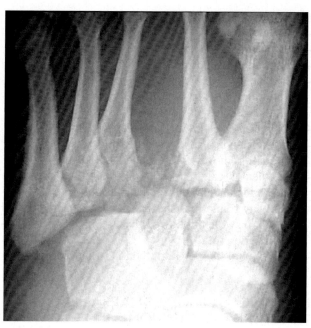

Presentation of an atypical Lisfranc injury. A: Initial radiographs show disruption of the tarsometatarsal joints with evidence of intra-articular fracture and fracture of the medial cuneiform. (From Bucholz RW, Heckman JD, eds. Rockwood and Green's Fractures in Adults, 5th ed. Philadelphia, PA: Lippincott Williams & Wilkins; 2001.)

- Stress films can be performed by applying supination/ pronation or abduction/adduction stress to the fore-foot on AP and lateral radiographs if the patient is unable to stand
- >2 mm of displacement represents an unstable joint
- Lateral radiograph with unbroken line between dorsum of first and second metatarsal with respective cuneiforms

Subtle Signs of Injury
- "Fleck sign"—avulsion of second metatarsal base
- Widening of base of first and second metatarsals
- CT scan can be utilized in patients who are unable to undergo stress radiographs and to further evaluate the injuries

Treatment
- Nondisplaced stable fracture
    - Patients can be treated with a short leg cast, non–weight bearing for 6 wk
- ORIF should be considered if >1–2-mm displacement
- Consider acute arthrodesis in significantly displaced injuries
- Avoid fusion of the fourth and fifth metatarsals due to a higher frequency of pseudoarthrosis and continued pain and discomfort

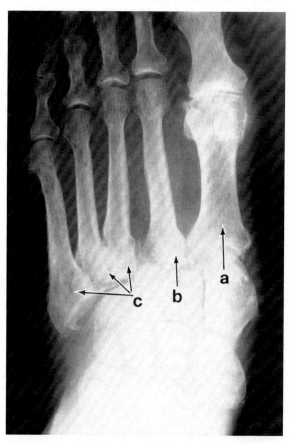

Radiograph of a Lisfranc dislocation. First metatarsal (A); second metatarsal (B); and third, fourth, and fifth metatarsals (C), which have been dislocated laterally. (From Harwood-Nuss A, et al. The Clinical Practice of Emergency Medicine, 3rd ed. Philadelphia, PA: Lippincott Williams & Wilkins; 2001.)

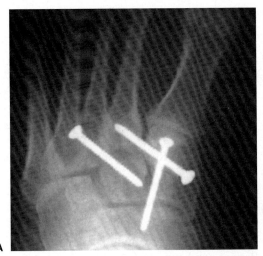
A

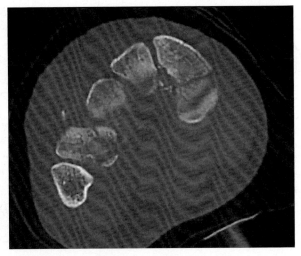
B

Presentation of an atypical Lisfranc injury. **A:** Reduction and fixation of the tarsometatarsal joints are accomplished with only medial column fixation. The medial cuneiform is fixed first with a lag screw, followed by the tarsometatarsal joints. The first joint was stable. The lateral joint required no fixation after reduction of the medial column. **B:** Computed tomography scan showing the longitudinal fracture of the medial cuneiform and the comminution of the second and third cuneiforms. (From Bucholz RW, Heckman JD, eds. Rockwood and Green's Fractures in Adults, 5th ed. Philadelphia, PA: Lippincott Williams & Wilkins; 2001.)

– Fixation can be performed utilizing mini-fragment plates or cortical screws from the medial cuneiform to the base of the second metatarsal
– Fixation should also be performed across the cuneiforms to prevent instability
– Screw removal should be performed at >4 mo to allow motion at the midfoot.
– Most common cause of suboptimal results is malreduction

Recommended Readings

Kuo R, et al. Outcome after open reduction and internal fixation of Lisfranc joint injuries. J Bone Joint Surg Am 2000;82:1609–1618.
Lee C, et al. Stabilization of Lisfranc joint injuries: a biomechanical study. Foot Ankle Int 2004;25:365–370.
Vuori J, Aro H. Lisfranc joint injuries: trauma mechanisms and associated injuries. J Trauma 1993;35:40–45.

FIFTH METATARSAL/JONES FRACTURE

Background
– Common injuries resulting from rotational injuries of the midfoot
– Patients complain of discomfort
– Essential to evaluate the fracture and fracture location as blood supply to the fifth metatarsal may involve watershed zone → nonunion

Anatomy
– Single nutrient artery enters from the medial cortex at the proximal and middle third junction of the metatarsal

Injury/Treatment
– Tuberosity avulsion
– Most common and most proximal injury
– Avulsion by lateral band of the plantar aponeurosis (not the peroneus brevis as commonly taught)

Treatment
– No operative intervention indicated
– Patient can be made weight bearing as tolerated in a cast shoe

Jones Fracture
– Zone 2 injury that extends into the fourth to fifth intermetatarsal facet joint
– Acute injuries usually result from adduction and of a plantar flexed foot
– Patient can be made non–weight bearing in a cast 8 wks but there is a risk of nonunion (>70%–90% union)
– In athletes and patients desiring early return to activity, an intramedullary cancellous screw is recommended to improve time to union
– Allows earlier return to activity

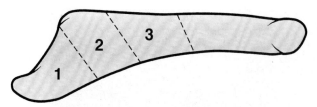

Three zones of proximal fifth metatarsal fracture. Zone 1: Avulsion fracture. Zone 2: Fracture at the metaphyseal–diaphyseal junction. Zone 3: Proximal shaft stress fracture. (From Bucholz RW, et al., eds. Rockwood and Green's Fractures in Adults, 6th ed. Philadelphia, PA: Lippincott Williams & Wilkins; 2006.)

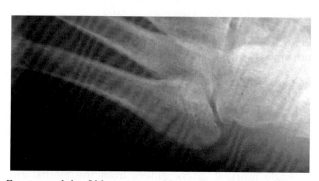

Fracture of the fifth metatarsal base. Zone 2 injury. (From Bucholz RW, Heckman JD, eds. Rockwood and Green's Fractures in Adults, 5th ed. Philadelphia, PA: Lippincott Williams & Wilkins; 2001.)

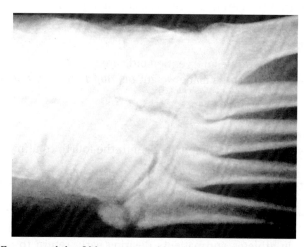

Fracture of the fifth metatarsal base. Zone 1 injury with comminution. (From Bucholz RW, Heckman JD, eds. Rockwood and Green's Fractures in Adults, 5th ed. Philadelphia, PA: Lippincott Williams & Wilkins; 2001.)

Diaphyseal Stress Fracture
- Zone 3 injuries
- Treatment is controversial as well
- I—acute: non–weight bearing in short leg cast in low-activity individuals
- Consider intramedullary screw fixation in patients with desire for early return to activity
- II—Delayed union: ORIF with intramedullary cancellous screw
- III–Nonunion: ORIF with intramedullary cancellous screw

Dancer's Fracture
- Long spiral fracture diaphysis
- Nonoperative treatment indication
- Patient can be made weight bearing as tolerated in a hard-soled shoe

Recommended Readings

Josefsson PO, et al. Jones fracture: surgical versus nonsurgical treatment. Clin Orthop Relat Res 1994;299:252–255.
Torg JS, et al. Fractures of the base of the fifth metatarsal distal to the tuberosity: classification and guidelines for nonsurgical and surgical management. J Bone Joint Surg 1984; 66(2):209–214.

NAVICULAR FRACTURE

Background
- The navicular is a crucial portion of the midfoot based on its articulation with the talus, the cuneiforms, and the cuboid
- Due to the multiple articulations, injury can lead to significant midfoot dysfunction
- Injury may result from direct or indirect forces
- Most often results from axial loading along the long axis of the foot
- Other midfoot injuries should be ruled out accordingly
- Patients may present with visible deformity or localized tenderness, which should be fully investigated

Imaging
- AP, lateral, and oblique standing films should be performed to evaluate ligamentous disruption
- CT scan may be required to further evaluate the injury

Classification
- Avulsion: Results from talonavicular or naviculocuneiform ligament avulsion
- Tuberosity: Results from tibialis posterior avulsion

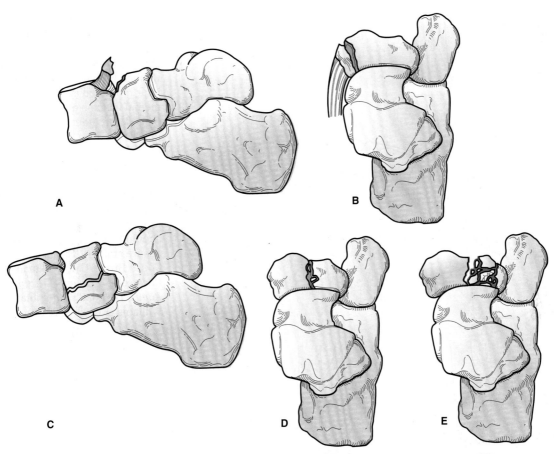

The present popular classification of navicular fractures is composed of three basic types with a subclassification for body fractures suggested by Sangeorzan. **A.** Avulsion-type fracture can involve either the talonavicular or naviculocuneiform ligaments. **B.** Tuberosity fractures are usually traction-type injuries with disruption of the tibialis posterior insertion without joint surface disruption. **C.** A type I body fracture splits the navicular into dorsal and plantar segments. **D.** A type II body fracture cleaves into medial and lateral segments. The location of the split usually follows either of the two intercuneiform joint lines. Stress fractures are usually be included in this group. **E.** A type III body fracture is distinguished by comminution of the fragments and significant displacement of the medial and lateral poles. (From Bucholz RW, Court-Brown CM, Heckman JD, et al. *Rockwood & Green's Fractures in Adults*, 7th ed. Philadelphia: Lippincott, Williams & Wilkins, 2010.)

- Body: See image below for further differentiation
- Stress fractures

Treatment
- Goals of treatment are to maintain medial column length and maintain talonavicular stability
- Nondisplaced fractures are treated nonoperatively with casting and 6 wk of non–weight bearing

Operative Treatment
- Limited to fractures that exhibit talonavicular instability or >2 mm of fragment displacement
- Fixation is limited to cortical screw fixation of the associated fragments

- Patients with >40% of the articular surface involved and irreparable should undergo acute talonavicular fusion
- External fixation can be considered in crush injuries with shortening of the medial column
- Graft can be utilized to fill any voids left by fracture comminution
- Dorsal lip avulsion medial column
- Tuberosity fracture from posterior tibial avulsion
  - Consider ORIF if intra-articular
- Navicular body fractures are intra-articular by definition
- Stress fracture, central one-third
- Short leg cast, non–weight bearing × 6 wk

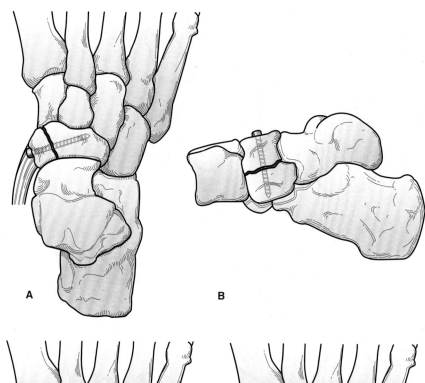

Suggested fixation methods for simple navicular fractures. **A.** Tuberosity fracture repaired with a 3.5-mm cortical lag screw and a soft tissue washer. **B.** Type I body fracture. The joint reduction is observed through a medial incision and lag screws are placed percutaneously dorsal to plantar. **C.** Type II body fractures are reduced with direct visualization of the fracture from a dorsal incision with percutaneous lag screws placed from either medial or lateral position. **D.** In the event that the lateral fragment is too small for stable fixation, the screws should be carried into the cuboid to ensure stability. (From Bucholz RW, Court- Brown CM, Heckman JD, et al. *Rockwood & Green's Fractures in Adults*, 7th ed. Philadelphia: Lippincott, Williams & Wilkins, 2010.)

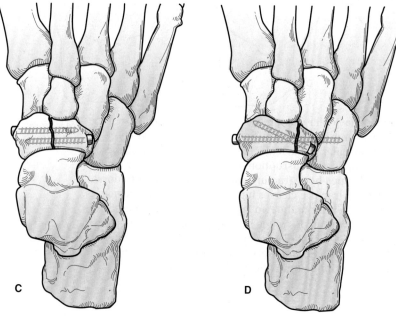

CUBOID FRACTURE

Background

- Uncommon isolated injury
- Injuries can be easily overlooked
- Patients present with lateral foot pain
- Structurally essential to maintenance of the lateral column of the foot
- Articulates independently with fourth and fifth metatarsals
    - This articulation provide the majority of the plantar and dorsal motion of the lateral column

Mechanism

- Fracture may occur in low-energy situations or as part of polytrauma
- Results from forced pronation of the midfoot combined with an axial force

Diagnosis

- AP, lateral, and oblique radiographs of the foot
- Stress views of the foot should be performed to rule out associated lisfranc or midfoot ligamentous injury
- CT scan will confirm injury

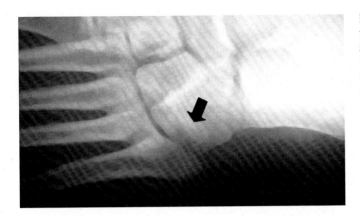

Radiograph of a cuboid fracture with impaction of the tarsometatarsal joint ~1 cm. The arrow marks the subchondral bone of the impacted articular surface. (From Bucholz RW, Heckman JD, eds. Rockwood and Green's Fractures in Adults, 5th ed. Philadelphia, PA: Lippincott Williams & Wilkins; 2001, with permission.)

Treatment

- Nonoperative treatment should be considered in fractures with <2 mm of displacement, stable calcaneocuboid and cuboid-metatarsal articulation, maintenance of the lateral column
- Non–weight bearing in cast for 4–6 wk
- Operative treatment should be considered if displaced or in the presence of instability

Recommended Reading

Weber M, Locher S. Reconstruction of the cuboid in compression fractures: short to midterm results in 12 patients. Foot Ankle Int 2002;23:1008–1013.

Pediatric Orthopaedic Trauma

CONSCIOUS SEDATION

- **Sedation should be performed by an appropriately credentialed physician**

Diazepam (Valium)

- Pediatrics: 0.1 mg/kg/dose, maximum 5 mg
- Onset 1–5 min
- Duration 4–6 hr
- Half-life 20–50 hr

Lorazepam (Ativan)

- Pediatrics: 0.05 mg/kg/dose every 4–8 hr
- Onset 15–30 min
- Duration 6–8 hr
- Half-life 16 hr

Meperidine (Demerol)

- Pediatrics: 2 mg/kg/dose IM 1 mg/kg/dose IV q4h, maximum 50 mg
- IV onset 5 min, peaks 15 min
- Half-life 3–4 hr

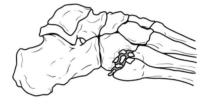

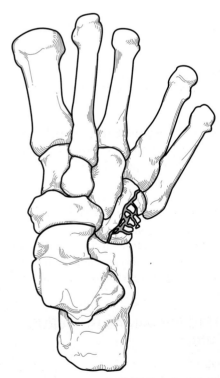

Restoration of a nutcracker fracture of the cuboid. Typical fracture appearance in anteroposterior and lateral plane. (From Bucholz RW, Heckman JD, eds. Rockwood and Green's Fractures in Adults, 5th ed. Philadelphia, PA: Lippincott Williams & Wilkins; 2001, with permission.)

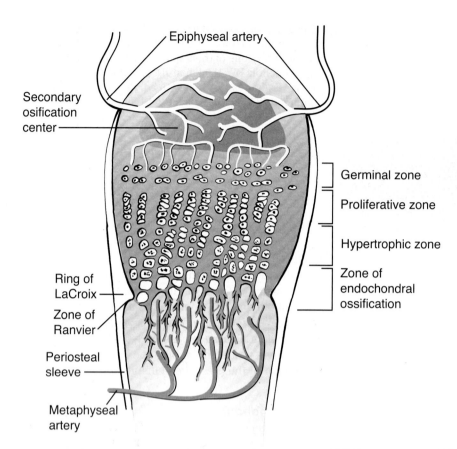

Schematic diagram of the organization of the physis. Four zones are illustrated: the germinal, proliferative, hypertrophic, and provisional calcification (or enchondral ossification) layers. Note also the groove of Ranvier and the perichondral ring of LaCroix. (From Beaty JH, Kasser JR. *Rockwood & Wilkins Fractures in Children*, 7th ed. Philadelphia: Lippincott, Williams & Wilkins, 2010.)

Midazolam (Versed)
- IV or IM, 0.15 mg/kg
- Onset 1–5 min
- Duration 20–60 min
- Half-life 1.5–4 hr

Morphine
- 0.1 mg/kg/dose
- Onset 1–5 min
- Duration 4–5 hr
- Half-life 1.5–2 hr

Ketamine
- 0.2–1 mg/kg over 2–3 min
- Onset 30 sec
- Duration 5–10 min
- Glycopyrrolate/atropine and Versed to decrease salivation and dreams

Naloxone (Narcan)
- 0.005–0.01 mg IV at 2-min intervals
- Onset 1 min
- Duration 45 min

- Half-life 30–60 min
- Noncardiogenic pulmonary edema

Flumazenil: Antagonist to Benzodiazepines
- <20 kg: 0.01 mg/kg, repeat doses of 0.005 mg/kg
- 20–40 kg: 0.2 mg, repeat doses of 0.005 mg/kg
- Onset 30–60 sec
- Duration 60 min
- Does not reverse respiratory effects: Be aware of the "blue and awake" patient
- An appropriate history and physical should be performed as flumazenil can cause seizures in patients with history of chronic benzodiazepine abuse

PEDIATRIC PROXIMAL HUMERUS FRACTURES

Background
- Uncommon pediatric injury
- 80% of humerus grows at proximal end, thus remodeling potential is huge
- May occur at birth

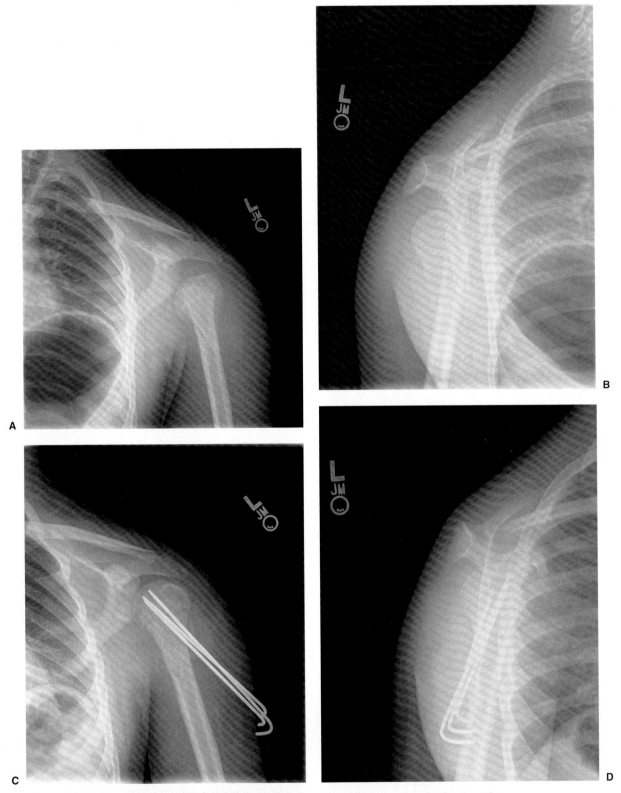

A. AP radiograph of displaced fracture of the proximal humeral metaphysis with shortening with inferior subluxation of the humeral head with respect to the glenoid. **B.** Scapular Y-view. **C, D.** Postoperative films after open reduction and fixation. The inferior subluxation has resolved. (From Beaty JH, Kasser JR. *Rockwood & Wilkins Fractures in Children*, 7th ed. Philadelphia: Lippincott, Williams & Wilkins, 2010.)

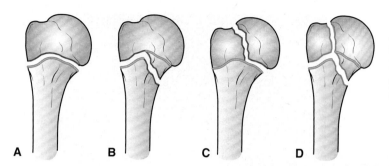

Physeal fractures of the proximal humerus. **A.** Salter-Harris I. **B.** Salter-Harris II. **C,** Salter-Harris III. **D.** Salter-Harris IV. (From Bucholz RW, Heckman JD, Court-Brown C, et al., eds. *Rockwood and Green's Fractures in Adults*, 6th ed. Philadelphia: Lippincott Williams & Wilkins, 2006.)

- Predominant mechanism in children and adolescents is direct trauma to the shoulder

History and Physical Examination
- Patient present with swelling and discomfort at the shoulder
- Infants may be irritable or refuse to use to injured extremity
- Neurovascular exam should be performed to rule out brachial plexus injury in newborns

Imaging
- True AP and Axillary images are necessary to provide treatment recommendations

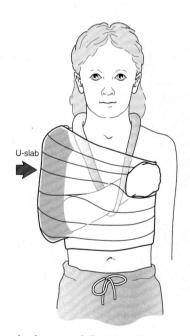

Sling and swathe for immobilization of proximal humeral fracture. (From Bucholz RW, Heckman JD, Court-Brown C, et al., eds. *Rockwood and Green's Fractures in Adults*, 6th ed. Philadelphia: Lippincott Williams & Wilkins, 2006.)

Classification
- Salter Harris classification is utilized for injuries involving the physis
- See image above

Treatment
- Due to the significant remodeling potential of the proximal humerus, most are treated nonoperatively
- Newborn proximal humerus fractures are treated by swath or attaching the extremity to the shirt with a safety pin as a means of immobilizing the extremity
- Those fractures heal within 1–2 wk

Acceptable Deformity
- 1–4 yr old: Up to 70 degrees of angulation will remodel
- 5–12 yr old: 45 degrees of angulation and 50% displacement
- 12–Maturity: 20 degrees of angulation and <30% displacement
- Closed reduction can be attempted in patients with unacceptable deformity
- If reduction cannot be maintained, closed reduction and percutanous pinning is utilized with at least two 0.62-mm K-wires from the lateral shaft to the humeral head
- Care should be taken to avoid penetrating the articular surface of the proximal humerus
- Pins are then left in place for 4 wk followed by removal and initiation of Codman's

Outcomes
- Patients recover with limited functional or cosmetic limitations
- Humerus varus is a rare complication that can occur in neonates and children <5 yr with significantly displaced/angulated fractures
  - May cause functional limitation requiring corrective osteotomy to prevent impingement and improve loss of motion
- Open reduction rarely indicated

PEDIATRIC ELBOW

Overview
- 8%–9% of all pediatric upper extremity fractures
- Most commonly in patients aged 8–10 yr
- Diagnosis is difficulty due to the multiple ossification centers of the pediatric elbow

Order of Ossification
- Capitellum: 6 mo to 2 yr
- Radial head: 4 yr old
- Medial epicondyle: 6–7 yr old
- Trochlea: 8 yr old
- Olecranon: 8–10 yr old
- Lateral epicondyle: 12 yr old

PEDIATRICS—TRANSPHYSEAL HUMERUS FRACTURE

Background
- 0–4 yr old, usually <2 yr old
- Distal fragment usually is translated posteromedially
- Results from hyperextension of the elbow in skeletally immature patients
- Injury most commonly related to child abuse
- Adequate child abuse workup should be performed as part of admission and treatment of the patients

History and Physical Examination
- Should be suspected in younger children with swollen extremity and refusal to use extremity under the age of 18 mo
- Clinical evaluation of bony landmarks may be limited

Imaging
- AP, lateral, and oblique views of the elbow should be performed
- Lateral condyle may displace in unison with the radius
- Metaphyseal flake on radiographs is pathognomonic
- Be aware that the proximal radius and ulna maintain adequate alignment with one another while being displaced posteromedially to the distal humerus
- May be confused for an elbow dislocation

Classification
Delee Classification
Group A
- Infants up to 12 mo old
- Prior to secondary ossification of the lateral condyle
- Salter-Harris I type physeal injuries

Group B
- 12 mo to 3 yr old
- Visible lateral condyle epiphysis
- May have a metaphyseal flake present on the distal fragment

Group C
- 3 –7 yr old
- Salter-Harris II injury

Treatment
- Long arm cast if nondisplaced
- Arthrogram can be performed to evaluate epiphysis
- Reduces easily but is unstable because of thin columns leading to varus and rotational deformity
- Closed reduction and percutaneous pinning of the distal fragment is then performed followed by arthrogram to confirm adequate reduction
- Patients are then casted for 4 wk followed by removal of pins and initiation of motion

Outcomes
- Cubitus varus is the most common complication
- Generally, patients recover without any functional limitation

SUPRACONDYLAR HUMERUS FRACTURES

Background
- The most common humeral facture in children presenting to orthopaedic surgeons
- Most commonly occur in children 5–6 yr old
- Result from low-energy falls from moderate height
- Range of injury severity and associated complications direct treatment accordingly

History and Physical Examination
- Most patients present following a fall from height with pain and deformity at the elbow
- Detailed neurovascular exam should be performed to document function
- Minimally displaced fractures may present with minimal swelling, slight loss of ROM
- Severe injuries may exhibit the "pucker sign"—sign of proximal fragment piercing the brachialis and contacting the dermis, but not piercing the epidermis
- Motor and sensory exam may be difficult in children, but it is essential to preoperative and postoperative evaluation (PIN, AIN, and ulnar nerve should be examined closely)
- Forearm swelling and pain with positive stretch should be examined closely
- Patient should be monitored for worsening pain or increasing pain medication requirement as verbal interaction may be limited
- Stryker pressure monitoring should be utilized in those patients with pain with passive stretch of the fingers, and progressive increases in pain medication requirements

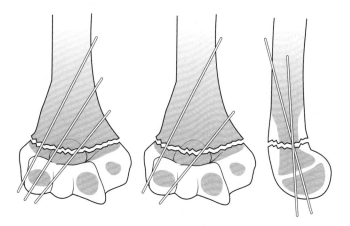

Properly placed divergent lateral entry pins. On the AP view, there should be maximal pin separation at the fracture site, the pins should engage both medial and lateral columns just proximal to the fracture site, and they should engage an adequate amount of bone proximal and distal to the fragments. On the lateral view, pins should incline slightly in the anterior to posterior direction in accordance with normal anatomy. (From Skaggs DL, Cluck MW, Mostofi A, et al. Lateral-entry pin fixation in the management of supracondylar fractures in children. J Bone Joint Surg Am 2004;86(4):702:707, with permission.)

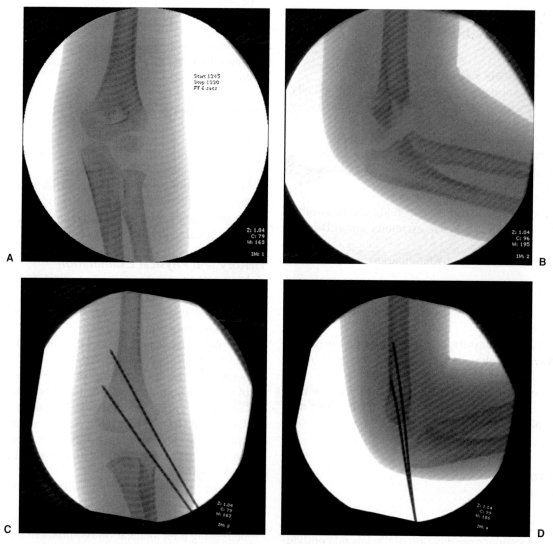

These intraoperative images are of a 4-year-old with a type II supracondylar humeral fracture that was closed reduced and pinned with two lateral entry pins according to the authors' preferred technique. (Reproduced with permission of Children's Orthopaedic Center, Los Angeles, CA.)

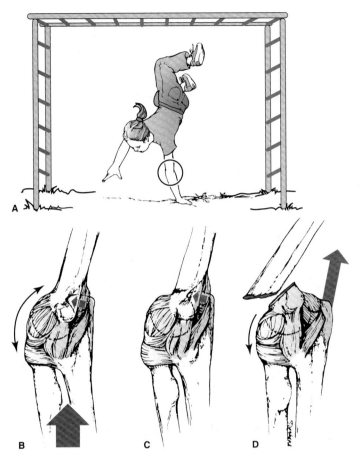

Mechanism of injury:elbow hyperextension. **A.** Most children attempt to break their falls with the arm extended. With hyperextension, the elbow falls into hyperextension. **B.** The linear applied force (large arrow) leads to an anterior tension force. Posteriorly, the olecranon is forced into the depths of the olecranon fossa (small arrow). **C.** As the bending force continues, the distal humerus fails anteriorly in the thin supracondylar area. **D.** When the fracture is complete, the proximal fragment can continue moving anteriorly and distally, potentially harming adjacent soft tissue structures such as the brachialis muscle, brachial artery, and median nerve. (From Beaty JH, Kasser JR. *Rockwood & Wilkins Fractures in Children*, 7th ed. Philadelphia: Lippincott, Williams & Wilkins, 2010.)

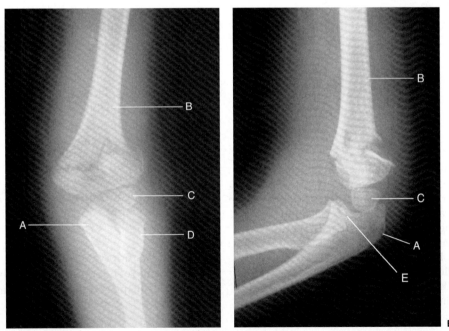

Supracondylar humerus fractures: operative management. Type II extension supracondylar humerus fracture (left elbow). **A.** Anterior-posterior. **B.** Lateral. A, ulna; B, humerus; C, capitellar epiphysis; D, radius; E, radial head. (From Koval KJ, Zuckerman JD. *Atlas of Orthopaedic Surgery: A Multimeidal Reference*. Philadelphia: Lippincott Williams & Wilkins, 2004.)

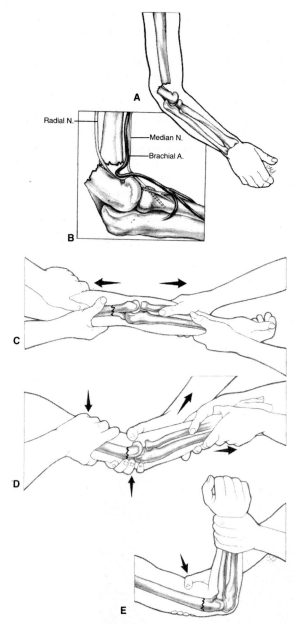

Reduction technique for supracondylar humeral fractures that occur with the elbow in flexion. **A.** Distal fragment is displaced posteriorly. **B.** The brachial artery may become entrapped at the fracture site. **C.** Restore length by applying traction against countertraction. **D.** With pressure directed anteriorly on the distal fragment, provide reduction. **E.** The reduction is generally stable with the elbow in flexion with the forearm pronated. (From Swiontkowski MF. *Manual of Orthopaedics*, 6th ed. Philadelphia: Lippincott Williams & Wilkins, 2006.)

Imaging
- AP, lateral, and oblique radiographs should be performed in all patients
- Due to pain or deformity, assistance may be necessary to get an accurate radiograph to truly evaluate the injury

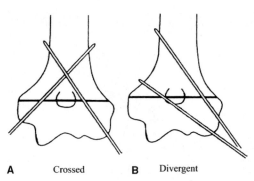

Pinning techniques in study by Lee et al. 123 **A.** Crossed: one medial and one lateral pin. **B.** Divergent: two divergent lateral pins. (From Beaty JH, Kasser JR. *Rockwood & Wilkins Fractures in Children*, 7th ed. Philadelphia: Lippincott, Williams & Wilkins, 2010.)

Classification
- 97%–99% of injuries result from falls onto an out-stretched extended elbow resulting in an extension-type supracondylar fracture

Flexion-type injuries
- Less common injury

Type 1
- Stable, nondisplaced injuries treated in a long arm cast

Type 2
- Minimally displaced fracture which may require reduction and casting in full extension

Type 3
- Completely displaced fracture requiring closed reduction and pinning followed by casting
- Open reduction can be considered if completely unstable or irreducible

Modified Gartland Classification
Type 1
- Nondisplaced

Type 2
- Hinged posteriorly
- Large range of injury from minimally displaced to significantly displaced requiring operative intervention

Type 3
- No cortical contact between proximal and distal fragment

Type 4
- Completely displaced with collapse of the medial column

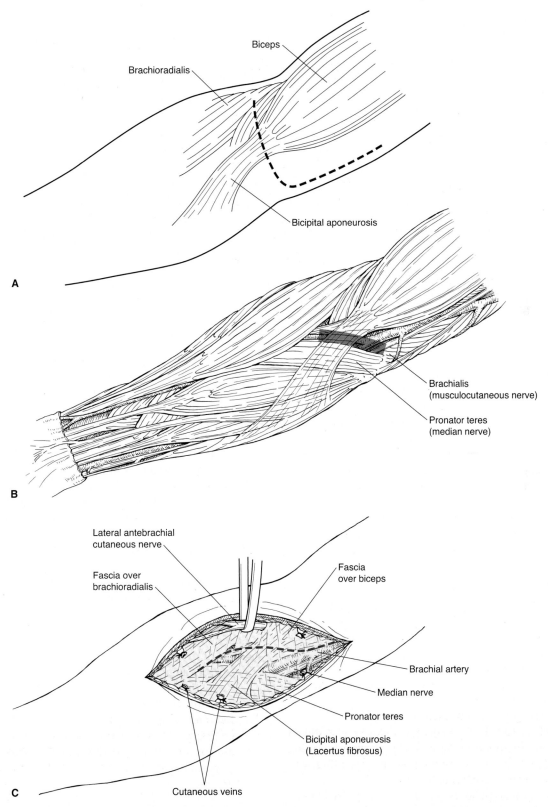

Anterior approach for open reduction and brachial artery and median nerve exploration. Most often, just the transverse part of the incision is needed for fracture reduction alone. (From Beaty JH, Kasser JR. *Rockwood & Wilkins Fractures in Children*, 7th ed. Philadelphia: Lippincott, Williams & Wilkins, 2010.) *(continued)*

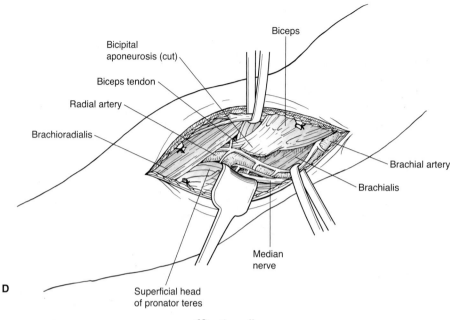

Bicipital aponeurosis (cut)

Biceps tendon

Radial artery

Brachioradialis

Biceps

Brachial artery

Brachialis

Median nerve

D

Superficial head of pronator teres

(Continued)

Neurologic Injury
- Extension-type injuries can result in neurovascular injury depending on the displacement of the fracture
- Displacement of the distal fragment leads to tension being placed on the surrounding neurovascular structures by the proximal fragment
- Medial displacement of the distal fragment is the most common pattern of injury (75% of patients)
- Medial displacement leads to tension on the radial nerve
- Lateral displacement leads to tension or entrapment of the median nerve (AIN) and brachial artery

Vascular Injury
- Vascular status of the patients should be monitored closely as the brachial artery is at risk with posterolateral displacement of the distal fragments
- Patients are separated into three categories that direct treatment
  - Palpable radial pulse
  - Warm perfused extremity with nonpalpable, but dopplerable pulse
  - Poorly perfused, pulseless extremity
- Choi et al. (2010) showed that majority of patients maintain adequate or improved perfusion following closed reduction and pinning when presenting with well perfused pulseless extremities
  - 57% of those patients regained distal pulses immediately postoperatively
- Of the nine patients with poorly perfused pulseless extremities
  - Four patients developed improved perfusion following closed reduction

- Three patients initially had improved perfusion following closed reduction, but two developed delayed compartment syndrome, while 1 required vascular intervention for repair
- At 8 wk follow-up, all 32 of their patients exhibited good extremity perfusion
- Current recommendations are for early closed reduction and percutaneous pinning in patients with pulseless extremities
- If perfusion is not improved, open exploration, and angiography should be initiated to evaluate for vascular injury
- If perfusion improves in the poorly perfused patients, postoperative management should consist of highly vigilant monitoring of neurovascular status and status of the patient's compartments

Treatment
- Based on classification of injury
- Goals of treatment
  - Correct alignment and rotation
  - Reduction performed with traction, flexion and pronation of the elbow
  - Bauman's angle can be utilized as a determinant of adequate fracture reduction (Angle between the line perpendicular to the humeral shaft and the physeal line of the lateral condyle: normal ≥10 degrees)

Gartland 1
- Diagnosis based on anterior or posterior fat pad and clinical exam
- Long arm cast placement for 3–4 wk followed by removal for initiation of ROM

- Periosteal reaction may be visualized at follow-up despite no early fracture lines

Gartland 2
- Treatment is dependent of amount of displacement of the distal fragment
- Nonoperative treatment is utilized if the capitellum is in line with the anterior humeral line on the lateral radiographs
- Closed reduction and percutaneous pinning is utilized in patients who do not fulfill that characteristic

Gartland 3, 4
- Following appropriate neurovascular evaluation, closed reduction and percutaneous pinning can be performed
- Percutaneous pinning is performed utilizing two divergent lateral pins to limit the need for medially placed pin
- No significant clinical difference in outcomes between lateral and cross-pinning, but cross-pins have been shown to have improved rotational control
- If still unstable, an additional lateral pin can be utilized or a medial pin can be placed through a mini open incision to avoid ulnar nerve injury
- Open reduction through anterior approach to the elbow can be considered in irreducible or highly unstable fractures
- A 5-cm transverse incision is made along the cubital fossa
- Most often, the injury has destroyed the intramuscular planes and the fracture fragments are visible
- Bicipital aponeurosis is incised
- Medial to the biceps tendon is the brachial artery then the median nerve
- Following visualization of the proximal and distal fragments, reduction should then be attempted once the neurovascular structures are protected

Outcomes/Complications
- Vascular injury was discussed in depth above
- Compartment syndrome occurs in 0.1%–0.3% of fractures
    - Diagnosis is difficult due to patient's inability to adequate express pain
    - Pain medication requirement should be monitored closely
    - Volkman's contracture is the risk of missed forearm compartment syndrome leading to loss of function and claw digits
- Neurologic deficit has been reported in between 10% and 29% of patients
    - AIN is the most commonly injured nerve
    - 2–6 mo of watchful waiting may be necessary before full recovery of function

- Cubitus varus (gunstock deformity)
    - Malunion leading to hyperextension and varus deformity of the distal humerus
    - Predominately a cosmetic deformity but can lead to progressive varus deformity, pain, posterolateoral rotatory instability or increased risk of lateral condyle fractures
    - Distal humeral corrective osteotomy can be considered

Recommended Readings

Blanco RG, et al. Medial and lateral pin versus lateral-entry pin fixation for type 3 supracondylar fractures in children: a prospective, surgeon-randomized study. J Pediatr Orthop 2010;30(8):799–806.
Choi PD, et al Risk Factors for vascular repair and compartment syndrome in the pulseless supracondylar humerus fracture in children. J Pediatr Orthop 2010;30(1):50–56.

Pediatric Lateral Condyle Fracture
- Most commonly occur in patients 5–10 yr old (peak age 6)
- Result from varus force in extension leading to "pull off" of lateral condyle by radius
- Forearm becomes displaced posterolaterally
- Blood supply to distal humerus is located posterior to lateral condyle and should be taken into account during fixation

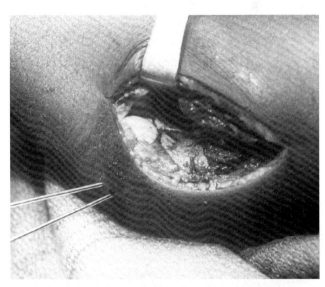

Lateral approach for open reduction and internal fixation of a lateral humeral condylar fracture of the left elbow. The approach is made through the brachioradialis:triceps interval; an anterior retractor is used to expose the joint surfaces, and the fracture is reduced and pinned percutaneously posterior to the incision. (From Beaty JH, Kasser JR. *Rockwood & Wilkins Fractures in Children*, 7th ed. Philadelphia: Lippincott, Williams & Wilkins, 2010.)

- Represents one of few pediatric fractures with high risk of nonunion
- High incidence of poor outcomes with loss of motion, trochlear avulsion if not treated appropriately

History and Physical Examination
- Patients may present with visible deformity and swelling of a painful elbow
- ROM is likely limited due to pain

Imaging
- AP, lateral, and oblique radiographs should be performed

- Internal oblique provides the best image to visualize displacement of the fracture (Song et al. 2007).

Classification
- **Milch I**
  - Lateral metaphysis through epiphysis to joint
  - Lateral trochlea attached to humerus
  - No ulnar displacement, ulnohumeral joint stable
- **Milch II**
  - Lateral metaphysis through physis to joint
  - Lateral trochlea attached to fractured lateral condyle
  - Ulna displaced laterally, ulnohumeral joint unstable

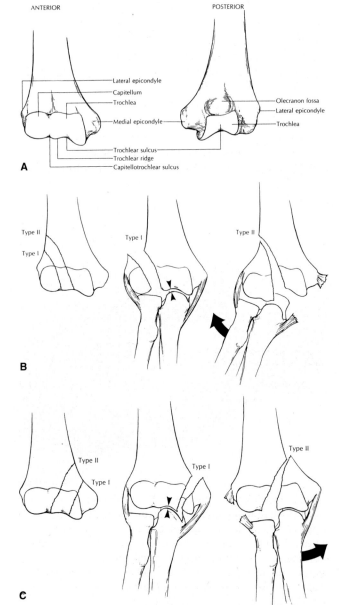

Classification of condylar fractures according to Milch and the location of the common fracture lines seen in Type I and II fractures of the lateral (**B**) and medial (**C**) condyles. (**A**) Anterior view of the anatomy of the distal articular surface of the humerus. The capitellotrochlear sulcus divides the capitellar and trochlear articular surfaces. The lateral trochlear ridge is the key to analyzing humeral condyle fractures. In type I fractures, the lateral trochlear ridge remains with the intact condyle, providing medial to lateral elbow stability. In type II fractures, the lateral trochlear ridge is a part of the fractured condyle, which may allow the radius and ulna to translocate in a medial to lateral direction with respect to the long axis of the humerus. (**B**) Fractures of the *lateral condyle*. In type I fractures, the lateral trochlear ridge remains intact, therefore preventing dislocation of the radius and ulna. In type II fractures, the lateral trochlear ridge is a part of the fractured *lateral condyle*. With capsuloligamentous disruption medially, the radius and ulna may dislocate. (**C**) Fractures of the medial condyle. In type I fractures, the lateral trochlear ridge remains intact to provide medial-to-lateral stability of the radius and ulna. In type II fractures, the lateral trochlear ridge is a part of the fractures medial condyle. With lateral capsuloligamentous disruption, the radius and ulna may dislocate medially on the humerus. (From Rockwood CA Jr, Green DP, Bucholz RW, et al., eds. Rockwood and *Green's Fractures in Adults*, 4th ed vol I. Philadelphia: Lippincott-Raven, 1996:954.)

Treatment

(Jakob, 1975)

Stage I

– Nondisplaced fracture with intact articular surface (<2 mm displaced)
– Ulnohumeral relationship OK
– Milch I or II but incomplete
– Long arm cast placed with weekly radiographs to monitor displacement

Stage II

– Moderately displaced (2–4 mm) with articular extension
– Varus stress views can be performed to visualize displacement
– Arthrogram can be performed to visualize the articular surface
– If displacement present, open reduction percutaneous fixation (2- × 1.6-mm or 2.0-mm K-wires) should be performed

Stage III

– Completely displaced and often rotated posteromedially
– Unstable fracture that cannot be reduced percutaneously
– Interval between brachioradialis and triceps used most commonly
– Kocher (anconeus and ECU) approach may be used as well
– Regardless of approach care should be taken to avoid stripping the posterior aspect of the epicondyle and risk damaging the blood supply
– Arthrogram should be performed following the procedure to confirm articular reduction
– Long arm cast placement for 4 wk followed by removal of K-wire
– Nonunion more common than in any other pediatric elbow fracture
    – Fix all nonunions to prevent late ulnar palsy and deformity
– Malunion
    – Cubitus varus most common in minimally or nondisplaced fractures (rate may be as high as 40%)
    – Cubitus valgus can also occur and is likely due to lateral physeal arrest
– Tardy ulnar palsy
    – Slow progressive ulnar neuritis
    – Occurs secondary to cubitus valgus
    – Late presentation, but can be debilitating
– Physeal closure
    – May result in fishtail deformity due to underdevelopment of the lateral crista of the trochlea
    – Can result in deformity, limb length discrepancy, decreased motion

Recommended Readings

Jakob R, Fowles JV, Rang M, Kassab MT. Observations concerning fractures of the lateral humeral condyle in children. J Bone Joint Surg Br 1975;57(4):430–436.

Song KS, et al. Internal oblique radiographs for diagnosis of nondisplaced or minimally displaced lateral condylar fractures of the humerus in children. J Bone Joint Surg Am 2007;89(1):58–63.

Pediatrics—Medial Epicondyle Fractures

– Peak age 11–12 yr
– 50% associated with elbow dislocations
– Motion is key (7–10 degrees) postinjury regardless of treatment
– 11.5% of all pediatric elbow fractures
– 15%–18% of patients have an incarcerated fracture fragment limiting motion

History and Physical Examination

– Most commonly result from acute injury
    – Direct trauma
    – Avulsion by flexor pronator wad with valgus stress
    – Secondary to dislocation

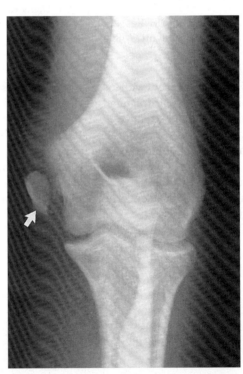

Medial Epicondyle Fracture. AP Elbow. Note that an avulsion fracture of the *medial epicondyle* has occurred (arrow). COMMENT: A similar injury in a developing child or adolescent has been called Little Leaguer's elbow and is usually associated with sports requiring strong throwing motions. (From Yochum TR, Rowe LJ. *Yochum and Rowe's Essentials of Skeletal Radiology*, 3rd Edition. Philadelphia: Lippincott Williams & Wilkins, 2004.)

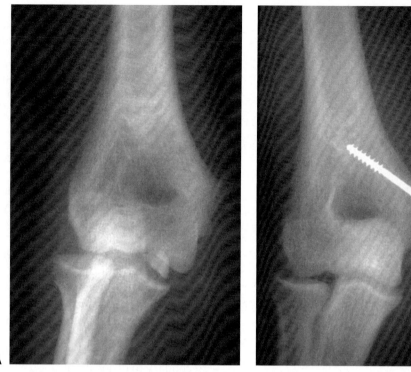

A. Entrapment of fracture fragment in medial epicondylar fracture with posterolateral elbow dislocation. **B.** After fragment extraction, open reduction, and screw fixation. (From Beaty JH, Kasser JR. *Rockwood & Wilkins Fractures in Children*, 7th ed. Philadelphia: Lippincott, Williams & Wilkins, 2010.)

– Patients may present with loss of motion in the setting of an intra-articular fragment
– Painful, swollen extremity
– Elbow instability should be evaluated in cases of dislocation and spontaneous reduction
– AP, lateral, and oblique radiographs should be performed
– Consider CT scan if concerned for intra-articular fragment

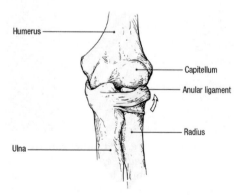

Nursemaid's elbow. Anatomy of injury to elbow joint; interposition of anular ligament between radial head and capitellum. (From LifeART Pediatrics 1, CD-ROM. Baltimore: Lippincott Williams & Wilkins. PED16011)

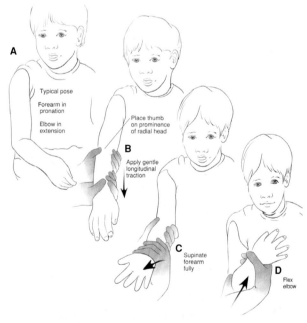

A–D: Supination–flexion maneuver for reduction of radial head subluxation (nursemaid's elbow).

Treatment

– The majority of these fractures are treated successfully nonoperatively (96%) with a long arm posterior

Open Reduction Internal Fixation Indications

– Incarcerated fragment
– Ulnar nerve entrapment
– Gross instability
– Displacement >5 mm
– Thrower's dominant arm

Excision Indications

– Comminution
– Delayed treatment
– Direct medial approach to the fracture site is taken
– Fracture site is cleared and periosteum is removed to expose fracture edges
– Following reduction, guide wire for 4.0 cannulated screw is inserted
– Patient is casted for 1 wk and following removal of cast, ROM is initiated

Complications

– Ulnar nerve dysfunction
    – 10%–16% of patients
    – Increases significantly with incarcerated fragment (50%)
– Unrecognized incarcerated fracture
    – Can result in severe loss of ROM
– Nonunion
    – Can occur in up to 50% of patients with significant displacement
    – Minimal functional implications in low activity children

Pediatrics—Nursemaid's

– Radial head subluxation
– 20% of all elbow injuries in under 10 yr old
– Mechanism is longitudinal traction in pronation; annular ligament gets stretched and caught in radiocapitellar joint
– Average age 2–4 yr
– Key is history of traction
– If positive history, then reduce and only treat if still painful after 24 hr
    – Radiographs should be performed prior to any attempts at manipulation

Reduction Maneuver

– Place thumb on radial head
– Hyperflex elbow in supination and then pronate at end of flexion

Sequelae

– No long- or short-term sequelae except another nursemaid's

Pediatrics—Radial Head and Neck Fractures

– 90% of proximal radius fractures affect the radial neck and proximal physis
– Age 4–14 yr, average 9 yr
– Radial neck fractures represent approximately 1% of pediatric fractures
– Annular ligament is primary stabilizer of proximal radioulnar joint
– Distal two-thirds of radial neck is extracapsular; thus, fracture may not produce fat pad

History and Physical Examination

– Patients may present with swollen extremity with limited ROM
– Palpable or visible effusion may be present
– Localized tenderness may be present at the radial head
– Diagnosis is difficult in minimally verbal patients

Imaging

– AP, lateral, and oblique views of the elbow should be performed

Classification

Chambers Classification

1. Head Displacement
    – Most result from valgus moment secondary to a fall onto outstretched hand
    – Associated with dislocation of elbow (either during reduction or dislocation)
    – Injuries may be Salter-Harris I, II, IV, or metaphyseal
2. Neck Displacement
    – Result from angular or rotational stresses
3. Stress Injuries
    – Result from repetitive stress at the radiocapitellar joint leading to disruption of radial head or radial neck growth

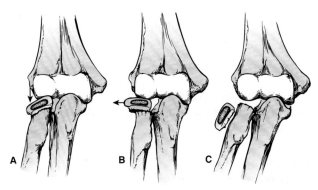

Displacement patterns. The radial head can be angulated **(A)**, translated **(B)**, or completely displaced **(C)**. (From Beaty JH, Kasser JR. *Rockwood & Wilkins Fractures in Children*, 7th ed. Philadelphia: Lippincott, Williams & Wilkins, 2010.)

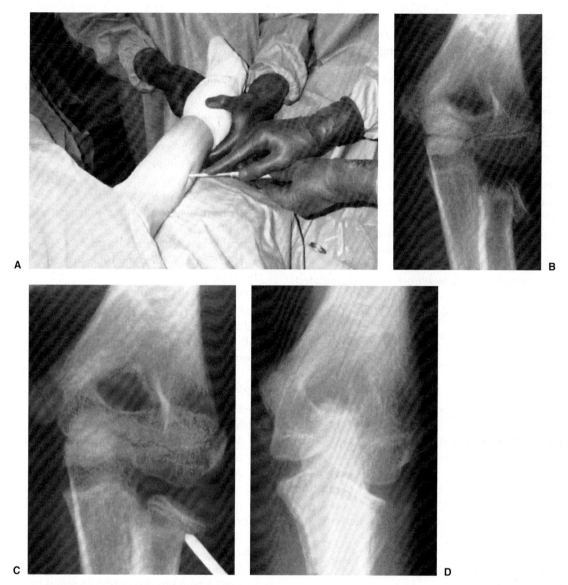

Percutaneous pin reduction. **A.** Image intensification shows the awl inserted next to the olecranon and directed proximally toward the radial head fragment. This is to avoid injury to the posterior interosseous nerve. **B.** Totally displaced valgus injury. **C.** Position of the Steinmann pin during reduction. **D.** Appearance 2 months after surgery. The patient has 60 degrees of supination and pronation with full elbow extension and flexion. (From Beaty JH, Kasser JR. *Rockwood & Wilkins Fractures in Children*, 7th ed. Philadelphia: Lippincott, Williams & Wilkins, 2010.)

The Salter-Harris classification for physeal fractures. The prognosis for growth disturbance worsens from type I through type V.

Treatment
– Dependent on the degree of angulation
– 0–30 degrees of displacement are treated with early immobilization and initiation of ROM
– 30–60 degrees of angulation—Closed reduction should be attempted (up to 45 degrees of angulation may be accepted without significant loss of function)

Techniques for reduction
– Supination allows one to position the radial head for direct contact
– Direct manipulation is then performed while traction is applied to the entire extremity

Operative Techniques
– Percutaneous reduction of the radial head/neck with a Steinman pin can be performed under sterile conditions and fluoroscopic guidance
– Open Reduction

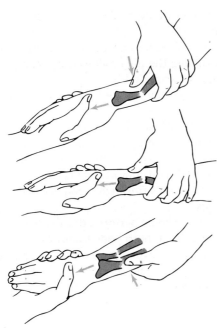

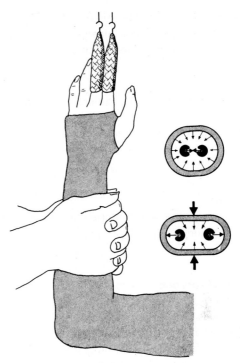

Top: Traction and counteraction of the thumb is used to increase the deformity. *Center:* With traction still maintained, the thumb slips farther distally to correct the angulation. It is best to avoid disrupting the periosteum, but on occasion this is necessary. *Bottom:* Ulnar or radial deviation can also be corrected by traction and thumb pressure. (Redrawn from Weber BG, Brunner C, Freuler F. *Treatment of Fractures in Children and Adolescents.* New York: Springer-Verlag, 1980.)

While the cast hardens, it is pressed together by both hands to form an oval. This increases the width of the interosseus space. Traction should be released gradually while this is done. (Redrawn from Weber BG, Brunner C, Freuler F. *Treatment of Fractures in Children and Adolescents.* New York: Springer-Verlag, 1980.)

- Often an adequate closed reduction provides better outcomes than perfect open reductions in pediatric patients
- Patients develop significant stiffness and loss of motion
- Fixation is performed with 2 small diameter K-wires across the fracture site into the radial head

Complications
- Malreduction
- Loss of motion
- Radial Head overgrowth
- Premature physeal closure
- Nonunion
- Osteonecrosis
- Radioulnar synostosis
- Missed diagnosis

PEDIATRICS—RADIUS AND ULNAR SHAFT FRACTURES

Background
- One of the most common injuries treated by orthopaedists

- Most common injury secondary to backyard trampoline use and second most common fracture secondary to monkey bar use
- When treated appropriately, lead to excellent outcomes, but poor treatment can lead to significant functional deficits
- Risk of injury increases exponentially until the age of 11, for both males and females
- After 11, the rate drops in females and continues to rise in males

History and Present Illness
- Most commonly results from a fall onto an outstretched hand
- Torsional injuries often lead to fractures at the same level
- High-energy trauma may result in some comminution
- Direct blows to the forearm usually lead to fracture of one forearm bone
- Patients present with pain, swelling, and visual deformity
- Forearm compartments may be full leading to significant discomfort
- Detailed neurovascular exam should be performed and documented

- Open fractures should be ruled out quickly
- Rule out any associated injuries as the risk of neurovacular injury increases significantly

Imaging

- AP and lateral forearm radiographs should be performed
- AP, lateral, and oblique views of the wrist and elbow should be performed in patients with pain at the associated joint

Treatment

- Fracture management is dependent on the location of injury, degree of displacement, and age of the patient

Acceptable Reduction

- <6 yr old: 15 degrees of angulation
- <10 yr old: 10 degrees of angulation
    - If >2 yr of growth remaining
        - 20 degrees of angulation in distal 3rd fractures
        - 15 degrees middle third
        - 10 degrees in proximal third
- Up to 100% apposition can be accepted if <1 cm of shortening
- Reduction is accomplished best with appropriate conscious sedation
- Finger traps with weight applied can provide adequate traction for reduction
- Rotation of the forearm should be performed to direct the thumb towards the apex of the fracture
- Distal fractures may require exaggeration of the deformity for adequate reduction
- Casting can be performed in one or two steps
- Appropriate IO molding should be performed to improve maintenance of reduction
- Cast index (Sagittal cast width/coronal width) at the level of the fracture should be ≤0.70
- Long arm cast should be applied to control rotation
- Appropriate supracondylar mold should be applied
- Casts should be univalved or bivalved to decrease risk of postreduction swelling and compartment syndrome

Open Treatment

- Limited to fractures failed closed reductions
- Plate fixation or flexible intramedullary nails are considered
- Closed reduction following by percutaneous insertion of intramedullary rods is the current treatment of choice
- Limits the need for extending open approaches with increased soft tissue stripping and repeat exposures

for later removal of hardware associated with plate fixation
- Single bone fixation can be performed by intramedullary nailing the ulna followed by manipulation of the radius for casting
- Radial nailing can be performed through two approaches
    - Direct lateral insertion proximal to the physis at the site of the first dorsal compartment
    - Dorsally near Lister's tubercle between the secnd and third dorsal compartments
- Ulna nailing is performed distal to the olecranon apophysis
- Plate fixation can be performed through the same approaches as adult both bone fractures
- Plating is accomplished through compression plating with 2.7 locking compression plates to confer adequate stiffness

Outcomes/Complications

- Loss of reduction occurs in 10%–25% of patients leading to need for operative intervention or repeat closed reduction
- Common causes
    - Poor cast placement
    - Patient compliance with cast restrictions
    - Poor molding
- Malunion
    - Can have cosmetic and functional implications
    - Significant malunion can lead to limited supination, pronation and functional outcome
- Refracture
    - Occurs more commonly than with other adolescent fractures
    - Most occur within 6 mo of injury
- Compartment syndrome
    - Less common in isolated closed fractures
    - Should be monitored closely in patients with associated injuries (supracondylar humerus fracture)

Growth Contributions

- Tibia: 60% proximal, 40% distal
- Femur: 30% proximal, 70% distal
- Humerus: 80% proximal, 20% distal
- Radius: 25% proximal, 75% distal
- DR contributes to 75% of longitudinal growth of radius; thus, excellent remodeling potential
- Physis is weaker than ligaments at 12 yr old
- Check stress radiographs in suspected MCL injury
- In proximal tibial metaphyseal fracture, 15% develop valgus deformity due to asymmetric stimulation of medial more than lateral

Pediatric Lower Extremity Injuries

PEDIATRIC PELVIC/ACETABULAR FRACTURES

Pelvic Fractures

Background
- 1%–2% of pediatric orthopaedic injuries
- Associated with high-injury mechanism or athletic activities
- Those associated with high-injury trauma require thorough trauma workup
  - Glasgow coma scale
  - Abdominal exam
  - Genitourinary system

Pediatric vs. Adults
- Lower mortality from pelvic injury
- Higher mortality from associated injuries (abdominal, CNS, etc.)
- High modulus elasticity increases the required force necessary for fracture and associated collateral damage
- Higher rate of lateral compression injuries and decreased risk if increasing pelvic volume.
- Higher incidence of single bone fractures due to the high elasticity and increased flexibility at the SI and pubic symphysis.

Physical Exam
- ABCs (airway, breathing, circulation)
- General ATLS principles
- Secondary survey
  - Morel-Lavallee lesions
  - Urethral injuries
  - Rectal exam to rule out open fracture

Imaging
- AP pelvis
- Inlet (60 degree caudal)
- Outlet (45 degree cephalad)
- Judet
- CT scan

Classification

Open vs. Closed Triradiate Cartilage
- Triradiate closes at 14 in boys and 12 in girls
- Open triradiate: increased risk of low-injury avulsion injuries
- Closed triradiate: increased rate of rami and acetabular fractures

Torode and Zieg Classification
- I. Avulsion injury: ASIS, AIIS, ischial tuberosity

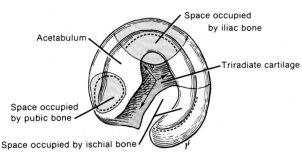

Triradiate-acetabular cartilage complex viewed from the lateral side, showing the sites occupied by the iliac, ischial, and pubic bones. **B.** Normal acetabular cartilage complex of a 1-day-old infant. The ilium, ischium, and pubis have been removed with a curette. The lateral view shows the cup-shaped acetabulum. (From Ponseti IV. Growth and development of the acetabulum in the normal child. Anatomical, histological, and roentgenographic studies. J Bone Joint Surg Am 1978;60(5):575–585, with permission.)

- II. Iliac Wing: Iliac wing fracture or iliac apophysis avulsion
- III. Simple ring: Fracture of pubic ramus and pubic symphysis disruption. Acetabular fracture without ring fracture.
- IV. Fractures producing an unstable segment

Treatment
- Types I and II
  - Treat symptomatically with protected weight bearing (2–4 wk)
  - Physical therapy
  - Return to play at 6 wk
- Type III
  - Weight bearing with crutches or walker as tolerated and pain management in compliant patients
  - Bed to chair restrictions in noncompliant patients
  - If acetabular extension: Non–weight bearing and traction in acute setting if necessary
  - Incongruity of joint with dislocation or triradiate cartilage displacement >2 mm requires evaluation of joint and ORIF
- Type IV
  - Increased risk for genitourinary injury
  - Focus on hemodynamic stability
  - Pelvic binder
  - External fixation
  - Bed rest if ring displacement <2 cm
  - Stabilization with external fixation, SI screw placement, pubic symphysis plating for >2-cm displacement

Acetabular Fractures

Classification
- 6%–17% of pediatric pelvic fractures

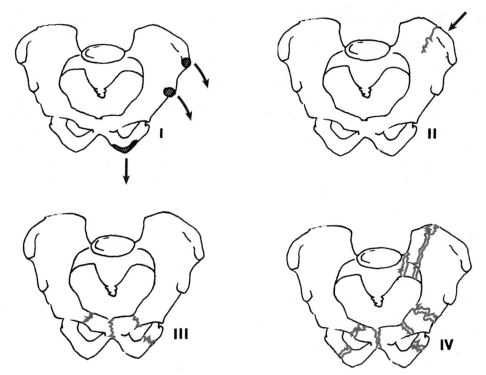

Torode and Zieg classification of pelvic fractures in children: type I, avulsion fractures; type II, iliac wing fractures; type III, simple ring fractures; type IV, ring disruption fractures; transverse with vertical component that exits out obturator foramen. (From Beaty JH, et al. *Rockwood & Wilkins Fractures in Childrens*, 7th ed. Philadelphia: Lippincott, Williams & Wilkins, 2010.)

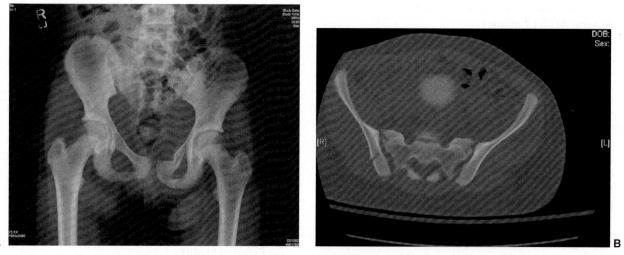

A potentially unstable pelvic fracture with anterior and posterior injury. **A:** The radiograph shows a left superior and inferior rami fractures. **B:** The CT scan shows a minimally displaced fracture adjacent to the SI joint. This is also an example where both CT and plan radiographs can be used to evaluate the injury and help decide on displacement and treatment. This patient was treated nonoperatively with follow-up making sure there was no displacement. (From Beaty JH, et al. *Rockwood & Wilkins Fractures in Children*, 7th ed. Philadelphia: Lippincott, Williams & Wilkins, 2010.)

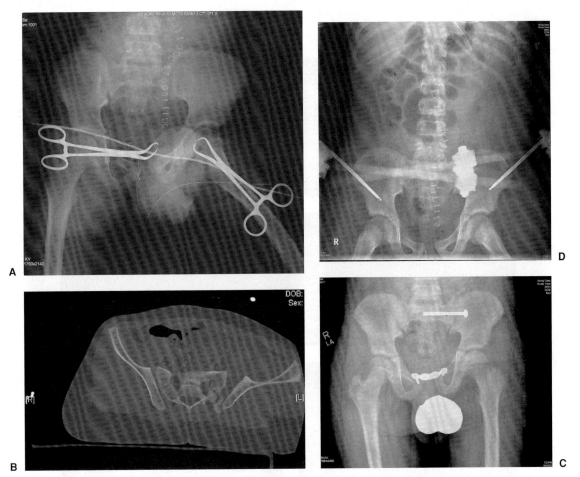

This radiographic series highlights treatment of an unstable pelvic fracture with hemodynamic instability. **A.** Anteroposterior pelvic radiograph of a 12-year-old boy who was a pedestrian hit by a car. There is a wide symphysis and a displaced fracture adjacent to the left SI joint. The towel clips seen on radiograph are to hold a sheet (sling) around the pelvis to help temporarily control hemorrhage. **B.** CT scan showing the displaced posterior injury. **C.** Pelvic radiograph after an anterior external fixation was placed urgently to stabilize the pelvis. This along with resuscitation stabilized the hemodynamic status. **D.** Once the patient was stabilized, the external fixation was converted to anterior internal fixation with a plate on the symphysis pubis and the posterior instability was treated with a SI screw. (From Beaty JH, et al. *Rockwood & Wilkins Fractures in Children*, 7th ed. Philadelphia: Lippincott, Williams & Wilkins, 2010.)

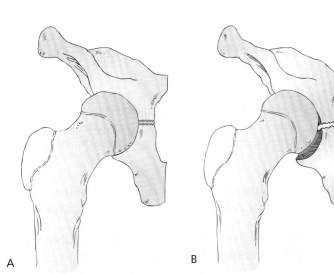

Types of triradiate cartilage fractures. **A.** Normal triradiate cartilage. **B.** Salter-Harris type I fracture. (From Beaty JH, Kasser JR, Skaggs DL, et al. *Rockwood & Wilkins Fractures in Children*, 7th ed. Philadelphia: Lippincott, Williams & Wilkins, 2010.)

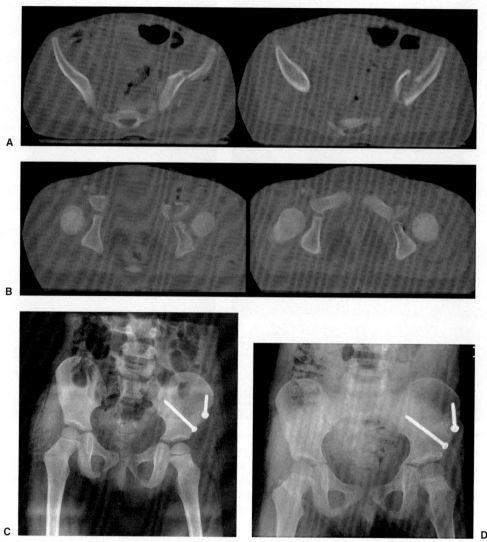

A. CT scan of a 7-year-old with a displaced pelvic wing fracture. **B.** CT scan showing the fracture propagation into the triradiate cartilage. **C.** Anatomic reduction of the triradiate cartilage with open reduction and internal fixation. **D.** Despite anatomic reduction, a medial osseous bar spans the triradiate cartilage. (From Beaty JH, Kasser JR, Skaggs DL, et al. *Rockwood & Wilkins Fractures in Children*, 7th ed. Philadelphia: Lippincott, Williams & Wilkins, 2010.)

- Fractures are usually the result of high-injury mechanisms
- Triradiate cartilage make the acetabulum a stress riser for force transmitted through the femur
- Children <10 yr old at greatest risk for posttraumatic acetabular dysplasia

Classification

Bucholz Classification
- Based on the prognosis of a triradiate cartilage injury
- Type 1: Physeal injury
- Type 2: Triradiate injury with metaphyseal bone fragment
- Type 5: Crushing injury

Watts Classification
- Type 1: Small fragments associated with hip dislocation
- Type 2: Linear fractures associated with pelvic fractures and minimal displacement (stable)
- Type 3: Linear fractures with joint instability
- Type 4: Central fractures due to central hip dislocation

Treatment
- Restoration of hip mechanics and congruity
- Triradiate cartilage alignment to prevent growth disturbances
- Nonoperative treatment if <1 mm displaced (non–weight bearing with crutches for 6–8 wk)

- ORIF if >1 mm displaced. Utilizing the same principles as adult acetabular fixation

Recommended Readings

Bucholz RW, et al. Injury to the acetabular triradiate physeal cartilage. J Bone Joint Surg Am 1982;64(4)L:600–609.
Watts HG. Fractures of the pelvis in children. Orthop Clin North Am 1976;7(3):615–624.

PEDIATRIC SEPTIC HIP

- Represents a surgical emergency in pediatric orthopedic surgery
- Requires early evaluation of patient and prompt intervention

- Care must be taken to rule out secondary causes of hip pain or discomfort
- Late diagnosis and intervention has terrible consequences including articular erosion, osteonecrosis of the proximal femur, sepsis, and poor functional outcomes
- Most commonly result from hematogenous bacterial dissemination

History and Physical Examination

- Patients present with pain, discomfort, and inability to bear weight on the extremity
- They may report previous localized bacterial infection including pneumonia, urinary tract infection, or abrasion
- Fevers (>38.5°C), chills and lethargy may be present

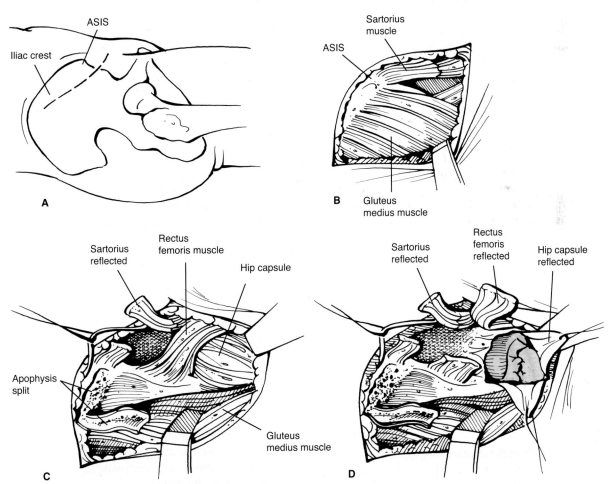

Smith-Petersen anterolateral approach to the hip joint. **A.** Skin incision. Incision is 1 cm below the iliac crest extends just medial to the anterior superior iliac spine. **B.** Skin is retracted, exposing the fascia overlying the anterior superior iliac spine. The interval between the Sartorius and the tensor fascia lata is identifiable by palpation. **C.** The Sartorius is detached from the anterior superior iliac spine. Splitting of the iliac crest apophysis and detachment of the rectus femoris (shown attached to anterior inferior iliac spine) will facilitate exposure of the hip capsule. **D.** The hip capsule is exposed. A T incision is made to reveal the femoral head and neck. (From Beaty JH, Kasser JR. *Rockwood & Wilkins Fractures in Children*, 7th ed. Philadelphia: Lippincott, Williams & Wilkins, 2010.)

- On physical exam, patients report pain with adduction, and internal rotation of the hip
- Patients can be found lying with the extremity flexed, externally, and abducted in an attempt to relax intra-articular pressure caused by the hip effusion

Laboratory Evaluation
- CBC
- Basic
- ESR
- CRP
- Blood cultures
- Lyme

Imaging
- AP and frog-leg pelvis films should be performed to evaluate location of the hip in the acetabulum or signs of effusion
- Ultrasound can be considered to evaluate joint for possible effusion or as part of diagnostic aspiration of the hip if there is high suspicion of infection
- MRI with and without gadolinium contrast provides a valuable means of diagnosing a joint effusion but may require patient sedation with anesthesiology assistance prior to undergoing the procedure

Diagnosis
- Kocher et al. (1999) (retrospectively) and Caird et al. (2006) (prospectively) evaluated clinical and laboratory data regarding patients presenting with signs and symptoms of septic arthritis and provided treatment recommendations for distinguishing septic arthritis from transient synovitis

Kocher Criteria
- Inability to bear weight
- ESR >45
- WBC >12
- Fever >38.5°C
0/4: <0.2%
1/4: 3%
2/4: 40%
3/4: 93.1%
4/4: 99.6

Caird: Included CRP in the evaluation (>2.0)
0/5: 16.9%
1/5: 36.7%
2/5: 62.4%
3/4: 82.6%
4/5: 93.1%
5/5: 97.5%

Treatment
Anterior (Smith-Petersen) Approach to the Hip
- Superficial interval: tensor fasciae latae (TFL: superior gluteal nerve) and sartorius (femoral nerve)

- Deep interval (rectus femoris: femoral nerve and gluteus medius: superior gluteal nerve)
- Expose and retract LFCN
- Avoid medial dissection and femoral vessels
- Expose rectus femoris tendon
- Direct head of the rectus may be taken down to allow improved exposure of the capsule
- Retract tendon medially
- "X"-shaped capsulotomy can be performed to allow for drainage of the joint
- Multiple cultures should be taken including aerobic, anaerobic, fungal, and AFB
- Close wound over Penrose
- Radiographs should be performed to confirm stability of the hip

Organisms
- Most common organisms are dependent on the age and characteristics of the patients
- Neonates should be covered for group B streptococcus, *Staphlyococcus aureus*, and gram-negative bacilli
- Patients in the 1-mo to 3-yr range should be treated for streptococcus pneumoniae, stroptococcus pyogenes
- Patients between 3 yr and adolescence should be evaluated for the above bacteria and the *Haemophilus influenzae* type B vaccine has cut down *H. influenzae* infections significantly
- Adolescents should be evaluated for *S. aureus* and *Neisseria gonorrhoeae*
- Infectious disease consult should be called form antibiotic regimen and time course
- Patients are usually treated with 1–2 wk of directed IV antibiotics followed by an additional 4 wk of oral antibiotics

Complications
- **Risk factors for poor prognosis**
  - Age <6
  - Delay in treatment >4 days
  - *S. aureus*/MRSA
  - Concomitant proximal femur osteonecrosis
  - Sequelae of missed or improperly treated septic arthritis are debilitating
  - Loss of articular cartilage
  - Proximal femur osteonecrosis
  - Acetabular dysplasia
  - Premature closure of the proximal femoral epiphysis or triradiate cartilage
  - Hip subluxation/dislocation
  - Limb length discrepancy

Recommended Readings
Caird MS, et al. Factors distinguishing septic arthritis from transient synovitis of the hip in children. J Bone Joint Surg 2006;88(6):1251–1257.

Kocher MS, et al. Differentiating between septic arthritis and transient synovitis of the hip in children: an evidence-based clinical prediction algorithm. J Bone Joint Surg 1999; 81(12):1662–1670.

PEDIATRIC HIP FRACTURES AND DISLOCATIONS

Background
- <1% of pediatric fractures
- Rare injury
- Result from high-energy accidents or falls
- Often associated with additional injuries including: abdominal trauma, CNS, other extremity injuries
- If associated with low-energy mechanism, metabolic or malignancy should be suspected

History and Physical Exam
- Traumatic
  - May present with the extremity shortened and externally rotated.
  - ABCs (airway, breathing circulation)
  - General ATLS principles
  - Secondary survey
    - GCS
    - Associated injuries
- Low energy
  - Patient may be able to ambulate with discomfort
  - Stress fracture vs. pathologic
  - Full exam including lymph nodes, abdominal exam
- Must rule out septic joint, slipped capital femoral epiphysis, Leg-Calve-Perthes

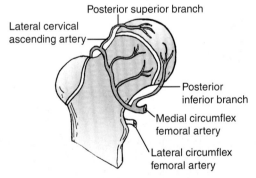

Arterial supply of the proximal femur. The capital femoral epiphysis and physis are supplied by the medial circumflex artery through two retinacular systems: the postero-superior and posteroinferior. The lateral circumflex artery supplies the greater trochanter and the lateral portion of the proximal femoral physis and a small area of the anteromedial metaphysis. (From Beaty JH, Kasser JR, Skaggs DL, et al. *Rockwood & Wilkins Fractures in Children*, 7th ed. Philadelphia: Lippincott, Williams & Wilkins, 2010.)

Imaging
- AP pelvis radiograph: with leg extended and internally rotated as much as patient is comfortable
- AP and cross table lateral hip films
- Consider CT vs. MRI for lesions for pathologic fractures or occult/stress fractures

Classification
Delbet Classification
- Both descriptive and prognostic
- Based on the anatomic location of the fracture
  - Type I: Transphyseal fracture: Through proximal femoral epiphysis (A: dislocation of proximal femoral epiphysis, B: without dislocation)
    - Equal proportion of type A and type B
    - Type B: better prognosis due to increased risk of osteonecrosis and high rate of physeal closure.
    - Improved prognosis with younger patients (<3 yr)
  - Type II: Transcervical fractures: Between physis with extension proximal to intertrochanteric line. Approximately 50% of pediatric fractures (most common)
    - Nondisplaced fractures with better prognosis
    - 28% risk of osteonecrosis
  - Type III: Cervicotrochanteric
    - At or above intertrochanteric line
    - Second most common (25%–30%)
    - Displaced fractures with worse prognosis.
    - Osteonecrosis rate of 18%
    - 25% with premature physeal closure
  - Type IV: Intertrochanteric fractures: Least common
    - Lowest complication rate
    - Osteonecrosis rate of 5%

Treatment
- Anecdotal evidence suggests fracture fixation within 24 hr to decrease risk of osteonecrosis
- Closed reduction can be performed with assistance of a fracture table, but excessive force should not be applied to prevent risk to the vasculature
- Closed reduction can performed in conjunction with capsulotomy to decrease capsular pressure theoretically limiting avascular necrosis.

Fracture Management
- Type I
  - <2 yr old
    - Closed reduction and spica casting if minimally displaced vs. smooth pinning
  - >2 yr old
    - Closed reduction and pinning (2 mm smooth)/spica casting
  - 2–4 yr old
    - Consider closed reduction, spica casting with close follow-up

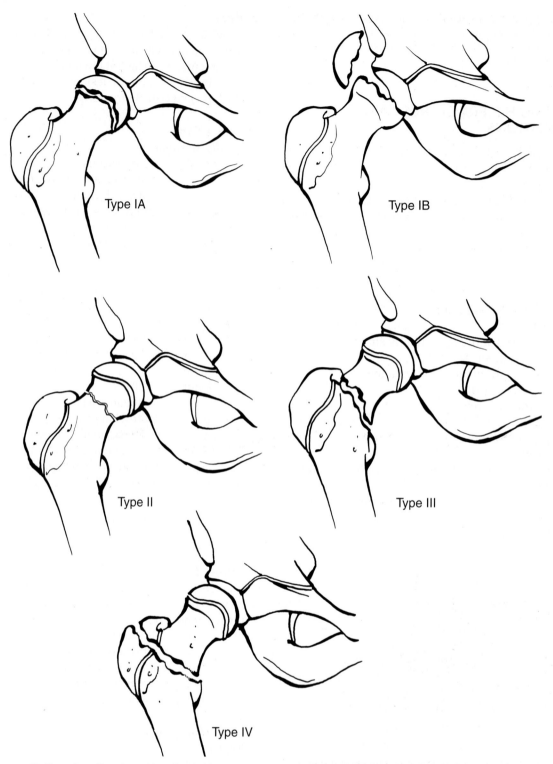

Delbet classification of hip fractures in children. I, transepiphyseal with (IB) or without (IA) dislocation from the acetabulum; II, transcervical; III, cervicotrochanteric; and IV, intertrochanteric. (From Beaty JH, Kasser JR, Skaggs DL, et al. *Rockwood & Wilkins Fractures in Children*, 7th ed. Philadelphia: Lippincott, Williams & Wilkins, 2010.)

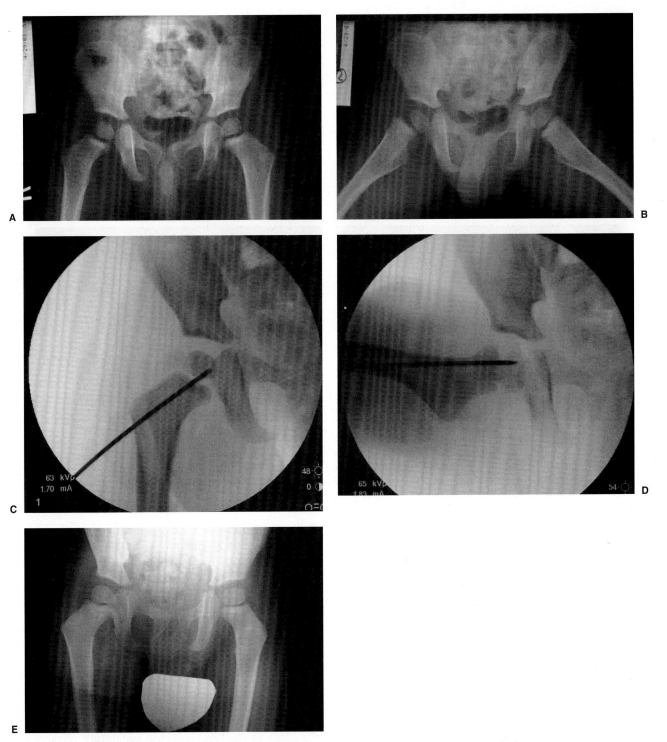

This 2-year-old boy fell on the trampoline and subsequently complained of right hip pain.
A. AP radiographs were not grossly abnormal. **B.** Frog lateral radiograph revealed a
transepiphyseal fracture. **C, D.** Closed reduction in the operating room was stabilized with
a percutaneous pin. **E.** At 8 months, he was asymptomatic and there was no evidence of
ON. (From Beaty JH, Kasser JR, Skaggs DL, et al. *Rockwood & Wilkins Fractures in Children*,
7th ed. Philadelphia: Lippincott, Williams & Wilkins, 2010.)

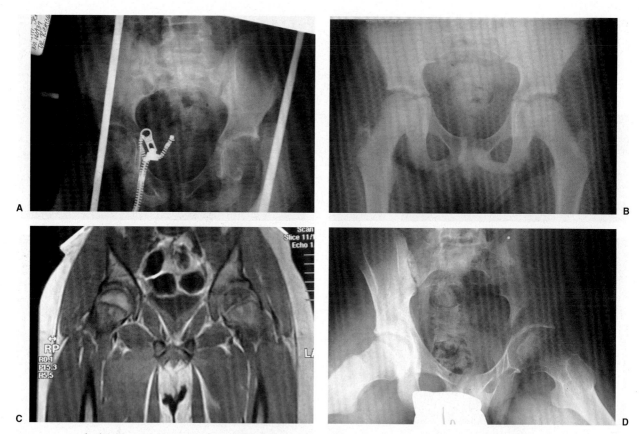

A. An 11-yr-old boy dislocated his left hip while wrestling. **B.** The hip was easily reduced. **C.** After 5 mo, hip pain led to an MRI, which shows ON of the capital femoral epiphysis. **D.** At 10 months after injury, there are typical changes of ON despite non–weight bearing. (From Beaty JH, Kasser JR, Skaggs DL, et al. *Rockwood & Wilkins Fractures in Children*, 7th ed. Philadelphia: Lippincott, Williams & Wilkins, 2010.)

- Type II
  - <5 yr old
    - If undisplaced and stable, consider spica casting with close follow-up
    - Must have <2 mm of cortical translation and <5 degrees of angulation with no malrotation
    - If not, open reduction (Watson-Jones) with 2 or 3 cannulated screws: 4.0 or 4.5 (<8), 6.5 (>8)
- Type III
  - <5 yr old
    - If undisplaced and stable, consider spica casting with close follow-up
  - <10 degrees of angulation
    - If not, open reduction (Watson-Jones) with 2 or 3 cannulated screws: 4.0 or 4.5 (<8), 6.5 (>8)
    - Close follow-up to prevent varus malalignment
- Type IV
  - Closed reduction and spica casting if stable (weekly follow-up)
  - If reduction not maintained, open reduction and pediatric sliding hip screw placement.

Complications
- AVN (Moon et al. 2006)
  - Rate of AVN by Delbet class: I (38%), II (28%), III (18%), IV (5%)
  - AVN present in 25% of displaced vs. 9% undisplaced fractures
  - Increased risk of AVN with each year of age (1.14 times as likely with each year of age)
- Chondrolysis
  - Usually secondary to AVN or hardware perforation
  - Rare
- Premature physeal closure
  - 28% of fractures develop premature physeal closure
  - Limited risk of leg length discrepancy due to low contribution to femoral growth
  - Increased risk with associated avascular necrosis
- Cox vara
  - Risk as high as 30% in fractures
  - Result from nonunion of fractures or loss of reduction in nondisplaced fractures

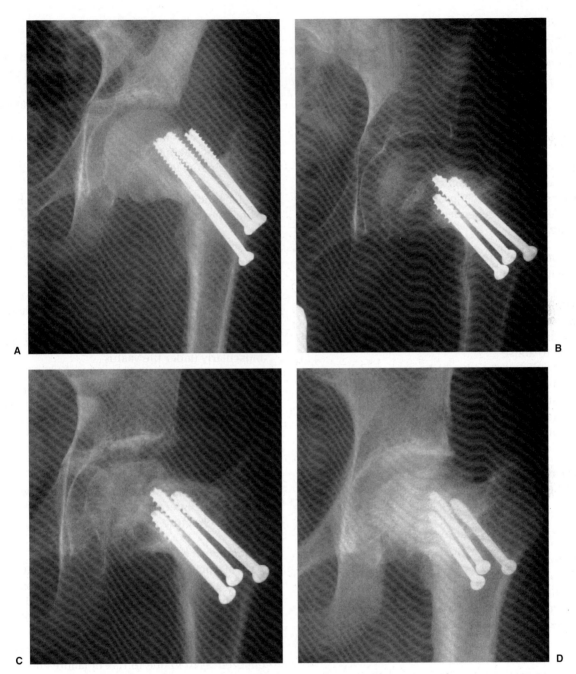

A. A 12-year-old boy with a type III left hip fracture. Poor pin placement and varus malposition are evident. **B.** The fracture united in mild varus after hardware revision. **C.** Fourteen months after injury, collapse of the weight-bearing segment is evident. **D.** Six years after injury, coxa breva and trochanteric overgrowth are seen secondary to osteonecrosis, nonunion, and premature physeal closure. (From Beaty JH, Kasser JR, Skaggs DL, et al. *Rockwood & Wilkins Fractures in Children*, 7th ed. Philadelphia: Lippincott, Williams & Wilkins, 2010.)

- – Diagnosis based on neck shaft angle <120 degrees
- – Consider subtroch valgus osteotomy or trochanteric physeal closure
- – Others
  - – Infection seen in <1% of patients
  - – Nonunion incidence as high as 7%

Recommended Readings

Boardman MJ. Hip fractures in children. J Am Acad Orthop Surg 2009;17(3):162–173.

Forlin E, et al. Complications associated with fracture of the neck of the femur in children. J Pediatr Orthop 1992;12:503–509.

Lam SF. Fractures of the neck of the femur in children. J Bone Joint Surg Am 1971;53-A:1165–1179.

Moon ES, Mehlman CT. Risk factors for avascular necrosis after femoral neck fractures in children: 25 Cincinnati cases and meta-analysis of 360 cases. J Orthop Trauma 2006;20(5):323–329.

PEDIATRIC FEMUR FRACTURES

- Represent 1%–2% of all pediatric fractures
- Age and mechanism of injury are often linked
- May result from low-energy or high-energy mechanism
- Treatment is also dependent on mechanism, age, and fracture

History and Present Illness

- Ambulatory status of patient is essential to mechanism
- Nonambulatory patients are concerning for child abuse
- Approximately 70% of fractures in patients <3 yr old are due to abuse
- High-energy injuries should be evaluated based on ATLS protocols
- Associated injuries should be ruled out as part of primary stabilization of the patient
- Adequate neurovascular examination should be performed and documented

Classification

- Primarily anatomic and descriptive classification

Imaging

- AP and lateral views of the femur should be performed

Treatment by Age

Age <6 mo

- Pavlik harness can be applied
- Stannard (1995) showed adequate alignment at 5 wk in his series of patients treated with pavlik harness

Age <6 yr, <60 LB

- Early spica casting is the treatment of choice
- Acceptable alignment
  - <10 degrees valgus/varus
  - <20 degrees sagittal bowing
  - <2 cm of shortening
  - <30 degrees of malrotation
- Care should be taken to avoid placement of short leg cast and utilization of the lower leg for traction to reduce the fracture as compartment syndrome is a real and severe consequence
- High-energy injuries may require repeat reduction or plating due to excessive shortening or angulation caused by tears of the periosteal sleeve in these injuries (Pollak and Thompson 1994)

Age 6–10 yr

- Flexible intramedullary nailing
- Titanium intramedullary nails are placed percutaneously through limited incisions proximal to the distal femoral physis
- Nail diameter should be 40% of the femoral shaft diameter
- Prior to insertion, rods are bent to allow for better interference fit in the shaft
- End 2 cm from femoral head physis and 1 cm from GT physis
- Eyelet should be 4 mm proximal to physis, bent away from bone to allow ease of removal

Submuscular Plating

- Gaining more popularity
- Can be performed on fracture table
- Following provisional reduction with traction, LC-DCP plate can be utilized and bent to accommodate the bend of the proximal and distal femur
- Through a small distal incision the plate is slide submuscularly under the vastus
- K-wires can be placed distally and proximally once adequate plate position and reduction is performed
- Six cortices should be utilized above and below the fracture

Age >10 yr or >110 LB

External Fixation

- Two to three pins above and below for 12 wk
- 8.5% pin site infection (Aronson)
- Highest refracture rate

Antegrade Intramedullary Nailing

- Lateral trochanter entry nails should be utilized
- Reaming can cause trochlear arrest and coxa valga
- Piriformis starting nails should not be used in adolescent or pediatric patients due to the risk of AVN due to hip vascularity at the starting point
- Flexible intramedullary nails should be avoided in children >110 lb due to risk of failure and loss of reduction

Compression Plating

- Utilized in polytrauma patients to advance rehab

Submuscular Plating

- Successful limited incision technique with low morbidity
- Overgrowth 0.9–1.5 cm in 2–10 yr old
- Weekly radiograph during first 3 wk
- Consider traction and delayed spic in multiply injured patients
- Multiply injured
- High energy (Pollak)
- If short >2 cm

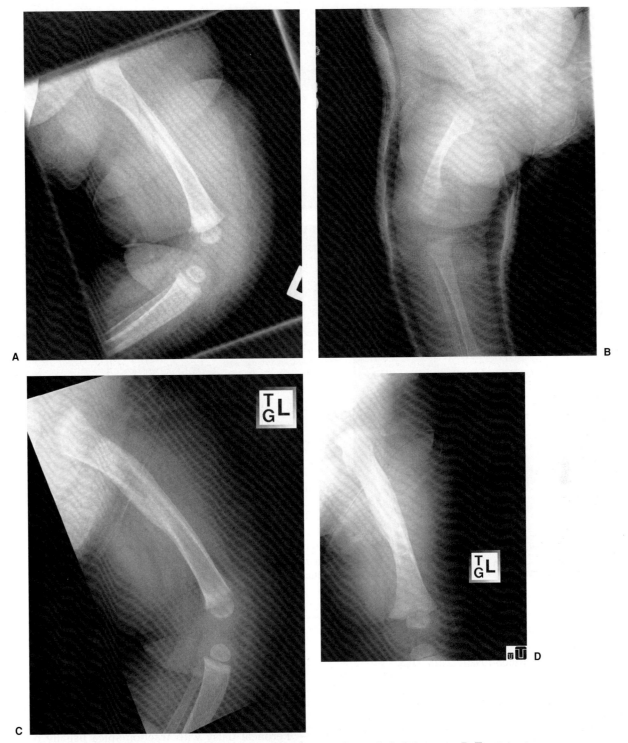

A. This 7-month-old sustained a low-energy spiral femoral shaft fracture. **B.** Treatment was in a spica cast. **C, D.** Excellent healing with abundant callus at only 4 weeks after injury. (From Beaty JH, Kasser JR. *Rockwood & Wilkins Fractures in Children*, 7th ed. Philadelphia: Lippincott, Williams & Wilkins, 2010.)

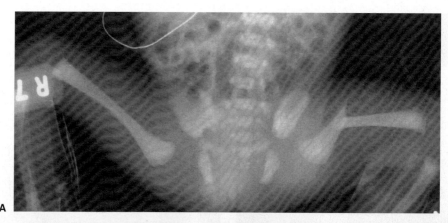

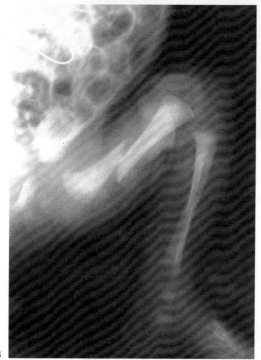

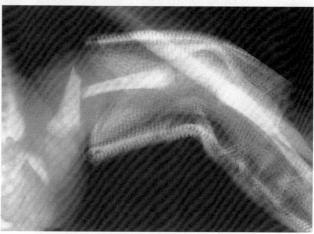

A. This infant had a birth-related left femoral fracture. **B.** An AP splint was used but ended at the fracture site, only increasing the angulation. **C.** A Pavlik harness reduced the fracture by flexing the distal fragment. (From Beaty JH, Kasser JR. *Rockwood & Wilkins Fractures in Children*, 7th ed. Philadelphia: Lippincott, Williams & Wilkins, 2010.)

Recommended Readings

Aronson J, Tursky EA. External fixation of femur fractures in children. J Pediatr Orthop 1992;12(2):157–163.

Beaty JH, Nichols L. Interlocking intramedullary nailing of femoral-shaft fractures in adolescents: preliminary results and complications. J Pediatr Orthop 1994;14(2): 178–183.

Pollack AN, Thompson GH. Spica Cast treatment of femoral shaft fractures in children–the prognostic value of the mechanism of injury. J Trauma 1994;37(2):223–229.

Stannard JP, Wilkins KE. Femur Fractures in infants: a new therapeutic approach. J Pediatr Orthop 1995;15(4):461–466.

Complications

- Leg length discrepancy
  - Most common in 2–10 yr old, with traction (Staheli)
  - 80% of overgrowth in first 18 mo
  - No overgrowth with rigid fixation including flexible nails
  - Average overgrowth 1.5 cm
- Angular deformity
- Rotational deformity rarely with symptoms
  - Rotate hips to check rotation
- Peroneal palsy with traction/spica usually resolves spontaneously
- AVN is a risk with piriformis entry intramedullary nail

DISTAL FEMORAL EPIPHYSEAL FRACTURES

- Uncommon pediatric injury
- Despite the low incidence, the probability of post injury complications and reoperation are as high as 4%–60%

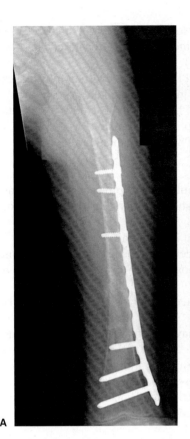
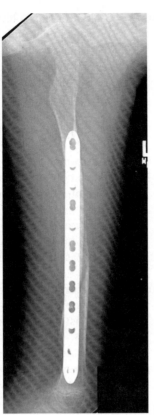

A. This child with an unstable femoral fracture in osteopenic bone was managed with a submuscular locking plate providing alignment and stability. **B.** The lateral bow of the femur may be partially preserved despite a straight plate. (From Beaty JH, Kasser JR. *Rockwood & Wilkins Fractures in Children*, 7th ed. Philadelphia: Lippincott, Williams & Wilkins, 2010.)

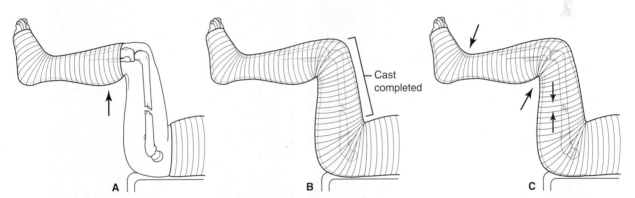

Application of the 90/90 spica and pathogenesis of the resulting problem. **A.** Below-knee cast is applied with the patient is on the spica frame. **B.** Next, traction is applied to the below-knee cast to produce distraction at the fracture site. The remainder of the cast is applied, fixing the relative distance between the leg and the torso. **C.** After the child awakens from general anesthesia, there is a shortening of the femur from muscular contraction which causes the thigh and leg to slip somewhat back into the spica. This causes pressure to occur at the corners of cast (arrows, proximal posterior calf and anterior ankle). (From Mubarak SJ, Frick S, Rathjen K, et al. Volkmann contracture and compartment syndromes after femur fractures in children treated with 90/90 spica casts. J Pediatr Orthop 2006;26(5):570.)

- Most often due to motor vehicle accidents or sports injuries
- Due to immaturity, loading leads to physeal injury rather than ligamentous disruption

History and Present Illness
- Lower extremity
  - Knee effusion
  - Physeal tenderness
  - Deformity may be apparent
  - Neurovascular exam essential in anteriorly or posteriorly displaced injuries

Imaging
- AP, lateral, and oblique knee radiographs
- Stress radiographs differentiate physeal separation from ligamentous injury
- MRI or CT may be essential in patients without apparent radiographic evidence of injury

Classification
- Salter-Harris classification is the most common
  - Salter-Harris I: Separation through the distal femoral physis. May not be detected due to lack of displacement

- Salter-Harris II: Most common injury. Includes physeal injury with metaphyseal extension (Thurston-Hollad fragment)
- Salter-Harris III: Physeal injury with epiphyseal extension. Usually involve the medial condyle
- Salter-Harris IV: Physeal injury includes both metaphyseal and diaphyseal extension
- Salter-Harris V: Physeal crush injury

Treatment
- Most common complication is physeal injury with associated growth disturbance leading to angular deformity
- Anatomic reduction is essential
- If <2 mm of displacement, closed reduction and long leg casting with close follow-up is the treatment of choice
- If >2 mm of displacement, closed reduction can be attempted
- Periosteal sleeve may prevent adequate closed reduction
- Consider closed reduction and percutaneous pinning (3.2-mm smooth wires) vs. cannulated screw (4.0, 4.5, or 6.5 mm partially threaded) placement perpendicular to the fracture line

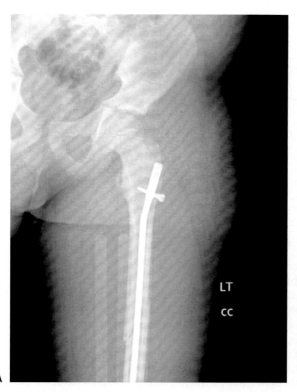 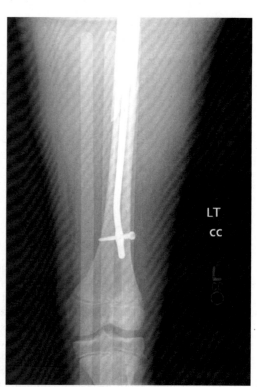

AP (**A**) and lateral (**B**) x-rays immediately after internal fixation of the midshaft femur fracture in a 13-year-old with a pediatric locking nail that permits easy lateral entry and requires minimal reaming of the child's proximal femur. (From Beaty JH, Kasser JR. *Rockwood & Wilkins Fractures in Children*, 7th ed. Philadelphia: Lippincott, Williams & Wilkins, 2010.)

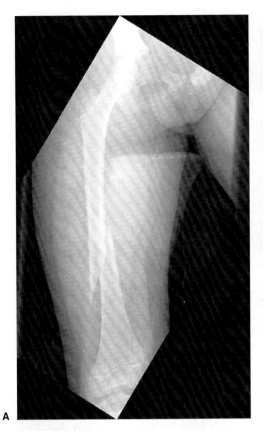

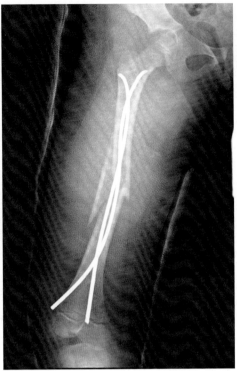

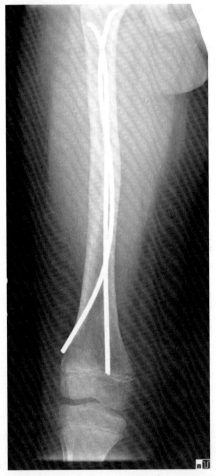

A. This high-energy, midshaft femur fracture was treated with titanium nails. **B.** A large butterfly fragment was dislodged during nail insertion. Because the fracture is now length-unstable, the surgeon wisely chose to protect the child for a few weeks in a one-leg spica cast. **C.** The fracture healed in excellent alignment. Note how the nails have wound around each other. This can make nail removal more difficult. (From Beaty JH, Kasser JR. *Rockwood & Wilkins Fractures in Children*, 7th ed. Philadelphia: Lippincott, Williams & Wilkins, 2010.)

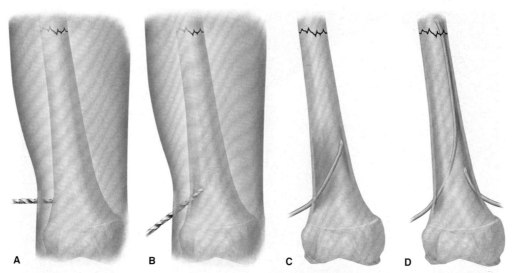

A. Once the incision has been made, the entry point for the nail is identified 2 cm superior to the growth plate at the midpoint of the femur anteroposteriorly. A 4.5-mm drill bit is used to make the starting point. **B.** Once the cortex has been entered the drill is angled obliquely to fashion a tract. **C.** The first nail is inserted until it reaches the fracture line. **D.** Once the first nail has reached the fracture line, the second nail is inserted in the same fashion. (From Beaty JH, Kasser JR. *Rockwood & Wilkins Fractures in Children*, 7th ed. Philadelphia: Lippincott, Williams & Wilkins, 2010.)

- Salter-Harris III and IV injuries will almost always require ORIF to prevent premature physeal closure

Complications
- Growth disturbance
    - Most common complication regardless of displacement (35 %–50% of patients)
    - Increased risk if displaced more than half the shaft diameter
    - High rate of growth at distal femur (1 cm/yr) increase the morbidity associated with this complication
    - Abnormal physeal closure can lead to angular deformity as well

Recommended Readings
Eid AM. Traumatic injuries of the distal femoral physis. A retrospective study on 151 cases. Injury 2002;33:251–255.
Thomson JS. Fractures of the distal femoral epiphyseal plate. J Pediatr Orthop 1995;4;409–415.
Zionts LE. Fractures around the knee in children. J Am Acad Orthop Surg 2002;10(5);345–355.

PEDIATRICS—TIBIAL EMINENCE FRACTURE

- Pediatric injury that occurs secondary to the relative strength of pediatric bone vs. ligamentous attachments
- Occur in children ages 8–14 and common result from rotational lower extremity injuries

- May lead to knee instability due to associated ligamentous injury

History and Physical Examination
- Patients present with swollen pain full extremity
- Effusion/hemarthrosis may be present
- Refusal to bear weight
- Positive Lachman/anterior or posterior draw
- Varus and valgus instability should be assessed

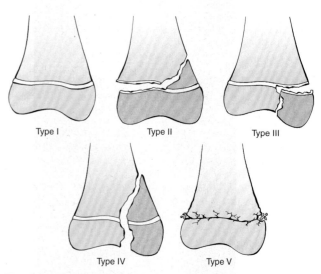

The Salter-Harris classification of fractures involving the distal femoral physis.

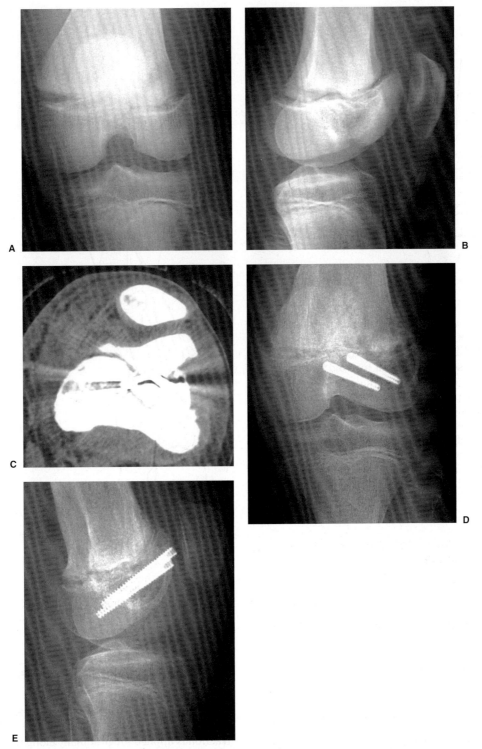

Complex fracture of the distal femur. There is a Salter-Harris type II fracture of the distal femoral physis. In addition, there is an additional coronal plane epiphyseal fracture of the major portion of the lateral femoral condyle, not involving the physis, which was not recognized at the time of initial treatment. The type II component was treated by closed reduction and cross-pinning. The epiphyseal fracture was treated separately and subsequently by open reduction and headless screw fixation. **A.** Initial anteroposterior radiograph showing what appears to be simple Salter-Harris type II fracture of the distal femur. **B.** Lateral radiograph after reduction appears acceptable; however, careful review demonstrates the coronal plane, intra-articular fracture of the lateral condyle. **C.** CT scan demonstrates the epiphyseal fracture of the lateral femoral condyle. **D, E.** Radiograph appearance after healing of the fractures. Patient was asymptomatic and recovered full knee motion. In follow-up, the patient developed symmetric distal physeal closure not requiring further treatment. (From Beaty JH, Kasser JR. *Rockwood & Wilkins Fractures in Children*, 7th ed. Philadelphia: Lippincott, Williams & Wilkins, 2010.)

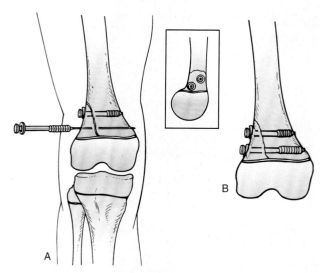

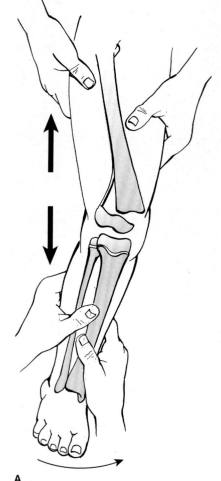

Screw fixation following closed or open reduction of Salter-Harris type II fracture with a large metaphyseal fragment. **A.** When using cannulated screws, place both guidewires before screw placement to avoid rotation of the fragment while drilling or inserting screw. Screw threads should be past the fracture site to enable compression. Washers help increase compression. Screws may be placed anterior and posterior to each other, which is particularly helpful when trying to fit multiple screws in a small metaphyseal fragment. **B.** This form of fixation is locally "rigid," but must be protected with long-leg immobilization or long lever arm.

Imaging

- AP, lateral, and oblique radiographs of the knee may easily diagnose the injury
- CT scan can provide insight into the exact location of the avulsion
- MRI can be utilized to evaluate associated ligamentous injuries and cartilage fragment displacement

Classification

Meyers & McKeever Classification of Tibial Spine Fractures

- I—minimal displacement, incomplete
- II—anterior displacement, posterior hinge
- III—complete separation

Treatment

Types I and II

- Type I and type II injuries are treated by closed with placement of a long leg cast
- Aspiration of the hemarthrosis may improve pain control in these patients, but the hemarthrosis will likely return
- Knee should be placed in 10–30 degrees of flexion and cast should remain in place for 4–6 wk before the initiation of physical therapy

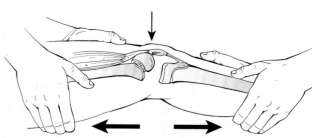

Closed reduction and stabilization of a Salter-Harris type I or II fracture. **A.** With medial or lateral displacement, traction is applied longitudinally along the axis of the deformity to bring the fragments back to length. **B.** For anterior displacement, the reduction can be done with the patient prone or supine. Length is gained first, then a flexion moment is added.

Type III

- ORIF or arthroscopically assisted fixation may be performed
- Care must be taken to rule out meniscal interposition, which can prevent adequate reduction

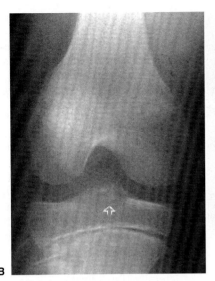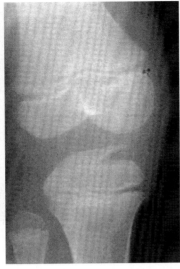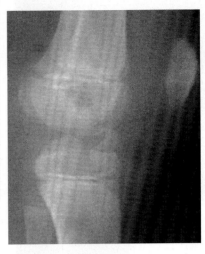

A,B   C

Stages of displacement of tibial spine fractures. **A.** Type 1 fracture, minimal displacement (*open arrow*). **B.** Type 2 fracture, posterior hinge intact. **C.** Type 3 fracture, complete displacement and proximal migration. (From Beaty JH, Kasser JR. *Rockwood & Wilkins Fractures in Children*, 7th ed. Philadelphia: Lippincott, Williams & Wilkins, 2010.)

- Screw fixation can be performed in skeletally mature patients
- Sutures through bone fragment and ACL brought through transepiphyseal drill holes should be performed in immature patients

Ligamentous Injuries
- Ligament–bone junction injuries occur in high energy, slow loading
- Midsubstance ligament injuries occur in low energy, rapid loading
- Due to varying viscoelastic properties

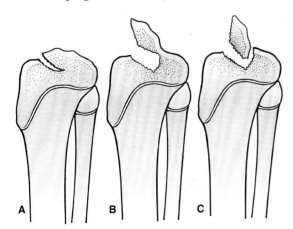

Classification of tibial spine fractures. **A.** Type I, minimal displacement. **B.** Type II, hinged posteriorly. **C.** Type III, complete separation. (From Bucholz RW, Heckman JD, Court-Brown C, et al., eds. *Rockwood and Green's Fractures in Adults*, 6th ed. Philadelphia: Lippincott Williams & Wilkins, 2006.)

- ACL undergoes irreversible plastic deformation before chondroepiphyseal failure
- >50% of patients with healed eminence fractures have residual laxity on examination but no complaints of instability and no pivot shift

Complications
- Most patients report good outcomes
- Loss of extension
- III malunion > impingement at extension in unrecognized
- ACL laxity, but low likelihood of instability or functional limitation

Recommended Readings
Meyers MG, McKeever FM. Fractures of the intercondylar eminence of the tibia. J Bone Joint Surg Am 1970;52(8):1677–1684.
Skak SV, Poulsen TD. Fracture of the proximal metaphysis of the tibia in children. Injury 1987;18(3):149–156.

PEDIATRIC TIBIAL TUBERCLE FRACTURES
- Usually occur in male patients between 12 and 17 yr old (peak 14 yr)
- Another common transitional fracture, which occurs due to relative strength of ligamentous attachments
- Commonly results from jumping or rapid quadriceps contraction

History and Physical Examination
- Present with pain, swelling, and tibial tubercle tenderness

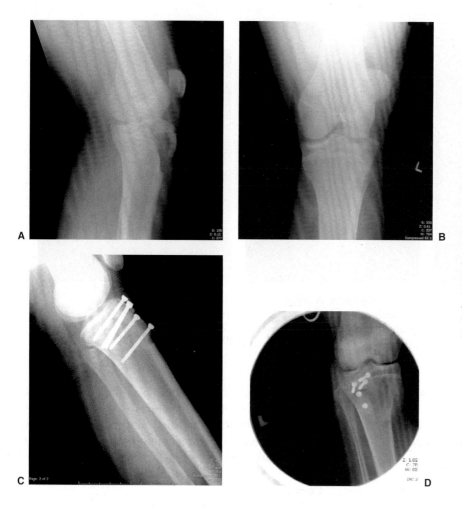

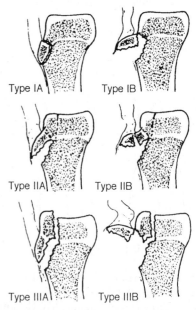

Type III tibial tuberosity avulsion in a 14-year-old girl sustained while landing after a jump in basketball. This is a very common mechanism of injury. **A.** Lateral view at injury. **B.** AP view at injury. **C.** Lateral view following open reduction and internal fixation with cannulated 4.5-mm screws. Note that screws are in compression with threads not crossing the fracture site. There is no significant growth left in this patient, so screw placement relative to the proximal tibial physis was not of concern. **D.** AP view of fixation. Note that screws are placed perpendicular to the plane of the fracture, which often leads to the screws directed laterally. (From Beaty JH, Kasser JR. *Rockwood & Wilkins Fractures in Children*, 7th ed. Philadelphia: Lippincott, Williams & Wilkins, 2010.)

- With increasing severity of injury, ability to perform a straight-leg raise decreases
- May have an effusion/hemarthrosis
- Compartments should be monitored closely as injury to the recurrent branch of the anterior tibial artery can increase CPs in the anterior compartment significantly
- Neurovascular exam should be performed and documented appropriately

Classification and Treatment
Watson Jones Classification as modified by Ogden
- A/B classification separates groups into severity of comminution

Type I—Distal to the junction of the ossification centers
- Able to extend actively
- Cylinder cast if able to fully extend

Type II—At the junction of the ossification centers of the proximal end of the tibia and the tibial tubercle
- Operative intervention is performed to limit further displacement of the fracture

Ogden classification of tibial tuberosity fractures in children. (From Ogden JA. *Skeletal Injury in the Child*, 2nd ed. Philadelphia: WB Saunders, 1990:808.)

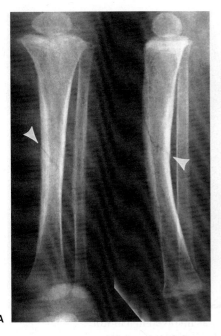
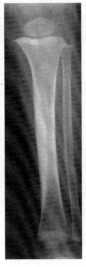

A. Anteroposterior and lateral radiographs of an 18-month-old child who presented with refusal to bear weight on her leg. Note the spiral middle one-third "toddler's" fracture (arrows). **B.** This fracture healed uneventfully after 4 weeks of immobilization in a cast. (From Beaty JH, Kasser JR. *Rockwood & Wilkins Fractures in Children*, 7th ed. Philadelphia: Lippincott, Williams & Wilkins, 2010.)

– Fixation accomplished through a 4.0 cancellous screws perpendicular to the fracture line

Type III—Fracture line extends into the articular surface
– Hemarthrosis is present
– Patella alta may be present
– Meniscal tear and meniscal interposition should be ruled out
– Admit, EHL palsy 3 mo
– Rule out meniscal tear
– Arthrotomy improves visualization of the articular portion of the fracture prior to screw fixation

Outcomes/Complications
– Very good prognosis for functional outcomes and return to activity
– Compartment syndrome should be monitored both pre- and postoperatively
– Bursitis may develop at screw sights necessitating hardware removal
– Growth posterior and anterior arrest leads to recurvatum—rare in >11 yr old

PEDIATRIC TIBIAL SHAFT FRACTURES

Background
– Common pediatric long bone injury
– Third behind radial/ulnar and femoral fractures in frequency
– Majority of fractures occur in the distal third of the tibia
– Child abuse should be ruled out in nonambulatory children with tibial fractures

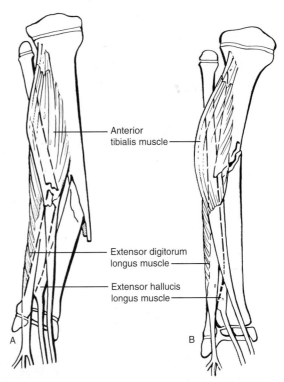

A. Fractures involving the middle third of the tibia and fibula may shift into a valgus alignment due to the activity of the muscles in the anterior and the lateral compartments of the lower leg. **B.** Fracture of the middle tibia without an associated fibular fracture tend to shift into varus due to the force created by the anterior compartment musculature of the lower leg and the tethering effect of the intact fibula.

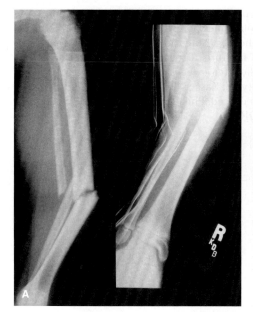 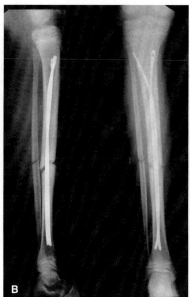 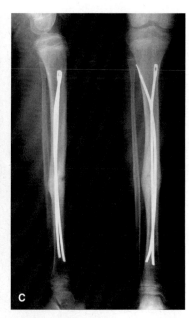

A. Anteroposterior and lateral radiographs of a 12-year-old who was involved in a motor vehicle accident sustaining a grade I open middle one third tibial and fibular fractures. **B.** This injury was treated with intramedullary nail fixation. **C.** At union, the patient has an anatomic alignment and no evidence of a growth disturbance.

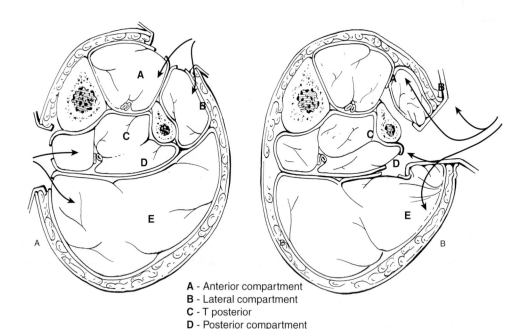

A - Anterior compartment
B - Lateral compartment
C - T posterior
D - Posterior compartment
E - Superficial posterior compartment

A. Decompressive fasciotomies through a two-incision approach. The anterior lateral incision allows decompression of the anterior and lateral compartments. The medial incision allows decompression of the superficial posterior and the deep posterior compartments. **B.** A one-incision decompression fasciotomy can be performed through a lateral approach that allows a dissection of all four compartments.

Mechanism
- Nearly 81% of isolated tibial fractures are secondary to rotational forces
- Tibia fractures with associated fibular fractures are likely secondary to high-energy mechanism

History and Present Illness
- Be aware of associated injuries to the ipsilateral ankle and foot
- Palpate the compartments for signs of CP
- In nonverbal and younger children, increasing pain medication requirements is concerning for compartment syndrome and pressures should be monitored

- Traumatic limping or pain should be concerning for infection (osteomyelitis or septic ankle)

Imaging
- AP and lateral radiographs of the tibia and fibula
- AP and lateral imaging of the knee, and AP, lateral, and oblique views of the ankle should be performed as well
- In atraumatic patients, MRI should be considered to rule out infectious causes

Laboratory
- ESR, CRP, WBC, UA, CXR should be considered in febrile patients, or patients with atraumatic cause of limp.

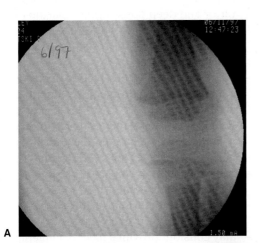
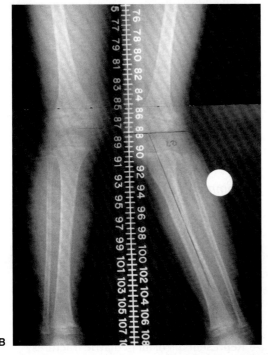
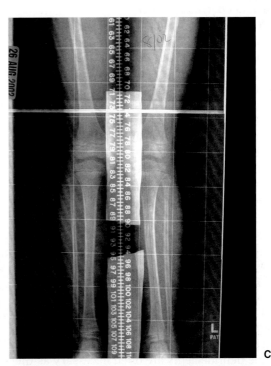

A–C. Anteroposterior radiographs demonstrating the development and subsequent spontaneous correction of post-fracture tibia valga.

Treatment

- Most pediatric tibial shaft fractures are treated with a long leg case following closed reduction
- Isolated tibial shaft fractures with intact fibula are at increased risk of varus malalignment
- Cast positioning should include knee flexion of 30–45 degrees with the foot in neutral position, limiting the risk of equinus contractures
- A slight degree of equinus may be necessary to maintain fracture reduction (20 degree for middle or distal third and 10 degrees for proximal third)
- Acceptable reduction
  - ≤8 yr old
    - May accept translation of the entire shaft
    - ≤10 degrees of varus or ≤ valgus deformity
    - ≤10 degrees of anterior angulation or ≤ of posterior angulation
    - ≤10 mm of shortening
    - ≤5 degrees of rotational malalignment
  - >8 yr old
    - Must have 50% apposition of the shaft
    - ≤5 degrees of varus or valgus deformity
    - ≤5 degrees of sagittal deformity
    - ≤5 mm of shortening
    - ≤5 degrees of rotation malalignment
- Close follow-up should be performed to monitor reduction
- Unstable fractures
- Intramedullary flexible nails
  - Increased frequency of operative treatment for unstable and open injuries
  - Most common treatment is flexible intramedullary titanium or stainless steel nails
  - Intramedullary nails can be inserted in the proximal or distal metaphysis of the tibia in unstable noncomminuted fractures to maintain rotation stability
- External fixation
  - Utilized for comminuted unstable fractures with associated soft tissue injury
  - Allows for closer evaluation of compartments in patients with suspicious exams
  - Must weigh risks of pin tract infection and refracture after frame removal in patients
  - Can be utilized in malunion and nonunions to improve fracture malalignment.
- Open fractures
  - 9% of pediatric tibial fractures
  - Most commonly result from high-energy mechanisms
  - Irrigation and debridement should be performed in a timely manner
  - Multiple debridements are often necessary as the soft tissue injury declares itself.
  - External fixation can be considered as the primary treatment mechanism
  - Consider internal fixation in grade 1 open injuries
  - Free flap or split thickness skin graft may be considered for definitive closure of the wounds

Complications

- Compartment syndrome
- **Please see section on compartment syndrome**
- No. 1 sign in pediatric patients is increasing pain medication requirements
- Diagnosis
  - Direct intracompartmental pressures at the fracture site for the anterior, lateral, superficial posterior and deep posterior compartments.
  - Consider in patients with pressures within 30 mm Hg of their diastolic pressures or absolute pressures >30 mm Hg
  - All casts should be bivalved to decrease the risk of compartment syndrome postreduction
- Cozen's fracture
  - Proximal tibial metaphyseal fractures can result in valgus malalignment regardless of initial angulation
  - Patients present at ages 3–6 yr old
  - Patients may develop late valgus deformity secondary to the trauma
  - Most valgus deformity will resolve without intervention
  - May consider proximal medial hemiepiphysiodesis in older patients with remaining growth
  - Early intervention may lead to recurrence of the deformity
- Malalignment and malrotation
  - Acceptable alignment (discussed above)
  - Malunion and malrotation may lead to significant functional impairment in pediatric patients
  - Corrective osteotomy or talar spatial frame placement can be considered as primary treatment options

Recommended Readings

Beaty JH, Kasser JR. Rockwood and Wilkins Fractures in Children, 7th ed. Philadelphia: Lippincott Williams & Wilkins, 2010.

Mashru RP, et al. Tibial shaft fractures in children and adolescents. J Am Acad Orthop Surg 2005;13(5):345–352.

PEDIATRIC ANKLE FRACTURES

Background

- Represent 5% of all pediatric fractures
- Most commonly occur between the ages of 8 and 15

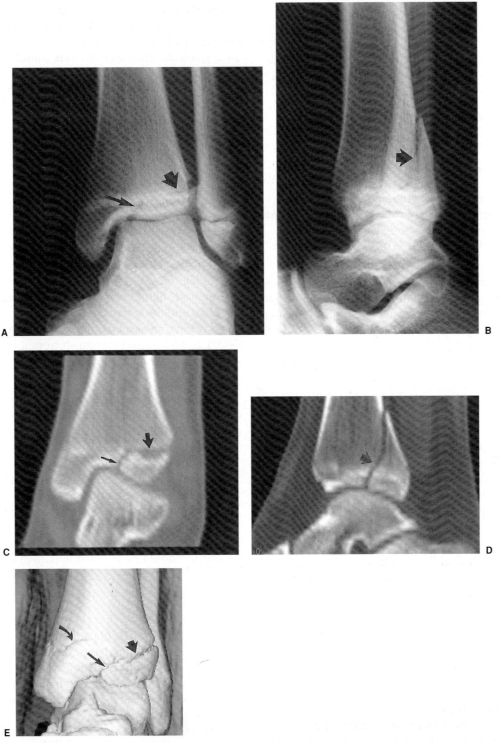

Triplane fracture of the distal tibia. **A.** Frontal radiograph shows fractures through the epiphysis (*thin arrow*) and the lateral physis (*fat arrow*). **B.** Lateral radiograph shows a coronal fracture of the posterior tibia (*arrow*). **C.** Coronal tomographic reconstructed CT image shows the epiphyseal (*thin arrow*) and the physeal (*fat arrow*) fractures. **D.** Sagittal tomographic reconstructed CT image shows the coronal fracture (arrow) actually extends to the joint surface. **E.** Three-dimensional reconstructed CT image shows the epiphyseal fracture (*thin arrow*) and physeal fracture (*fat arrow*) as well as the normal physis medially (*curved arrow*). (From Daffner RH. *Clinical Radiology: The Essentials*, 3rd ed. Philadelphia: Lippincott Williams & Wilkins, 2007.)

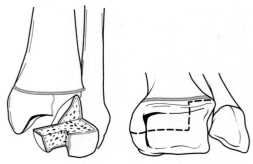

Anatomy of a three-part lateral triplane fracture (left ankle). Note the large epiphyseal fragment with its metaphyseal component and the smaller anterolateral epiphyseal fragment. (From Bucholz RW, Heckman JD, eds. *Rockwood and Green's Fractures in Adults*, 5th ed. Baltimore: Lippincott Williams & Wilkins, 2002.)

– Ligamentous attachments are stronger than physes-the physis in pediatric patients patient them at risk for physeal fractures as a result of low-energy trauma
– Increasing frequency of injuries with increase early sports participation
– Goals of treatment are to achieve adequate reduction, minimize physeal injury, and restore articular congruity

Anatomy
– Distal tibial physis closes at age 15–17 yr
– Closure takes 18 mo
– Physeal closure begins centrally travelling anteromedially, posteromedially, and laterally (CML)
– The anterolateral aspect of the physis is the last portion to close

History and Physical Examination
– Injuries commonly result from low-energy mechanisms including athletics
– Neurovascular exam should be monitored closely
– If part of a polytrauma evaluation, ATLS protocols should be utilized

Imaging
– AP, lateral, and Mortise views of the ankle should be performed for all patients
– Contralateral imaging can be considered in patients with minimal or questionable findings due to open physis
– CT scan provides a valuable diagnostic tool in pediatric ankle fractures
– Articular congruity can be evaluated closely to confirm adequate reduction or need for operative intervention
– Provides valuable information for preoperative planning

Classification
– Salter-Harris classification most commonly utilized
– Type I: Physeal separation
– Type II: Fracture line extends from the physis to the metaphysis
– Type III: Fracture line extends from the physis to the epiphysis
– Type IV: Fracture line passes from the epiphysis to the metaphysic
– Type V: Physeal Crush injury

Specific Pediatric Ankle Fractures: Description/Treatment
Juvenile Tillaux Fracture
– Age 12–14 yr
– Represent 3%–5% of pediatric ankle fractures
– Transitional type ankle fracture
– Supination external rotation mechanism
– Anterior tibiofibular ligament avulses anterolateral tibial epiphysis fragment
– May have an associated distal fibula fracture
– CT is utilized to distinguish from a triplane fracture and evaluate amount of displacement

Treatment
– Nondisplaced fractures are treated with a long leg cast for 4 wk followed by a short leg walking cast for an additional 2 wk
– Fractures with >2 mm of displacement can undergo an attempt at closed reduction under conscious sedation
– >2 mm of displacement on CT or articular step-off warrants open reduction and internal fixation
– Anterolateral approach to the ankle can be taken for reduction of the fragment followed by placement of a 4.0 cannulated screw across the fragment
– Physis should be avoided in patients with remaining growth

Triplane Fracture
– Average age 13
– Account for 5%–7% of pediatric ankle fractures
– Another transitional type fracture in pediatric patients with closing growth plates
– Result from supination external rotation mechanism
– Fracture lines are present in coronal, sagittal, and transverse plane
– Classified as:
  – Two part: Coronal fragment either posteromedial or posterolateral
  – Three part: With anterolateral "Tillaux" fragment, epiphysis, and tibial metaphysis
  – Four part

Treatment
– Closed reduction can be attempted followed by CT scan

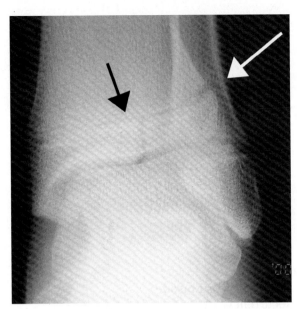

Tillaux fracture of the distal tibia. The medial aspect of the epiphysis is closing. The fracture line runs vertically through the epiphysis (*small arrow*) and then laterally along the open and slightly widened physis (*large arrow*). (From Fleisher GR, Ludwig S, Baskin MN. *Atlas of Pediatric Emergency Medicine*. Philadelphia: Lippincott Williams & Wilkins, 2004.)

- If >2 mm displacement, open reduction should be performed
- Anterolateral approach or anteromedial approach can be utilized depending on the location of the major fracture fragment
- Posterior fragment is captured following reduction with cannulated A to P screw
- Distal screw should be placed in the epiphysis from either medially or laterally with care taken to avoid the physis

Outcomes/Complications
- Growth arrest is most common complication in Salter-Harris III and IV fractures
  - May present as limb length discrepancy or angular deformity
  - Low likelihood in patients who undergo adequate reduction and fixation of their injuries
- Generally patients return to functional without limitation

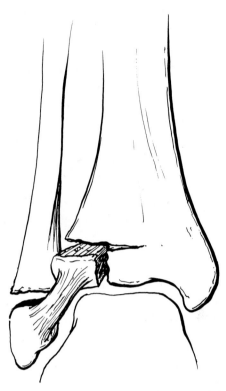

Juvenile Tillaux, Salter-Harris type III fracture of the distal tibial physis; the medial part of the tibial physis is fused.

Recommended Readings
Ertl JP, Barrack RL. Triplane fracture of the distal tibial epiphysis. Long-term follow-up. JBJS Am 1988;70(7):967–976.
Jarvis JG, Miyanji F. The complex triplane fracture: ipsilateral tibial shaft and distal triplane fracture. J Trauma 2001;51(4):714–716.
Pollock FH, et al. The isolated fractures of the ulnar shaft. Treatment without immobilization. J Bone Joint Surg Am 1983;65(3):339–342.

PEDIATRICS—PHYSEAL INJURIES
Background
- 50% incidence of growth arrest in fracture through distal femoral physis due to mammillary processes
- 32% in distal tibia
- 4% in distal radius
- Very low likelihood of growth arrest at the proximal or distal humerus

CHAPTER 5

General/Basic Science

Matthew E. Cunningham, Joseph M. Lane

Alkaptonuria
Amyotrophic Lateral Sclerosis
  (ALS)
  Differential Diagnosis
Anion Gap (AG)
Ankylosing Spondylitis
  (AS)
Antibiotics
  Surgical Prophylaxis
  Dental Prophylaxis for Total Joint Arthroplasty
    (TJA) Patients
  Surgical Treatment(s)
  Bone and Joint Infections
Anticoagulation
  Stop These Preop
  Venous Thromboembolism
  Virchow Triad
  Aspirin
  Warfarin
  Heparin
  Heparinoids
Bisphosphonates
Bone Grafts
  Synthetic
  Allografts
  Autografts
  Demineralized Bone Matrix
  BMP (Bone Morphogenetic Protein)
  Allografts (structural)
C-Reactive Protein (CRP)
Diffuse Idiopathic Skeletal Hhyperostosis (DISH;
  Forestier)
Diabetes Mellitus (DM)
Epidemiology/Study Types
Frostbite
Gentamicin
  Nephrotoxicity
  Ototoxicity
  Dosing

Gout
  Acute Arthritis Episode
  Recurrent Gout
Guillain-Barré
Hemophilia
  Other Causes
Hyperparathyroidism
  Parathyroid Hormone (PTH)
  Calcitonin
  Hyper-PTH
  Osteomalacia
  Differential Diagnosis: Giant Cells
Lyme
Malnutrition
  Lab Studies
  Clinical Determinants
Material Science
  CoCr
  Titanium
  Stainless Steel
Metabolic Bone Diseases
Nerve Conduction Velocity/Electromyography
  (NCV/EMG)
  Nerve Conduction Velocity
    (Surface Electrodes)
  EMG (Intramuscular Electrodes)
Osteoarthritis (OA)
  Risk Factors
  Knee
Osteopetrosis
Osteoporosis
  Workup
  Dual Energy X-Ray Absorptiometry (DEXA)
  World Health Organization (WHO) Criteria
    (Using Z Score)
  Hip Protectors
  Exercise
  Calcium
  Estrogen

Bisphosphonates
PTH
Physiology—Bone
Osteoblasts
Osteoclasts
Osteocalcin (Classical Cross Talk)
RANKL/OPG
Physiology—Cartilage
Zones
Physiology—Muscle
Physiology—Nerve Endings
Meissner Corpuscle
Merkel Cells
Pacinian Corpuscle
Ruffini End Organs
Polio
Polio-Associated Scoliosis (Spine)
Pseudogout (Calcium Pyrophosphate Dihydrate [CPPD])
Renal Osteodystrophy/-Malacia
Rhabdomyolysis (RML)
Treatment
Rheumatoid Arthritis
RA in Hand
Rickets (Osteomalacia)
Vitamin D
Causes
Sarcoidosis
Scurvy
Sensitivity/Specificity
Sensitivity ("See What *Is* There")
Specificity ("See What *Is Not There*")
Positive Predictive Value (PPV)
Negative Predictive Value (NPV)
Precision
Accuracy
Seronegative Arthropathies (Seronegative Spondyloarthropathies)
Sickle Cell
Crisis
Pain: Infarction vs Osteomyelitis
Somatosensory-Evoked Potential (SSEP), EMG
Acetabulum
Spine
Neuromuscular Scoliosis
Statistics
Steroids
National Acute Spinal Cord Injury Studies (NASCIS)
Systemic Lupus Erythematosus (SLE)
Temporal Arteritis
Transfusion
Vancomycin
X-rays and Radiation Doses

Alkaptonuria

(Bullough, 2004)
– Homogentisic acid excess, from HG oxidase deficiency
– Deposits in joints, and can cause chondrocalcinosis
– Classically turns cartilage black (joints, ears, nose); may also affect other tissues (heart valves)
– Progressive joint destruction of spine

Reference

Bullough PG. Orthopaedic Pathology, 4th ed. Philadelphia: Mosby/Elsevier; 2004.

Amyotrophic Lateral Sclerosis (ALS)

(See also Guillain-Barré and Polio)
(Simon et al., 1999)
– Most common adult progressive motor neuron disease
– Affects upper and lower motor neurons (UMN and LMN)
– Denervation leads to atrophy
– Loss of fibers in corticospinal and corticobulbar tracts
– Entirely spares sensory system
– Parasympathetic and ocular motor neurons spared
– Cognition spared
– Presents with insidious asymptomatic weakness
– Atrophy and fasciculations (LMNs), hyperreflexia and spasticity (UMNs)
– Eventually global involvement and becomes symmetric

Reference

Simon RP, et al. Clinical Neurology, 4th ed. Stamford, CT: Appleton & Lange; 1999.

DIFFERENTIAL DIAGNOSIS

– Cervical cord compression leading to weak and atrophic upper extremity (UE) and spastic lower extremity (LE) can be mistaken for ALS
– Median survival 3–5 yr
– No effective treatment exists

Anion Gap (AG)

(Marino, 1998)

$$AG = (Na) - (Cl) - (HCO_3)$$

– Normal AG is 12 mEq/L
– Useful in differential diagnosis of metabolic acidosis
– Indirectly measures plasma (protein) anions, which are not measured directly by routine labs

- Increased AG with metabolic acidosis can be from diabetic ketoacidosis or lactic acidosis (organic acids or chronic renal failure [CRF] accumulation of H+ causing HCO_3 to be lost)
- Normal AG with metabolic acidosis can be from HCO_3 loss via gastrointestinal (GI) or renal (acute) causes (HCO_3 loss is balanced by Cl retention—by physiologic mechanisms to balance charge)

Reference

Marino PL. The ICU Book, 2nd ed. Baltimore: Williams & Wilkins; 1998.

Ankylosing Spondylitis (AS)

(Also see Seronegative Arthropathies and DISH)
(Hochberg et al., 2007)
- Males 20–40
- Begins with bilateral sacroiliitis and progresses to severe deformity
- 90% HLA-B27 positive (North America)
  - Other nationalities with different rates of being positive and different markers (i.e., Japanese HLA-B27 less prevalent)
- For HLA-B27 in general population, they have 10%–25% chance of getting ankylosing spondylitis
  - Positive rates in the at-risk group also differ by nationality (i.e., Native Americans with HLA-B27 (+) have higher rates of AS than all comers).
- Involves annulus, so early x-ray (XR) sign is squaring off of vertebral body leading to marginal syndesmophytes and bamboo spine
- In contrast, diffuse idiopathic skeletal hyperostosis (DISH) involves anterior longitudinal ligament (ALL) so you see nonmarginal syndesmophytes
- Anterior uveitis, conjunctivitis
- Prostatitis
- Pulmonary fibrosis
- Aortic insufficiency
- Plantar fasciitis, Achilles tendonitis, costochondritis (all enthesitis)
- Hips with protrusio lead to heterotopic ossification (HO) in total hip replacement (THR)
- Vertical syndesmophytes
- Chin on chest due to kyphosis at thoracolumbar (TL) and cervicothoracic (CT) junctions
- Limitation of chest wall expansion is most sensitive test for AS (<3 cm)
- MRI—early findings of high signal intensity on anterior corners of vertebral bodies on T2 at TL junction. Caused by inflammation of Sharpey fibers of ALL as they insert
- These correspond to "shiny corners" of vertebral bodies on plain XR lateral

- Severe acute back pain with negative XRs must be admitted for occult fracture with ascending epidural hematoma
- High risk c-spine fracture with minimal trauma
- High risk of delayed neurologic deficit
- Needs more aggressive operative or or nonop immobilization due to osteopenia
- Worse prognosis with younger onset and lower extremity involvement

Reference

Hochberg MC, et al., eds. Rheumatology, 4th ed. Philadelphia: Mosby/Elsevier; 2007.

Antibiotics

(Also see Gentamicin and Vancomycin)
(Levinson and Jawetz, 1998; and citations noted)
- Five basic mechanisms for efficacy
  1. Inhibit cell wall synthesis
     - Penicillins, cephalosporins, vancomycin, bacitracin, aztreonam, imipenem
  2. Increase cell wall permeability
     - Polymyxin, nystatin, amphotericin
  3. Inhibit ribosome function
     - Bacteriostatics (reversibly bind ribosome): tetracycline, chloramphenicol, macrolides (e.g., erythromycin and clindamycin)
     - Bacteriocidals (cause misreading): aminoglycosides (gentamicin, streptomycin, tobramycin, amikacin, neomycin)
  4. Interfere with DNA metabolism
     - Quinolones (DNA gyrase inhibitors—nalidixic acid, ciprofloxacin, ofloxacin, levofloxacin), rifampin, metronidazole
  5. Act as antimetabolites
     - Sulfonamides (Bactrim)

SURGICAL PROPHYLAXIS

Antibiotics given to patients without obvious infection in the surgical field

Organisms: *Staphylococcus aureus*, *S. epidermitis*, aerobic and anaerobic cocci

Antibiotics chosen should be appropriate to cover the above skin flora, or an organism that the patient is known to harbor (e.g., methicillin-resistant *S. aureus* [MRSA])
- Try to use a narrow-spectrum intravenous (IV) agent (Ancef is standard)

Predose antibiotics (up to 1 hr, or "on call") to have the drug *in the tissues* when incision is made

Duration of postop antibiotics is controversial. Standard is 24.

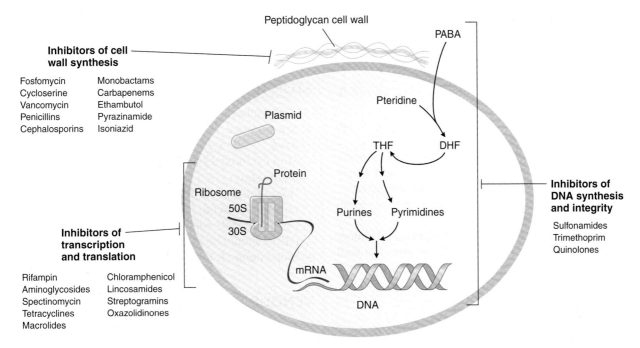

Sites of action of antibacterial drug classes. Antibacterial drug classes can be divided into three general groups. Drugs in one group inhibits pecific enzymes involved in DNA synthesis and integrity: sulfonamides and trimethoprim inhibit the formation or use of folate compounds that are necessary for nucleotide synthesis; quinolones inhibit bacterial type II topoisomerases. Drugs targeting transcription and translation inhibit bacterial processes that mediate RNA and protein synthesis: rifampin inhibits bacterial DNA-dependent RNA polymerase; aminoglycosides, spectinomycin, and tetracyclines inhibit the bacterial 30S ribosomal subunit; macrolides, chloramphenicol, lincosamides, streptogramins, and oxazolidinones inhibit the bacterial 50S ribosomal subunit. A third group of drugs inhibits specific steps in bacterial cell wall synthesis: fosfomycin and cycloserine inhibit early steps in peptidoglycan monomer synthesis; vancomycin binds to peptidoglycan intermediates, inhibiting their polymerization; penicillins, cephalosporins, monobactams, and carbapenems inhibit peptidoglycan cross-linking; ethambutol, pyrazinamide, and isoniazid inhibit processes necessary for synthesis of the cell wall and outer membrane of Mycobacterium tuberculosis. There are several clinically useful antibacterial drugs that do not fit into one of these three groups; one recent example is daptomycin. The development of resistance is a problem for all antibacterial agents. Many bacteria carry plasmids (small, circular segments of DNA) with genes that confer resistance to an antibacterial agent or class of agents. PABA, para-aminobenzoic acid; DHF, dihydrofolate; THF, tetrahydrofolate. From Golan DE, Tashjian AH, Armstrong EJ. Principles of Pharmacology The Pathophysiologic Basis of Drug Therapy, 2nd Edition. Baltimore: Wolters Kluwer Health, 2008 with permission.

DENTAL PROPHYLAXIS FOR TOTAL JOINT ARTHROPLASTY (TJA) PATIENTS

Standard is amoxicillin (500 mg), four pills 2 hr before dental work

No clear requirement for routine prophylaxis has been proven, but certain high bacteremic load procedures within the first 2 years from TJA should be covered (ampicillin)

Others for prophylaxis: malnourished, immunocompromised, rheumatoid arthritis (RA), systemic lupus erythematosus (SLE), diabetes mellitus (DM), prior TJA sepsis, hemophilia, end stage renal disease (ESRD)

References

Levinson W, Jawetz E. *Examination and Board Review: Medical Microbiology and Immunology*, 5th ed. Stamford, CT: Appleton & Lange; 1998.

AAOS guidelines for Antibiotic Prophylaxis for Bacteremia in Patients with Joint Replacements. http://www.aaos.org/about/papers/advistmt/1033.asp retrieved July 1, 2011.

SURGICAL TREATMENT(S)

Open Fractures
Gustilo Classification (1976, 1984)
- Also Veliskakis (1959)

Start with tetanus, iodine dressing to open wound in emergency room (ER)

Grade I (<1 cm, minimal stripping) and grade II (>1 cm, minimal/moderate stripping)
- Classically given first-generation cephalosporin preop and for 48–72 hr postop; may add single dose of aminoglycoside if highly contaminated

Grade III (large open wound, possible tissue loss, extensive periosteal stripping)
- Dual antibiotic therapy (cephalosporin and aminoglycoside) continuously until 72 hr after the final débridement. For barnyard or similarly contaminated wounds add penicillin (PCN)

References
Gustilo RB, Anderson JT. Prevention of infection in the treatment of one thousand and twenty-five open fractures of long bones. *J Bone Joint Surg* 1976; 58A(4):453–458.

Gustilo RB, et al. Problems in the management of type III (severe) open fractures: a new classification of type III open fractures. *J Trauma* 1984; 24(8):742–746.

Veliskakis KP. Primary internal fixation in open fractures of the tibial shaft; the problem of wound healing. *J Bone Joint Surg* 1959; 41B(2):342–354.

BONE AND JOINT INFECTIONS

Get an aspirate prior to starting antibiotics

Prefer sterile cultures from operating room (OR) than by other means

Joint infections should have initial management of arthroscopic or open irrigation and débridement followed by appropriate antibiotic therapy

Provide empiric therapy (against *S. aureus*) until cultures return, or antibiotics to treat a known prior (at the site) or concurrent infection (upper respiratory infection/urinary tract infection [URI/UTI])

Typically duration of treatment is 4–6 wk

Can follow progress with C-reactive protein (CRP) (or erythrocyte sedimentation rate [ESR])

TJA infections are special
- Early infections (<3 mo from surgery) may be salvaged (incision and drainage [I&D]—no removal) and 6 wk IV antibody therapy (ABX). Follow *closely*
- Late infections will require two-stage replantation. Removal of components and placement of antibiotic spacers (vancomycin/gentamicin or vancomycin/tobramycin), IV antibiotics for 6 wk. Possible biopsy of TJA bed with intraop cultures, and if all show no infection, then replant.

Anticoagulation

(HSS experience; and references cited)

STOP THESE PREOP

- Acetylsalicylic acid (ASA; aspirin) 7–10 days
- Nonsteroidal anti-inflammatory drugs (NSAIDS) 4–7 days
- Stop cyclooxygenase (COX) 2s to reduce hypercoagulable state
- Hold biologics for RA preop and start 2 wk postop if no infection seen
- Birth control and hormone replacement therapy (HRT) should be stopped 1 mo prior to surgery
- Stop vitamin E 1 wk prior to surgery

VENOUS THROMBOEMBOLISM

Untreated 1%–3% fatal pulmonary embolisms (PEs) (old data)
- Versus 0.1%–0.2% (newer data)

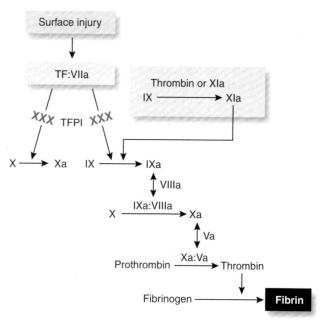

Coagulation cascade. The coagulation cascade is initiated by endothelial injury, which releases tissue factor (TF). The latter combines with activated factor VII (VIIa) to form a complex that activates small amounts of X to Xa and IX to IXa. The complex of IXa with VIIIa further activates X. The complex of Xa with Va then catalyzes the conversion of prothrombin to thrombin, after which fibrin is formed from fibrinogen. TFPI = tissue factor pathway inhibitor From Raphael Rubin, David S. Strayer, Rubin's Pathology: Clinicopathologic Foundations of Medicine, Fifth Edition. Philadelphia: Lippincott Williams & Wilkins, 2008 with permission.

Prophylaxis for deep vein thrombosis (DVT)/PE warranted
- Several options exist
- Typically maintained for 6 wk

VIRCHOW TRIAD

Stasis
Intimal injury
Hypercoagulable state
- Including genetic abnormalities, including factor V-Leiden, deficiencies in protein C or S, etc.

ASPIRIN

Irreversibly binds and inactivates cyclooxygenase (COX 1 and 2) and thus production of thromboxane A_2
Poisons platelets (irreversibly) and prevents their activation
Also has an antiheterotopic ossification effect
Many studies to support/refute benefit of ASA (Westrich et al., 1999; Ryan et al., 2002)
Currently being used for healthy and younger patients status post (s/p) total hip arthroplasty (THA) (325 mg orally [PO] twice daily [BID])

WARFARIN

Inhibits vitamin K metabolism and production of vitamin K–dependent clotting factors (II, VI, IX, X) and endogenous anticoagulants (C and S)
48–72-hour delay from dosing to effect
Follow with prothrombin time (PT) and/or international normalized ratio (INR)
Prophylaxis INR 1.8–2.5
Treatment INR 2.0–3.0
Used for total knee arthroplasty (TKA) and THA patients with comorbidities
Typical doses 2.5–5 mg/day

HEPARIN

Sulfated mucopolysaccharide
Various lengths (average unfractionated is 15 KDa)
Pentasaccharide sequence in heparin chain binds antithrombin-III and activates it (exposes active site)
- Activated AT-III then can deactivate factor Xa (with less clot formation)
Given either subcutaneously (5,000 units BID) or IV by continuous drip
- Subcutaneous has shown in the orthopaedic literature to be less effective than other agents

- IV administration, in the orthopaedic literature, is associated with unacceptably high wound complications (hematoma, hemarthrosis, etc.)
Not extensively used at our institution

HEPARINOIDS

Shorter chain length heparins
- (Lovenox and others)
Mechanism is similar to heparins, but the shorter chain length does not allow activated AT-III to inhibit thrombin
- This results in less severe anticoagulation effect and fewer bleeding complications
Not extensively used at our institution
Typically held for 12–18 hrs postop to prevent bleeding complications and wound problems.

References

Westrich GH, et al. The incidence of venous thromboembolism after total hip arthroplasty: a specific hypotensive epidural anesthesia protocol. *J Arthroplasty* 1999; 14(4):456–463.
Ryan MG, et al. Effect of mechanical compression on the prevalence of proximal deep venous thromboses as assessed by magnetic resonance venography. *J Bone Joint Surg* 2002; 84A(11):1998–2004.

Bisphosphonates

(See also Metabolic Bone Disease and Osteoporosis)
(Lin JT et al., 2003)
- Formerly called diphosphonates
- Analogs of inorganic pyrophosphate where the high-energy P-O-P bond has been modified to the nonhydrolyzable P-C-P bond
- Identity of individual bisphosphonates determined by their structure (the "C")
  - Clinical behaviors *very* different
- Have their desired effect by osteoclast inhibition
Increase bone density
Decrease bone turnover (decrease amount of NTX—a marker of turnover)
Decrease fractures, but may delay healing
  - First generation bisphosphonates were also known to prevent mineralization (hydroxyapatite crystal formation), specifically with etidronate in higher doses
Oral meds include alendronate (Fosamax) in widespread use for antiosteoporosis regimen; typical dosing 70 mg PO every wk, and risedronate is 35 mg PO every wk
IV meds include pamidronate 30 mg IVSS (in 250 mL D5W—given over 2 hr on a Q3mo basis), and Zometa 4 mg IVSS (in 100 mL D5W—given over 30 min on an annual basis)
Bisphosphonates also used for Paget, certain hypercalcemic states, metastatic disease states,

prophylaxis against corticosteroid bone wasting, vertebral body collapse (compression fractures), rickets, osteomalacia, and renal osteodystrophy

Reference

Lin JT, Lane JM. Bisphosphonates. *J Am Acad Orthop Surg.* 2003; 11:1–4.

Bone Grafts

(HSS experience; Browner, 2009; and references cited)

SYNTHETIC

- Calcium phosphate (CaPO$_4$)
  Osteoconductive (scaffold on which bone forms)
  Biodegrades slowly, at a rate between hydroxyapatite (HA) and calcium sulfate
  Slower replacement by normal trabecular bone, lower mechanical strength than HA: e.g., Norian
- Calcium carbonate (CaCO$_3$), and calcium sulfate (CaSO$_4$)
  Both are osteoconductive
  Fastest of the grafts to resorb, but only very limited mechanical strength
- Coralline hydroxyapatite (Interpore)
  CaCO$_3$ converted to CaPO$_4$ by thermoexchange
  Hydroxyapatites are slowest to resorb, but have good osteoconduction
  Limited utility in osteoporotic bone, due to limited remodeling potential

ALLOGRAFTS

- Fresh—high antigenicity
- Fresh frozen
  - Lower antigen
  - Preserves bone morphogenetic proteins (BMPs)
- Freeze dried
  - Much lower antigen
  - No BMP
  - Purely osteoconductive
  - "Croutons"

AUTOGRAFTS

- Bone is necrotic, few living osteoblasts survive transfer
- Cancellous graft first gets layer of new bone on its trabeculae, then later resorbed; most allograft is replaced
- Cortical graft first gets vascular invasion (weakening it for up to years), then bone resorbed in Haversian remodeling, then new bone follows, leaving necrotic intralamellar bone
- These processes are called creeping substitution
- Vascularized graft strong in 1–2 yr versus 4–5 yr for nonvascularized autografts

DEMINERALIZED BONE MATRIX

- Grafton
- Osteoconductive and
- Osteoinductive (induces mesenchymal cells to turn into bone)
- BMP is bonded to cortical matrix, thus demineralization allows BMP release

BMP (BONE MORPHOGENETIC PROTEIN)

- Huge doses of rBMP2, equal to extraction from 200 skeletons
  Number of receptors decreases with highest species
  Not a growth factor. It is a *differentiation* factor
  Collagen 1 sponge as carrier (anterior spinal fusion [ASF] cages)
  Containment of BMP is issue
  Also stimulates remodeling
  Can be complete bone graft substitutes
  Collagen carrier does not work in posterior spine fusions
- A newer agent is BMP-7 (OP-1)
  Published reports with utility in spinal fusions, fracture healing (tibiae)

ALLOGRAFTS (STRUCTURAL)

- Weakest in 6–12 mo
- Takes 18 mo to heal
- 15% nonunion
- 15% infection
- 15% fracture
- Only 3% of allograft is replaced by creeping substitution
  Hornicek (2001)
- 163/945 allograft nonunions (17%)
- 11% without chemo
- 27% with chemo
- Worst nonunion to best
  - Alloarthrodesis (worst)
  - Intercalary
  - Osteoarticular
  - Alloprosthesis (best)

References

Browner BD, et al., eds. Skeletal Trauma, 4th ed. Philadelphia: Saunders/Elsevier; 2009.
Hornicek FJ, et al. Factors affecting nonunion of the allograft-host junction. *Clin Orthop Relat Res* 2001; 382:87–98.

C-Reactive Protein (CRP)

(HSS experience; Gardner, 2003)
- Three to six times normal values in osteoarthritis (OA)
- Normal value, 0.1 mg/dL
- Increasing/increased CRP predicts XR progression of knee OA
- 40 times normal values in RA
- 200 times in septic joint
  - 8-hr doubling time
  - Peaks in 2 days with treatment
  - Back to normal by 7 days with treatment
  - ESR not normal at up to 1 mo
- In RA septic joint, no change in CRP from baseline RA
- In TJA, nine times early in postop, back to normal in 7–10 days
  - No differences seen in revision or primary total joints
  - 100 times normal values in TJA infections

Reference

Gardner GC, Kadel NJ. Ordering and interpreting rheumatological laboratory tests. *J Am Acad Orthop Surg.* 2003; 11: 60–67.

Diffuse Idiopathic Skeletal Hhyperostosis (DISH; Forestier)

(See also Ankylosing Spondylitis)
- Elderly males
- Prevalence 28%
- Associated with lower back pain (LBP)
- Associated with DM and gout
- Flowing ossification along anterolateral aspect of four or more contiguous vertebrae
- No vacuum phenomenon or end plate sclerosis
- Most common in thoracic spine
- Nonmarginal osteophytes because ALL affected
- In contrast, ankylosing spondylitis affects annulus and has marginal osteophytes within border of vertebral bodies
- High risk for HO after THR

Diabetes Mellitus (DM)

(HSS experience; Lieberman, 1996)
- Insulin effects
  Net anabolic effect on muscle
  Helps cells store carbohydrates, fatty acids, amino acids.
  Increases glucose uptake into cells
  Increases glycogen synthesis, amino acid uptake, triglyceride and protein synthesis

- DM estimated at 4.5% of U.S. population
- Broadly categorized by
  Type I (deficient secretion)
  - Typically young
  Type II (target resistance)
    - Typically associated with hypertension (HTN), cholesterol (CHL), coronary artery disease (CAD)
    - Can assess glycemic control with hemoglobin (Hgb) A1C, which is abnormal when >6%
- Classical diagnosis requires fasting glucose >126 mg/dL or glucose challenge with 2-hr residual >200
- Glucose intolerance also seen with steroid use, sepsis, Cushing, acromegaly, pheochromocytoma, etc.
- Osteoporosis associated typically secondary in DM I and primary in DM II
- Thiazide diuretics may cause further renal insulin spilling, and beta-blockers may mask or blunt symptoms of glucose intolerance
- Hospital management
- American Diabetes Assocciation (ADA) diets
- Hold oral DM meds until tolerating POs
- Fasting serum glucose (FSG) checks Q6h with sliding scale
  Sliding scale insulin (SSI): regular (Humulin) subcutaneous
  0–60—4 oz juice and call resident
  60–200—no coverage
  201–250—2 units
  251–300—4 units
  301–350—6 units
  351–400—8 units
  401 and greater—10 units and call resident
- For really low or high obtain chem-10
- Chem-10 is needed because FSG readers tend to be inaccurate at higher glucose values. Prior to aggressively treating a very high FSG value, it is best to have a chem-10 glucose to reassure yourself that the reading is accurate

Reference

Lieberman S. Diabetes mellitus. In Fishman MC, et al., eds. *Medicine*, 4th ed. Philadelphia: Lippincott-Raven Publishers; 1996: 203–216.

Epidemiology/Study Types

(See also Sensitivity/Specificity and Statistics)
(Wright, 2003)
- Prevalence
  - Total number affected at single point in time divided by total number at risk
- Incidence
  - New cases during specified time interval

– Prospective cohort
  a group (cohort) of disease-free subjects is followed over time (prospective) to identify onset of disease. Identifies incidence, helpful in establishing relative risk
– Case series
  Presentation of a disease or condition (case) that occurred in multiple patients (series). Generates speculative associations, which can be further tested by analytical studies
– Case control
  Subjects in the study group (cases) are chosen for the presence of an injury or the presence of a disease. Controls are then chosen from the population with certain variables normalized (age, gender, medical comorbidities) and others allowed to fluctuate (smoking status, weight, occupation) to aid in answering the research question regarding the effect of the non-normalized variables on the condition of interest. The groups are then analyzed to identify associated clinically relevant information. By definition these studies begin with a population and its disease and cannot be evaluated prospectively

Reference

Wright JG, Swiontkowski MF, Heckman JD. Introducing levels of evidence to the Journal. *J Bone Joint Surg* 2003; 85A:1–3.

Frostbite

(Golant, 2008)
– If acute (<24 hr), rapidly warm in 106°F (41°C) for 30 min
– Traditionally, observation with delayed amputation
– Now, triple-phase bone scan to determine salvageable tissue and early operation to provide blood supply to at-risk tissue

Reference

Golant A, Nord RM, Paksima N, Posner MA. Cold exposure injuries to the extremities. *J Am Acad Orthop Surg.* 2008; 16: 704–15.

Gentamicin

(See also Antibiotics and Vancomycin)
(Levinson and Jawetz, 1998)
– Blocks protein synthesis by binding the 30S ribosome and blocks formation of initiation complex; causes mRNA misreading
– Bactericidal versus gram positive, gram negative, and mycobacteria
– Not active in poor oxygen, thus bad for abscesses and anaerobes

– Bactericidal effects are concentration dependent
– Efficacy related to serum peak level (4–8 μg/mL). Alter with dose
– Toxicity related to serum trough (<2 μg/mL). Alter with interval

NEPHROTOXICITY

– 20% of patients will get some amount
– Onset 3–7 days after therapy
– Early
  – Casts
  – Proteinuria
  – Inability to concentrate urine
– Later
  – Rising creatinine
– Worse in elderly, hypovolemia, chronic renal impairment (CRI)
– Usually nonoliguric
– Reversible

OTOTOXICITY

– Dose (peak level) related
– Irreversible loss for high-frequency sounds
– Audiometry needed because these frequencies are above range in normal human conversation

DOSING

– 5–7 mg/kg IV q24hr
– Once-daily dosing gives equal efficacy, less costly, less nephrotoxicity
  To adjust for renal insufficiency with q8hr dosing, give normal first dose, then divide usual dose by serum Cr for the remainder of the day

Gout

(See also Pseudogout)
(Hochberg et al., 2007)
– Abnormal nucleic acid, purine metabolism with overproducers (10%) or undersecretors (90%) of uric acid
– Monosodium urate crystals
– Thin, tapered, negative birefringent crystals
– Negative means yellow in crystals that are parallel to light
– Podagra (gout in big toe)
  – 50%–75% of first attack in first metatarsophalangeal (MTP) joint
– Tophi from chronic gout
  – Destructive bony lesions away from articular surface
– Giant inflammatory reaction
– Three forms—asymptomatic, acute, recurrent

ACUTE ARTHRITIS EPISODE

- Attack precipitated by dehydration, surgery, binge eating, ethanol (EtOH) binge, chemotherapy for round cell malignancies (i.e., leukemia)
- Usually subsides over several days, but prompt treatment can abort attack
- Serum uric acid level is normal in 30% with acute gout and should not be manipulated until attack resolved
- NSAIDs are drug of choice
  - Easy and lower toxicity profile
  - Clinical response in 12–24 hr
  - High dose, then taper
  - Indocin 50 mg q6h for 2 days, then q8h for 3 days, then 25 mg q8h for 3 days
- Colchicine for acute attack
  - Limits production of inflammatory mediators
  - Most effective within 12–24 hr of attack and response in 6–12 hr
  - 0.6 mg PO q1–2hr or 1.2 mg PO q2hr until symptoms abate, GI toxicity develops, or maximum dose of 6 mg in 24-hr period is reached. Then no more than 1.2 mg/day thereafter with that attack
- IV colchicine has less GI toxicity and is faster but can cause severe myelosuppression and IV infiltration can cause tissue necrosis
- Intra-articular or PO steroids if NSAID and colchicine contraindicated
  - Prednisone 20–50 mg PO QD then rapid taper

RECURRENT GOUT

- Avoid ASA, diuretics, EtOH, sweetbreads, anchovies, sardines, livers, and kidneys
- Prophylaxis with colchicine 0.6 mg PO QD to BID is usually okay but watch for GI toxicity
- Serum uric acid level should be manipulated if arthritis frequent, renal damage, or serum or urine uric acid levels consistently elevated
- Maintenance colchicine 0.6 mg BID should be given a few days before manipulation to prevent acute attack
- Discontinue colchicine if no attacks after normal uric level maintained for 6–8 wk
- Allopurinol—inhibits xanthine oxidase
  - To prevent/treat tophaceous gout
  - Never for acute gout
  - 300 PO QD but lower by 100 mg every 2–4 wk to maintain minimum dose that keeps uric acid level normal
  - Watch for hypersensitivity
- Probenecid—blocks renal tubular reabsorption of urate
  - Get 24-hr Cr clearance and urine urate before starting because ineffective if glomerular filtration rate (GFR) <50 mL/min and high urine urate can cause stones
  - Start 500 mg PO QD and raise 500 mg every wk until normal urate levels or urine urate >800 mg/day. Maximum dose 3 g daily. Most need 1–1.5 g/day in 2–3 divided doses.
- Salicylates and probenecid antagonistic

Guillain-Barré

(See also Amyotrophic Lateral Sclerosis and Polio)
(Simon et al., 1999)
- Acute autoimmune demyelinating polyradiculoneuropathy
- Seen after infections, inoculations, surgery
- Usually proximal symmetric weakness begins in legs, then arms, then face
- Can affect breathing and swallowing
- Distal dysesthesias
- Radicular or neuropathic pain
- Autonomic disturbances
- Rule out infectious and metabolic neuropathies—porphyria, diphtheria, botulism, heavy metals, tick
- Pyramidal signs, markedly asymptomatic motor deficit, sharp sensory level, and early sphincter involvement suggest focal cord lesion
- Most (70%–75%) recover, but takes months
- 10%–20% with residual disability
- 5% mortality (respiratory)
- Steroids ineffective
- Plasmapheresis helps but only if within few days of onset and is in setting of shock to cardiovascular system
- Intravenous immunoglobulin (IVIG) is best
- Consider intensive care unit (ICU), intubation
- Crystalloid volume or pressors for autonomic dysfunction
- 3% get relapses similar to initial symptoms

Hemophilia

(Gordeuk, 1996a)

A—X-linked recessive (XR), decreased VIII (estimated 10,000 in U.S.)
vWD (Von Willebrand disease)—autosomal dominant/recessive (AD/R), abnormal VIII and platelet function
B—XR, decreased IX, Christmas disease
- Males
- Hemarthrosis
- Intramuscular bleeding
- Blood cysts—pseudotumor

- Squaring patella and condyles
  - Wide notch
- Before orthopaedic surgery, get factor level 100% preop and maintain >50% for 10 days postop
- Antibody inhibitors are relative contraindications to surgery; treat with large amounts of VIII
- Synovectomy for recurrent synovitis
- P32 radioisotope injections for ablation synovectomy

OTHER CAUSES

- Von Willebrand disease
  - Autosomal dominant inheritance, reduced amounts of factor VIII antigen or factor VIII coagulation activity
  - Von Willebrand factor (vWF) is a protein that mediates platelet adhesion and is deficient or defective
  - Another function of vWF is to bind to and protect activated factor VIII
  - Diagnosed by abnormal values of vWF, or combinations of prolonged prothrombin time (PTT), sensitivity to ASA, diminished factor VIII, etc.

References

Gordeuk V. Abnormalities of hemostasis. In Fishman MC, et al., eds. *Medicine*, 4th ed. Philadelphia: Lippincott-Raven Publishers; 1996a: 355–363.
Gordeuk V, Anemia. In Fishman MC, et al., eds. *Medicine*, 4th ed. Philadelphia: Lippincott-Raven Publishers; 1996b: 341–353.

Hyperparathyroidism

(See also Metabolic Bone Diseases)
(Buckwalter et al., 2000)

PARATHYROID HORMONE (PTH)

- Releases Ca^{++} and PO_4 from bone by direct effects on oblasts, indirect effects on osteoclasts
- Retains Ca^{++} and excretes PO_4 from kidney (this is net effect)
- Increased synthesis of 1,25-vitD
- Stimulated by low Ca^{++}
- Made in parathyroid chief cells

CALCITONIN

- Stimulatess osteoblasts, inhibits osteoclasts and bone resorption
- Decreased calcium levels via effects on bone, kidney, GI tract
- From parafollicular cells of thyroid

HYPER-PTH

- Sixth decade, F >M (3:1)
- Solitary parathyroid adenoma most common cause (80%)
- High Ca^{++}, low PO_4 (typically no symptoms)
- Poor mineralization due to low PO_4
  - Primary: high PTH, high Ca^{++}
  - Secondary: high PTH, low Ca^{++}
    - Associated with osteomalacia
  - Tertiary: high PTH, high Ca^{++}

OSTEOMALACIA

- Decreased 25(OH) vitamin D
- Increased alkaline phosphatase
- Decreased urinary Ca^{++}

DIFFERENTIAL DIAGNOSIS: GIANT CELLS

- Hyper-PTH—surrounding red blood cells (RBCs)
- Giant cell tumor (GCT)—evenly distributed
- Tuberculosis (TB)—giants at periphery
- sarcoid, any granulomatous disease, necrosis
- Osteopenia, subperiosteal bone loss
- Salt-pepper skull
- Osteitis fibrosa cystica (fibrous replacement of marrow)
- Multiple destructive metaphyseal lytic lesions, or lytic nonmetaphyseal lesions (brown tumors)
- Subperiosteal bone resorption in radial aspect of middle phalanges is pathognomonic. Also common are tuft erosions
- Rugger jersey spine
- High Ca^{++} leads to kidney stones (20%)
- Chondrocalcinosis
- Metastatic calcifications
- Peptic ulcer disease, pancreatitis
- Treatment: parathyroidectomy versus medical management (hydration and low Ca^{++} diet) with consideration of osteoclast inhibiting agents (estrogen and bisphosphonates)

Reference

Buckwalter JA, et al., eds. *Orthopaedic Basic Science: Biology and Biomechanics of the musculoskeletal System*, 2nd ed. Rosemont, IL: AAOS Press; 2000.

Lyme

(Levinson and Jawetz, 1998)
- Gram negative *Borrelia burgdorferi*
- *Ixodes dammini* and *I. pacificus* tick transport the bacteria between humans and their animal reservoirs: deer and rodents

- Targets nervous system, joints (medial compartment of knee), heart
- Stage 1 is the early localized infection. The skin lesion erythema migrans occurs within 3–32 days
- Stage 2 is the early disseminated infection stage. It is the first stage with musculoskeletal involvement. Transient migratory arthralgias, swelling
- Stage 3 is the persistent infection phase. This stage is characterized by persistent and migratory arthritis of the body's large joints.
- Takes 2–6 wk to seroconvert
- Takes 2–4 mo for true arthritis to develop (infection in summer but seen by MD in October and November)
- Oral amoxicillin for 10–30 days for stage 1
- Doxycycline or amoxicillin for 30 days for stage 2. Ceftriaxone is needed for nonresponders
- Intravenous antibiotics for neurologic involvement
- For severe cases, intra-articular steroid or synovectomy can be performed

Malnutrition

(See also Metabolic Bone Diseases)
(HSS experience)

LAB STUDIES

- Albumin <3.5 g/dL
- Serum transferrin <150 μg/dL
- Absolute lymphocyte count <800/mL
- 24-hr urine creatinine excretion of <10.5 mg in men and <5.8 mg in women associated with negative nitrogen balance indicates malnutrition
- Also with decreased sodium clearance
- There is a formal association of malnutrition and osteomalacia
- Also seen secondary to bariatric surgery, sprue, Crohn disease, alcoholism, etc.
- Therefore osteomalacia requires a full workup (4.7% of osteomalacia patients have sprue, a reversible nutritional condition)

CLINICAL DETERMINANTS

- Triceps skin fold
- Midarm muscle circumference
- Body mass index: weight (in kg)/height^2 (in meters), with normal 20–25 kg/m^2

Material Science

(HSS experience; Buckwalter et al., 2000)
Young's modulus of elasticity in decreasing order (higher = more brittle)

- Ceramic
- Cobalt-chromium (CoCr)
- Stainless steel (20 times bone)
- Titanium (10 times bone)
- Cortical bone
- Polymethylmethacrylate (PMMA)
- Polyethylene
- Cancellous bone

CoCr

- Less metal debris
- Stiffer, higher modulus

TITANIUM

- Poor wear resistance, more debris
- Higher notch sensitivity
- Surface hardness of titanium is low, can be scratched, increased wear and debris, lysis, loosening in TJA
- Low modulus
- More biocompatible (forms oxide coat)

STAINLESS STEEL

- Most likely to corrode
- Worst galvanic corrosion between steel and CoCrMo (cobalt/chrome/molybdenum alloy)
- Stress = force/surface area
- Strain = change in length/original length
- Young's modulus of elasticity—E = stress/strain. It is key in load-sharing capacity. Linear in elastic range of material
- Hooke's law—stress-strain relationship is linear (below the yield point)
- Yield point—where linear (elastic) behavior changes to nonlinear (plastic) behavior
- Ultimate strength—maximum strength obtained by material = highest point on stress/strain curve
- Toughness—ability of material to absorb energy prior to failure = strain energy = area under stress/strain curve
- Brittle materials only undergo elastic deformation (return to original shape)
- Ductile materials undergo a large amount of plastic deformation prior to failure
- Viscoelastic materials (i.e., bone) exhibit stress-strain behavior that is rate-load dependent (modulus increases with increases in rate). Faster rates cause bone to behave more elastically
- Bending rigidity/stiffness of cylinder is related to 4th power of radius
- Bending rigidity/stiffness of plate is related to 3rd power of thickness

- Stiffness (resistance to load) is related to geometry, area, and modulus
- Cannot measure stress within bone cortex because stress relieved as bone is cut to measure
- Loads—axial, bend, torsion
- Fatigue = cyclic stress versus number of cycles
- Load shared proportional to stiffness like flowing water
- Torsion leads to spiral fracture because bone fails first in tension and tension forces are 45 degrees to axis of torsion
- Torque at a point inside cylinder is related to radius and moment, i.e., $T = (M)(r)/I$
- Polar moment is proportional to 4th power of radius
- Maximal torque is oriented 45 degrees to long axis of cylinder

Metabolic Bone Diseases

(Buckwalter et al., 2000)
(See also Physiology—Bone and topics mentioned below)
- Multiple broad categories of etiology for altered hormonal control, poor bone production/growth, deficient mineralization, or insufficient maintenance (remodeling)
- Too numerous to concisely and completely summarize. Here are some of the highlights
- Matrix disturbances
  Genetic
  - Osteogenesis imperfecta AD/AR defect in type I collagen
  Nutritional
  - See Scurvy: deficiency of vitamin C, defect in collagen synthesis (secondary to an inability to hydroxylate proline, a required collagen synthesis step).
  - See Malnutrition
- Mineral homeostasis disturbances
  See Rickets, Osteomalacia
  Primary renal, GI disturbance (ESRD, sprue); see Renal Osteodystrophy
  - Hypophosphatasia inborn error of tissue nonspecific alkaline phosphatase
  - Hypophosphatemic rickets (vitamin D-resistant) inborn error in phosphate transport (renal most likely)
  Signaling dysregulation (PTH, vitamin D, calcitonin, estrogen, corticosteroids)
  - See Hyperparathyroidism
  - Menopause
  - Corticosteroid osteodystrophy through decreasing absorption and decreasing collagen synthesis
  - Hereditary vitamin D–dependent rickets—deficiency of a vitamin D receptor

- Albright hereditary osteodystrophy has an absence of renal PTH effect
- Mixed
  Osteopenia – relative decrease in bone amount
  "Osteoporosis" – quantified definition of bone loss
  "Osteopetrosis" – altered bone turnover (osteoclast defect) resulting in increased bone mass (poor quality)
- Nutritional syndromes
  See Malnutrition
  - Vitamin D intoxication
  - Vitamin D–deficiency rickets
  - Calcium-deficiency rickets
  - Phosphate-deficiency rickets
  - Iatrogenic
    - Ca^{++} chelators (diet: spinach)
    - Aluminum-containing antacids
  Sprue
  Postgastrectomy/short bowel syndrome
  Liver/biliary disease
  Inflammatory bowel disease
- Others
  Malignancy
  Anticonvulsants (phenytoin)
  Heavy metal intoxication
  Hypercalcemic: including hyper-PTH, hyperthyroid, sarcoid, milk alkali syndrome, myeloma, metastatic diseases, and lab error

Nerve Conduction Velocity/ Electromyography (NCV/EMG)

(See also SSEP, EMG)
(Buckwalter et al., 2000)

NERVE CONDUCTION VELOCITY (SURFACE ELECTRODES)

- Distance/latency (time)
- Age effects by 0.1 m/sec/decade
- Temperature effects 2.4 m/sec/degree
- "Normal" usually >50 m/sec (45–70)
- A function of myelin
- Usually in sensory nerves
- Onset latency uses the first/initial spike, which is caused by the fastest fibers in nerve
- Peak latency is caused by all fibers, but this method has problems
- Temporal dispersion is widening of wave due to a portion of fibers being slowed/injured
- Amplitude can be decreased by dispersion or by block

- Area under curve (AUC) should be equal if it is just temporal dispersion, but AUC is less if there is complete block of (some) fibers

Distal Latency

- Time to get to the most distal point/response
- Can be motor or sensory
- For motor, it is a function of nerve, NMJ, and muscle because it is measured over motor unit. For sensory, it is pure nerve action potential
- Normal responses 1–2 wk postinjury (with no function at time of injury) suggest neuropraxia

EMG (INTRAMUSCULAR ELECTRODES)

Spontaneous Activity

- Fibrillations
- Positive sharp waves
- Abnormal recruitment patterns
- All show denervation of muscle fiber.
- Seen 4 wk after injury

Fasciculation

- Single motor unit activity
- Indicates neuromuscular disorder (anterior horn cell level), typically denervating

Recruitment Rate

- Changes seen right away after injury
- Increased in myopathy
- Decreased in neuropathy

Osteoarthritis (OA)

(Hochberg et al., 2007)

RISK FACTORS

- Males
- Genetic
  First-degree relative: three times increased risk
- Mechanical
  Valgus or varus: six times increased risk
- Obesity
  BMI 27 (upper third): 11 times risk
  11-lb weight loss in women decreases risk of OA by 50%
- Posttraumatic
  Intra-articular fracture (FX)

KNEE

- Semiflexed posteroanterior (PA) view best assesses posterior femur-tibia joint space (rolls condyle)

Osteopetrosis

(See also Metabolic Bone Diseases)
(Buckwalter et al., 2000; and reference cited)
- Excellent review in Tolar et al. (2004)
- Failure of osteoclastic resorption
  - Loss of ruffled border
- Defect in thymus (immune system abnormality)
- Mild adult form AD, severe infantile form AR
- Marble bone
- Rugger jersey spine
- Erlenmeyer flask proximal humerus
- Normal labs (increased acid phosphatase)
- Wide zone proliferating cartilage
- Pathologic fracture, healing normal
- Marrow filled with necrotic calcified cartilage
- Anemia due to no space for marrow
- Blindness due to pressure on optic nerve
- Bone marrow transplant
- High-dose calcitriol and steroids

Reference

Tolar J, et al. Osteopetrosis. *N Engl J Med* 2004; 351(27):2839–2849.

Osteoporosis

(See also Metabolic Bone Diseases and Bisphosphonates)
(HSS experience)
- Quantity, quality, and distribution
- Base for >1 million fractures/yr
- Anorexia, smokers, EtOH, Dilantin users, sedentary, breast-fed children, low Ca^{++}/vitamin D diets
- Fair skin, freckles, red/blonde
- 45% incidence in women >50 years old
- With diagnosis, 40% lifetime risk of fracture
- Osteoporotic fractures pose same lifetime risk of death as breast cancer
- 5% of osteoporosis patients have sprue
- Peak bone mass at 25–30 yr
- 2%–3% loss per year for 5–10 yr after menopause
- Trabecular bone affected more in postmenopausal type
- Trabecular and cortical affected in age-related type (>75 years old)
- Bone shifted outward (thinner cortex but wider diameter) leads to increased bend and torsional strength but no effect on axial strength
- Associated with short fifth finger, which does not go beyond ring finger's distal crease
- Two-thirds of osteoporotic vertebral compression fractures painless
- XRs only positive if >30% loss of mass

7-dehydrocholesterol

Skin ↓〜〜〜 UV

Vitamin D₃
(cholecalciferol)

Circulation

Dietary
Vitamin D₃
(animal sources)
Vitamin D₂
(plant sources)

Side-chain of Vitamin D₂
(ergocalciferol)

Vitamin D storage

25-hydroxylase

Liver

25-hydroxy vitamin D
(calcifediol)

1α-hydroxylase ← PTH

Kidney

1,25-dihydroxy vitamin D
(calcitriol)

Photobiosynthesis and activation of vitamin D. Both endogenous and exogenous vitamin D are converted to 25-hydroxy vitamin D in the liver and then to calcitriol in the kidney. Calcitriol is the active metabolite of vitamin D. Endogenous vitamin D_3 is synthesized in the skin from 7-dehydrocholesterol, in a reaction that is catalyzed by ultraviolet light. Exogenous vitamin D can be provided as D_3 (from animal sources) or as D_2 (from plant sources); D_3 and D_2 have the same biological activity. Parathyroid hormone (PTH) increases the activity of 1 α-hydroxylase in the kidney and thereby stimulates the conversion of 25-hydroxy vitamin D to calcitriol. From Golan DE, Tashjian AH, Armstrong EJ. Principles of Pharmacology The Pathophysiologic Basis of Drug Therapy, 2nd Edition. Baltimore: Wolters Kluwer Health, 2008 with permission.

WORKUP

1. Rule out multiple myeloma (MM)
   - Complete blood count (CBC), smooth muscle actin (SMA) 12, liver function tests (LFTs)
   - ESR
   - Urine protein electrophoresis (UPEP), serum protein electrophoresis (SPEP)
   UPEP picks up extra 20% MM
2. Rule out endocrine disorder
   - T3, T4, thyroid-stimulating hormone/immunoradiometric assay (TSH/IRMA)
   - PTH, glucose (type I DM), steroid history
3. Rule out osteomalacia
   - Alkaline phosphatase high, PTH high, Ca^{++} low, PO_4 low, 25-vitD low
4. Others
   - 24-hr urine Ca^{++}
   - Hydroxyproline
   - Nephrogenic cAMP
   - Vitamin D, PTH, osteocalcin
   - GI malabsorption studies (sprue)

- Bone resorption markers
  - N- or C-telopeptides, pyridinoline
- Bone formation markers
  - Bone alkaline phosphatase, osteocalcin

DUAL ENERGY X-RAY ABSORPTIOMETRY (DEXA)

- Poor precision in spine if osteophytes or scoliosis, then must use hip
- In hip, generally worse than spine because of lack of rotational control
- T—compares with 25-year-old Austrian F, relates to ideal bone mass, flat line on graph
- Z—compares with age-matched, sloping line on graph

WORLD HEALTH ORGANIZATION (WHO) CRITERIA (USING Z SCORE)

- >1.0 standard deviation (SD)—osteopenia
  - No medication yet
- 1.0–2.5 SD—osteoporosis
- >2.5 SD—severe osteoporosis, medication needed
- Risk for fracture if absolute bone mineral density (BMD) is
  - 0.8—spine
  - 0.6—hip
  - 0.4—wrist

HIP PROTECTORS

- Toby Hayes—they work, but compliance is known to be poor

– For patients that get out from bed, or fall from bed at night, a mattress on the floor next to their bed has been suggested

EXERCISE

– Falls are most important in hip fracture and increase hip fracture risk by five times. Tai Chi decreases falls by 47%, more effective than endurance and balance training
– Vitamin D/Ca^{++} and starting exercise in post-menopause each do not increase BMD but decrease fractures 25% because better bone quality

CALCIUM

Daily Requirements
– 1 cup milk = 250 mg Ca^{++}
– Child, 700 mg
– Teen, 1,300 mg
– Adult man, 750 mg
– Adult woman, 1,200 mg
– Pregnant, 1,500 mg
– Lactating, 2,000 mg
– Postmenopause, 1,500 mg
– Fracture, 1,500 mg
– Ca^{++} citrate dissolves in all solutions and decreased risk of kidney stones
– Ca^{++} carbonate has highest Ca^{++} but caused constipation, gas; needs acidity to dissolve (H2 blockers)

ESTROGEN

– HRT decreased all fractures by 30%–50%
– Increased breast cancer up to 40% after 10 yr
– Tamoxifen 70% as effective but increases risk of uterine cancer
– Evista (raloxifene) has no uterine or breast effects, has partial cardiolipid protection, decreased spine fractures 40%, but had no effect on hip fractures
– Calcitonin decreased spine fractures 37%, no data on hip fractures, 2% nasal inflammation, ideal for painful osteoporosis

BISPHOSPHONATES

– Alendronate (Fosamax) has half-life of 10 years versus only 3 years for risedronate (Actonel)
– Actonel has possibly fewer GI symptoms
– Fracture rate 8% (compared to placebo 20%) during 1–3 yr of drug, 7–10 yr of drug, and during yr 5–10 without drug after taking it first 5 years. Thus, continued protection even after being off it 5 yr
– Intravenous pamidronate has effects within 72 hr versus several months for oral meds

– Long-term effects unknown
– Fractures heal but do not remodel

PTH

– Anabolic and paradoxically builds bone if pulsatile (given subcutaneously) in low-turnover osteoporosis
– Dosing is 20 μg/day/subcutaneous for 2 yr
  Provides 8%–13% increase in bone mass, speeds FX healing, and decreases fracture rates
– Contraindications: children, women with breast cancer history, patients with Paget disease

Physiology—Bone

(See also Metabolic Bone Diseases)
(Buckwalter et al., 2000)
– Type I collagen

OSTEOBLASTS

– Produce alkaline phosphatase
– Produce osteocalcin when stimulated by 1,25-D
– Form bone, collagen I
– Respond to PTH (sends second messenger to activate osteoclasts), 1-25 Vitamin D (stimulates), glucocorticoids (suppresses), estrogen (stimulates)

OSTEOCLASTS

– Produce tartrate-resistant acid phosphatase (TRAP)
– Resorb bone (Howship lacunae)
– Stimulated by interleukin (IL)-1, suppressed by IL-10
– Respond to calcitonin (suppressor),
– Not PTH (indirect effect)
– Attach to bone via integrins

OSTEOCALCIN (CLASSICAL CROSS TALK)

– Produced by osteoblasts
– Attracts osteoclasts
– Most abundant noncollagenous matrix in bone
– Levels in urine/serum as mark of bone turnover
– Levels high in Paget disease, hyperPTH, renal osteodystrophy

RANKL/OPG

– Osteoblast-osteoclast coupling is a complicated matter and involves cell signaling
– Osteoblasts produce an osteoclast differentiation factor as a membrane-associated ligand (RANKL). RANKL can be bound by osteoclast cell surface receptors

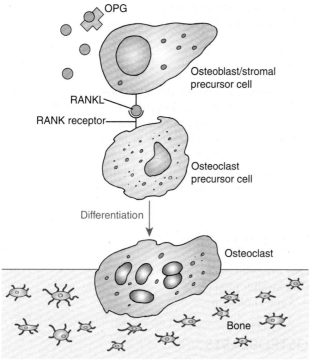

RANK ligand (RANKL), RANK receptor, and osteoprotegerin (OPG) interactions in the activation of osteoclasts and subsequent resorption of bone. RANKL, which is produced by osteoblasts and their stromal precursors, binds to the RANK receptor on osteoclast precursor cells, promoting osteoclast differentiation and proliferation. The soluble OPG molecule, which is produced by a number of tissues, acts as a decoy receptor, blocking the action of RANKL From Porth CM. Essentials of Pathophysiology Concepts of Altered Health States, 2nd Edition. Philadelphia: Lippincott Wiliams & Wilkins, 2007 with permission.

- (RANK) to drive differentiation/activation and anti-apoptosis
- Osteoprotegerin (OPG) is basically a soluble (non-membrane bound) form of RANK, and inhibits signaling of RANKL to RANK.
- Research to date has demonstrated the OPG/RANK/RANKL system to be integral but not sufficient for osteoclast production

Physiology—Cartilage

(Buckwalter et al., 2000)
- Type II collagen

ZONES

- Calcified
- Tidemark—deepest, tangential, resists shear
- Deep—radial, vertical, resists compression
- Middle—transitional, oblique, resists compression
- Superficial—tangential, resists shear, highest collagen concentration, greatest tensile strength
- Proteoglycans in cartilage retain fluid

Physiology—Muscle

(Buckwalter et al., 2000)
- Type I (red, slow twitch, slow oxidative, small motor unit, low strength, high fatigue resistance, high aerobic capacity, lots of mitochondria, higher fat content)
- Type IIA (white, fast twitch, fast oxidative glycolytic, large motor unit, high strength, low fatigue resistance, low aerobic capacity)
- Type IIB (fast glycolytic)
- Concentric—firing, shortening
- Eccentric—firing, lengthening
- Isotonic—shortens with constant load
- Isometric–firing, same length
- Isokinetic—load adjusted to maintain constant velocity of shortening or lengthening

Physiology—Nerve Endings

(Junqueira et al., 1989)

MEISSNER CORPUSCLE

- Rapidly adapting
- Small discrete field
- Located within interdermal ridges (dermal papillae), typically in hairless skin areas (palms and soles)
- Function: moving two-point discrimination, light touch

MERKEL CELLS

- Slow adapting
- Small discrete field
- Specialized epithelial cells in proximity to unmyelinated nerve fibers (collectively, Merkel disks)
- Function: static two-point discrimination, deeper touch

PACINIAN CORPUSCLE

- Rapid adapting
- Large field
- In subcutaneous tissue, layers of fibroblasts and fluid layers surrounding an unmyelinated nerve ending
- Function: pressure sensation (but rapidly adapts), vibration

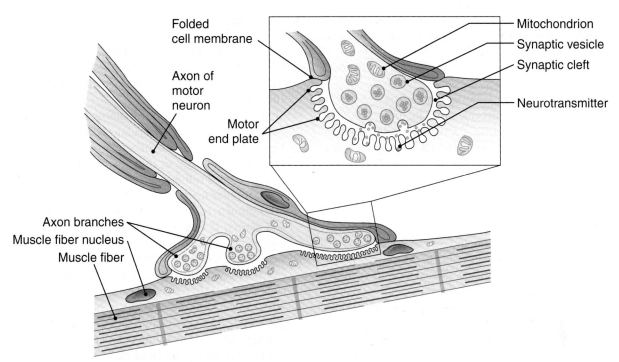

Neuromuscular junction. **(A)** The branched end of a motor neuron makes contact with the membrane of a muscle fiber (cell). **(B)** Enlarged view. (Reprinted with permission from Cohen BJ, Wood DL. Memmler's The Human Body in Health and Disease. 9th Ed. Philadelphia: Lippincott Williams & Wilkins, 2000.)

RUFFINI END ORGANS

- Spindle shaped and encapsulated
- Appear in joints and dermis
- Thin capsule surrounds myelinated fiber that branches repeatedly to form a dense cluster of endings
- Function: pressure, vibration

Reference

Junqueira LC, et al. Basic Histology, 6th ed. Norwalk, CT: Appleton & Lange; 1989.

Polio

(See also Amyotrophic Lateral Sclerosis and Guillain-Barré)
(Simon et al., 1999)
- Infection of anterior horn cells
- Unpredictable in location or severity
- Most recovery occurs between 6 mo and 2 yr after initial onset
- Surgical treatment after that time is dependent on affect muscles

- Postpolio syndrome presents 30 yr after initial onset with progressive weakness and fatigue
- Increased weakness affects both the paretic and the previously normal muscles
- Joint pain, atrophy of muscles, respiratory insufficiency, dysphagia, and sleep apnea also seen
- Due to chronic overuse of weak muscles, latent reactivation of virus, or progression of disease to an ALS form
- Gentle PT and modification of lifestyle recommended

POLIO-ASSOCIATED SCOLIOSIS (SPINE)

- Deformity type and severity variable
- Lateral abdominal and quadratus function critical
- Intercostal paralysis leads to thoracic scoliosis
- Nonoperative treatment usually not successful

Pseudogout (Calcium Pyrophosphate Dihydrate [CPPD])

(See also Gout)
(Hochberg et al., 2007)
- Crystalline pyrophosphate deposition disease
- Short, rhomboid, positive birefringent crystals

- Positive shown by blue in crystal pointed parallel to polarized light, and yellow perpendicular to light direction
- Increased rates of pseudogout associated with hyper-PTH
- Most common cause of chondrocalcinosis
- Other causes of chondrocalcinosis include
  Ochronosis (alkaptonuria, deposition of dark melanotic deposits, dark urine, OA, and fusions in spine or other joints)
  Hyperparathyroidism
  Hypothyroidism
- Abrupt onset
- Pain milder than gout
- Knee most commonly affected
- Talonavicular and subtalar joints in foot
- Ca^{++} in soft tissues, cartilage, meniscus, and synovial fluid
- Hand metacarpophalangeal (MCP) joints, wrist joints involved in CPPD
- Acute onset due to stress
- Symptomatic treatment with NSAIDs

Renal Osteodystrophy/-Malacia

(See also Metabolic Bone Diseases)
(Buckwalter et al., 2000)
- High turnover (chronic high PTH)
  Can induce secondary hyper-PTHism
  Decreased renal PO_4 excretion
    - low Ca^{++} (direct effect of high PO_4)
    - PO_4 impairs one-position hydroxylation of 25-vit D (with resultant low Ca^{++})
    - PO_4 may directly increase PTH production
  All three above can induce hyper-PTH
- Low turnover (aluminum (Al) deposition in bone with normal PTH)—quite rare today
  Aluminum-containing phosphate-binding antacids used to control phosphate accumulation contribute
    - Al impairs differentiation of osteoblasts
    - Al impairs proliferation of osteoblasts
    - Al impairs PTH release
    - Al disrupts mineralization process
  May see rugger jersey spine and/or soft tissue calcifications
- Chronic dialysis leads to accumulation of beta$_2$ macroglobulins, which leads to amyloidosis, which leads to carpal tunnel, arthropathy, path fractures
- Very slow healing of fractures
- Amyloid is pink with Congo red stain
- Slipped capital femoral epiphysis (SCFE) through metaphyseal spongiosa
- Physial disturbance in children

Rhabdomyolysis (RML)

(Cervellin et al., 2010; and references cited)
- Skeletal muscle injury—widespread
- RML classically creatine phosphokinase (CPK) >50 K–100 K IU/L
- Myoglobin overloads haptoglobin-binding capacity, gets filtered across glomerular membrane
- Myoglobin can be reabsorbed in renal tubules (causing direct damage), or may form distal tubule casts, blocking renal tubules. Either mechanism can lead to acute tubular necrosis (ATN)
- In addition to trauma ("real" trauma, or "sleeper arm") and burns, it can be caused by ETOH, cholesterol-lowering drugs
- Uric acid (UA) with myoglobin (hemoglobin as a cross-reaction), typically dark in color, positive dip, no red cells at Urine Microscopic exam
- With muscle injury may also have hyperkalemic, hyper-PO_4, hyperuricemic, and elevated blood urea nitrogen (BUN), creatinine (Cr), creatine kinase (CK) alkaline phosphatase, aldolase
- Acute renal failure (ARF) associated with CK >16,000
- 15% of all ARF due to rhabdomyolysis

TREATMENT

- Hydration (intravenous fluids [IVF] until CK <1,000) (worse ATN with hypovolemia)
- Alkalinize urine, mannitol/osmotic diuretics
- Follow K, PO_4
  - See Malinoski et al. (2004)
- Do not correct hypocalcemia unless symptomatic because expect Ca^{++} increase in recovery phase

References

Cervellin G, Comelli I, Lippi G. Rhabdomyolysis: historical background, clinical, diagnostic and therapeutic features. *Clin Chem Lab Med.* 2010; 48:749–56.
Malinoski DJ, et al. Crush injury and rhabdomyolysis. 2004; *Crit Care Clin* 2004; 20(1):171–192.

Rheumatoid Arthritis

(See also Systemic Lupus Erythematosus)
- F >M (3:1)
- Most common in third to fifth decade
- HLA-DR4
- Positive rheumatoid factor (RF) (RF is IgM reacting against native IgG)
- IL-1 and tumor necrosis factor (TNF) implicated
- Shortens lifespan 7 yr in men, 3 yr in women
- Need four of seven to make diagnosis (American Rheumatology Association [ARA])
  - Morning stiffness >1 hr
  - At least three joints total

- At least one of wrist, MCP, or proximal interphalangeal (PIP) joints
- Symmetry
- Rheumatoid nodules
- Positive RF
- XR changes on hand or wrist
- Hand, wrist, feet first
- Then c-spine, knee, elbow, hip, shoulder
- Fatigue, malaise, soft tissue pain
- Pericarditis
- Pulmonary fibrosis
- Splenomegaly/leukopenia (Felty)
- X-rays
  Osteoporosis
  Joint erosions
  No osteophytes
- NSAIDs, COX-2 s only symptomatic relief
- Disease-modifying drugs
  - Steroids decrease joint erosions
  - Enbrel inhibits TNF
    - Soluble TNF-R
    - Do not use if getting a live virus vaccine (immunosuppressant)
  - Methotrexate (MTX)
    - Drug of choice
    - Do not use in patients with HIV or those taking sulfonamide antibiotics
    - Liver, marrow toxicity
  - Remicade

RA IN HAND

- EPL rupture (Vaughn-Jackson)
- MCP joints involved in hand with ulnar deviation. PIPs typically spared
- MCP arthroplasty
- PIP fusion for radial digits and arthroplasty for ulnar digits—to maintain power grip
  C-Spine (in up to 90%)
- *Check before any surgery!*
- Pain is typical, but may have no symptoms
- Rule out myelopathic changes
- Anteroposterior (AP)/lateral (Lat)/flex-extend/open mouth
  Many radiographic criteria: Ranawat index, anterior atlantodens interval (AADI), Space Available for the Cord/posterior atlantodens interval (SAC/PADI)
- Classic pathology patterns
  Atlantoaxial subluxation
  Atlantoaxial impaction (settling)
  Subaxial subluxation
- Space available for cord (PADI) is most predictive of surgical outcome. Boden et al. (1993) suggested stabilizing for PADI less than 14 mm (atlantoaxial subluxation [AAS])

Reference

Boden SD, et al. Rheumatoid arthritis of the cervical spine. A long-term analysis with predictors of paralysis and recovery. *J Bone Joint Surg* 1993; 75A(9):1282–1297.

Rickets (Osteomalacia)

(See also Metabolic Bone Diseases)
(Buckwalter et al., 2000)
- Is basically a deficient or impaired mineralization of bone
- *Many* causes in broad categories, including nutritional deficiency, GI absorption, renal tubule defects (PO_4 leak), renal osteodystrophy, miscellaneous
  Approximately 40% of diagnoses made after workup done in setting of hospital admission for fracture, and another 20% made in workup prior to arthroplasty. Very commonly unrecognized disease state
- Rickets typically with the following: hypo/normal Ca^{++}, hypo-PO_4, hyper–alkaline phosphatase, normal/hyper-PTH, hypo/normal urine Ca^{++}
- *Osteomalacia* in adults
- *Rickets* in children

VITAMIN D

- Diet and skin (D3), liver (25-vitD), kidney (1,25-vitD). Increased GI absorption, stimulated osteoclast resorption of bone, results in increased serum Ca^{++} and PO_4 (this is net effect)
- Stimulated by high PTH, low Ca^{++}, low PO_4

CAUSES

- Nutritional (vitamin D)
- Renal osteodystrophy
- Renal tubular acidosis (PO_4 leak)
- Vitamin D–resistant (hypophosphatemic)
- GI absorption defects (irritable bowel disease)
- Iatrogenic (Dilantin blocks vitamin D metabolism, which leads to osteomalacia—treated with vitamin D supplementation)

Nutritional (Vitamin D Deficient)—

- Normal or low Ca^{++}, low PO_4 (from PTH)
- High PTH, high alkaline phosphatase
- Low 25-vit D (diet, sprue, total parenteral nutrition)
- Bow legs, swollen joints
- Prolonged breast feeding, vegan mom
- Can tell time of onset by knees
  - Rickets at birth leads to bowing
  - Later onset rickets leads to valgum
- 31% of African Americans with hip fractures have osteomalacia
- Brittle bones
- Physial cupping, widening
- Looser lines

- Large costal cartilage (rachitic rosary)
- Dorsal kyphosis (cat back)
- Wide osteoid seams
- Expansion of hypertrophic zone of physis
- Swiss cheese trabeculae
- Open fontanels
- Flaring radial metaphyses
  Treatment—5,000I U vitamin D daily, calcium

Vitamin D–Resistant Hypophosphatemic

- X-linked dominant
- Most common type of rickets in United States
- Impaired renal tubular resorption of PO_4
- Normal GFR, impaired vitamin D3 response
- 10th percentile height (stunted)
- Low phosphorus levels (marked)
- Lower limb deformities
- Treat with PO_4 and high-dose 1,25(OH) vitamin D (need both to prevent iatrogenic low-Ca^{++} and resultant hyper-PTH syndrome)
  - Use of the 1,25(OH) vitamin D is recommended due to 4-hr turnover of the agent and less likelihood of vitamin D toxemia/overload
  - Treatment course is for rest of patient's life—not just until full recovery from episode
- Growth hormone before ambulating to prevent bowing

	Ca^{++}	PO_4	Alkaline Phosphatase
Porosis	Normal	Normal	Normal
hPTH	High	Normal/low	Normal/high
Malacia	Low/normal	High/low	High
Paget	Normal	Normal	Very high

Sarcoidosis

(Wilson et al., 1991)
- Deposition of granulation tissue anywhere in body, most commonly lungs (90%)
- Most commonly 20–40-yr-old black versus northern European whites
  Of African American patients women >men
- Insidious malaise, fever, dyspnea
  Or erythema nodosum, uveitis, parotid enlargement, peripheral nerves, hepatic, renal, cardiac presentation, versus no symptoms and pickup on routine chest x-ray exam (CXR)
- Workup may show leucopenia, eosinophilia, high ESR, hyper-Ca^{++} (serum and/or urine)
- A key test is to assess if the angiotensin-converting enzyme (ACE) is high—present in 40%–80% of patients with active disease
- Skin test anergy present in 70%
- Differential diagnosis—TB, histoplasmosis, cancer, lymphoma

- Diagnosis made by transbronchial biopsy (or biopsy of skin lesion) demonstrative of noncaseating granulomas
- ACE levels are supportive but not diagnostic
- CXR with bilateral hilar lymphadenopathy ± parenchymal involvement, or with parenchymal involvement alone (diffuse reticular infiltrates). Pleural effusions uncommon (10%)
- Arthritis in approximately 10%–35%
- Most common in knees/ankles, but can be anywhere; typically symmetric and self-limiting (but can be chronic or recurrent)
- Hands with multiple lytic destructive lesions, which are lacelike most prominently in short tubular bones
- Hand XR differential diagnosis—hyper-PTH or multicentric reticulohistiocytosis (cutaneous xanthomas with mutilating arthritis of hands, rare, similar to RA with erosion and bilateral symmetry but lacks osteoporosis)
- Affects distal tuft, which enchondromas do not affect because tufts are formed by membranous ossification
- Many go into remission without treatment. Patients in remissions tend not to relapse
- Low-dose steroids usually for patients with progressive disease. These patients tend to relapse
  ACE levels tend to drop with successful treatment(s)

Reference

Wilson JD, et al., eds. Harrison's Principles of Internal Medicine, 12th ed. New York: McGraw-Hill; 1991.

Scurvy

(See also Metabolic Bone Diseases)
(Buckwalter et al., 2000)
- Vitamin C deficiency
- Decrease in chondroitin sulfate synthesis, leads to defective collagen growth and repair
- Decreased/impaired hydroxylation of collagen peptides is biochemical deficiency
- Fatigue, gum bleeding, ecchymosis
- Joint effusions, iron deficiency
- Thin cortices, thin trabeculae
- Metaphyseal clefts (corner)
- Greatest effect on bone formation at metaphysis
- Histologically: replacement of primary trabeculae with granulation tissue, widening of provisional zone of calcification
- White line of Frankel at metaphyseal-physis junction
- Ringed epiphysis—Wimberger sign
- Labs normal

Sensitivity/Specificity

(See also Epidemiology/Study Types and Statistics)

SENSITIVITY ("SEE WHAT *Is* THERE")

- True positive/ all specimens with disease
- Ability to identify truly positive

SPECIFICITY ("SEE WHAT *Is Not There*")

- True negatives/all specimens without the disease
- Ability to identify truly negative
- Sensitivity and specificity are inherent qualities of any test

POSITIVE PREDICTIVE VALUE (PPV)

- All positive with the disease (true positive)/(all positive test results)
- Probability of having disease if the test is positive
- Higher PPV with higher prevalence

NEGATIVE PREDICTIVE VALUE (NPV)

- All (true negatives)/(all negative test results)
- PPV and NPV are affected by prevalence

Disease

Test	Pos	Neg
Pos.	a	b
Neg	c	d

Sensitivity = $a/(a + c)$
Specificity = $d/(b + d)$
PPV = $a/(a + b)$
NPV = $d/(c + d)$

PRECISION

- Ability to repeat measurements exactly
  Basically: *repeat* data with *low scatter*

ACCURACY

- Tests the issue of data differentiation. Perfectly accurate data points are on the mark, are true measurements of the system, and different data values represent differences in the *system* (not error in the data collection, etc.)
  Basically: Are your data *correct*?

Seronegative Arthropathies (Seronegative Spondyloarthropathies)

(See also Ankylosing Spondylitis)
(Buckwalter et al., 2000)
- Heterogeneous group of diseases characterized by inflammatory axial spine involvement (sacroiliitis, spondylitis)

- Also see asymmetric peripheral arthritis, enthesopathy, inflammatory eye disease, and mucocutaneous symptoms
- All in *absence of* rheumatoid factor
- Includes ankylosing spondylitis, reactive arthritis, psoriatic arthritis, arthritis of inflammatory bowel disease, juvenile spondyloarthropathy, and undifferentiated spondyloarthropathy

Three relatively common types
- Ankylosing spondylitis (70 cases/100 K)
  Diagnosis: >3 mo LBP/stiffness better with exercise, limitation of spine range of motion ROM), limitation of chest wall expansion, XRs with sacroiliitis
  Men >women 5:1, usually in 20s
  Uveitis, pulmonary fibrosis, cardiac, mucosa, etc. Fatigue, fevers, anorexia, weight loss
  90% HLA-B27 (+) *not diagnostic*, mild elevations ESR, CRP, CPK
  XRs: fusions (spine, hips), marginal syndesmophytes, fractures (spine) common
- Psoriatic arthritis
  Several subtypes
  Arthritis years before skin lesions in 20%, M = F, typically young at onset
  Symmetric involved hands and feet (peripheral and symmetric)
  Cuticle and *nail* changes, "sausage digits"
  "Cup and saucer" or "pencil in cup" from proximal phalanx destruction
  Only 40%–55% HLA-B27, also associations with HLA-DR3/DR4
- Reactive arthritis (Reiter)
  Approximately 4 cases/100 K
  - Conjunctivitis, urethritis, symmetric arthritis
  - GI infection—*Campylobacter*, *Yersinia*, *Salmonella*
  - Lower extremity usually involved
  - "Sausage toes" (or fingers)
  - Can present with heel pain (plantar fasciitis), myalgias, mucocutaneous lesions, stiffness, asymmetric arthritis
  - Typically young males, 40%–80% HLA-B27

Sickle Cell (Gordeuk, 1996b; and references cited)

- 1% of African Americans
- Trait in 8% of African Americans

CRISIS

- Typically begins in patients at 2–3 yr old
- Crises usually last 3–5 days
- Pain from infections lasts longer

- High ESR during crisis and with infections (although not as high as would be expected for osteomyelitis in a "normal" patient)
- Bone infarcts
- Avascular necrosis (AVN) femoral heads
- Osteomyelitis of diaphysis
- *Salmonella* is characteristic but *Staphylococcus aureus* is most common organism of osteomyelitis
- Exchange transfusions and oxygenation for preop patients
- Hydroxyurea for crisis

PAIN: INFARCTION VS OSTEOMYELITIS

- Skaggs et al. (2001)
- Sequential bone marrow and bone scan within 24 hr to diagnose children with acute bone pain
- Bone infarct leads to decreased uptake on marrow and increased uptake on bone
- Osteomyelitis shows normal uptake on marrow and increased uptake on bone

Reference

Skaggs D, et al. Differentiation between infarction and acute osteomyelitis in children with sickle-cell disease with use of sequential radionuclide bone-marrow and bone scans. *J Bone Joint Surg* 2001; 83A(12):1810–1813.

Somatosensory-Evoked Potential (SSEP), EMG

(See also NCV/EMG)
(Buckwalter et al., 2000; and reference cited)

ACETABULUM

- For acetabular fractures, leads are placed in common peroneal nerve, posterior tibial nerve, tibialis anterior muscle, peroneal muscle, abductor hallucis, flexor hallices brevis (FHB), and a ground in heel
- EMG is instantaneous and gets signals when nerve is injured. More reliable/accurate than SSEP
- SSEP is time averaged, thus takes longer to detect changes. Signals are impaired/lost when nerves are injured. Requires complex interpretation
- Evoked potentials are stimulated peripherally (in characteristic nerve distributions) and recorded with scalp electrodes

SPINE

- EMG indicates only nerve root injury and not cord. Thus, for L3 down, for *cord* monitoring (above surgi-

cal field) SSEP is useful (retrograde) or transcranial motor-evoked potentials (tcMEP) (antegrade)

NEUROMUSCULAR SCOLIOSIS

- Concern over cord injury versus getting spinal balance
- Even in nonambulatory and incontinent patients, monitoring needed to prevent further motor loss and sensibility (late decubitus ulcers a risk)
- Upper extremity monitoring needed to avoid brachial plexopathy in a patient who is totally dependent on upper extremities for function
- In setting of neuromuscular blockers, halogenated agents, nitric oxide, and controlled hypotension, obtaining baseline monitoring potentials may be very difficult or impossible, or may have small amplitude
- Total IV anesthesia technique may give better recordings (DiCindio et al., 2003)
- Transcranial motor-evoked potentials is a good option but may be contraindicated in patients with seizure history (kindling phenomenon). However, anesthesia may protect patient from potential seizure activity induced by transcranial stimulation

Reference

DiCindio S, et al. Multimodality monitoring of transcranial electric and somatosensory-evoked potentials during surgical correction of spinal deformity in patients with cerebral palsy and other neuromuscular disorders. *Spine* 2003; 28(16):1851–1855.

Statistics

(See also Epidemiology/Study Types and Sensitivity/ Specificity)
- Research hypothesis: that possibility one theorizes to be true
- Null hypothesis: that possibility one hopes to statistically reject
- Type I alpha error
  Rejecting a true null hypothesis
  P-value is probability of having type I error or the probability that the study arrived at conclusion by chance alone
- Type II beta error
  Accepting a false null hypothesis
  Power is the probability of rejecting null hypothesis when it is actually false or the probability that a difference would be found between two groups given that a difference truly did exist
- Confidence interval
  Range of values that includes the true value within a given probability (usually 95% for two SDs from mean)

- Discrete data
  Noncontinuous
  Categorical
  Qualitative
  Can be placed in specific categories
  Data evaluated for differences (with p-values given)
    - Chi-square test (frequency of observation)
    - Fisher exact test (typically with smaller sample sizes)
  Chi-square test compares frequencies or proportions within two or more groups
  Fisher exact test is same as chi-square except it puts out exact p value. Thus, easier to use over chi-square if possible
- Continuous data
  Vary over continuous range
  Parametric: normal distribution
  Evaluated for central tendency, variation, and distribution
    - One-sample t-test
    - Independent two-sample t-test
    - Paired t-test
    - Analysis of variance (ANOVA)
- Student's t-test (small sample sizes)
  Difference between two means
- One-sample t-test
  Compares sample mean to a known mean or hypothetical value
- Two-sample t-test
  Compares means of two independent groups
- Paired t-test
  Compares means of two *dependent* groups
- Analysis of variance (ANOVA) –
  Difference among means of more than two samples with normal distribution
- The Wilcoxon two-sample test
  Equality of medians rather than means
- Regression analysis
  Calculates approximate values of a variable from known values of another variable
  Differentiates the slope between two variables and the effect of one on the other
- Correlation analysis
  Used to assess extent to which two sets of data or variables are related
  Mean—average value of observations
  Median—middle-most observation
  Mode—most frequent observation
- Variance and SD
  Variance is a measure of how much the typical member of a group deviates. High variance indicates that data are more spread out. It is the average of the squares of each observation's deviation from the mean
  Standard deviation (SD) is square root of variance

95% of observations within two SDs
Two-thirds of observations within one SD of mean
- SEM (standard error of mean)—SD divided by square root of N
  SEM quantifies how accurately you know the true population mean. As you take a bigger sample size, the SEM gets smaller. SD, however, does not depend on N
- Reliability—precision, ability to repeat the same result/measurement
- Validity—accuracy, extent to which an experimental value represents a true value

Steroids

(Herkowitz et al., 2011; and references cited)
Stress dose steroids: when to use?
- Most common setting: if patient has had >2 wk of steroids in the past year
- Give 100 mg hydrocortisone on call and then q8hr for two doses
- Osteoporosis prevention in setting of steroid administration
  Dietary Ca^{++} supplementation of 1,200 mg daily
  Vitamin D 50,000 units every 1–2 wk
  Bisphosphonate treatment (see bisphosphonate section)

NATIONAL ACUTE SPINAL CORD INJURY STUDIES (NASCIS)

- Steroids for cord injury based in time
  Less than 3 hr 30 mg/kg methylprednisolone bolus over 15 minutes, and then, beginning 45 minutes later, a 23-hr continuous infusion of 5.4 mg/kg
  Patients 4–8 hours from injury get same bolus followed by 47-hr continuous infusion at 5.4 mg/kg

Reference

Herkowitz HN, et al., eds. Rothman-Simeone The Spine, 6th ed. Philadelphia: Saunders/Elsevier; 2011.

Systemic Lupus Erythematosus (SLE)

(See also Rheumatoid Arthritis)
(Hochberg et al., 2007)
- Malar butterfly rash ± fever
- Pericarditis, pleuritis, arthritis
- Vasculitis, Raynaud phenomenon, pancytopenia
- Glomerulonephritis with renal failure
- Joint laxity, deformity
- Positive antinuclear antibody (ANA), anti-DNA antibodies, HLA-DR2/DR3, possible RF/CRP/ESR

- Women >men
- Symmetric arthralgia and synovitis
- Easily confused with RA early in course
- Jaccoud arthropathy
  - MCP ulnar deviated, flexed, subluxated
  - PIP hyperextension
  - Distal interphalangeal (DIP) flexion
- Hitchhiker's thumb
- Carpometacarpal (CMC) subluxation
- Treatment is similar to RA—disease-modifying antirheumatatic drugs (DMARDs) in pyramid fashion
- AVN secondary to steroids is most common cause of orthopaedic intervention
- Soft tissue procedures classically with poor outcome (stretch out); fusions are most reliable surgical intervention

Reference

Bullough PG. Orthopaedic Pathology, 4th ed. Philadelphia: Mosby/Elsevier; 2004.

Temporal Arteritis

(Wilson et al., 1991; and references cited)
- Idiopathic systemic vasculitis of medium to large arteries
- 1 case in 500 in patients >50 yr old
- F:M ratio is approximately 5:1
- Jaw or tongue claudication
- Extremity stiffness
- Scalp/temporal tenderness
- Visual changes with anterior ischemic optic neuropathy ("window shade")

American College of Rheumatology (three of five for diagnosis)—Hunder (2000)
- >50 yr old
- New-onset localized headache
- Temporal artery tender or decreased pulse
- ESR >50
- Arterial biopsy with necrotizing arteritis with mononuclear cell infiltrates or granulomatous process
- Treatment started as soon as suspected to prevent blindness
- Prednisone 60 mg/day for 2–4 wk, taper
- Osteoporosis prevention in setting of steroid administration

  Dietary Ca^{++} supplementation of 1,200 mg daily

  Vitamin D 50,000 units every 1–2 wk

  Bisphosphonate treatment (see bisphosphonate section)

Reference

Hunder GG. Classification/diagnostic criteria for GCA/PMR. *Clin Exp Rheumatol* 2000; 18(4 Suppl 20):S4–5.

Transfusion

(HSS experience)
- Virus transmission rates

  HIV—1/200 K–1/2 million per unit

  Hepatitis A—very rare (1/1 million)

  Enteric transmission

  Vaccine available

  No chronic liver disease

  Hepatitis E—very rare

  Enteric transmission

  No vaccine

  No chronic liver disease

  Hepatitis B—1/30 K–1/250 K

  Hepatitis C—1/30 K–1/150 K

  Cytomegalovirus (CMV)—1/2,500

  HTLV1/2—1/250 K–1/2 million
- Fatal hemolytic reaction <1:600,000
- Fever, allergic reaction 1/100
- transfusion (TFN) and total joint arthroplasty (TJA)

  30% need allogeneic TFN if baseline hemoglobin (Hb) 10–13 prior to surgery

  10% need TFN if Hb >14

  Total knee replacement (TKR) average Hb drop 3.9

  bilateral TKR average Hb drop 5.4

  THR average Hb drop 4.1
- Trigger point for transfusion

  Optimal trigger point unknown

  2,000 Jehovah's Witness patients having various surgeries

  Odds of death increased from 1.1 at Hb 11–12 to 1.4 at Hb 6–7 if no cardiovascular (CV) disease and blood loss <1 L

  Odds of death increased from 1.5 to 12.3 if previous history of CV disease
- TFN immunosuppression

  Due to graft versus host disease (GVHD)

  Leads to higher infection rate, faster return of tumor (in oncology surgery)

  Not seen in autologous donations

  May be eliminated by leukocyte depletion of allogeneic blood by X-ray treatment
- massive TFN is defined as replacement of total blood volume within 24-hr period (5 L for 70-kg patient), leading to depletion of platelets and clotting factors
- Factor replacement therapy guided by *labs* and *clinical evidence* of bleeding. *Avoid using ratios* of fresh frozen plasma (FFP) to red cells
- Prevention of need for TFN

  Hypotensive anesthesia

  Preoperative normovolemic hemodilution requires skilled anesthesiologist

  Indicated if baseline Hb >10 and >20% blood volume loss expected

- Cell saver indicated if blood loss >1 L expected, contraindicated in surgeries being done for infection or tumor
- Postop reinfusion associated with fibrin degradation products, free Hb, activated clotting factors and may lead to disseminated intravascular coagulation (DIC), respiratory distress
- Both methods reinfuse dilute blood
- Preop autologous donation (PAD)
  Not crossed over into general blood supply in most places
  Discard rates of 50%
  British consensus guidelines suggest donation if risk of TFN >50%
  Journal of the American Academy of Orthopedic Surgeons—if >10% risk for TFN and Hb >13
  Should begin 3–5 wk before schedule surgery
  2 U unilateral TJA, 3 U bilateral TJA
  Can still get fever from endotoxin (bacterial contamination)
  Relative contraindication if >80 yr old due to falls risk versus infection risk
- Donor-directed donation
  Can speed up time of blood availability for surgery but not proven to decrease infection risks; may be more dangerous because different pool (somewhat less strict screening)
  Takes 5 working days
  Higher incidence of GVHD
- Erythropoietin
  Patients mildly anemic with Hb 10–13 getting 300 units/kg daily for 10 days preop then 4 days postop, or alternately, 600 units/kg weekly for 3 wk preop (cheaper). Either method tends to reduce TFN need by 1 U per patient and most patients do not require TFN
  Theoretical increased risk of thrombosis in patients with CV disease if HCT raised too fast
  Must have adequate iron stores (supplement)
  Loss of positive DVT prophylaxis of thin blood during surgery

Vancomycin

(See also Antibiotics and Gentamicin)
(Levinson and Jawetz, 1998)
- Tricyclic glycopeptide
- Inhibits cell wall mucopeptide formation (binds a cell wall precursor)
- Bactericidal versus Gram-positive cocci (including MRSA)
- Bacteriostatic versus enterococci
- *Not* absorbed from the GI tract (PO doses will treat *Clostridium difficile*, not septic joints)

- Rapid infusion causes "red man" with flushing and sometimes hypotension
- Levels need to be monitored
  For "normal" patients a single 1-g IV dose will produce a serum concentration of 15–30 μg/mL 1 hr after infusion, which is well into the therapeutic range
- Ototoxicity
  Rare, frequently but not always permanent
  Usually after prolonged therapy, and with high serum concentrations
- Nephrotoxicity
  Occurs in 5%
  Reversible
  No strict relationship to dose, but more common in higher serum concentrations
  Higher incidence if given in combination with aminoglycosides
  Not clearly associated with current preparations
- Renal excretion mainly
  ARF/CRF patients may have vancomycin half-lives up to 8 days!
  Dose accordingly (at hemodialysis [HD])

X-rays and Radiation Doses

(HSS experience)
- DEXA spine posteroanterior (PA)—10 micro-Sieverts (Sv)
- DEXA femur—2 microSv
- CXR—60 microSv
- Lumbar spine XR—1.3 milliSv
- Transatlantic flight—60 microSv
- Background daily—7 microSv
- Background annually—3 milliSv
- 1 milliSv = 100 cigarettes (estimate for relative cancer risk)
- 10 milliSv = increases fatal cancer risk by 1/2,000
- Sievert (Sv) is a measurement that reflects effective dose in that it has a built-in factor that incorporates the sensitivity of that tissue
- cGy is absorbed dose where 1 Gy is 1 joule per kg
- 1 Gy roughly equals 1 Sv
- Deterministic or acute health effects occur only after a threshold dose, and severity is related to dose (i.e., cataracts)
- Stochastic effects have no threshold and severity is independent of dose although probability of occurring proportional to dose (i.e., leukemia)

Reference

Fishman MC, et al., eds. *Medicine*, 4th ed. Philadelphia: Lippincott-Raven Publishers; 1996.

CHAPTER 6

Tumors

Moe R. Lim, John H. Healey

Benign Lytic Bone Lesions
  Mnemonic—"FEGNOMASHIC"
  Rule Out if Older Than 30 Years
  Rule Out if Pain or Periostitis (Without Fracture)
  Epiphyseal
  Multiple
  Sequestrations
  Expansile, Lytic, Posterior Spine
  Differential Diagnosis, Sclerosis, Age 20–40 Yr
  Sacral Lesions
Biopsy Principles
  High Complication Rate
  Types of Biopsy
  Practical Biopsy Tips
  Indications for Primary Excisional Biopsy
  No Need for Biopsy
  Biopsy and Shape of Bone Hole
  Biopsy and Size of Bone Hole
Fibrous Lesions
  Nonossifying Fibroma
  Benign Fibrous Histiocytosis (BFH)
  Fibrous Cortical Defect
  Desmoplastic Fibroma
  Chondromyxoid Fibroma
  Malignant Fibrous Histiocytoma (MFH)
  Fibrosarcoma
Malignant Bone Tumors
  X-Ray (XR) Signs of Malignancy/Aggressiveness
  Mimics Malignant Bone Tumor
  Malignant Bone Tumor and Age
  Tumors With Bone Edema
Metastatic Carcinoma
  Bone Metastases
Musculoskeletal Tumors
  Bone Dysplasia
  Benign Bone
  Malignant Bone
  Benign Cartilage
  Synovial Tumors

  Benign Soft Tissue
  Malignant Soft Tissue
  Nerve Sheath Tumors
  Nontumors
Pathological Fracture
  Mortality and Prognosis
  After Resection of Soft Tissue Sarcoma
Skeletal Metastases of Unknown Origin
  Protocol
  Recommendations From This Study
Soft Tissue Sarcomas
  Types
  Grading
  Treatment
  Chemotherapy
  Prognosis
Spine Tumors
  Age, Location, and Differential Diagnosis
Spine Metastatic Tumors
  General
  Imaging
  Treatment
  Surgery Principles
Staging, Types of Excisions
  Musculoskeletal Tumor Staging
  Benign Enneking System
  Malignant Enneking System
  Malignant Bone (AJCC-6)
  Soft Tissue Tumor Staging (AJCC-5)
  Soft Tissue (AJCC-6)
  Types of Excisions
Radiation Therapy
  High Sensitivity
  Moderate Sensitivity
  Low Sensitivity
  Complications
  Brachytherapy (Intraoperative Radiation Therapy)
  Preoperative versus Postoperative Radiation
    Therapy for Soft Tissue Sarcoma

Aneurysmal Bone Cyst
General
History and Physical Examination
Imaging
Pathology
Differential Diagnosis
Treatment
Adamantinoma
General
X-Ray
History and Physical Examination
Pathology
Treatment
Bone Island (Enostosis)
General
History and Physical Examination
Imaging
Treatment
**Chemotherapy—Adriamycin
(Doxorubicin)**
General
Myocardial Toxicity
Extravasation
Chemotherapy—Cisplatin
General
Adverse Effects
Chemotherapy—Ifosfamide
General
Adverse Effects
Chemotherapy—Vincristine
General
Adverse Effects
Chondroblastoma (Codman Tumor)
General
History and Physical Examination
Imaging
Differential Diagnosis
Pathology
Natural History
Treatment
Chondromyxoid Fibroma
General
History and Physical Examination
Imaging
Pathology
Treatment
Chondrosarcoma
General
History and Physical Examination
Imaging
Chondrosarcoma (versus
Osteochondroma)
Chondrosarcoma (versus
Enchondroma)
Chondrosarcoma in Situ

Five Histologic Subtypes of
Chondrosarcomas
Pathology
Differential Diagnosis
Metastasis
Treatment
Chordoma
General
History and Physical Examination
Imaging
Pathology
Differential Diagnosis
Treatment
Prognosis
Clear Cell Sarcoma
General
Pathology
Treatment
Desmoid (Fibromatosis)
General
History and Physical Examination
Imaging
Pathology
Treatment
Enchondroma
General
History and Physical Examination
Imaging
Pathology
Natural History
Treatment
Ollier Disease
Maffucci Syndrome
**Eosinophilic Granuloma (Langerhans Cell
Histiocytosis)**
Eosinophilic Granuloma
Hand-Schüller-Christian Disease
Letterer-Siwe Disease
Peripheral Neuroectodermal Tumor
General
History and Physical Examination
Imaging
Pathology
Metastases
Small Round Cell Tumors and Age
Treatment
Chemotherapy
Radiation Therapy
Prognosis
Histologic Response to Chemotherapy
Fibrous Dysplasia
General
Imaging
Pathology
Treatment

Giant Cell Tumor
General
History and Physical Examination
Imaging
Histology
Differential Diagnosis of Giant Cell Tumor
Differential Diagnosis of Giant Cells
Treatment
Prognosis
Metastases
Glomus Tumor
General
History and Physical Examination
Differential Diagnosis
Treatment
Hemangioma
General
Imaging
Pathology
Treatment/Prognosis
Intramuscular Hemangioma
Hemipelvectomy
Internal Hemipelvectomy
Reconstruction Options
Hinge Total Knee Replacement (TKR)
Indications
Leukemia (Acute Lymphocytic Leukemia [ALL])
History and Physical Examination
Laboratory Values
Treatment
Prognosis
Lipoma
General
History and Physical Examination
Imaging
Pathology
Treatment
Variants
Intramuscular Lipoma
Liposarcoma
General
Subtypes With Differing Courses
Imaging
Pathology
Metastases
Treatment and Prognosis
Lymphoma of Bone
General
History and Physical Examination
Imaging
Pathology
Treatment
Malignant Fibrous Histiocytoma
General
History and Physical Examination

Subtypes
Pathology
Metastases
Treatment (for Soft Tissue Sarcomas)
Prognosis
Malignant Fibrous Histiocytoma of Bone
General
Histologic Subtypes
Treatment
Prognosis
Metastatic Renal Cell Carcinoma (RCC)
General
Prognosis
Treatment
Metastatic Thyroid Cancer
General
Prognosis
Multiple Hereditary Osteochondromas (MHO)
General
Presentation
Natural History
Differential Diagnosis
Surgery
Multiple Myeloma
General
Clinical Variants
Presentation
Laboratory Values
Imaging
Diagnosis
Pathology
Staging
Treatment
Prognosis
Myositis Ossificans
Imaging
Pathology
Treatment
Nerve Sheath Tumors
Neurilemoma (Schwannoma)
Neurofibroma
Malignant Peripheral Nerve Sheath Tumor (MPNST)
Nonossifying Fibroma
General
History and Physical Examination
Imaging
Differential Diagnosis
Histology
Natural History
Treatment
Ossifying Fibroma
General
Differential Diagnosis
Treatment

Osteoblastoma
  General
  Imaging
  Pathology
  Differential Diagnosis
  Treatment
Osteochondroma
  General
  Imaging
  Differential Diagnosis
  Pathology
  Natural History
  Treatment
Osteogenic Sarcoma—Classic
  High Grade
  General
  History and Physical Examination
  Imaging
  Pathology
  Differential Diagnosis
  Metastases
  Treatment
  Prognosis
  Molecular Staging
Osteogenic Sarcoma—Subtypes
  Primary Osteosarcoma
  Secondary Osteosarcoma
Osteoid Osteoma
  General
  Prostaglandins
  History and Physical Examination
  Imaging
  Pathology
  Differential Diagnosis
  Treatment
Paget Disease
  General
  History and Physical Examination
  Laboratory Values
  Imaging
  Differential Diagnosis
  Pathology
  Oncologic Problems
  Medical Treatment
  Surgical Treatment
Periosteal Chondroma
  General
  Imaging
  Natural History
  Pathology
  Treatment
Postradiation Sarcoma of Bone
Pigmented Villonodular Synovitis/Giant Cell
  Tumor of Tendon Sheath
  General
  Imaging
  Pathology
  Treatment
  Giant Cell Tumor of Tendon Sheath
Rhabdomyosarcoma
  General
  History and Physical Examination
  Subtypes
  Pathology
  Differential Diagnosis
  Treatment
Unicameral Bone Cyst
  General
  Imaging
  Differential Diagnosis
  Pathology
  Prognosis
  Treatment
Synovial Chondromatosis
  General
  History and Physical Examination
  Imaging
  Pathology
  Treatment
Synovial Sarcoma
  General
  Imaging
  Metastases
  Pathology
  Treatment
  Prognosis
Tumoral Calcinosis
  General
  History and Physical Examination
  Imaging
  Pathology
  Treatment

Benign Lytic Bone Lesions

MNEMONIC—"FEGNOMASHIC"

Fibrous Dysplasia
- Can be mixed sclerotic
- Ground glass, expansile
- Long lesion in long bone
- Monostic lesion in proximal femur
- If in tibia, think of adamantinoma

Enchondroma
- Calcification a must, except in fingers
- Stippled or popcorn calcification
- Most common in phalanges
- Ollier disease—multiple, benign, uncommonly malignant

- Maffucci syndrome—multiple, with hemangiomas, can denerate to malignant

Eosinophilic Granuloma (EG)
- <30 yo
- Diaphyseal
- Waveform layer of new bone
- Not expansile
- No soft tissue mass
- No sclerotic border early, sclerosis with healing

Giant Cell Tumor (GCT)
- Closed epiphysis
- Epiphyseal
- Abuts articular surface
- Eccentric
- No sclerotic border

Nonossifying Fibroma (NOF)
- <30 yo
- Eccentric, elongated
- Scalloped thin sclerotic border

Osteoblastoma
- Think of this whenever you think of aneurysmal bone cyst
- Posterior spine
- Even if >30 yo

Myeloma, Metastases
- >40 yo
- Renal cell cancer with bubble lesions
- Metastases usually medullary, not cortical
- Lung cancer metastases can be cortical

Aneurysmal Bone Cyst (ABC)
- <30 yo
- Expansile, anywhere, eccentric
- Magnetic resonance imaging (MRI) fluid/fluid level

Simple Bone Cyst/Unicameral Bone Cyst (UBC)
- <30 yo
- **Central**

Hyperparathyroidism (HyperPTH)
- Other evidence of hyperPTH
- Periosteal erosion
- Brown tumor

Infection
- Adjacent to joint
- Percolates through cortex
- Mixed lytic-sclerotic

Chondroblastoma
- <30 yo, epiphyseal
- Intralesional calcification

Chondromyxoid Fibroma (CMF)
- Similar in appearance to NOF
- Cortical buttressing

RULE OUT IF OLDER THAN 30 YEARS
- EG
- ABC
- NOF
- Chondroblastoma
- UBC

RULE OUT IF PAIN OR PERIOSTITIS (WITHOUT FRACTURE)
- Fibrous dysplasia
- Enchondroma
- NOF
- UBC

EPIPHYSEAL
- Chondroblastoma
- Clear cell chondrosarcoma
- GCT
- Infection
- Geode
- Metastases/myeloma

MULTIPLE
- Fibrous dysplasia
- Enchondroma
- Metastases, myeloma
- HyperPTH
- Infection

SEQUESTRATIONS
- Osteomyelitis
- EG
- Fibrosarcoma
- Lymphoma
- Osteoid osteoma

EXPANSILE, LYTIC, POSTERIOR SPINE
- ABC
- Osteoblastoma
- Tuberculosis (TB)

DIFFERENTIAL DIAGNOSIS, SCLEROSIS, AGE 20–40 Yr
- NOF
- EG

- UBC
- ABC
- Chondroblastoma

SACRAL LESIONS

- GCT
- Chordoma
- Osteoblastoma
- Chondrosarcoma
- Metastases

Reference

Helms CA. Fundamentals of Skeletal Radiology. Philadelphia: Saunders; 2004.

Biopsy Principles

HIGH COMPLICATION RATE

(Mankin et al., 1996)
- 600 malignant tumors
- 8% biopsies inadequate
- Biopsies led to 18% inaccurate diagnosis
- Led to 20% change in treatment
- Led to 10% change in outcome
- Error 2–12 times more likely when biopsy done at referring facility

TYPES OF BIOPSY

- Fine-needle aspiration
  - 21G needle
  - Stab tumor with 5 mL of fluid
  - Put on glass slide
- Needle biopsy (Skrzynski et al., 1996)
  - 84% accurate
  - 93% accurate for malignancy
- Open biopsy
  - 96% accurate

Frozen Sections

- At Memorial Sloan-Kettering, diagnosis changes from frozen to final pathological in 15% of cases

PRACTICAL BIOPSY TIPS

- Biopsy is last step of evaluation
  - Chest computed tomography (CT) affected by general anesthesia
  - Biopsy may affect MRI
- Talk to pathologist before biopsy
- Hold antibiotics
- No Esmarch to avoid fracture, tumor embolization
- Longitudinal incision based on incision for definitive procedure

- Go through muscle
- Biopsy the most aggressive part of lesion
- Biopsy periphery of lesion
- Biopsy soft tissue component of bone mass
- Do frozen biopsy to confirm adequacy
- Consider polymethylmethacrylate (PMMA) over hole in diaphysis to control hematoma and tumor contamination
- Drain inline with skin incision
- Careful hemostasis

INDICATIONS FOR PRIMARY EXCISIONAL BIOPSY

- Osteoid osteoma (must remove all of it)
- Soft tissue sarcoma <3 cm (easy to get wide margins)
- Fibular head mass (avoid contamination of peroneal nerve)

NO NEED FOR BIOPSY

- Radiographic diagnosis, assuming classic signs:
  - Enchondroma
  - Fibrous cortical defect
  - NOF
  - Bone infarct
  - Osteochondroma
  - Fibrous dysplasia
  - Proven metastases

BIOPSY AND SHAPE OF BONE HOLE

(Clark et al., 1977)
- 23 pairs of human femora
  - 1—Rectangular, square corners
  - 2—Rectangular, rounded corners
  - 3—Oblong hole with rounded ends
- 1 and 2 were equal
- Oblong hole withstood 44% more torque before failure and stored 83% more energy
- Increasing the width of the hole weakened the bone, whereas increasing the length did not
- Parallel straight-down cut increased amount of bone removed but did not change strength of bone compared to cuts perpendicular to bone surface

BIOPSY AND SIZE OF BONE HOLE

- 1/4-in. hole leads to 50% decreased torsion strength (Burstein et al., 1972; Edgerton et al., 1990)
- Paired sheep femora
- Circular defects from 10% to 60% of diameter created and torqued

- Small defect of 10% caused no significant decrease in torsional strength
- 20% defect led to 34% decreased strength
- 50% defect led to 62% decreased strength
  - Led to 88% decreased energy to failure
- Defects of 20%–60% decreased strength linearly; thus, there was no "open section" where there was a sudden decrease in strength

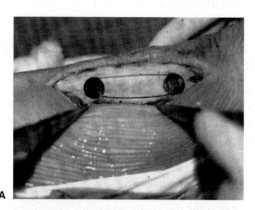

An oblong window made by connecting two circular holes lessens the chance of a pathologic fracture. **A:** Photograph of a biopsy of the tibia following the fashioning of two circular holes connected by straight saw lines.
B: Photograph of the tibia following removal of the window. Note the curved, narrow window. (From Simon MD, Springfield DS. Surgery for Bone and Soft-Tissue Tumors. Philadelphia: Lippincott Williams & Wilkins; 1998, with permission.)

References

Burstein AH, et al. Bone strength: the effect of screw holes. J Bone Joint Surg Am 1972; 54:1143–1156.

Clark CR, et al. The effect of biopsy-hole shape and size on bone strength. J Bone Joint Surg Am 1977; 59:213–217.

Edgerton BC, et al. Torsional strength reduction due to cortical defects in bone. J Orthop Res 1990; 8:851–855.

Mankin HJ, et al. The hazards of the biopsy, revisited. Members of the Musculoskeletal Tumor Society. J Bone Joint Surg Am 1996; 78:656–663.

Skrzynski MC, et al. Diagnostic accuracy and charge-savings of outpatient core needle biopsy compared with open biopsy of musculoskeletal tumors. J Bone Joint Surg Am 1996; 78:644–649.

Fibrous Lesions

- Fibroblasts have pointed nuclei

NONOSSIFYING FIBROMA

- <30 yo

BENIGN FIBROUS HISTIOCYTOSIS (BFH)

- BFH is NOF in patient >30 yo
- Fibrocytes
- Giant cells
- Lipid-laden, foam histiocytes

FIBROUS CORTICAL DEFECT

- Same histology as NOF but smaller at 1–2 cm

DESMOPLASTIC FIBROMA

- Benign, fibroblasts in collagen
- Purely lytic, expands, metaphysis
- Average age 25 yr (12–56 yr)
- Locally destructive
- Often recurs if excision incomplete
- Metastases never been reported
- Curettage to wide resection, depending on affected bone

CHONDROMYXOID FIBROMA

MALIGNANT FIBROUS HISTIOCYTOMA (MFH)

- Spindle cells
- Atypical, pleomorphic nuclei
- Essentially the same as fibrosarcoma

FIBROSARCOMA

- Very similar to MFH but more organized
- Herringbone pattern

References

Cheng EY. Benign soft tissue tumors. In: Craig EV, ed. Clinical Orthopaedics. Philadelphia: Lippincott Williams & Wilkins; 1999:998–1003.

Cheng EY. Malignant soft tissue tumors. In: Craig EV, ed. Clinical Orthopaedics. Philadelphia: Lippincott Williams & Wilkins; 1999:1004–1012.

Malignant Bone Tumors

X-RAY (XR) SIGNS OF MALIGNANCY/ AGGRESSIVENESS

- Cortical destruction
- periostitis
- Zone of transition
  - Only with lytic lesion on XR

MIMICS MALIGNANT BONE TUMOR

- Eosinophilic granuloma
- Infection

MALIGNANT BONE TUMOR AND AGE

- *Note:* Using age only, diagnosis can be made in 80% of cases
- <30 yo
  - Ewing sarcoma
  - Osteosarcoma
- 30–40 yo
  - Fibrosarcoma and MFH
  - Malignant giant cell tumor
  - Lymphoma
  - Parosteal sarcoma
- >40 yo
  - Metastases
  - Myeloma
  - Chondrosarcoma

TUMORS WITH BONE EDEMA

- Pathological fracture
- Osteoblastoma
- Osteoid osteoma
- Chondroblastoma
- Various other cancers

Reference

Helms CA. Fundamentals of Skeletal Radiology. Philadelphia: Saunders; 2004.

Metastatic Carcinoma

BONE METASTASES

- "BLT with Kosher Pickle": Breast, Lung, Thyroid, Kidney, Prostate
- Most common place for bony metastases is spine
- Majority is breast and prostate
- Metastases uncommon to elbows and knees
- Most common metastasis to hand is lung

Presenting Symptoms

- Pain (75%)
- Fracture (25%)
- Cord compression (10%)
- Hypercalcemia (10%–30%)

Blastic versus Lytic

- 75% of prostate metastases are blastic
  - Multifocal, axial first
- 50% of breast metastases are blastic
- 25% of lung metastases are blastic

Acrometastases

(Healey et al., 1986)
- 29 patients, 41 acrometastases
- Five patients mimicked benign condition and wrong treatment given
- 11 patients had acrometastases as first indication of malignant disease

Biopsy

- Should be performed at first appearance of lesion to confirm metastases as diagnosis, except for anatomically difficult locations

Metastatic Breast

- 85% of BRCA have bone metastases at death

Metastatic Bladder

- Bone is most common metastasis second to within pelvis
- 30% patients have bone metastases at autopsy

Metastatic Colon

- Rare to bone (1%–6%)
- When to bone, 80% patients also had metastases to other systems
- Bone metastases only—38% 5-yr survival
- Bone and other metastases—16% 5-yr survival

Metastatic Lung

- 8% positive bone scan after resection of stages I and II
- Lesion is often cortical
- More bone metastases with adenocarcinoma
- Median survival after diagnosis of metastases to hand is 6 mo

Better Survival Associated With the Following

(Bohm & Huber, 2002)
- No visceral metastases
- No pathological fracture
- >3 yr from diagnosis to first metastasis

References

Bohm P, Huber J. The surgical treatment of bony metastases of the spine and limbs. J Bone Joint Surg Br 2002; 84:521–529.

Healey JH, et al. Acrometastases: a study of twenty-nine patients with osseous involvement of the hands and feet. J Bone Joint Surg Am 1986; 68:743–746.

Musculoskeletal Tumors

BONE DYSPLASIA

- Fibrous dysplasia
- Osteogenesis imperfecta
- Osteopoikilosis
- Melorheostosis
- Paget disease

BENIGN BONE

- UBC
- NOF
- Langerhans cell histiocytosis (LCH; EG)
- GCT
- ABC
- Osteoid osteoma
- Osteoblastoma

MALIGNANT BONE

- Osteosarcoma
- Ewing sarcoma
- Chondrosarcoma
- Lymphoma
- Adamantinoma

BENIGN CARTILAGE

- Enchondroma
- Osteochondroma
- Chondroblastoma
- Chondromyxoid fibroma

SYNOVIAL TUMORS

- Pigmented villonodular synovitis (PVNS)
- Synovial chondromatosis

BENIGN SOFT TISSUE

- Lipoma
- Hemangioma
- Desmoid

MALIGNANT SOFT TISSUE

- MFH
- Liposarcoma
- Synovial cell sarcoma
- Rhabdomyosarcoma
- Malignant peripheral nerve sheath tumor

NERVE SHEATH TUMORS

- Schwannoma
- Neurofibroma
- Neurilemoma
- Myeloma
- Metastases

NONTUMORS

- Avascular necrosis (AVN)
- Rheumatoid arthritis (RA)
- Gout
- Calcium pyrophosphate dihydrate deposition disease (CPPD)
- Osteomalacia/rickets
- Osteoporosis
- Gaucher disease
- Bone infarct
- Bone island (enostosis)
- Intraosseous ganglion

Pathological Fracture

- Functional pain = loss of mechanical strength

(Mirels, 1989)
- Retrospective on 78 lesions that were given radiation therapy (XRT) in 38 patients with 6-mo follow-up

Score	1	2	3
Site	UE	LE	Peritroch
Pain	Mild	Moderate	Functional
Lesion	Blastic	Mixed	Lytic
Size	<1/3	1/3–2/3	>2/3

- 35% fractured within 6 mo—mean score 10
- Remaining 65% did not fracture—mean score 7
- Score and fracture prognosis
  - 7–4% fracture, do not do open reduction and internal fixation (ORIF)
  - 8–15% fracture, get CT to evaluate size
  - 9–33% fracture, ORIF
- Breast—lowest fracture risk
- Lung—highest fracture risk

MORTALITY AND PROGNOSIS

- After pathological fracture, lung cancer has 100% 6-mo mortality
- After pathological fracture, breast cancer has 50% 6-mo mortality

- Mean patient survival after pathological fracture of long bone or pelvis
  - Prostate 29 mo
  - Breast 23 mo
  - Kidney 12 mo
  - Lung 4 mo

AFTER RESECTION OF SOFT TISSUE SARCOMA

(Lin et al., 1998)
- Risk factors
  - Female, lower extremity
  - Bone or periosteal resection
  - Irradiation
- Occurs late, often >6 mo
- Nonunions common

(Gainor & Buchert, 1983)
- Retrospective of 130 pathological fractures
  - Multiple myeloma—67% union
  - Renal cell—44% union
  - Breast—37% union
  - Lung—0% union
  - Overall 35% healing
    - 74% union in those living >6 mo
    - Total XRT <3,000 cGy did not affect callus
    - ORIF improved healing rates 23%

References

Gainor BJ, Buchert P. Fracture healing in metastatic bone disease. Clin Orthop 1983; (178):297–302.
Lin PP, et al. Pathologic femoral fracture after periosteal excision and radiation for the treatment of soft tissue sarcoma. Cancer 1998; 82:2356–2365.
Mirels H. Metastatic disease in long bones: a proposed scoring system for diagnosing impending pathologic fractures. Clin Orthop 1989; (249):256–264.

Skeletal Metastases of Unknown Origin

- (Rougraff et al., 1993)
- Prospective study of ability of protocol to identify primary tumor in 40 consecutive patients

PROTOCOL

- History and physical—8% found
- Chest XR (CXR)—+43% found
- CT chest—+15%
- CT abdominal/pelvis—+13% found
- Biopsy—+8% found
- Bone scan
- 85% of primary tumor identified with this protocol
- 75% identified with CT chest/abdomen/pelvis alone

RECOMMENDATIONS FROM THIS STUDY

- Do not start with biopsy because only additional 8% identified with biopsy

- Unable to identify primary in 65% with biopsy alone
- Do not mammogram unless history and physical abnormal because breast is uncommon cause of skeletal metastases of unknown origin
- Rule out multiple myeloma
- Most common skeletal metastases of known origin
  - Breast
  - Prostate
- Most common skeletal metastases of unknown origin
  - Lung (63%)
  - Kidney (10%)

Reference

Rougraff BT, et al. Skeletal metastases of unknown origin: a prospective study of a diagnostic strategy. J Bone Joint Surg Am 1993; 75:1276–1281.

Soft Tissue Sarcomas

- Superficial tumors have 1:100 chance of being malignant
- Deep tumors have 1:10 chance of being malignant

TYPES

- Malignant fibrous histiocytoma—most common
- Liposarcoma—second most common
- Synovial sarcoma—third most common (most common in foot; however, most common in hand at Memorial Sloan-Kettering [MSKCC])
- Rhabdomyosarcoma (most common in children)
- Leiomyosarcoma
- Clear cell sarcoma (most common lymph node spread)
- Epithelioid (most common soft tissue sarcoma in hand)
- Fibrosarcoma
- Angiosarcoma
- Hemangiopericytoma
- Hemangioendothelioma

Soft Tissue Sarcomas That Spread Through Lymph Nodes
- Clear cell
- Epithelioid
- Synovial
- Rhabdomyosarcoma

Soft Tissue Sarcomas of Hand
- Most common was synovial sarcoma at MSK versus epithelioid sarcoma on Orthopaedic In-Training Examination (OITE)
- Compared with <5-cm lesions elsewhere, lesions in hand have worse prognosis

Soft Tissue Sarcoma, Metastases Workup

- Metastases to lungs
- Rare to bones (thus, usually no bone scan needed for systemic workup)
- Physical exam
- CXR and CT

GRADING

- Considered high grade if >15% of tumor is high grade

TREATMENT

- All generally treated the same except rhabdomyosarcoma and synovial sarcoma, which are sensitive to chemotherapy
- Treatment is surgical ± XRT
- XRT usually if high grade ± positive margins
  - Usually total ~6,000 cGy in 200-cGy fractions
- Chemotherapy usually for metastatic disease (high-dose Adriamycin and ifosfamide is most effective)

CHEMOTHERAPY

(Sarcoma Meta-Analysis Collaboration, 1997)
- Meta-analysis of randomized controlled trials for adjuvant Adriamycin-based drugs with surgery
- Improved time to local and distant recurrence
- Absolute 10% improvement of overall recurrence-free survival at 10 years
- Trend toward absolute 4% improvement of 10-year survival (Frustaci et al., 2001)
- Randomized controlled trial of doxorubicin/ifosfamide versus no chemotherapy
- 50 patients with spindle cell sarcoma in each arm
- Disease-free survival 48 mo versus 16 mo
- Overall survival 72 mo versus 46 mo
- No toxic deaths from chemotherapy

PROGNOSIS

- Size is more important than depth or histologic subtype for prognosis
- Margin status most important for local recurrence
- Grade most important for risk of metastases

References

Frustaci S, et al. Adjuvant chemotherapy for adult soft tissue sarcomas of the extremities and girdles: results of the Italian randomized cooperative trial. J Clin Oncol 2001; 19:1238–1247.

Mankin HJ, Hornicek FJ. Diagnosis, classification, and management of soft tissue sarcomas. Cancer Control 2005; 12: 5–21.

Sarcoma Meta-Analysis Collaboration. Adjuvant chemotherapy for localised resectable soft-tissue sarcoma of adults: meta-analysis of individual data. Lancet 1997; 350:1647–1654.

Spine Tumors

AGE, LOCATION, AND DIFFERENTIAL DIAGNOSIS

- >40 yo—think metastases
- <40 yo, posterior elements
  - Usually benign
  - Osteoid osteoma, osteoblastoma
  - ABC
  - Excisional biopsy or intralesional resection
- <40 yo, anterior elements
  - Think malignant
  - Ewing sarcoma or osteosarcoma, if younger
  - Lymphoma, myeloma
  - Hemangioma
  - Giant cell tumor
  - Eosinophilic granuloma

Spine Tumor Pearls

- Craniocervical or sacral location:
  - Think chordoma
  - Primary bone tumors rare in C-spine

Hemangioma

- "Jailhouse," "honeycomb"
- Striations, stippled
- Bright on T1 and T2 images

Paget Disease

- Dense at edges
- "Picture window" vertebra

Lymphoma

- "Ivory vertebrae"
- Entire vertebral body is dense, no change in shape

Eosinophilic Granuloma

- "Vertebra plana"

Osteomyelitis

- Destroys disc space
- Crosses joint space

"Rugger Jersey Spine"

- Renal osteodystrophy
- Osteomalacia
- Osteopetrosis

Vertebral Body With Increased Radiodensity

- Lymphoma
- Metastatic breast or prostate cancer
- Paget disease

Thalassemia

- Distal femur, Erlenmeyer flask shape
  - Due to increased marrow

- Unlike sickle cell, no infarctions
- Vertebral body with vertical striations
  - Due to increased marrow, decreased trabecula

Reference

Helms CA. Fundamentals of Skeletal Radiology. Philadelphia: WB Saunders; 1995.

Spine Metastatic Tumors

GENERAL

(Harrington, 1993)
- Most common site of bony metastases
- Vertebral body usually affected first (90%) due to blood supply (via Batson valveless plexus), then spreads to pedicles
- Avascular disc is spared (if disc affected, think infection)
- Tumor lysis weakens bone, body collapses, progressive kyphotic deformity, and extrusion of tumor/bone/disc into canal
- Motor deficits typically precede sensory deficits due to anterior location of compression
- Rapidity of onset of weakness associated with worst prognosis because sudden onset is likely caused by vascular compromise of cord

IMAGING

- XR normal until one-third of vertebral body is destroyed
- Loss of pedicle is early XR sign (owl wink)
- Myeloma can be falsely negative on bone scan
- **Disc spared** on every cut on MR
  - Dark on T1 (fatty marrow replaced)
  - Bright on T2 (edema)

TREATMENT

- Steroids (especially for lymphoma, leukemia)
- XRT alone if life expectancy <4 mo
  - Consider radiosensitivity of primary cancer

Indications for Surgery
- Progressive neurologic compromise
- Intractable mechanical pain

Consider Surgery Before Radiation Therapy If:
- Instability—any translation is unstable
- **Circumferential radioinsensitive** tumor
- Bone in canal

SURGERY PRINCIPLES

- Posterior laminectomy without stabilization is only as effective as XRT (Gilbert et al., 1978)

- Anterior compression must be decompressed anteriorly, followed by anterior stabilization (if posterior elements remain intact)
- Combined anterior and posterior "napkin ring" compression must be decompressed anteriorly and posteriorly and stabilized anteriorly and posteriorly
- Anterior-posterior procedure usually necessary for disease at cervicothoracic or thoracolumbar junctions, or translational deformity
- No role for laminectomy alone
- Consider achieving instant stability with PMMA because bone grafts not likely to incorporate in setting of postoperative XRT
- Bone grafting and fusion indicated if life expectancy >6 mo

Posterolateral Transpedicle Approach (PTA)
(Bilsky et al., 2000)
- Anterior approach alone usually suffices for body and anterior epidural tumor
- Anterior-posterior procedure needed for:
  - Three-column disease
  - Multilevel body or epidural tumor
  - Bilateral or circumferential cord compression
  - Major deformity
- PTA avoids the morbidity of anterior approach in patients who need circumferential decompression and fusion
- Allows maximal decompression and immediate stability with circumferential fusion

References

Bilsky MH, et al. Single-stage posterolateral transpedicle approach for spondylectomy, epidural decompression, and circumferential fusion of spinal metastases. Spine 2000; 25:2240–2249; discussion 250.

Gilbert RW, et al. Epidural spinal cord compression from metastatic tumor: diagnosis and treatment. Ann Neurol 1978; 3(1):40–51.

Harrington KD. Metastatic tumors of the spine: diagnosis and treatment. J Am Acad Orthop Surg 1993; 1(2):76–86.

Khan SN, Donthineni R. Surgical management of metastatic spine tumors. Orthop Clin North Am 2006; 37:99–104.

Staging, Types of Excisions

MUSCULOSKELETAL TUMOR STAGING

- Grade (histology)
  - T—size
  - N—nodes (essentially equals distant metastases)
  - M—metastases (most important for prognosis)

BENIGN ENNEKING SYSTEM

- 1—Latent (enchondroma, fibrocartilaginous dysplasia [FCD])

- 2—Active (ABC, eroded cortex)
- 3—Aggressive (GCT, breaks through cortex, soft tissue component)

MALIGNANT ENNEKING SYSTEM

- I—low grade
  - A—intracompartmental
  - B—extracompartmental
- II—high grade
  - A—intracompartmental
  - B—extracompartmental
- III—any metastases or nodes

MALIGNANT BONE (AJCC-6)

- I—low grade
  - A—<8 cm
  - B—≥8 cm
- II—high grade
  - A—<8 cm
  - B—≥8 cm
- III—skip metastases (same bone)
- IV—distant metastases
  - A—lung metastases
  - B—other than lung

SOFT TISSUE TUMOR STAGING (AJCC-5)

- IA—low grade, small, superficial or deep
- IB—low grade, large, superficial
- IIA—low grade, large, deep
- IIB—high grade, small, superficial or deep
- IIC—high grade, large, superficial
- III—high grade, large, deep
- IV—metastases

SOFT TISSUE (AJCC-6)

- AJCC-5 grouped together to I, II, III, and IV

TYPES OF EXCISIONS

- Intralesional
- Marginal (in pseudocapsule)
- Wide (with cuff of normal tissue)
- Radical (entire compartment)

References

Peabody TD, et al. Evaluation and staging of musculoskeletal neoplasms. J Bone Joint Surg Am 1998; 80:1204–1218.

Scarborough MT. Musculoskeletal neoplasms: staging, biopsy, and surgical margins. In: Craig EV, ed. Clinical Orthopaedics. Philadelphia: Lippincott Williams & Wilkins; 1999:972–975.

Radiation Therapy

HIGH SENSITIVITY

- Myeloma
- Lymphoma
- 2,500–5,000 cGy adequate

MODERATE SENSITIVITY

- Colon
- Breast
- Prostate
- Lung
- Squamous cell

LOW SENSITIVITY

- Renal
- Thyroid
- Melanoma
- Metastatic sarcoma

COMPLICATIONS

(Threshold 3,000–3,500 cGy)
- Destruction of microvasculature
- Myelopathy
- Transverse myelitis
- Radiation osteitis
- Wound healing
- Graft incorporation
- Osteochondromas on edge of field

BRACHYTHERAPY (INTRAOPERATIVE RADIATION THERAPY)

- Allows high doses to limited tissue volume
- Reduced XRT treatment time
- Less expensive than external XRT
- Reduced local recurrence for high-grade soft tissue sarcomas in randomized trial
- Advantageous if flap needed
- Logistically complex

PREOPERATIVE VERSUS POSTOPERATIVE RADIATION THERAPY FOR SOFT TISSUE SARCOMA

(O'Sullivan et al., 2002)
- Randomized controlled trial, about 100 patients each arm
- Wound complications 35% for preop versus 17% for postop
- Survival slightly better in preop group

Reference

O'Sullivan B, et al. Preoperative versus postoperative radiotherapy in soft-tissue sarcoma of the limbs: a randomised trial. Lancet 2002; 359:2235–2241.

Aneurysmal Bone Cyst

GENERAL

- Fast-growing vascular blow-out lesion
- Common

- F = M
- <30 yo, usually in second decade
- Most common in distal femur, proximal tibia
- **Metaphysis of long bone, posterior elements of spine**
- Can be anywhere

HISTORY AND PHYSICAL EXAMINATION

- Mild pain and swelling

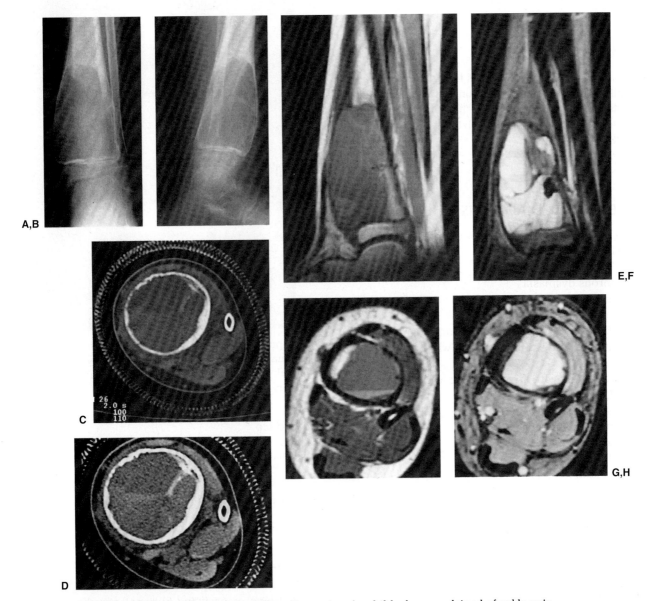

A,B

C

D

E,F

G,H

Anteroposterior **(A)** and lateral **(B)** radiographs of a child who complained of ankle pain and swelling for 6 mo show an eccentric, expansile, well-marginated stage II lesion of the metaphysis of the distal tibia without intralesional mineralization. Computed tomography scans of the lesion **(C, D)** confirmed that this was a stage II lesion without intralesional mineralization, and demonstrated a possible fluid–fluid level. Magnetic resonance images of the lesion **(E–H)** show fluid–fluid levels most compatible with an aneurysmal bone cyst. (From Simon MD, Springfield DS. Surgery for Bone and Soft-Tissue Tumors. Philadelphia: Lippincott Williams & Wilkins; 1998, with permission.)

IMAGING

- XR
  - Ballooned, soap bubble (multicyst)
  - Eggshell cortical rim
  - Eccentric
  - Expansile
  - Most commonly diaphyseal
- MRI—gray on T1, bright on T2
- CT—*fluid/fluid levels*
- Bone scan shows increased uptake

PATHOLOGY

- Blood-filled cavity with villous lining
- Wall composed of fibrous connective tissue, **giant cells,** mononuclear cells, and "blue" bone (much busier and cellular compared with UBC)
- Slitlike lumen
- Lumen **hemorrhagic**

DIFFERENTIAL DIAGNOSIS

- It is a diagnosis of exclusion. Must rule out:
  - GCT
  - Telangiectatic sarcoma
  - Fibrous dysplasia
  - Osteoblastoma
  - Chondroblastoma
  - UBC (UBC is narrower than width of growth plate, whereas ABC is wider than the width of the growth plate)
- Other tumors with areas of cystic ABC-like tissue
  - GCT
  - Osteoblastoma
  - Chondroblastoma
  - Osteosarcomas
  - Fibrous dysplasia
  - Vascular neoplasms

TREATMENT

- Significant bleeding from axial lesions; therefore, consider embolization
- Curettage and graft
  - Recurrence 20%–70%
  - Recurrence 8% with cryotherapy
  - Recurs usually within 6 mo, rare after 2 yr
- Higher recurrence if growth plate open
- Adjuvant therapy to avoid recurrence
- May want to radiate anatomically dangerous lesions because of reported degeneration to MFH or osteosarcoma

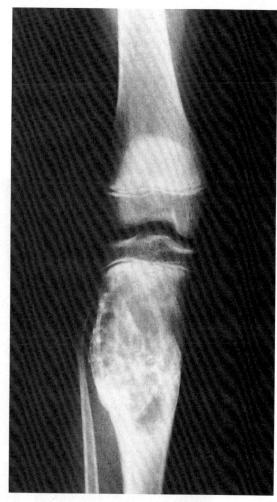

Anteroposterior view of the knee and proximal tibia of a 12-yo male, showing an aneurysmal bone cyst. (From Craig EV, et al. Clinical Orthopedics. Philadelphia: Lippincott Williams & Wilkins; 1999, with permission.)

Reference

Ramirez AR, Stanton RP. Aneurysmal bone cyst in 29 children. J Pediatr Orthop 2002; 22:533–539.

Adamantinoma

GENERAL

- Rare, low-grade malignant bone tumor
- 20–40 yo
- **Osteofibrous dysplasia** (also known as Campanacci syndrome or ossifying fibroma) may be the benign precursor to adamantinoma

X-RAY

- Exclusively in tibia, usually no bowing
- Starts anterior cortex then invades canal
- Bubbly symmetric lytic lesion

HISTORY AND PHYSICAL EXAMINATION

- Pain for months to years
- Angular deformity, mass

PATHOLOGY

- Squamouslike cells in sheets (epithelial)
- Osteofibrous dysplasia (looks like fibrous dysplasia but with bone also)
- Has mesenchymal and epithelioid components

TREATMENT

- Wide resection needed
- Risk of metastases is <20%

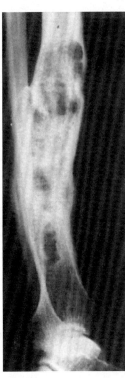

Lateral plain radiograph of a patient with an adamantinoma. This lesion has been present for more than a year. Adamantinoma needs to be resected with a wide surgical margin. This one requires an intercalary resection of the tibia with a small cuff of normal tissue. (From Simon MD, Springfield DS. Surgery for Bone and Soft-Tissue Tumors. Philadelphia: Lippincott Williams & Wilkins; 1998, with permission.)

Reference

Kahn LB. Adamantinoma, osteofibrous dysplasia and differentiated adamantinoma. Skeletal Radiol 2003; 32:245–258.

Bone Island (Enostosis)

GENERAL

- Mature compact cortical bone within cancellous bone
- Cause unclear
    - Tumor?
    - Hamartoma?
    - Failure of resorption during endochondral ossification?

HISTORY AND PHYSICAL EXAMINATION

- Asymptomatic
- Pelvis, femur, other long bones

IMAGING

- Dense sclerotic focus within cancellous bone
- "Thorny radiation" is brushlike border that blends into host trabeculae
- On CT and MR, looks cortical
- Usually cold on bone scan, but mass shows blastic activity on pathology

TREATMENT

- Observation

Reference

Cerase A, Priolo F. Skeletal benign bone-forming lesions. Eur J Radiol 1998; 27(Suppl 1):S91–97.

Chemotherapy—Adriamycin (Doxorubicin)

GENERAL

- An anthracycline
- Intercalating agent
- Interacts with topoisomerase II

MYOCARDIAL TOXICITY

- Irreversible
- Congestive heart failure
- Occurs during or up to years after therapy
- Cumulative dose and infusion rate dependent
- **Rare if <450 mg/m^2**
- Preexisting heart disease increases risk
- Kids at particular risk for delayed cardiac toxicity as drug impairs myocardial growth
- (Steinherz et al., 1995)
    - Onset median 12 yr after chemotherapy
    - Described clinical course in 15 patients

- One death from congestive heart failure (CHF), three sudden deaths
- Hypertrophy, fibrosis, dysrhythmia
- (Lipshultz et al., 1991)
    - Impairs myocardial growth
    - 115 kids with acute lymphoblastic leukemia (ALL) treated with doxorubicin
    - 60% with cardiac abnormality
    - Cumulative dose biggest risk factor
    - Decreased contractility
        - Associated with cumulative dose
    - Increased afterload due to thin left ventricular wall
        - Associated with age <4 yo at treatment
- Electrocardiogram (ECG) and echocardiography (echo) pretreatment and periodically
- Cumulative cardiotoxicity among anthracycline class of drugs
- Red coloration of urine for 1–2 days

EXTRAVASATION

- Leads to tissue necrosis
- Drug is unable to be cleared from subcutaneous tissue, thus spreads progressively
- **Prompt débridement is required**
- No nephrotoxicity
- Death from myelosuppression and subsequent infection

References

Lipshultz SE, et al. Late cardiac effects of doxorubicin therapy for acute lymphoblastic leukemia in childhood. N Engl J Med 1991; 324:808–815.

Steinherz LJ, et al. Cardiac failure and dysrhythmias 6–19 years after anthracycline therapy: a series of 15 patients. Med Pediatr Oncol 1995; 24:352–361.

Chemotherapy—Cisplatin

GENERAL

- Cross-links DNA

ADVERSE EFFECTS

- Cumulative ototoxicity
    - Tinnitus
    - High-frequency loss
    - Can be unilateral
    - May not be reversible
- Cumulative nephrotoxicity
    - Tubular damage
    - Appears 2 wk after first dose
    - Pretreatment hydration
    - Only once per 3–4 wk

- Bone marrow suppression
- Hepatotoxicity
- Peripheral neuropathies reported
- Incompatible with aluminum in needles/IVs

Reference

Ferrari S, et al. Neoadjuvant chemotherapy with high-dose ifosfamide, high-dose methotrexate, cisplatin, and doxorubicin for patients with localized osteosarcoma of the extremity: a joint study by the Italian and Scandinavian Sarcoma Groups. J Clin Oncol 2005; 23:8845–8852.

Chemotherapy—Ifosfamide

GENERAL

- Becomes active by hydroxylation in liver
- Alkylating agent
- Cross-links DNA
- Oncogenic

ADVERSE EFFECTS

- Uropathy
    - Hemorrhagic cystitis
    - Mesna interacts with ifosfamide in renal tubules and detoxifies it
    - Reduces urinary tract complications from 40% to 3%
    - Resolves with cessation of drug
- Nephropathy
    - Parenchymal and tubular necrosis reported
    - Fanconi syndrome (renal tubular acidosis) with electrolyte disturbance
    - Risk factor is prior kidney disease or cisplatin
- Coagulopathy
    - Enhances effects of Coumadin
- Central nervous system
    - Somnolence, hallucinations, confusion, coma
    - Increase in brain metastases or cerebral atherosclerosis
- Myelosuppression
- Alopecia
- Sterility

Reference

Eilber FC, et al. Advances in chemotherapy for patients with extremity soft tissue sarcoma. Orthop Clin North Am 2006; 37:15–22.

Chemotherapy—Vincristine

GENERAL

- Inhibits spindle formation during mitosis
- Inhibits RNA synthesis

ADVERSE EFFECTS

- No consistent significant bone marrow suppression at recommended doses
- Adverse reactions are dose related, reversible
  - Most common is hair loss
  - Most troublesome is neuromuscular
    - Sensory impairment
    - Paresthesias occur first
    - Motor impairment and neuritic pain develop later
  - Syndrome of inappropriate secretion of antidiuretic hormone (SIADH)
- Upper colon fecal impaction (colic but with empty rectum) diagnosed with XR
- Paralytic ileus can occur
- Reactions lessen with decreased dosage
- Overdosage can be fatal
- Fatal if given intrathecally

Reference

Kolb EA, et al. Long-term event-free survival after intensive chemotherapy for Ewing's family of tumors in children and young adults. J Clin Oncol 2003; 21:3423–3430.

Chondroblastoma (Codman Tumor)

GENERAL

- Benign proliferation of immature cartilage
- Less common than giant cell tumor
- 10–20 yo
- 50% in skeletally immature
- <10% in >40 yo
- M > F
- Most common proximal humerus, then distal femur and proximal tibia
- Periacetabular lesion in young patient is commonly chondroblastoma; in old patient, it is commonly chondrosarcoma

HISTORY AND PHYSICAL EXAMINATION

- **Pain**
- Local muscle atrophy
- Joint effusion if cartilage involved

IMAGING

- Lytic
- **Ring of sclerotic bone**
- Open physis

- Unlike GCT, it is usually in skeletally immature but is difficult to tell in a child with chondroblastoma that goes on to close physis with lesion remaining
- **Most common in epiphysis and apophysis**
- Rarely only in metaphysis
- Fine calcification best seen on CT
- Typically central
- Narrow transitional zone
- Classic for bone edema
- Blow-out features with secondary ABC in 20% (this feature is most common in tarsal bones)

DIFFERENTIAL DIAGNOSIS

- CMF—same age group but usually metaphyseal
- GCT—usually in skeletally mature
- EG
- Intraosseous ganglion
- ABC
- UBC
- Clear cell chondrosarcoma
  - Epiphyseal lesion in older patients
  - More calcification

PATHOLOGY

- Chondroblasts (monos with pink cytoplasm) packed like cobblestones
- Fine calcification between cells looks like chicken wire
- Multinucleated giant cells common
- Positive S-100 and vimentin

NATURAL HISTORY

- If left alone, destroys bone and invades joint
- Has <5% metastatic potential
- Follow-up with serial CXRs

TREATMENT

- Biopsy, curettage, bone graft ± PMMA
  - 10% local recurrence
- Second curettage if locally recurs
- Benign lung implants have been reported
- Large intra-articular lesions need joint reconstruction

Reference

Bloem JL, Mulder JD. Chondroblastoma: a clinical and radiological study of 104 cases. Skeletal Radiol 1985; 14:1–9.

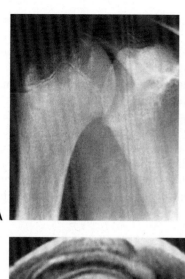
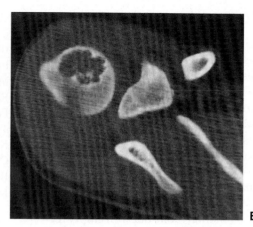
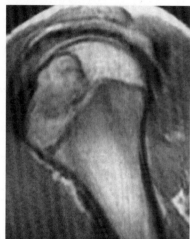

Anteroposterior radiograph **(A)**, computed tomography (CT) scan **(B)**, and sagittal magnetic resonance image **(C)** of the right humerus of an adolescent with vague shoulder pain show a well-marginated epiphyseal lesion, with calcification, best seen on CT. This is a typical example of a chondroblastoma. (From Simon MD, Springfield DS. Surgery for Bone and Soft-Tissue Tumors. Philadelphia: Lippincott Williams & Wilkins; 1998, with permission.)

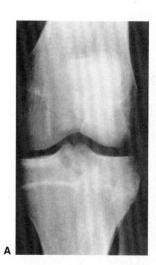
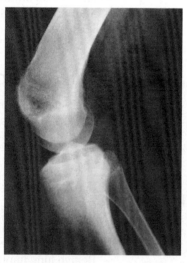
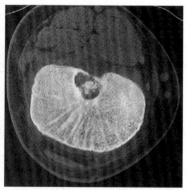

Anteroposterior **(A)** and lateral **(B)** radiographs of the knee in an adolescent boy show a well-marginated central epiphyseal lesion compatible with either a chondroblastoma or giant cell tumor. Computed tomography scan of the lesion **(C)** shows intralesional calcification, substantiating the likely diagnosis of a chondroblastoma. (From Simon MD, Springfield DS. Surgery for Bone and Soft-Tissue Tumors. Philadelphia: Lippincott Williams & Wilkins; 1998, with permission.)

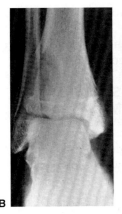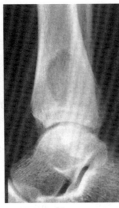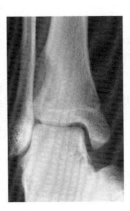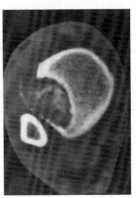

A,B   **C,D**

Anteroposterior **(A)**, lateral **(B),** and oblique **(C)** radiographs of the distal tibia in an
adolescent with ankle pain show a well-marginated eccentric metaphyseal lesion without
any obvious matrix mineralization. This radiographic appearance is most likely compatible
with a nonossifying fibroma, an aneurysmal bone cyst, or chondromyxoid fibroma.
Computed tomography scan of the lesion **(D)** shows calcification in the lesion most
compatible with a chondromyxoid fibroma, instead of the more common nonossifying
fibroma or aneurysmal bone cyst. A magnetic resonance imaging scan would not have
detected this mineralization. (From Simon MD, Springfield DS. Surgery for Bone and
Soft-Tissue Tumors. Philadelphia: Lippincott Williams & Wilkins; 1998, with permission.)

Chondromyxoid Fibroma

GENERAL

– Rare
– 0–20 yo
– More common in males
– Long bones

HISTORY AND PHYSICAL EXAMINATION

– Pain

IMAGING

– Lytic, **eccentric,** buttressing
– Cortical destruction
– Thin periosteal reaction
– Looks like ABC on XR
– **Soap bubble calcification**
– Classic in proximal ulna

PATHOLOGY

– Fibroblasts
– Myxoid tissue
– Nodular chondroid matrix

TREATMENT

– Marginal excision
  – 20%–60% recurrence
  – Recurrence higher in young
– Curette if excision would take away too much bone

Recommended Reading

Lersundi A, et al. Chondromyxoid fibroma: a rarely encountered
  and puzzling tumor. Clin Orthop 2005; 439:171–175.

Chondrosarcoma

GENERAL

– Second most common primary bone tumor
– Malignant cartilage-producing tumor
– Central or peripheral
– Primary or secondary from prior benign cartilage le-
  sion (multiple hereditary exostosis)
– 25% of all chondrosarcomas are those that trans-
  formed from something else
– >50 yo
– M > F
– Less common in Asians
– Chinese patients present younger than Japanese or
  Americans

HISTORY AND PHYSICAL EXAMINATION

– **Pain in hip and buttock**
– Most common in pelvis, proximal femur, and proximal
  humerus
– Common near triradiate cartilage

IMAGING

– XR usually diagnostic
– Bony destruction

- Associated soft tissue mass
- Thick periosteal reaction
- Small foci of calcifications, "popcorn"
- MRI—cartilage is gray on T1, bright on T2

CHONDROSARCOMA (VERSUS OSTEOCHONDROMA)

- Large size
- Growing
- Cartilage cap >2 cm in skeletally mature

CHONDROSARCOMA (VERSUS ENCHONDROMA)

- Size >2 in., older patient, painful
- Growth
- Adaptive changes
  - Cortical thickening
  - Cortical expansion
- Aggressive changes
  - Cortical disruption
  - Soft tissue mass
- If intramedullary canal filled >90% by tumor, then 75% chance of being chondrosarcoma

CHONDROSARCOMA IN SITU

- Premalignant
- **Usually symptomatic**
- No signs of adaptive or aggressive XR changes

- Enchondroma or grade I chondrosarcoma on histology
- 0 of 57 local recurrence after 5 yr from curettage ± liquid nitrogen (Marco et al., 2000)

FIVE HISTOLOGIC SUBTYPES OF CHONDROSARCOMAS

- Dedifferentiated
  - Becomes high-grade osteosarcoma or MFH
  - 10% 5-yr survival, worst prognosis
- Clear cell
  - 85% long-term survival
  - Teens to 30s
  - Secondary ossification centers (epiphyseal)
  - Most common proximal humerus and proximal femur
  - Differential diagnosis—chondroblastoma
- Mesenchymal
  - 30% long-term survival
  - Most common in mandible and vertebrae
  - Chemotherapy may help survival
- Round cell
- Myxoid
  - t(9:22) EWS:TEC(CHN) in extraskeletal

PATHOLOGY

- Histology varies from benign looking to very malignant
- Chondrocytes in lacunae
- Cartilage invading trabeculae and eroding endosteum

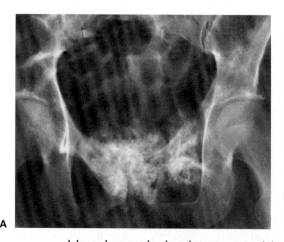
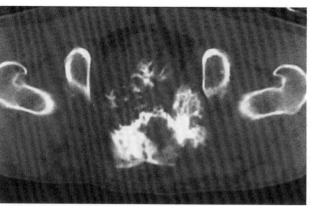

A large low-grade chondrosarcoma originating from the pubis bilaterally in a 45-yo man whose tumor was discovered by rectal palpation during a urologic examination and diagnosed by transrectal needle biopsy of what was thought to be an enlarged prostate. The plain radiograph **(A)** and computed tomography scan **(B)** show the extensive extraosseous soft tissue component of this tumor, characterized by dense, speckled, and popcornlike calcifications characteristic of chondrosarcoma. (From Simon MD, Springfield DS. Surgery for Bone and Soft-Tissue Tumors. Philadelphia: Lippincott Williams & Wilkins; 1998, with permission.)

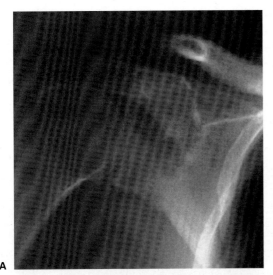

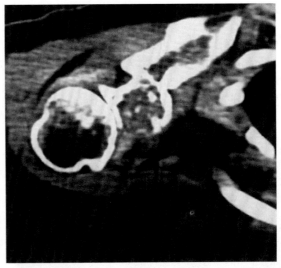

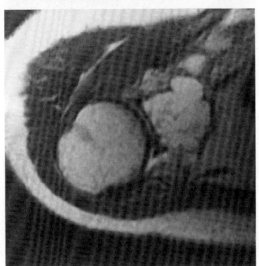

This moderate-grade chondrosarcoma with high-grade areas involved the glenoid and corticoid region of the scapula in an elderly patient. Plain radiograph **(A)** demonstrates a predominantly lytic component with what appears to be some lower-grade findings of pseudotrabeculated endosteal cortical erosion and cortical expansion. However, the computed tomography (CT) scan **(B)** and magnetic resonance imaging **(C)** show an area of cortical destruction and extension of tumor into the surrounding soft tissues, where higher-grade histologic features were identified. The speckled calcifications, which are difficult to appreciate on plain film, are readily apparent on the CT scan. (From Simon MD, Springfield DS. Surgery for Bone and Soft-Tissue Tumors. Philadelphia: Lippincott Williams & Wilkins; 1998, with permission.)

- Histologic grade most important for prognosis and metastases prediction
- Even high-grade chondrosarcoma is not as likely to metastasize as osteosarcoma or Ewing' sarcoma
- S-100 stains for cartilage

DIFFERENTIAL DIAGNOSIS

- Bone infarct, AVN
- Infection
- Enchondroma

METASTASIS

- 3% in low grade
- Up to 60% in high grade
- Must NOT needle biopsy lung mass if chondrosarcoma metastasis is suspected (unlike carcinoma, cartilage does not need much oxygen to survive; thus, needle biopsy seeds pleura and turns potentially resectable disease into incurable disease)

TREATMENT

- Chemotherapy and XRT not very effective
- All, except in situ, need wide resection
- In pelvis, even if pathology is very low grade, needs wide excision because recurrence rate is high
- Low grade—90% cure with wide resection
- High grade—50% cure with wide resection
- Genetic markers not very useful

Reference

Marco RA, et al. Cartilage tumors: evaluation and treatment. J Am Acad Orthop Surg 2000; 8:292–304.

Chordoma

GENERAL

- Arises from notochordal rests
- Slow malignant, locally aggressive
- >50 yo
- M > F
- Practically never in African Americans
- Less common in Asians than Americans
- Fourth most common primary malignancy bone tumor (after osteosarcoma, chondrosarcoma, Ewing sarcoma)

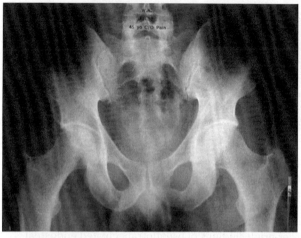

A

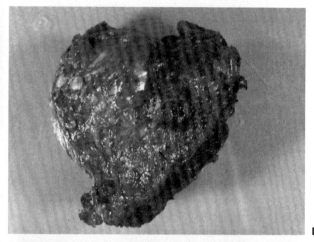

D

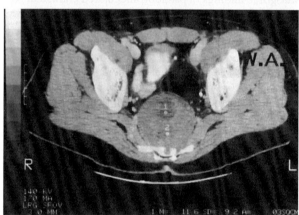

B

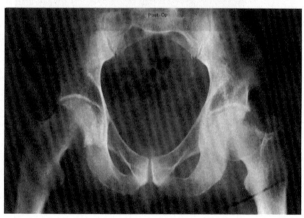

E

Illustrative case of a 45-yo man who presented with complaints of sacral pain associated with bike riding and was subsequently diagnosed as having a chordoma.
A: Anteroposterior radiograph of the pelvis demonstrates subtle loss of definition of the lower sacral foramina.
B: Axial computed tomography scan demonstrates a destructive sacral tumor with a large ventral soft tissue mass. **C:** Sagittal magnetic resonance image again demonstrates the destructive tumor and illustrates the relationship of the tumor mass to the sigmoid colon and other pelvic viscera. **D:** The gross tumor specimen immediately after resection, showing the upper resection level through the inferior aspect of S2. A continence-sparing resection was possible in this case.
E: Postoperative anteroposterior radiograph of the pelvis. (From Simon MD, Springfield DS. Surgery for Bone and Soft-Tissue Tumors. Philadelphia: Lippincott Williams & Wilkins; 1998, with permission.)

C

- Essentially always axial
- 50% are sacrococcygeal and 35% in spheno-occipital region
- Most common tumor of sacrum

HISTORY AND PHYSICAL EXAMINATION

- Pain
- Compresses sacrococcygeal nerves
- **One-half palpable on rectal exam**

IMAGING

- Lytic
- Possible intralesional calcification
- Grows from vertebral body into dura
- Lobulated, low signal on T1, enhances on T2
- Negative on bone scan

PATHOLOGY

- DO NOT do transrectal biopsy
- Vacuolated cells
- Myxoid intracellular matrix
- **Physaliphorous cell (vacuoles encircling nucleus) is hallmark**
- Coexpresses S-100 and epithelial markers (cytokeratins [CKs], epithelial membrane antigen [EMA])
- Cytokeratins (also seen in synovial sarcoma, epithelioid sarcoma)
- Positive carcinogenic embryonic antigen (CEA), periodic acid–Schiff stain (PAS)

DIFFERENTIAL DIAGNOSIS

- Chondrosarcoma—likely to be negative for epithelial markers
- Chondromyxoid fibroma—rarely axial
- Metastatic adenocarcinoma—mistaken for adenocarcinoma because of clear cells and signetlike cells

TREATMENT

Wide Excision

- Laparoscopic assisted ± colostomy (Conlon & Boland, 1997)
  - Laparoscopic rectal mobilization off sacrum
  - Hypogastric arterial isolation
  - Ureter isolation
  - Posterior coccygectomy
  - For large proximal chordomas
- Posterior approach alone if small and does not extend above S3

- Sequential laparotomy and posterior sacrectomy
- Synchronous abdominosacral approach
- XRT possible

PROGNOSIS

- Mean survival 4 yr
- Death from compression of vital structures near axial skeleton
- >10-yr survival is rare due to age
- 10% distant metastases, to lungs
- 40% regional metastases
- High rate of local recurrence

References

Conlon KC, Boland PJ. Laparoscopically assisted radical sacrococcygectomy: a new operative approach to large sacrococcygeal chordomas. Surg Endosc 1997; 11:1118–1122.

Papagelopoulos PJ, et al. Chordoma of the spine: clinicopathological features, diagnosis, and treatment. Orthopedics 2004; 27:1256–1263; quiz 1264–1265.

Clear Cell Sarcoma

GENERAL

- Related to melanoma but behaves like soft tissue sarcoma
- Metastases most common to lymph nodes
- Young adults (15–35 yo)
- Common in foot and ankle, associated with tendons and aponeuroses

PATHOLOGY

- Histologically related to melanoma
  - Neural crest origin
  - Contains melanin
  - Stains for melanoma HMB-45
- EWS:ATF (12:22) translocation

TREATMENT

- Wide excision or amputation
  - Average survival 10 yr
- Marginal or intralesional excision
  - Average survival 6 yr
- Worse prognosis if >5 cm; thus, offer adjuvant therapy with doxorubicin
- Survival—5 yr 67%, 10 yr 33%, 20 yr 10%
  - Need lifelong surveillance
- Potential role for immunotherapy with interferon (IFN)-α2b, like melanoma

References

Bos GD, et al. Foot tumors: diagnosis and treatment. J Am Acad
Orthop Surg 2002; 10:259–270.

Jacobs IA, et al. Clear cell sarcoma: an institutional review. Am
Surg 2004; 70:300–303.

Desmoid (Fibromatosis)

GENERAL

- Also known as desmoid, especially if from abdominal
wall
- A benign but locally invasive neoplasm
- Older children, young adults
- F:M is 2:1
- In abdominal desmoid, F:M is 7:1
- Natural history unpredictable
- No metastatic potential unless radiated
- NOT a low-grade fibrosarcoma
- Associated with Gardner syndrome

HISTORY AND PHYSICAL EXAMINATION

- Painless enlarging mass
- "Rock hard" multiple lesions
- XR nonspecific

IMAGING

- On MRI, low signal intensity (SI) on T1 and T2

PATHOLOGY

- Uniform paucicellular spindle-shaped cells sur-
rounded and separated by collagen fibers
- Dense fibrous tissue
- Myofibroblasts like Dupuytren contracture
- Extremely infiltrative
- In contrast, dermatofibrosarcoma protuberans is
storiform and more superficial

TREATMENT

- Surgery is mainstay
- If wide resection not possible, then marginal resection
with XRT
- Most resected cases have positive margins
- One-half of those with positive margins will recur
- Anti-inflammatories may decrease local recurrence
- 25% local recurrence overall
- Difficult to control once it recurs

Reference

Hosalkar HS, et al. Desmoid tumors and current status of management. Orthop Clin North Am 2006; 37:53–63.

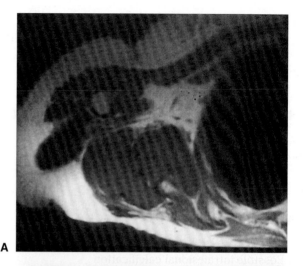

A

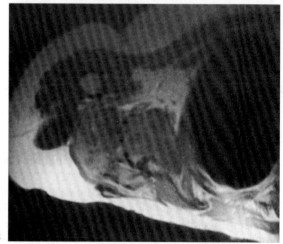

B

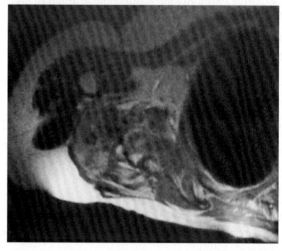

C

Desmoid tumor of the axilla demonstrated on axial
magnetic resonance images. T1-weighted (TR 533, TE 20)
(A), proton density (TR 2000, TE 30) **(B)**, and T2-weighted
(TR 2000, TE 60) **(C)** images. Note heterogeneous low
signals in all pulse sequences. (From Simon MD, Springfield
DS. Surgery for Bone and Soft-Tissue Tumors. Philadelphia:
Lippincott Williams & Wilkins; 1998, with permission.)

Enchondroma

GENERAL

- Solitary benign intramedullary cartilage lesion
- M = F
- Second decade
- Rarely seen in children
- Growth during adulthood
- Most common lytic lesion in hand (short tubular bones)
- Distal femur, proximal humerus

HISTORY AND PHYSICAL EXAMINATION

- **Asymptomatic**
- Presents as incidental finding or pathological fracture
- If pain without fracture, think low-grade chondrosarcoma

IMAGING

- Should not enlarge once growth completed, although calcification may increase
- Intramedullary, **metaphyseal**
- Narrow transition zone

- Punctate calcification, except in hands
- Calcification in adults, usually not in children
- If scalloping and cortical destruction, think chondrosarcoma
- Never in distal phalanx because it forms by membranous ossification
- Scalloping and expansion acceptable if in hand
- On bone scan, shows mild increased uptake but bone infarcts do not

PATHOLOGY

- Nodules of bland chondrocytes, rims of lamellar bone formation, minimal cellularity
- Calcifications are due to necrosis, whereas ossification is more organized
- Enchondromas from hand are allowed to be more cellular than from other sites before being called chondrosarcoma

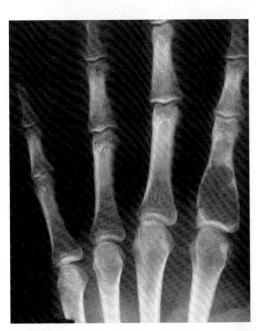

Anteroposterior radiograph of the hand of a young woman with acute pain in the index finger after a trivial injury. The proximal phalanx of the index finger has a well-marginated stage II lesion with intralesional calcification and a pathologic fracture, typical of an enchondroma. (From Simon MD, Springfield DS. Surgery for Bone and Soft-Tissue Tumors. Philadelphia: Lippincott Williams & Wilkins; 1998, with permission.)

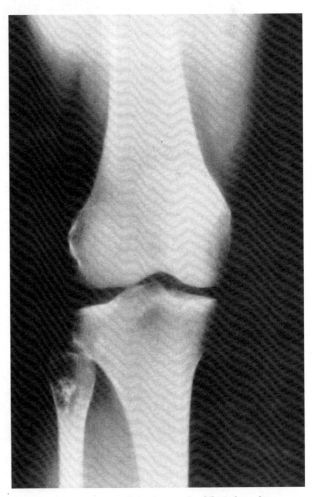

Anteroposterior view of the knee of a 35-yo female, showing an enchondroma. (From Craig EV, et al. Clinical Orthopedics. Philadelphia: Lippincott Williams & Wilkins; 1999, with permission.)

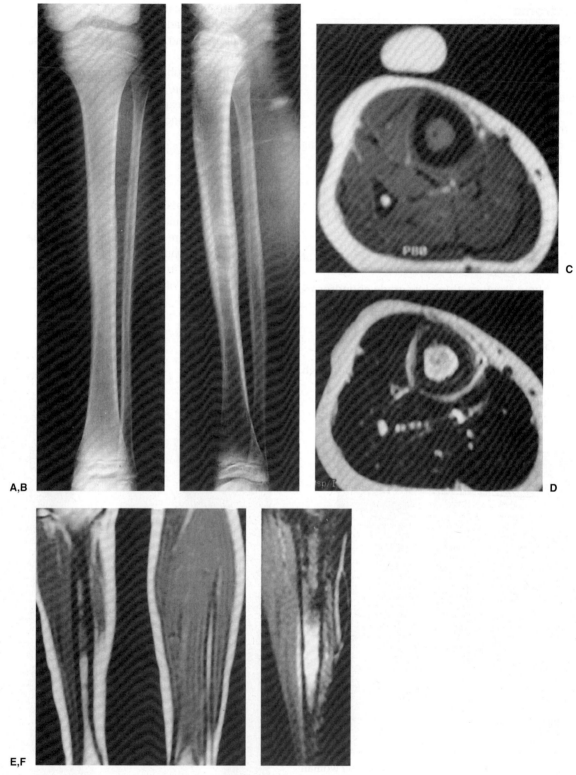

Anteroposterior **(A)** and lateral **(B)** radiographs of the tibia of a child with leg pain for 6 wk show an apparently focal central diaphyseal lesion without intralesional mineralization, which was diagnosed as eosinophilic granuloma. Axial **(C, D)** and coronal **(E, F)** magnetic resonance images of the lesion show a more diffuse process with nonspecific signal characteristics that is more extensive than the lesion on the plain radiographs. (From Simon MD, Springfield DS. Surgery for Bone and Soft-Tissue Tumors. Philadelphia: Lippincott Williams & Wilkins; 1998, with permission.)

NATURAL HISTORY

- 10% chance of growth
- Solitary enchondroma has <1% risk of malignant transformation

TREATMENT

- Usually observation
- Biopsy usually not indicated
- If performing biopsy, do excisional, not incisional
- Patient should have CT/MRI and bone scan
- Small chance of becoming chondrosarcoma
- If pathological fracture, allow to heal, then observe or curette/bone graft

OLLIER DISEASE

- Multiple enchondromas
- Usually on one side of body
- Increased chance of becoming chondrosarcoma
- 30% malignant transformation

MAFFUCCI SYNDROME

- Multiple enchondromas
- Systemic hemangiomas
- Higher rate of malignancy but usually not in the musculoskeletal system
- 60%–100% malignant transformation

Reference
Marco RA, et al. Cartilage tumors: evaluation and treatment. J Am Acad Orthop Surg 2000; 8:292–304.

Eosinophilic Granuloma (Langerhans Cell Histiocytosis)

- Three syndromes with same histology:
  - Eosinophilic granuloma
  - Hand-Schüller-Christian disease
  - Letterer-Siwe disease

EOSINOPHILIC GRANULOMA

- Usually around 7–9 yo, rare >30 yo
- Two-thirds affected are male
- Usually have pain at site
- Pelvis and scapula most common

X-Ray Findings
- Radiolucent
- Waveform layer of new bone
- Soft tissue mass is rare
- Nonexpansile, nonsclerotic border
- Can be permeative—differential diagnosis infection
- **Vertebral plana—collapse of vertebral body**
- If vertebral plana seen, must biopsy for diagnosis

Histology
- Langerhans histiocytes—**fuzzy cells with kidney-shaped nuclei**
- Eosinophils (pink, bilobed nuclei)

Differential Diagnosis
- Ewing sarcoma
- Infection
- If bone pain, constitutional symptoms; with multiple lytic lesions, think leukemia, metastases neuroblastoma, or EG

Treatment
- Often heals spontaneously
- Curettage ± bone grafting at time of biopsy sufficient
- XRT for spine tumor, recurrent tumor, and soft tissue mass (~1,000 cGy)

HAND-SCHÜLLER-CHRISTIAN DISEASE

- Diabetes insipidus
- Exophthalmos
- Bone lesions
- Diagnosis with urine-specific gravity after midnight fast
- Treat with systemic chemotherapy
- Good prognosis

LETTERER-SIWE DISEASE

- Skin, brain, liver, skeleton lesions
- Presents before age 3 yr
- Potentially lethal
- Systemic chemotherapy

Reference
Garg S, Dormans JP. Tumors and tumor-like conditions of the spine in children. J Am Acad Orthop Surg 2005; 13:372–381.

Peripheral Neuroectodermal Tumor

GENERAL

- t(11:22) EWS/FLI1 translocation
- 5–25 yo, 80% of patients <20 yo
- M > F
- Most common in femur, otherwise in flat bone and associated with soft tissue mass
- Rare in African Americans
- Less common in Asians than Americans

– No difference in treatment or prognosis between skeletal and extraskeletal EWS

HISTORY AND PHYSICAL EXAMINATION

– Pain
– Low-grade fever (the only sarcoma with systemic symptoms)
– High erythrocyte sedimentation rate (ESR), white blood cell (WBC) count

IMAGING

– Most common in metaphysis, but diaphysis is characteristic for EWS
– Mottled, permeative destruction
– Periosteal reaction, "onion skin"
– **Extraosseous soft tissue mass**

PATHOLOGY

– During biopsy, must check frozen for adequacy because necrosis is common
– Looks like purulent material on biopsy
– Round undifferentiated cells
– No cytoplasm
– **Monomorphic**
– Necrosis
– "Sheets of small blue cells"
– Intracytoplasmic glycogen on PAS
– MIC2 glycoprotein positive
  – 95% sensitivity for Ewing sarcoma
  – O13 antibody stains MIC2
– Primitive neuroectodermal tumor (PNET) is slightly more differentiated with rosettes (in girls, chest wall)

METASTASES

– Most common metastasis is to lung, then to bone marrow
– 10% patients with disease at multiple bone marrow sites
– Metastases workup is CXR, chest CT, bone scan, bone marrow aspirate

SMALL ROUND CELL TUMORS AND AGE

– <5—neuroblastoma
– 15—Ewing sarcoma, alveolar rhabdomyosarcoma
– 30—B-cell lymphoma
– 50—multiple myeloma
– >60—metastases, usually primary lung
  – Round cell–type liposarcoma

TREATMENT

– Chemotherapy and definitive local treatment with surgery, XRT, or both

CHEMOTHERAPY

– Multidrug chemotherapy is mainstay
– With chemotherapy, 65% 5-yr survival
  – Intermittent high-dose VACA
    – *V*incristine
    – *A*ctinomycin D
    – *C*yclophosphamide
    – *A*driamycin (doxorubicin)
  – + Ifosfamide, + etoposide
– Previously, surgery only for expendable bones
– Recent studies show surgery improves survival

RADIATION THERAPY

– XRT without surgery has unacceptable 28% recurrence

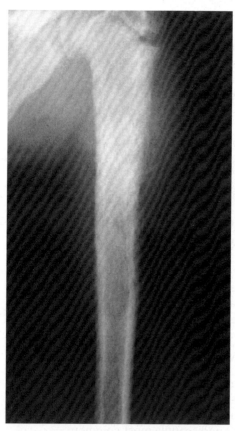

A humeral metaphysodiaphyseal Ewing sarcoma demonstrating Codman triangles distally, irregular areas of cortical destruction with "half-on-end" periosteal spiculations, and a poorly defined osteolysis and osteosclerosis. (From Simon MD, Springfield DS. Surgery for Bone and Soft-Tissue Tumors. Philadelphia: Lippincott Williams & Wilkins; 1998, with permission.)

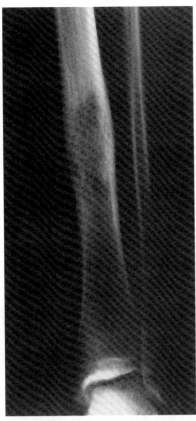

An ill-defined cortical osteolysis in a diaphyseal Ewing sarcoma with a maturation of periosteal layering, giving an appearance of cortical expansion. (From Simon MD, Springfield DS. Surgery for Bone and Soft-Tissue Tumors. Philadelphia: Lippincott Williams & Wilkins; 1998, with permission.)

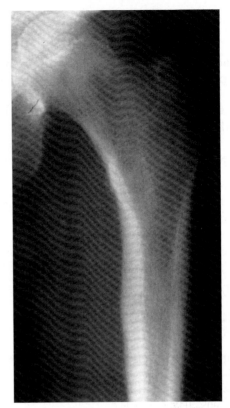

A proximal femur Ewing sarcoma with only the vaguest of permeative patterns, and yet producing a markedly thickened cortex as a result of concentric layerings of periosteal reaction. (From Simon MD, Springfield DS. Surgery for Bone and Soft-Tissue Tumors. Philadelphia: Lippincott Williams & Wilkins; 1998, with permission.)

A purely lytic Ewing sarcoma with an extensive "ratty" or "moth-eaten" destructive pattern, lacking any reactive sclerosis, cortical thickening, or periosteal reaction. (From Simon MD, Springfield DS. Surgery for Bone and Soft-Tissue Tumors. Philadelphia: Lippincott Williams & Wilkins; 1998, with permission.)

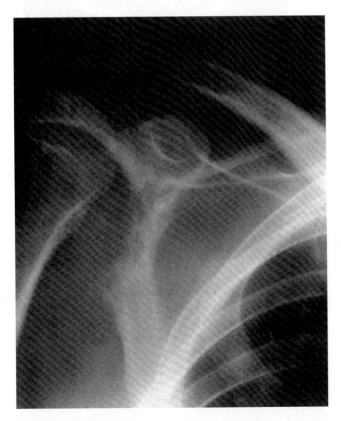

- Consider preoperative XRT (lowest recurrence rates with preoperative XRT in studies from European centers)
- Consider postoperative XRT if margin <1 cm, surrounding edema seen intraoperatively

PROGNOSIS

- Worse prognosis if:
  - Metastases
  - In pelvis
  - Large tumor volume
- EWS:FLI fusion type 1 most common and associated with better prognosis (de Alava et al., 1998; Wunder et al., 1998)

HISTOLOGIC RESPONSE TO CHEMOTHERAPY

- 74 patients, two-thirds had postoperative XRT
  - I—<50% necrosis—0% 5-yr survival
  - II—50%–90% necrosis—38% 5-yr survival
  - III—90%–99% necrosis
  - IV—100% necrosis
  - III and IV—84% 5-yr disease-free survival
- <8 cm—79% 5-yr disease-free survival
- >8 cm—38% 5-yr disease-free survival

References

de Alava E, et al. EWS-FLI1 fusion transcript structure is an independent determinant of prognosis in Ewing's sarcoma. J Clin Oncol 1998; 16:1248–1255.

Wunder JS, et al. The histological response to chemotherapy as a predictor of the oncological outcome of operative treatment of Ewing sarcoma. J Bone Joint Surg Am 1998; 80:1020–1033.

Fibrous Dysplasia

GENERAL

- Replacement of normal bone with fibrous tissue containing spicules of woven bone
- Activating mutation of Gs-α
- Most commonly monostotic
- Variants
  - McCune-Albright syndrome (polyostotic, precocious puberty, café au lait spots)
  - Mazabraud syndrome (myxomas)
  - Cherubism
- Polyostotic form with coast of Maine spots and endocrinopathy
- First or second decade
- **Most commonly proximal femur,** tibia, rib, and humerus
- Does not deform tibia
- Uncommon in spine and sacrum

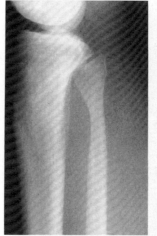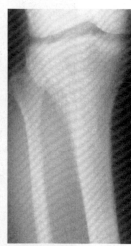

A,B

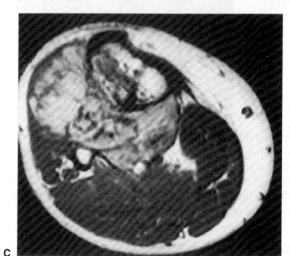

C

A, B: Plain radiographs demonstrate an eccentric proximal tibial Ewing sarcoma with cortical destruction and an area of "saucerization" on the lateral aspect of the metaphysis. It is difficult to identify a soft tissue mass or the intraosseous extent of tumor. **C:** Only through magnetic resonance imaging can the true anatomic extent of the intraosseous tumor as well as the large accompanying soft tissue mass be determined, along with the relationship of adjacent neurovascular structures. (From Simon MD, Springfield DS. Surgery for Bone and Soft-Tissue Tumors. Philadelphia: Lippincott Williams & Wilkins; 1998, with permission.)

IMAGING

- Ground-glass discrete lesion
- Thinned cortex
- **Shepherd crook deformity**
- If cortical, in deformed tibia, think ossifying fibroma (also known as Campanacci syndrome or osteofibrous dysplasia, possible precursor to adamantinoma)
- Hot bone scan
- Low signal on MRI (fibrous)

PATHOLOGY

- Abundant collagen matrix
- Bland fibrous background
- Chinese letters of woven bone, "c"s and "o"s
- Unlike reactive bone, woven bone of fibrous dysplasia has no rimming by osteoblasts and osteoclasts

TREATMENT

- Generally, if no symptoms, no treatment
- Treat intertrochanteric and subtrochanteric lesions to prevent deformity
- Most monostotic lesions involute or remain indolent
- If symptomatic, curettage and grafting versus resection
- Cortical grafts better than cancellous
- If <18 yo, internal fixation to prevent deformity

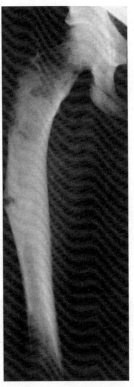

Anteroposterior radiograph of the right proximal femur in an adolescent girl with groin and thigh pain for 1 yr shows a long metaphyseal, diaphyseal lesion, with a well-marginated border and fine intralesional mineralization with deformity and a stress fracture. This radiograph is compatible with fibrous dysplasia. (From Simon MD, Springfield DS. Surgery for Bone and Soft-Tissue Tumors. Philadelphia: Lippincott Williams & Wilkins; 1998, with permission.)

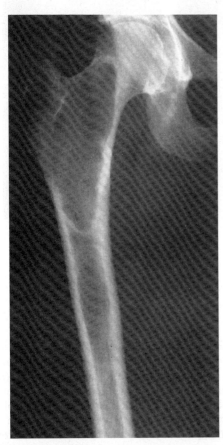

Anteroposterior radiograph of the proximal femur of a young adult with mild groin and thigh pain shows a central, well-marginated metaphyseal and diaphyseal lesion that has intralesional mineralization of granular appearance, typical of fibrous dysplasia. (From Simon MD, Springfield DS. Surgery for Bone and Soft-Tissue Tumors. Philadelphia: Lippincott Williams & Wilkins; 1998, with permission.)

Reference

DiCaprio MR, Enneking WF. Fibrous dysplasia: pathophysiology, evaluation, and treatment. J Bone Joint Surg Am 2005; 87:1848–1864.

Giant Cell Tumor

GENERAL

- Benign but locally aggressive
- One of the only bone tumors where F > M
  - Lesion grows during pregnancy
  - Other F > M tumor is parosteal osteogenic sarcoma (OGS)
- More common in Asians than Americans
  - most common bone tumor in China
- Most common in 20–40 yo
- Most common site is distal femur, then proximal tibia and distal radius

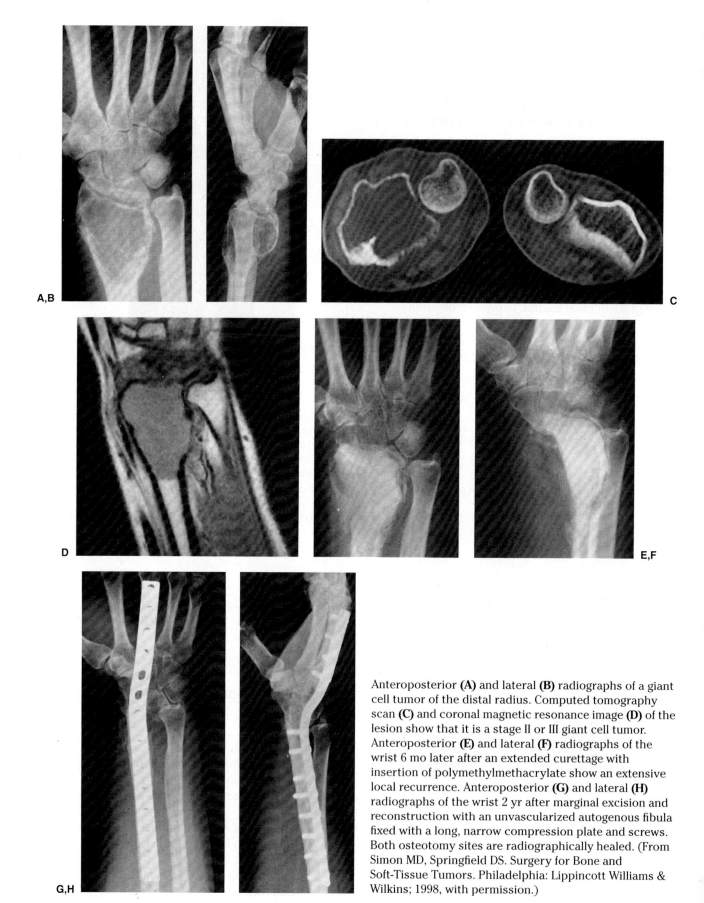

Anteroposterior **(A)** and lateral **(B)** radiographs of a giant cell tumor of the distal radius. Computed tomography scan **(C)** and coronal magnetic resonance image **(D)** of the lesion show that it is a stage II or III giant cell tumor. Anteroposterior **(E)** and lateral **(F)** radiographs of the wrist 6 mo later after an extended curettage with insertion of polymethylmethacrylate show an extensive local recurrence. Anteroposterior **(G)** and lateral **(H)** radiographs of the wrist 2 yr after marginal excision and reconstruction with an unvascularized autogenous fibula fixed with a long, narrow compression plate and screws. Both osteotomy sites are radiographically healed. (From Simon MD, Springfield DS. Surgery for Bone and Soft-Tissue Tumors. Philadelphia: Lippincott Williams & Wilkins; 1998, with permission.)

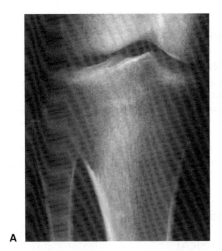
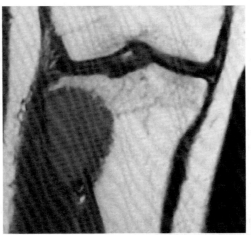
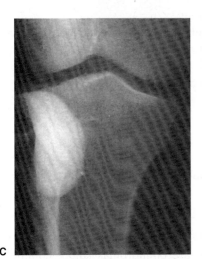
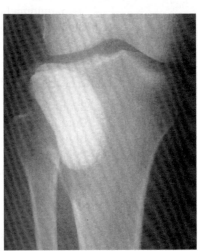
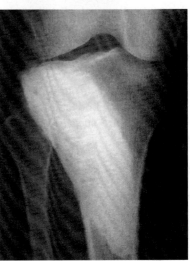

A: Anteroposterior radiograph of the proximal tibia of a 20-yo man with a small giant cell tumor of the proximal lateral tibia. **B:** Coronal magnetic resonance image of the proximal tibia shows the intraosseous extent of the tumor. **C:** Postoperative anteroposterior radiograph of the knee after extended curettage and insertion of polymethylmethacrylate (PMMA). In retrospect, the extent of the curettage may have been insufficient; note the initial lesion and the contour of the PMMA. **D:** Anteroposterior radiograph of the proximal tibia 6 mo later, showing recurrence of the tumor distal to the PMMA. **E:** Postoperative anteroposterior radiograph after repeat extended curettage and insertion of PMMA. Note the more extensive surgical procedure, as indicated by the amount of PMMA used. (From Simon MD, Springfield DS. Surgery for Bone and Soft-Tissue Tumors. Philadelphia: Lippincott Williams & Wilkins; 1998, with permission.)

HISTORY AND PHYSICAL EXAMINATION

- Patient localizes pain to adjacent joint
- Often patient mistaken to have intra-articular pathology and undergoes arthroscopy

IMAGING

- Radiolucent
- Eccentric
- Well-defined transition
- No sclerotic border unless there is secondary ABC

- Epiphyseal, extending into metaphysis
- Closed physis (open in 2%)
  - If open physis, location is metaphysis
- Abuts articular surface, subchondral
- Usually does not penetrate joint

HISTOLOGY

- Vascular
- Multinucleated giant cells in background of mononuclear cells
- **Nuclei of giant and background cells are identical**

- Necrosis is common
- One-third of GCTs associated with ABC in same lesion; these have higher recurrence because they bleed more with subsequent inadequate curetting

DIFFERENTIAL DIAGNOSIS OF GIANT CELL TUMOR

- Telangiectatic osteosarcoma
  - This is the reason to do biopsy to confirm diagnosis

DIFFERENTIAL DIAGNOSIS OF GIANT CELLS

- Hyperparathyroidism (Brown tumor)—giant cells have surrounding red blood cells
- GCT—giant cells evenly distributed
- TB—giant cells at periphery
- Sarcoid, any granulomatous disease, necrosis
- ABC
- EG
- If multiple lesions, rule out Brown tumor; in Brown tumor, the rest of the body must be osteopenic because Brown tumors are seen in end-stage hyperparathyroidism

TREATMENT

- Intralesional curettage
- Local adjuvant such as liquid nitrogen or PMMA if close to cartilage (Marcove et al., 1978)
- PMMA for:
  - Structural support
  - Extra kill from heat
  - Easy to see recurrence
- Embolize before surgery in sacrum
- XRT if surgery contraindicated
  - XRT can cause malignant transformation

PROGNOSIS

- Local recurrence rates (Campanacci et al., 1987)
  - 27% in intralesional (curettage)
  - 8% in marginal
  - 0% in wide
- Local recurrence 2% with cryotherapy (Malawer et al., 1999)
- Local recurrence successfully treated with recurettage

METASTASES

- 2%–5% distant embolic events
  - Most common in lungs
    - Follow CXRs
  - Benign distant implants caused by surgical curettage?

- GCTs of hand have 25% metastases and higher malignant potential

References

Campanacci M, et al. Giant-cell tumor of bone. J Bone Joint Surg Am 1987; 69:106–114.
Malawer MM, et al. Cryosurgery in the treatment of giant cell tumor: a long-term followup study. Clin Orthop 1999; (359):176–188.
Marcove RC, et al. Cryosurgery in the treatment of giant cell tumors of bone: a report of 52 consecutive cases. Clin Orthop 1978; (134):275–289.

Glomus Tumor

GENERAL

- Hemangioma family
- Glomus is a regulatory neurovascular body that controls perfusion to dermal vascular plexus

HISTORY AND PHYSICAL EXAMINATION

- Exquisite point tenderness
- Cold intolerance
- Bluish subungual lesion is pathognomonic
- Benign
- **Digits, subungual**

DIFFERENTIAL DIAGNOSIS

- Most common cystic and pseudocystic lesions of the distal phalanges are chondromas (more commonly proximal phalanx) and epidermoid inclusion cysts
- epidermal inclusion cysts arise from traumatic implantation of epithelial cells into the underlying soft tissue or bone

TREATMENT

- Local excision is curative
- 20% recurrence

References

Carroll RE, Berman AT. Glomus tumors of the hand: review of the literature and report on twenty-eight cases. J Bone Joint Surg Am 1972; 54:691–703.
Phillips CS, Murphy MS. Vascular problems of the upper extremity: a primer for the orthopaedic surgeon. J Am Acad Orthop Surg 2002; 10:401–408.

Hemangioma

GENERAL

- Benign lesion of veins and/or arteries
- Also known as "arteriovenous malformations"

- **Most common benign soft tissue tumor in children**
  - In children, spontaneously regress
- Painless or pain from thrombosis

IMAGING

- Small, smooth, round **phleboliths**
- CT—striated on sagittal view, stippled on axial view

- MRI is diagnostic
  - **Dark round signal voids within fat**
  - Bright on T1 and T2 in spine

PATHOLOGY

- Vessels within normal fat
- Infiltrates local tissue
- No respect for fascial boundaries

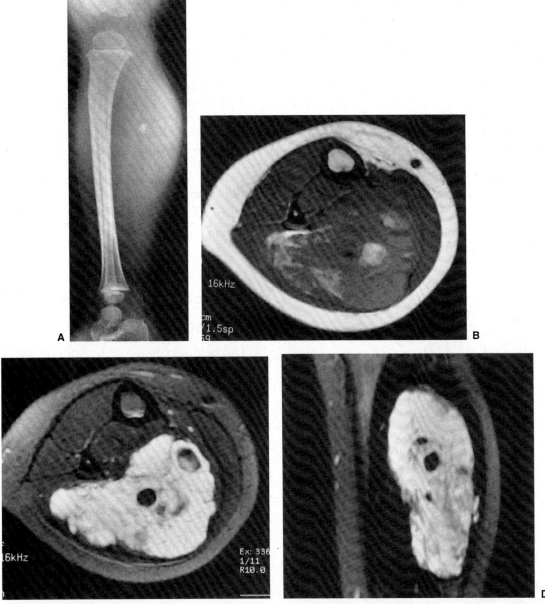

Lateral radiograph **(A)** of a 3-yo girl with a large painful mass of the right calf shows a water density mass with a phlebolith consistent with a hemangioma. Axial **(B, C)** and sagittal **(D)** magnetic resonance images of the leg show a large mass in the soleus muscle. On T1-weighted images, there is high signal intensity, and the phlebolith is best seen by a signal void on T2-weighted images. These images are very consistent with a hemangioma. (From Simon MD, Springfield DS. Surgery for Bone and Soft-Tissue Tumors. Philadelphia: Lippincott Williams & Wilkins; 1998, with permission.)

TREATMENT/PROGNOSIS

- No malignant potential
- Best left alone unless symptomatic
- Recurs after limited excision

INTRAMUSCULAR HEMANGIOMA

- Lower limb, quads
- Usually painful
- Size and pain fluctuates with venous stasis
- Phleboliths on plain XR are pathognomonic
- On MRI
  - On T1, intermediate between fat and muscle
  - Bright on T2, fibrous septa

Reference

Fox MW, Onofrio BM. The natural history and management of symptomatic and asymptomatic vertebral hemangiomas. J Neurosurg 1993; 78:36–45.

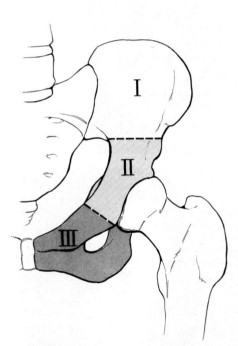

The basic types of pelvic resections. The ilium is I, the acetabulum is II, and the ischium and pubis are III. The sacrum is not shown, but is numbered IV. Further classification can be done using these Roman numerals. "P" is sometimes used to indicate that the Roman numerals refer to the pelvis. Some surgeons use an "A" to indicate that only the bone was removed and "B" to indicate that adjacent soft tissue was removed. This system does permit more accurate comparison of data between surgeons. (From Simon MD, Springfield DS. Surgery for Bone and Soft-Tissue Tumors. Philadelphia: Lippincott Williams & Wilkins; 1998, with permission.)

Hemipelvectomy

INTERNAL HEMIPELVECTOMY

(Enneking & Dunham, 1978; modified by Musculoskeletal Tumor Society)
- I—iliac wing resection
- II—periacetabular resection
- III—ischiopubis resection
- A—removal of only bone
- B—removal of bone and adjacent soft tissue
- H—proximal femur excision

RECONSTRUCTION OPTIONS

- Enneking I
  - No graft
  - Allograft femur
  - Autograft fibula
  - Vascularized fibula—best anecdotal results

Reference

Enneking WF, Dunham WK. Resection and reconstruction for primary neoplasms involving the innominate bone. J Bone Joint Surg Am 1978; 60:731–746.

Hinge Total Knee Replacement (TKR)

INDICATIONS

- Ligamentous failure
- Bone loss
(Westrich, 2000)
- 24 consecutive knees (1994–1997)
- Average follow-up 33 mo
- Knee Society rating system score: preop 44 points to postop 83 points
- Improved pain and function comparable to standard TKR revision
(Kawai et al., 1999)
- 2- to 7-yr follow-up on 25 Finns
- Seven underwent prosthetic exchange
- 88% 5-yr prosthetic survival for distal femoral replacements
- 58% 5-yr survival for proximal tibia replacements

References

Kawai A, et al. A rotating-hinge knee replacement for malignant tumors of the femur and tibia. J Arthroplasty 1999; 14:187–196.

Westrich GH, et al. Rotating hinge total knee arthroplasty in severely affected knees. Clin Orthop 2000; (379):195–208.

Leukemia (Acute Lymphocytic Leukemia [ALL])

- ALL is most common cancer in children
- ALL usually in 2–5 yo
- ALL accounts for 25% of cancer in <15 yo
- Whites > blacks
- Incidence highest among Hispanics

HISTORY AND PHYSICAL EXAMINATION

- Fever, lethargy, anemia, bleeding
- Down syndrome has increased risk of ALL and acute monocytic leukemia (AML)
- 6% have back pain

LABORATORY VALUES

- WBC count can be high, normal, or low
- Hematocrit (HCT) and platelets (PLT) always low
- Blasts seen on peripheral smear
- Bone marrow biopsy confirms diagnosis

TREATMENT

- Induction chemotherapy
  - Allopurinol for tumor lysis
- Consolidation chemotherapy
- Maintenance chemotherapy
- XRT to brain and testes
- Intrathecal chemotherapy for meningeal metastases
- If relapse, high-dose chemotherapy with allogenic stem cell transplantation is best hope for cure

PROGNOSIS

- Nearly 80% cure in children
- Best prognosis in 3–7 yo

Reference

Pui CH, Evans WE. Treatment of acute lymphoblastic leukemia. N Engl J Med 2006; 354:166–178.

Lipoma

GENERAL

- Adults
- Most common in back or shoulder

HISTORY AND PHYSICAL EXAMINATION

- Painless
- Smooth, soft, mobile if subcutaneous

- Smooth, firm, less mobile if deep to superficial fascia
- Deep lipomas tend to be bigger and get confused with sarcoma

IMAGING

- XR usually normal
- Diagnosis by CT or MRI
  - Because lipoma has normal fat, it has same signal as normal fat on CT/MRI
  - If only fat density seen, safe to make diagnosis based only on CT/MRI
  - Lipomas can have nonfat density but if any nonfat density seen, perform biopsy to prove diagnosis
  - Liposarcoma does not look like lipoma at all on CT/MRI

PATHOLOGY

- Normal fat cells

TREATMENT

- Marginal excision or left alone

VARIANTS

- Angiolipoma
- Spindle cell lipoma
- Lipoblastoma
- Hibernoma

INTRAMUSCULAR LIPOMA

- Infiltrates muscle
- Some density within mass on CT/MRI
- No abnormal vascularity with contrast study
- Must excise some muscle
- High local recurrence

Reference

Murphey MD, et al. From the archives of the AFIP: benign musculoskeletal lipomatous lesions. Radiographics 2004; 24:1433–1466.

Liposarcoma

GENERAL

- Second most common soft tissue sarcoma
- Retroperitoneum, pelvis, thigh, popliteal fossa

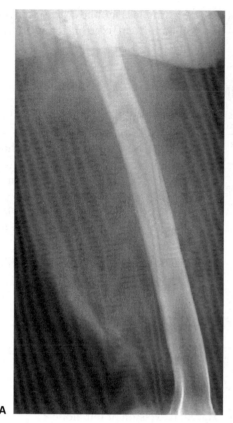

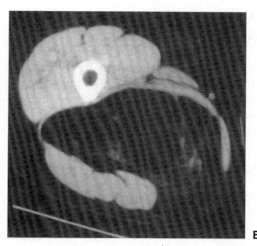

A: Low-grade liposarcoma. Lateral view of the thigh reveals a large soft tissue mass, mostly composed of low-attenuation tissue, suggesting fat. **B:** On computed tomography scan, it can be observed that the mass is not entirely composed of fat, but contains a variable amount of higher-attenuation tissue, indicating that the lesion is not a simple lipoma. (From Simon MD, Springfield DS. Surgery for Bone and Soft-Tissue Tumors. Philadelphia: Lippincott Williams & Wilkins; 1998, with permission.)

SUBTYPES WITH DIFFERING COURSES

- Well differentiated (hard to differentiate from atypical or larger lipoma)
- Myxoid (most common type, metastases to spine)
- Round cell (looks like Ewing sarcoma)
- Pleomorphic (metastases to lungs)
- Dedifferentiated

IMAGING

- Soft tissue calcifications can be seen

PATHOLOGY

- **Lipoblast** (signet ring cells) with mitotic figures
- Fine vascularity
- More fat, fewer cells indicate better prognosis
- Well-differentiated subcutaneous liposarcoma is considered atypical lipoma
- t12:16 CHOP-FUS translocation in 95% of myxoid/round cell liposarcoma (both considered poorly differentiated)

METASTASES

- Unusually high rate of nonpulmonary initial metastases

TREATMENT AND PROGNOSIS

- Similar to other soft tissue sarcomas
- Wide resection
  - Add XRT, depending on margins
- Wide resection and XRT if high grade, >5 cm
- If low grade, problem is local recurrence, not metastases
- Low grade in retroperitoneum has bad prognosis due to local recurrence and compression of bowels

Recommended Reading

Antonescu CR, et al. Specificity of TLS-CHOP rearrangement for classic myxoid/round cell liposarcoma: absence in predominantly myxoid well-differentiated liposarcomas. J Mol Diagn 2000; 2:132–138.

Wolfe SW, et al. Computed tomographic evaluation of fatty neoplasms of the extremities: a clinical, radiographic, and histologic review of cases. Orthopedics 1989; 12:1351–1358.

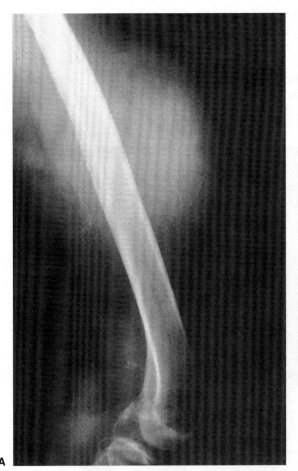

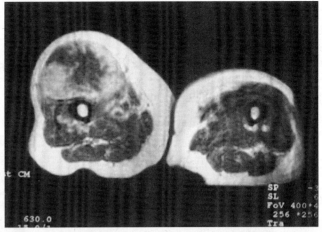

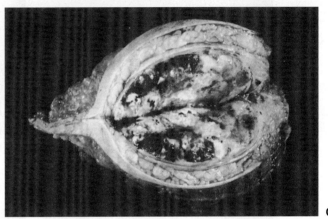

Lateral radiograph of the thigh **(A)** of a 70-yo woman with a mass in the midthigh for 4 mo shows a water density mass without bone erosion. Axial magnetic resonance image of the thigh **(B)** shows a heterogeneous mass in the quadriceps muscle adjacent to the femur. A biopsy showed this mass to be a liposarcoma. After preoperative radiation therapy, a wide excision was performed. An intraoperative photograph **(C)** of surgical specimen shows the heterogeneous appearance. (From Simon MD, Springfield DS. Surgery for Bone and Soft-Tissue Tumors. Philadelphia: Lippincott Williams & Wilkins; 1998, with permission.)

Lymphoma of Bone

GENERAL

- Most bone lymphomas are non-Hodgkin lymphoma
- <10% of extranodular lymphomas are bone
- 30–60 yo

HISTORY AND PHYSICAL EXAMINATION

- Bony destruction causes pain
- Adenopathy
- Suspect in young patient with pathological fracture
- One-half in long bone
- One-half in skull, face, spine, rib, or pelvis

IMAGING

- Usually lytic
- Ivory vertebra (entire body dense without change in shape)

PATHOLOGY

- Can have myelofibrosis diffusely in bone
- Diagnosis from biopsy difficult because of crush artifact and spontaneous necrosis
- Dense round cells with clear cytoplasm and prominent nucleoli
- Cells bigger than Ewing sarcoma
- Pleomorphic nuclei with differing sizes
- Reticulin fibers in matrix

TREATMENT

- Local stereotactic radiotherapy (SRT) for solitary lesion
- CHOP chemotherapy for extensive disease
  - *C*yclophosphamide
  - *H*ydroxy doxorubicin (Adriamycin)
- *Vincristine (Oncovin)*
- *P*rednisone
- Good prognosis, most living >5 yr

Reference

Gill P, et al. Primary lymphomas of bone. Clin Lymphoma Myeloma 2005; 6:140–142.

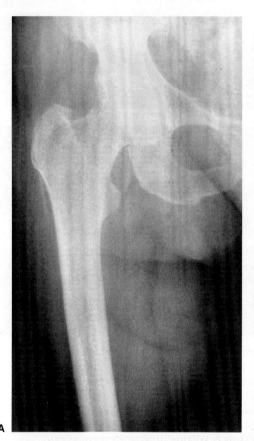

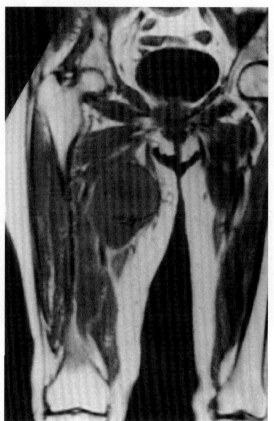

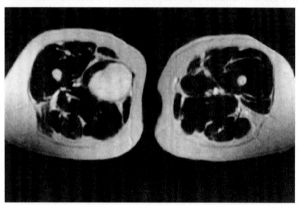

An anteroposterior radiograph **(A)** of the thigh of a 50-yo woman with a large mass in the medial proximal thigh for 6 mo shows a water density mass without bone erosion. Coronal T1-weighted **(B)** and axial T2-weighted **(C)** magnetic resonance images of the thigh show a large soft tissue mass in the adductor compartment with nonspecific signal characteristics. The patient had a biopsy that disclosed this to be a malignant fibrous histiocytoma. (From Simon MD, Springfield DS. Surgery for Bone and Soft-Tissue Tumors. Philadelphia: Lippincott Williams & Wilkins; 1998, with permission.)

Malignant Fibrous Histiocytoma

GENERAL

- Most common soft tissue sarcoma in adult
- MFH and liposarcoma make up 80% of all soft tissue sarcomas in adults
- Fibrosarcoma is essentially MFH, which is a bit more organized, with **herringbone** pattern
- Histiocyte = fibroblast, which is fatter and can phagocytose
- High-grade spindle cell sarcoma with storiform pattern
- MFH is not histiocytic; pleomorphic sarcoma not otherwise specified (NOS) is better term

HISTORY AND PHYSICAL EXAMINATION

- 30–80 yo
- M > F
- Pelvis, buttock, thigh
- Presents with enlarging mass
- Minimal symptoms
- No constitutional symptoms

SUBTYPES

- *Note:* No difference in treatment or prognosis
  - Pleomorphic—most common, giant cell rich
  - Myxoid—low grade, upper extremity, locally recurs, increases grade with each recurrence
  - Giant cell
  - Inflammatory
  - Histiocytic
  - Angiomatoid

PATHOLOGY

- Cartwheel pattern of collagen
- Storiform "starry night" pattern with background of malignant histiocytic cells
- Necrosis, mitoses

METASTASES

- Most common to lung, then nodes, liver, and bone

TREATMENT (FOR SOFT TISSUE SARCOMAS)

- Surgery is mainstay
  - 76% 5-yr survival with wide margin
  - 52% 5-yr survival with lesser margins
- Local recurrence increases mortality
  - Intralesional resection
    - 90% local recurrence for low grade
    - 100% local recurrence for high grade
  - Marginal resection
    - 70% local recurrence for low grade
    - 90% local recurrence for high grade
  - Wide resection and XRT
    - 15% local recurrence
- Brachytherapy if >5 cm, high grade
- External XRT if >5 cm, low grade
- ? Chemotherapy on an individual basis (high-dose Adriamycin)

PROGNOSIS

- Depends on:
  - Grade
  - Size
    - >5 cm—46% 5-yr survival
    - <5 cm—63% 5-yr survival
  - Deep to fascia
  - Proximal
  - Age
  - Metastases (mostly pulmonary)
  (Salo et al., 1999)
    - 719 patients with lung metastases
    - Overall 15-mo median, 25% 3-yr survival
    - Complete resection of metastases
    - 33-mo median, 46% 3-yr survival
  - Nonoperative treatment
    - 11-mo median survival
    - Metastasis resection most important for outcome

References

Billingsley KG, et al. Pulmonary metastases from soft tissue sarcoma: analysis of patterns of diseases and postmetastasis survival. Ann Surg 1999; 229:602–610; discussion 610–612.
Salo JC, et al. Malignant fibrous histiocytoma of the extremity. Cancer 1999; 85:1765–1772.

Malignant Fibrous Histiocytoma of Bone

GENERAL

- Occurs at any age, unlike soft tissue MFH
- Average age 40 yr
- 21% are <21 yo
- 10 times less common than osteosarcoma
- 72% primary
- 28% secondary (most commonly from Paget disease)

HISTOLOGIC SUBTYPES

- Fibrous
- Histiocytic/xanthomatous
- Malignant giant cell

TREATMENT

- Same as MFH

PROGNOSIS

- Depends on:
  - Grade
  - Patient's age
  - Secondary MFH of bone worse
  - 71% 3-yr survival
  - 53% 5-yr survival

Reference

Huvos AG, et al. The pathology of malignant fibrous histiocytoma of bone: a study of 130 patients. Am J Surg Pathol 1985; 9:853–871.

Metastatic Renal Cell Carcinoma (RCC)

GENERAL

- Clear cells on pathology

PROGNOSIS

- Metastatic disease with <10% 5-yr survival
- Average life expectancy 12–24 mo

- 50% of patients with metastases get skeletal disease

(Althausen et al., 1997)
- 38 patients with RCC and solitary bony metastases
- Almost one-half had metastases already at RCC diagnosis
  - One-half of those presented with bone pain
- Variety of treatments
- Surprising 40% 10-yr survival
- Good prognosis associated with:
  - Presentation without metastases
  - Longer time between nephrectomy and metastases
  - Peripheral location
  - Solitary metastasis

TREATMENT

- Preoperative embolization is key
- PMMA to achieve stability with fixation
- Aggressive resection of solitary metastasis may improve survival
- Interferon therapy
- Experimental mismatched bone marrow transplant with graft-versus-host disease to fight metastases

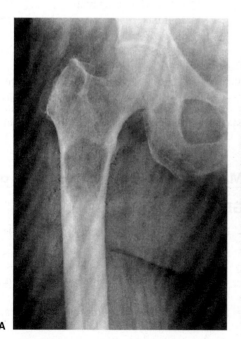 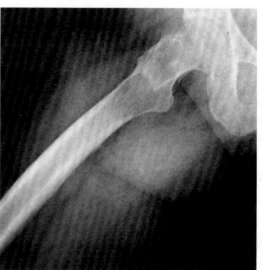

Anteroposterior **(A)** and lateral **(B)** roentgenograms of the right hip and proximal femur in a 61-yo woman with metastatic renal carcinoma. A destructive permeative lesion with ill-defined margins is noted in the subtrochanteric region. (From Simon MD, Springfield DS. Surgery for Bone and Soft-Tissue Tumors. Philadelphia: Lippincott Williams & Wilkins; 1998, with permission.)

Reference

Althausen P, et al. Prognostic factors and surgical treatment of osseous metastases secondary to renal cell carcinoma. Cancer 1997; 80:1103–1109.

Metastatic Thyroid Cancer

GENERAL

- Follicular cells with colloid on pathological

PROGNOSIS

(Pittas & Robbins, 2000)
- MSKCC's thyroid cancers with metastases to bone
- 47% with bone metastases at diagnosis of thyroid cancer
- Most common to vertebrae, pelvis, ribs, and then femur
- 53% with multiple lesions
- 35% 10-yr survival from time of thyroid cancer diagnosis
- 13% 10-yr survival from time of bone metastasis diagnosis
- Better prognosis if:
  - No nonosseous metastases
  - Iodine-125 uptake
  - Hürthle cell type

Reference

Pittas AG, et al. Bone metastases from thyroid carcinoma: clinical characteristics and prognostic variables in one hundred forty-six patients. Thyroid 2000; 10:261–268.

Multiple Hereditary Osteochondromas (MHO)

GENERAL

- 10 times less frequent than solitary
- Autosomal dominant
- M:F is 2:1
- Abnormal cartilage growth that goes through endochondral ossification
- Mutations in EXT1, 2, 3, 7, 11, 18, which encode glycosyl transferases in synthesis of cell surface heparin proteoglycans
- EXT1 associated with worse disease and higher malignant transformation

PRESENTATION

- At the end of a tubular bone that contributes to greatest growth
- Bone with smaller cross-sectional area of physis more severely affected
- Most commonly present with forearm deformity (pseudo-Madelung)
- Shoulder, hip (coxa valga), knee, ankle (valgus due to short fibula)
- Short stature from lower extremity involvement

NATURAL HISTORY

- 0.5% malignant degeneration to secondary chondrosarcoma
- Increases to 1.3% in those >21 yo
- Higher rate than solitary

DIFFERENTIAL DIAGNOSIS

- Madelung deformity
  - In MHO, ulnar shortening leads to radial bowing with radial tilt to distal radial physis and ulnar translation of carpus
  - In Madelung deformity, ulna longer and dorsally subluxated

SURGERY

- Most common indication is progressive ankle valgus
  - Supramalleolar osteotomy
- Excise symptomatic exostoses
- Extracapsular dissection with removal of cartilage cap and adjacent periosteum
- Reconstructive procedures

Reference

Stieber JR, Dormans JP. Manifestations of hereditary multiple exostoses. J Am Acad Orthop Surg 2005; 13:110–120.

Multiple Myeloma

GENERAL

- Malignant tumor of plasma cells
- When localized without systemic increase in plasma cells in bone marrow, it is called plasmacytoma
- Most common primary malignant bone tumor in adults
- Exposure to ionizing radiation is strongest single risk factor

CLINICAL VARIANTS

- Solitary myeloma
- POEMS
  - *P*olyneuropathy
  - *O*rganomegaly
  - *E*ndocrinopathy
  - *M* protein (IgM)
  - *S*kin changes

PRESENTATION

- >50 yo, median age 68 yo
- Presents with fatigue, weight loss, and anemia
- Can cause amyloidosis
- Waldenström macroglobulinemia in myeloma that produces immunoglobulin M (IgM) leads to blood hyperviscosity (maintain high suspicion in patient with paraproteinemia and mental status change or shortness of breath because plasmapheresis can relieve symptoms and prevent irreversible organ damage)
- Recurrent bacterial infection from deficiency of humoral and cellular responses
- Coagulopathy as paraprotein interferes with normal coagulation cascade

LABORATORY VALUES

- Anemia
- Increased creatinine in 50%—Bence-Jones proteinuria leads to renal compromise
- High ESR from paraproteinemia
- One-third with hypercalcemia (present with mental status change, lethargy, constipation, and vomiting; measure ionized calcium because patients get low albumin)
- At risk for hypercalcemia due to bone breakdown by osteoclasts
- Abnormal serum protein electrophoresis (SPEP), urine protein electrophoresis (UPEP) from monoclonal gammopathy

IMAGING

- Radiolucent punched-out lesions
- 30% of lesions are lytic
- Vertebral body
- **Diffuse osteoporosis**
- Usually **cold** bone scan, hot in 30%
- Sternum pathological fracture is pathognomonic
- MRI with short tau inversion recovery (STIR) reveals tumor burden best

DIAGNOSIS

- Usually one major and one minor, or three minor
- Major criteria
  - Plasmacytoma on tissue biopsy
  - Bone marrow >30% plasma cells
  - Ig spike on SPEP
- Minor criteria
  - Bone marrow with 10%–30% plasma cells
  - Small Ig spike on SPEP
  - Multiple lytic bone lesions
  - Suppression of uninvolved Igs

PATHOLOGY

- Sheets of plasma cells
- Pink cytoplasm with prominent nuclei with clock face appearance

STAGING

- I—low tumor burden
  - Hemoglobin (Hb) >10
  - Normal calcium, normal skeletal survey
  - 49-mo survival with standard chemotherapy
- III—high tumor burden
  - Hb <8.5
  - Calcium >12
  - Three or more advanced lytic bone lesions
  - 25-mo survival with standard chemotherapy

TREATMENT

- Local XRT for true solitary plasmacytoma
  - 20% eradication and long-term survival
- Bisphosphonates for indolent myeloma to delay bone-related complications
- **Palliative chemotherapy** for multiple myeloma
  - Alkylating melphalan and steroids
- Bone marrow transplant
- Most plasmacytomas become multiple myelomas

PROGNOSIS

- **β-Microglobulin very important**
  - light chain of major histocompatibility complex I (MHC-I) antigen
  - Renally excreted
  - Level reflects tumor burden and renal function
  - >2.5 associated with poor prognosis
- High C-reactive protein (CRP), low PLT, low Hb, large tumor burden associated with poor prognosis
- Variable disease course
- Median survival 2 yr
- 5-yr survival <30%

Reference

Kyle RA, Rajkumar SV. Multiple myeloma. N Engl J Med 2004; 351:1860–1873.

Myositis Ossificans

- After single or repetitive trauma
- Most common in midaspect of muscle bellies (over diaphysis)

IMAGING

- Peripheral mineralization with central lucency
- This radiographic "zoning" best seen on CT
- Usually not attached to underlying bone

PATHOLOGY

- Histologic "zoning" phenomenon with peripheral mature trabecular bone with less mature central spindle cells

TREATMENT

- Wait for bone scan to normalize
- Repeat XR to confirm maturation of ossification with radiographic zoning phenomenon
- Consider perioperative XRT

Reference

Beiner JM, Jokl P. Muscle contusion injuries: current treatment options. J Am Acad Orthop Surg 2001; 9:227–237.

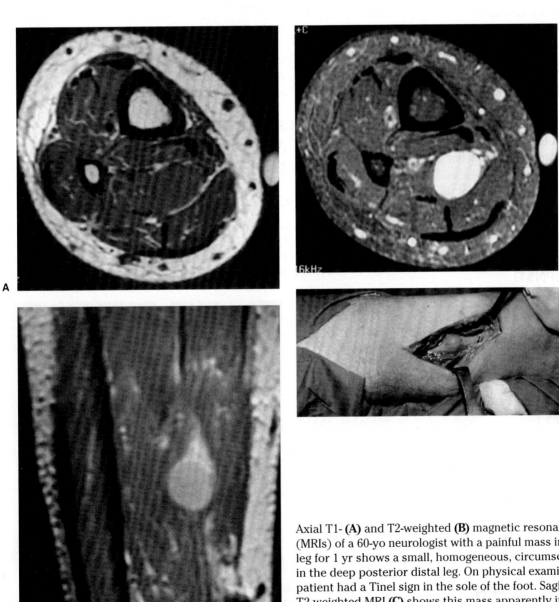

Axial T1- **(A)** and T2-weighted **(B)** magnetic resonance images (MRIs) of a 60-yo neurologist with a painful mass in the right leg for 1 yr shows a small, homogeneous, circumscribed mass in the deep posterior distal leg. On physical examination the patient had a Tinel sign in the sole of the foot. Sagittal T2-weighted MRI **(C)** shows this mass apparently in continuity with the posterior tibial nerve. Intraoperative photograph **(D)** shows the mass to be in continuity with the posterior tibial nerve. (From Simon MD, Springfield DS. Surgery for Bone and Soft-Tissue Tumors. Philadelphia: Lippincott Williams & Wilkins; 1998, with permission.)

Nerve Sheath Tumors

NEURILEMOMA (SCHWANNOMA)

- Benign tumors that arise from nerve sheath
- Typical Antonio A and B components
  - A—highly ordered, cellular
  - B—loose myxoid
- **Positive S-100** differentiates it from neurofibroma
- Bright on MRI T1 and T2
- Not associated with neurofibromatosis
- Rarely becomes malignant
- Almost always solitary
- Usually well encapsulated
- Simple marginal excision adequate

NEUROFIBROMA

- Associated with neurofibromatosis (NF), solitary or multiple
- Teardrop nuclei
- Bright on MRI T1 and T2
- Occurs within nerve fascicles and hard to separate from nerve
- Look for signs of systemic NF
- Can degenerate to malignant form
- Tends to recur if excision not complete

MALIGNANT PERIPHERAL NERVE SHEATH TUMOR (MPNST)

- Also known as neurofibrosarcoma, malignant schwannoma, or neurosarcoma
- De novo or from neurofibroma
- Higher incidence (2%–30%) in NF
  - Presents at young age if NF
  - Worse prognosis if NF
- Looks like fibrosarcoma on pathology
- High grade
- Treated like other high-grade sarcomas

References

Cheng EY. Benign soft tissue tumors. In: Craig EV, ed. Clinical Orthopaedics. Philadelphia: Lippincott Williams & Wilkins; 1999:998–1003.

Cheng EY. Malignant soft tissue tumors. In: Craig EV, ed. Clinical Orthopaedics. Philadelphia: Lippincott Williams & Wilkins; 1999:1004–12.

Nonossifying Fibroma

GENERAL

- Most common bone tumor in children
- 27% of children have this based on fluoride/H_2O studies

- Fibrous cortical defect (FCD) is identical histologically but cortical and smaller (<2 cm); FCD tends to heal more than NOF
- Histology same as benign fibrous histiocytoma of adults

HISTORY AND PHYSICAL EXAMINATION

- Rare in <5 yo and >20 yo
- Most common in distal femur and distal tibia
- Usually asymptomatic prior to pathological fracture

IMAGING

- XR is diagnostic
  - Eccentric, metaphyseal
  - Radiolucent
  - Well-defined margin, scalloped
  - On tibia, usually lateral near syndesmosis

DIFFERENTIAL DIAGNOSIS

- Chondromyxoid fibroma
- If multiple, think Campanacci-Jaffe syndrome

HISTOLOGY

- Dense fibrous storiform pattern
- Hemosiderin deposits
- Foam cells
- Multinucleated giant cells

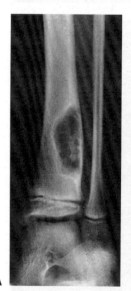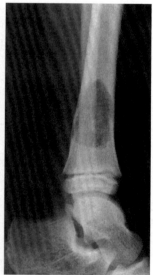

A   B

Anteroposterior **(A)** and lateral **(B)** radiographs of the distal tibia of a child who underwent radiography for an injury to the ankle show an eccentric stage II metaphyseal lesion without intralesional mineralization, compatible with a nonossifying fibroma. (From Simon MD, Springfield DS. Surgery for Bone and Soft-Tissue Tumors. Philadelphia: Lippincott Williams & Wilkins; 1998, with permission.)

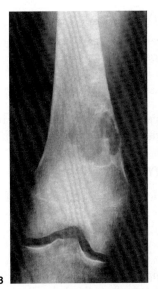 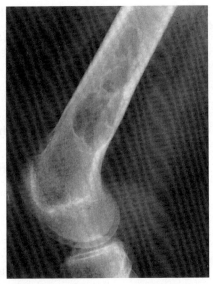 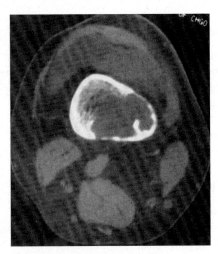

A,B   C

Anteroposterior **(A)** and lateral **(B)** radiographs and computed tomography scan **(C)** of the distal femur of a young woman with spontaneous pain in the distal thigh show a large, eccentric, well-marginated lesion of the metaphysis without mineralization but with cortical perforation. This patient had a biopsy-confirmed stage III nonossifying fibroma. (From Simon MD, Springfield DS. Surgery for Bone and Soft-Tissue Tumors. Philadelphia: Lippincott Williams & Wilkins; 1998, with permission.)

NATURAL HISTORY

– Resolves over a period of years

TREATMENT

– XR other long bones because there is 20% incidence of another lesion elsewhere
– Pathological fracture will heal with or without surgery
– 75% refracture rate
– Some recommend surgery for size >3.3 cm or involvement of >50% of diameter of bone on both anteroposterior (AP) and lateral XRs, persistent pain, with or without repeated pathological fracture (Arata, 1981)
– Activity restrictions if >25% of diameter involved
– Curettage and grafting leads to 100% healing

Reference

Arata MA, et al. Pathological fractures through non-ossifying fibromas. Review of the Mayo Clinic experience. J Bone Joint Surg Am. 1981; 63(6):980–988.
Marks KE, Bauer TW. Fibrous tumors of bone. Orthop Clin North Am 1989; 20:377–393.

Ossifying Fibroma

GENERAL

– Young, <10 yo
– Bowed tibia
– Cortical

– Possible precursor to adamantinoma
– Also known as Campanacci syndrome, osteofibrous dysplasia, or cortical fibrous dysplasia

DIFFERENTIAL DIAGNOSIS

– Adamantinoma
– Fibrous dysplasia
– Congenital tibial pseudoarthrosis of neurofibromatosis

TREATMENT

– Usually conservative treatment

Reference

Marks KE, Bauer TW. Fibrous tumors of bone. Orthop Clin North Am 1989; 20:377–393.

Osteoblastoma

GENERAL

– Benign bone-forming tumor
– Same histology as osteoid osteoma except bigger (>2 cm) and pain not as intense
– Less common than osteoid osteoma
– Most common in spine (posterior elements)
– Vertebral body and epiphysis spared
– Common in talus
– Twice as common in M than F

- Most common in 10–30 yo
- Radicular symptoms in 50% of those involving spine

IMAGING

- Eccentric, circumscribed
- Bone destruction with new reactive bone formation
- Can appear moth eaten, permeative
- Blastic when in spine
- Lytic when in long bone
- Surrounding bone edema on MRI
- Bone scans positive

PATHOLOGY

- Mixture of fibrous and bony tissue
- Should have no cartilage unless there was fracture

DIFFERENTIAL DIAGNOSIS

- Giant cell tumor
- Osteosarcoma

TREATMENT

- Will continue to grow, so should be excised when technically feasible
- May be locally aggressive form
- Marginal resection (curette, nitrogen)
- If metastases, then it should be considered an osteosarcoma

Recommended Reading

White LM, Kandel R. Osteoid-producing tumors of bone. Semin Musculoskelet Radiol 2000; 4:25–43.

Osteochondroma

GENERAL

- Arises from malfunction of physis
- Cartilage cap that undergoes enchondral ossification
- Common
- 5–20 yo
- Growth in childhood, stops in adulthood
- Presents with painless, hard, fixed mass
- Pain from fracture

IMAGING

- Diagnosis made by plain XR
- Pedunculated or sessile
- Near physis
- Medullary canals of host bone and lesion are connected
- If solitary, no risk of malignant degeneration

DIFFERENTIAL DIAGNOSIS

- Often difficult to differentiate sessile osteochondroma from parosteal osteosarcoma

PATHOLOGY

- Normal-appearing cartilage cap undergoing nearly normal endochondral ossification

NATURAL HISTORY

- Solitary osteochondroma has <1% risk of malignant degeneration

TREATMENT

- Removal if local symptoms
- If large, growing, and cap >2 cm (in skeletally mature), then it is a chondrosarcoma and needs wide excision

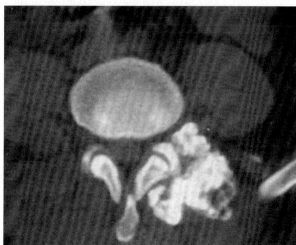

A

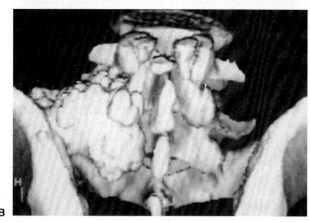

B

Osteochondroma arising from the transverse process of L5. **A:** Computed tomography (CT) scan. **B:** Three-dimensional CT scan. (From Simon MD, Springfield DS. Surgery for Bone and Soft-Tissue Tumors. Philadelphia: Lippincott Williams & Wilkins; 1998, with permission.)

Recommended Reading

Murphey MD, et al. Imaging of osteochondroma: variants and complications with radiologic-pathologic correlation. Radiographics 2000; 20:1407–1434.

Osteogenic Sarcoma—Classic High Grade

GENERAL

- Most common primary malignant bone tumor in children
- Second most common primary bone malignancy (multiple myeloma is most common)
- Third most common malignancy in children (leukemia and lymphoma are most common)
- Called osteogenic sarcoma by James Ewing
- Called osteosarcoma by World Health Organization
- 75% of patients between 10 and 25 yo
- More common in Chinese and Japanese
- Second peak in 60s with Paget disease
- M = F
- One-half of all cases in distal femur and proximal tibia
- Third most common is proximal humerus

HISTORY AND PHYSICAL EXAMINATION

- Dull ache
- No constitutional symptoms
- Patients are taller than average
- Think Ewing sarcoma if lesion is in flat bone and associated with soft tissue mass
- Usually presents at stage IIB

IMAGING

- Usually arises in **metaphysis of long bones**
- Bone destruction, new bone formation
- Periosteal reaction
- In contrast to myositis ossificans, center of lesion is more heavily mineralized
- Usually has extraosseous component
- MRI indications
  - To determine local and marrow extent
  - To define viable area for biopsy
  - To define necrosis after neoadjuvant chemotherapy
- CT better for pelvic tumor to define normal versus tumor in fat planes
- Bone scan to look for skip metastases (in same bone but outside reactive zone) and stage local and distant extent

PATHOLOGY

- Bone formation by spindle cells
- Osteoblasts, mitosis, necrosis
- Invasion into normal bone
- May have fibrous or cartilage tissue
- Low-grade central and parosteal types are less cellular; thus, fibrous dysplasia is in their differential diagnosis
- Periosteal type is mainly cartilaginous; thus, differential diagnosis is chondrosarcoma

DIFFERENTIAL DIAGNOSIS

- Old patient—think metastases, chondrosarcoma
- Young patient—think fibrous lesion

METASTASES

- 80% of OGS presents with stage IIB
- 20%–30% have skip lesion
- Most common site of metastases is lung; second is bone
- Chest CT can only see a nodule of ≥3 mm
- Lymphatic spread uncommon

TREATMENT

- 65% 5-yr survival with wide resection and chemotherapy
- XRT not used for OGS (unless it is in the spine)
- If pathological fracture occurs, must resect all regions contaminated by hematoma

Wide Resection

- If you can get a wide margin, survival as good as amputation
- Nerve function needed for limb sparing

Reconstructive Options

- Osteoarticular allograft
- Intercalary allograft
- Metal end prosthesis
- Allograft–prosthesis composite
- Arthrodesis
- Rotationplasty
- Free fibular vascularized transfer

Adjuvant Chemotherapy

- Doxorubicin (Adriamycin)
  - Cumulative cardiotoxicity
- Methotrexate
- Cisplatin
- Ifosfamide
- Surgery plus chemotherapy
  - >60% 5-yr survival
- Surgery alone
  - <20% 5-yr survival
- Do chemotherapy within 21 days of surgery
- Low grades do not require chemotherapy

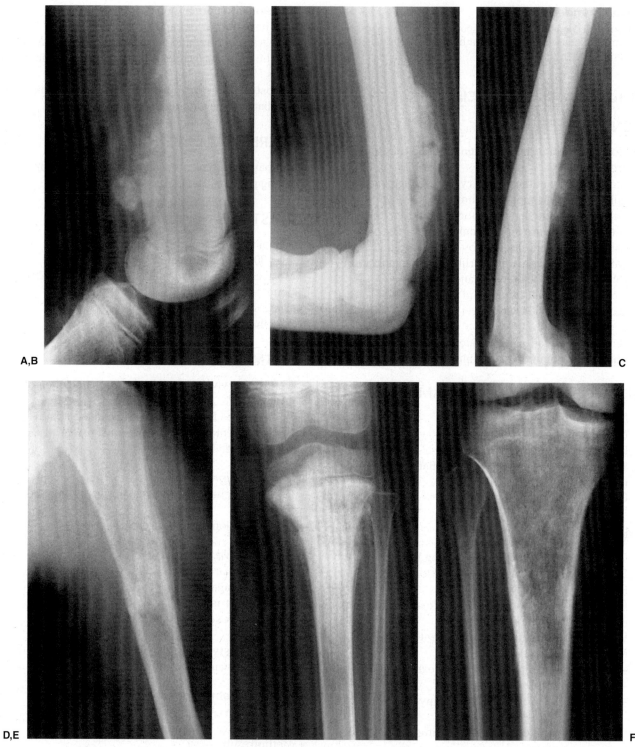

Various radiographs demonstrating the great heterogeneity of osteosarcomas. The three key diagnostic features are (1) a poorly mineralized bone lesion, (2) a soft tissue mass, and (3) matrix production. (From Simon MD, Springfield DS. Surgery for Bone and Soft-Tissue Tumors. Philadelphia: Lippincott Williams & Wilkins; 1998, with permission.) *(continued)*

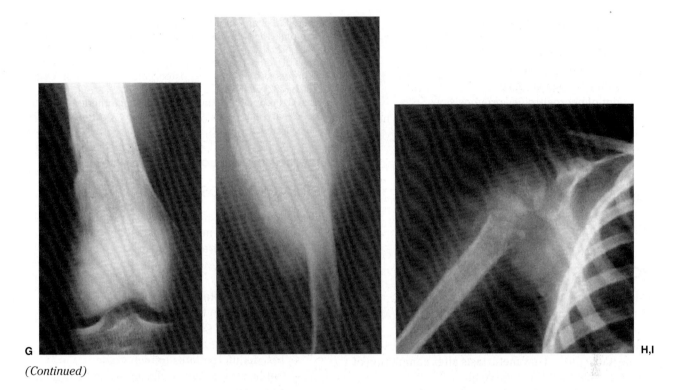

G   H,I

(Continued)

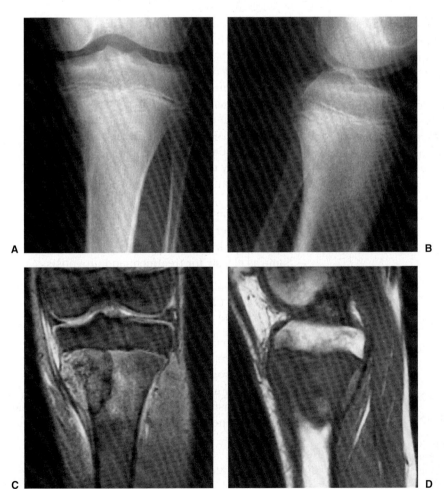

A

B

C

D

Plain radiographs **(A, B)** demonstrate a small osteolytic lesion of the proximal tibia in an immature patient with a poorly defined intramedullary margin and evident cortical destruction, but without obvious periosteal reaction or matrix production. Magnetic resonance imaging with a T2-weighted anteroposterior view **(C)** and a T1-weighted lateral view **(D)** demonstrates with particularly accurate detail and clarity the intramedullary extent of the tumor and the precise relationship of the extraosseous tumor mass to the periosteum and the adjacent periarticular soft tissue structures. (From Simon MD, Springfield DS. Surgery for Bone and Soft-Tissue Tumors. Philadelphia: Lippincott Williams & Wilkins; 1998, with permission.)

Neoadjuvant Chemotherapy

(Rosen, 1985)

- Prevents resistant clones
- Kills micrometastases
- Gives time to plan surgery
- Amount of necrosis gives prognosis
- No large series that show survival advantage of neoadjuvant therapy

(Goorin et al., 2003)

- Randomized controlled trial of neoadjuvant versus adjuvant chemotherapy
- 50 patients each arm
- No difference in event-free survival
- Earlier surgery may prevent metastases

PROGNOSIS

- Most important is detectable metastases
- Undetectable metastases—76% 5-yr survival (Memorial Sloan-Kettering)
- Metastases at presentation—10%–20% 5-yr survival
- Resectable pulmonary metastasis after completion of therapy—20%–40% 5-yr survival
- True skeletal metastasis (not skip lesion) associated with worst prognosis
- >90% necrosis (responders) after neoadjuvant chemotherapy associated with good prognosis (87% 8-yr survival vs. 52% 8-yr survival in nonresponders)
- In nonresponders, <15% long-term survival if chemotherapy regimen is not changed
- African American race, high lactate dehydrogenase (LDH), high alkaline phosphatase, and proximal site associated with poor prognosis (Meyers et al., 1992)
- Absence of telomere maintenance mechanism associated with favorable prognosis
- Chemotherapy dose does not affect prognosis

MOLECULAR STAGING

- p53 and Rb tumor suppressors
- MDM2 inhibits p53
- c-myc, c-fos transcription factors
- Her2/ErbB-2 growth factor receptors (Morris et al., 2001)
- MDR1 (multidrug resistance)
- Vascular endothelial growth factor (VEGF) for angiogenesis of metastases

References

Gibbs CP Jr, et al. Malignant bone tumors. Instr Course Lect 2002; 51:413–428.

Goorin AM, et al. Presurgical chemotherapy compared with immediate surgery and adjuvant chemotherapy for non-metastatic osteosarcoma: Pediatric Oncology Group Study POG-8651. J Clin Oncol 2003; 21:1574–1580.

Meyers PA, et al. Chemotherapy for nonmetastatic osteogenic sarcoma: the Memorial Sloan-Kettering experience. J Clin Oncol 1992; 10:5–15.

Morris CD, et al. Human epidermal growth factor receptor 2 as a prognostic indicator in osteogenic sarcoma. Clin Orthop 2001; (382):59–65.

Rosen G. Preoperative (neoadjuvant) chemotherapy for osteogenic sarcoma: a ten year experience. Orthopedics. 1985; 8(5):659–64.

Osteogenic Sarcoma—Subtypes

PRIMARY OSTEOSARCOMA

- I—classic (high grade central)
  - More common, more metastases
- II—low grade central
- III—juxtacortical (surface)
  - A—parosteal
    - Posterior distal femur >50%
    - Cleft between tumor and bone
    - Older, **F > M (2:1)**
    - Usually low grade (60%), less cellular
    - 10% dedifferentiates to high grade
    - Duplication of part of chromosome 12, ring chromosomes
    - Wide excision
    - **No chemotherapy if low grade**
    - 93% long-term survival
  - B—periosteal
    - Diaphysis of long bone
    - Adolescents
    - Intermediate grade
    - Osteoid in **chondroid background**
    - Wide excision ± chemotherapy
  - C—high grade surface
    - Extremely rare
- IV—telangiectatic
  - High grade
  - Hemorrhagic, little tissue
  - "Bag of blood," >90% vascular channels
  - Differential diagnosis ABC
  - Same as classic for treatment and prognosis

SECONDARY OSTEOSARCOMA

- Paget disease
- After irradiation, 60% are around pelvis
- Both aggressive, destructive
- Both dismal prognosis
- Chemotherapy may be beneficial
- Malignant transformation of fibrous dysplasia, bone infarct, and bone cyst

Reference

Gibbs CP, Jr, et al. Malignant bone tumors. Instr Course Lect 2002; 51:413–428.

Osteoid Osteoma

GENERAL

- Benign bone-forming tumor
- <1 cm in diameter by definition
- Neoplastic versus inflammatory process
- Most common in 5–30 yo, 13% >30 yo
- Most in proximal femur and posterior spine

PROSTAGLANDINS

- Intense pain via prostaglandin effects on vasodilation and bradykinin system
- Prostaglandin F stimulates bone production
- Cortical hyperostosis in cyanotic congenital heart caused by treatment with prostaglandin E

HISTORY AND PHYSICAL EXAMINATION

- Most common cause of painful scoliosis in children
- Exertional pain if lesion intracapsular with synovitis
- Warmth/erythema unusual
- Pain worse at night
- Relieved with acetylsalicylic acid (ASA) in 73%

IMAGING

- Radiolucent lesion <1 cm, surrounded by reactive bone of varying size
- Intracapsular lesions do not have sclerosis but have synovitis
- Lucency is cherry red nidus
- High signal on T2, edema in surrounding bone on MRI

PATHOLOGY

- Identical to osteoblastoma
- Nidus with vessels, "trabecular" osteoid, and osteoblasts
- "Cherry red" = vascular
- Nidus surrounded by reactive woven bone

DIFFERENTIAL DIAGNOSIS

- Stress fracture
- Avascular necrosis
- Osteochondritis desiccans
- Rheumatoid arthritis
- Brodie abscess, osteomyelitis
- Osteoblastoma
- Osteosarcoma

TREATMENT

- Tends to disappear
- **Surgical excision is treatment of choice, especially if causing scoliosis**
- ? Surgical or radiofrequency ablation for those not relieved by nonsteroidal anti-inflammatory drugs (NSAIDs)
- Intraoperative radioisotope scanning to locate tumor and confirm removal

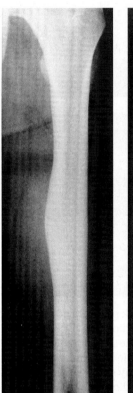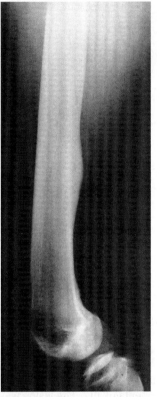

A   B

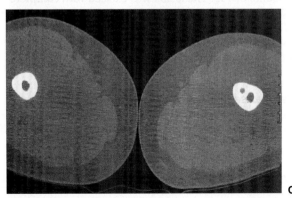

C

Anteroposterior (**A**) and lateral (**B**) radiographs of the femoral diaphysis in an adolescent boy show an intracortical or surface lesion most compatible with an osteoid osteoma. Computed tomography scan of the lesion (**C**) shows a well-marginated intracortical lesion diagnostic of an osteoid osteoma. (From Simon MD, Springfield DS. Surgery for Bone and Soft-Tissue Tumors. Philadelphia: Lippincott Williams & Wilkins; 1998, with permission.)

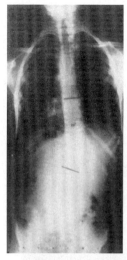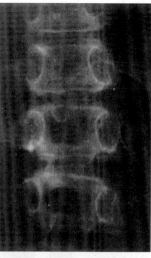

A,B

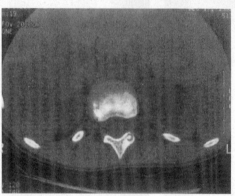

C

A 13-yo boy presented with back pain caused by osteoid osteoma. **A:** Anteroposterior radiograph demonstrates thoracolumbar scoliosis. **B:** Coned-down radiograph demonstrates a probable nidus in the posterior elements of T12. **C:** Computed tomography scan demonstrates a nidus consistent with an osteoid osteoma in the posterior elements of T12. The lesion was excised with complete relief of pain and resolution of the scoliosis. (From Simon MD, Springfield DS. Surgery for Bone and Soft-Tissue Tumors. Philadelphia: Lippincott Williams & Wilkins; 1998, with permission.)

Reference

Healey JH, Ghelman B. Osteoid osteoma and osteoblastoma: current concepts and recent advances. Clin Orthop 1986; (204):76–85.

Paget Disease

GENERAL

- "Osteitis deformans"
- 3%–4% of people >50 yo
- Increased in family members, Europeans
- ? Due to infection by paramyxovirus in genetically susceptible osteoclast leading to osteoclast hyperactivity with reactive osteoblast hyperactivity

- Juvenile Paget disease associated with hyperphosphatemia, diaphyseal location, diffuse lesions, and tibias
- Three phases:
  - Lytic
  - Mixed
  - Sclerotic

HISTORY AND PHYSICAL EXAMINATION

- Usually asymptomatic
- Mono- or polyostotic
- Increased bone size with deformity
- Cardiomegaly due to hypervascularity
- CHF due to high output via atrioventricular (AV) shunts
- Bone weakened from increased vascularity
- Arthritis
- Bone tenderness
- Dental loosening
- Hearing loss caused by narrowing canal
- Spinal stenosis
- Pathological and fissure fractures

LABORATORY VALUES

- Increased alkaline phosphatase, normal calcium, and normal phosphate
- Increased urine pyridoxamine cross-links
- Increased urine hydroxycholine
- Urolithiasis
- Hyperuricemia leads to gout

IMAGING

- Epiphysis
- Lytic versus sclerotic, depends on phase
- **Coarse trabeculae**
- **Increased bone size**
- Hot bone scan
- Arthritis
- **Picture-window vertebra**
- Blade of grass, advancing flame
- Pagetic bone has fat signal on MRI

DIFFERENTIAL DIAGNOSIS

- Myelofibrosis without cortical thickening and deformity
- Giant cell tumor

PATHOLOGY

- Disorganized mosaic of woven and lamellar bone
- Increased osteoblast and osteoclast activity

- Giant osteoclasts with viral inclusions
- Cement lines

ONCOLOGIC PROBLEMS

- Paget disease associated with primary GCTs
- Can cause secondary tumors
  - Osteosarcoma, >70 yo, 1% incidence
  - Chondrosarcoma
  - Fibrosarcoma
  - Mixed tumors

MEDICAL TREATMENT

- Calcitonin, bisphosphates, mithramycin
- Indicated if:
  - Elevated alkaline phosphatase
  - Skull lesions
  - Spine lesions
  - Deforming long bone
  - Periarticular lesion (prevent arthritis)

SURGICAL TREATMENT

- Deformity—intramedullary rod
- Arthritis—total hip replacement (THR)
- Fracture—open reduction and internal fixation (ORIF) ± osteotomy

Reference

Roodman GD, Windle JJ. Paget disease of bone. J Clin Invest 2005; 115:200–208.

Periosteal Chondroma

GENERAL

- Benign cartilage tumor that forms under periosteum
- Rare
- 30s, 40s
- M > F
- Most common in humeral or femoral diaphysis

IMAGING

- Saucerlike erosions
- Well-defined rim, underlying reactive bone

NATURAL HISTORY

- Malignant transformation not reported

PATHOLOGY

- Lobules of immature cartilage, but unlike chondrosarcoma, surface bound by mature fibrous capsule without vascular proliferation
- Looks very much like chondrosarcoma on pathology

TREATMENT

- Wide/marginal excision
- If asymptomatic, can follow with serial XRs

Reference

Lewis MM, et al. Periosteal chondroma: a report of ten cases and review of the literature. Clin Orthop 1990; (256):185–192.

Postradiation Sarcoma of Bone

- Modified criteria of Arlen et al. (1971):
  - Primary lesion devoid of osteoblastic activity
  - Irradiation must have been given and sarcoma developed in path of beam
  - Latent period >3 yr
  - Secondary sarcoma must be proven histopathologically

Reference

Arlen M, et al. Radiation-induced sarcoma of bone. Cancer 1971; 28:1087–1099.

Pigmented Villonodular Synovitis/Giant Cell Tumor of Tendon Sheath

GENERAL

- Benign neoplasia of synovium
- Young adult
- Most common in knee; second is ankle/foot
- Swollen joint, little pain
- Joint fluid is dark old blood

IMAGING

- XR usually normal, possible joint erosions
- Joint space usually not narrowed until late
- **No calcification**
- On MRI
  - Thick synovium
  - Hemosiderin is dark on T1 and T2
  - Solid portion of mass is dark on all sequences
- Thallium scan positive
- On arthroscopy, synovium looks like "seaweed"

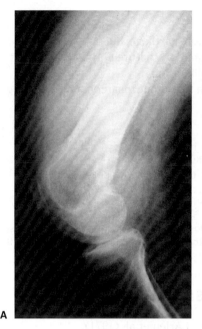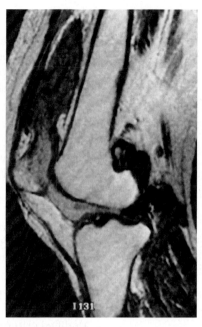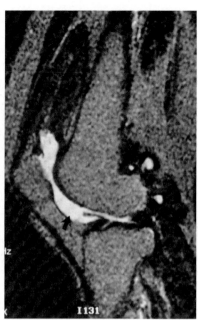

A   B,C

Magnetic resonance imaging (MRI) features of pigmented villonodular synovitis. **A:** Lateral radiograph of knee shows a soft tissue mass with water density in the anterior distal femur. **B:** MRI sagittal T1-weighted view shows low-signal, heterogeneous soft tissue mass in the suprapatellar area and posterior knee. **C:** A sagittal T2-weighted MRI shows low-signal mass in suprapatellar area and posterior knee with intra-articular high signals characteristic of joint effusion (*arrow*). (From Simon MD, Springfield DS. Surgery for Bone and Soft-Tissue Tumors. Philadelphia: Lippincott Williams & Wilkins; 1998, with permission.)

PATHOLOGY

- Can get false-positive pathology from recurrent hemarthrosis of shoulder
- Hypertrophic synovial cells, histiocytes, multinucleated giant cells with hemosiderin in cytoplasm, villi
- **Lipid-laden macrophages**

TREATMENT

- Synovectomy
- Injection of dysprosium radionuclide
- Recurrence common

GIANT CELL TUMOR OF TENDON SHEATH

- Histologically identical to PVNS
- Clinically different
- Well encapsulated
- Solid nodule attached to tendon sheath, usually in hand or feet
- Usually on volar surface
- Excision is curative

Recommended Reading

Rao AS, Vigorita VJ. Pigmented villonodular synovitis (giant-cell tumor of the tendon sheath and synovial membrane): a review of eighty-one cases. J Bone Joint Surg Am 1984; 66:76–94.

Rhabdomyosarcoma

GENERAL

- Malignant tumor of striated muscle
- Almost exclusive to children
- 50% in <5 yo
- **Most common soft tissue sarcoma in children**

HISTORY AND PHYSICAL EXAMINATION

- Mild pain and mass
- In gastrourinary tract, head and neck, and extremities
- Lower extremity more commonly involved than upper extremity

SUBTYPES

- Alveolar—t(2:13), metastasizes to nodes, round blue cells, less chemotherapy sensitive

- Embryonal—metastasizes to lungs, looks like muscle
- Pleomorphic
- Botryoid—embryonal type in hollow organ such as bladder
- Nodal spread common

PATHOLOGY

- Small round blue cells with septations in alveolar type
- **Striations due to contractile elements**
- Positive **desmin stain**
- Intensely eosinophilic, filamentous, and granular cytoplasm
- Multinucleated giant cells
- Racquet-shaped cells

DIFFERENTIAL DIAGNOSIS

- Alveolar type must be differentiated from Ewing sarcoma

TREATMENT

- Chemotherapy with surgery or XRT
  - Unlike other soft tissue sarcomas, it responds to chemotherapy
  - 65% survival with chemotherapy versus 20% without chemotherapy

Recommended Reading

Thomas F, et al. Primary rhabdomyosarcoma of the humerus: a case report and review of the literature. J Bone Joint Surg Am 2002; 84:813–817.

Unicameral Bone Cyst

GENERAL

- Also known as simple bone cyst
- Serous-filled fluid cavity lined with thin layer of synovial cells
- ? Due to physeal disturbance
- M > F, two-thirds of patients are male
- Usually 5–15 yo, must be <30 yo
- One-half are in proximal humerus
- In proximal long bone—humerus, femur, tibia
- Seen in pelvis and calcaneus

IMAGING

- Must be central
- **Abuts physis from metaphysis**
- Can be away from physis, but patient must be old enough so that it has been pushed away

- "Fallen fragment" sign
- Narrow transition zone
- Bone does not expand wider than physis
- Hard to differentiate from fibrous dysplasia in proximal femur by radiology alone
- MRI—gray on T1, bright on T2

DIFFERENTIAL DIAGNOSIS

- ABC
- Fibrous dysplasia

PATHOLOGY

- **Just single cell layer without giant cells, mononuclear cells, or blood as seen in ABC**

PROGNOSIS

- If it abuts physis, then it is active
- If normal bone intervenes, then it is latent
- Heals at skeletal maturity, usually by age 10 yr

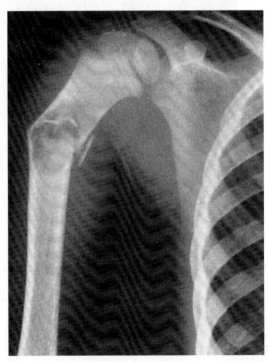

Anteroposterior radiograph of a child with acute pain in the arm after a fall shows a well-marginated, centrally placed lesion in the upper humerus with bone fragments in the area of radiolucency, indicative of a cystic lesion. (From Simon MD, Springfield DS. Surgery for Bone and Soft-Tissue Tumors. Philadelphia: Lippincott Williams & Wilkins; 1998, with permission.)

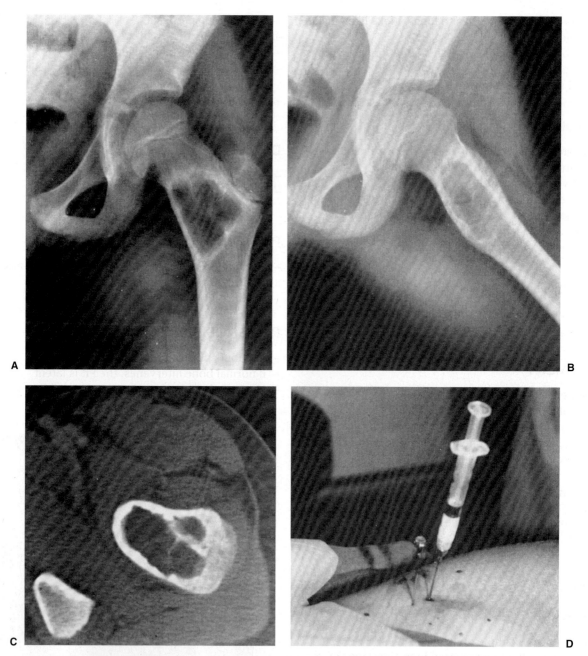

Anteroposterior **(A)** and lateral **(B)** radiographs and computed tomography scan **(C)** of a child with groin pain and a limp show a central, well-marginated lesion in the metaphysis of the proximal femur without matrix mineralization. Intraoperative photograph **(D)** shows two large-gauge needles introduced into the lesion. (From Simon MD, Springfield DS. Surgery for Bone and Soft-Tissue Tumors. Philadelphia: Lippincott Williams & Wilkins; 1998, with permission.)

TREATMENT

- Most do not need treatment because spontaneously resolves
- Treat femoral neck lesion to decrease fracture risk
- If pathological fracture, treat fracture routinely without regard for cyst
- If needed, treat only after healing of fracture
- Aspirate (if bloody, get formal biopsy to determine whether it is ABC or other tumor)
  - Inject contrast and suspect something else if not fully filled
  - Inject with **steroids or marrow** because it is as effective as curettage/graft
- Curettage/graft in high-stress regions

Recommended Reading

Wilkins RM. Unicameral bone cysts. J Am Acad Orthop Surg 2000; 8:217–824.

Synovial Chondromatosis

GENERAL

- Benign primary synovial tumor
- Synovial cells extrude small nodules of cartilage into the joint
- 20–50 yo
- 80% in knee, then elbow and hip

HISTORY AND PHYSICAL EXAMINATION

- Pain, swelling, locking

IMAGING

- Plain XR normal or small calcification flecks
- MRI can easily see nodules
- Must have loose body

PATHOLOGY

- Cellular nodules of cartilage with synovial lining, embedded in edematous synovium
- No synovitis, joint fluid is clear
- If this type of lesion seen in bone, it would be considered low-grade chondrosarcoma

TREATMENT

- Synovial excision
- Recurrence common

Recommended Reading

Coles MJ, Tara HH, Jr. Synovial chondromatosis: a case study and brief review. Am J Orthop 1997; 26:37–40.

Synovial Sarcoma

GENERAL

- Third most common soft tissue sarcoma
- Makes up 6%–10% of all soft tissue sarcomas
- Most common in lower extremities
- Most common soft tissue sarcoma of hand
- Classic soft tissue mass in sole of **foot**
- Rarely within a joint but usually periarticular
- Occurs in younger patients than other sarcomas, usually in 30s and 40s

IMAGING

- **Most common soft tissue sarcoma with calcifications on XR (50% calcify)**
- Bone scan with increased uptake

METASTASES

- To lungs
- 25% metastases to regional nodes

PATHOLOGY

- Almost always high grade, extracompartmental
- Highly cellular, vascular, biphasic pattern
- **Cytokeratins** positive (marker of epithelioid cells)
- All sarcomas have mesenchymal origin (indicated by positive vimentin)
- However, synovial sarcoma and adamantinoma have epithelial and mesenchymal components
- Monophasic
  - Only spindle cells
- **Biphasic**
  - Glandular epithelial differentiation
  - Positive EMA
  - Background of spindle cells
(Kawai et al., 1998; Ladanyi et al., 2002)
- SYT(chr18)-SSX(chrX) fusion
- If metastases at diagnosis (*n* = 25), 0% survival at 4 yr
- SYT-SSX1 associated with biphasic, worse prognosis
  - More common
  - Overall survival median 6 yr, 53% 5-yr survival
  - More likely to present with metastases
  - If local at diagnosis, median 9 yr, 61% 5-yr survival
- SYT-SSX2 associated with monophasic type and better prognosis
  - Overall survival median 14 yr, 73% 5-yr survival
  - If local at diagnosis, median 14 yr, 77% 5-yr survival
(Lewis et al., 2000)
- Age of patient and histology did not affect prognosis
- Local recurrence related to site being proximal
- Distant recurrence related to size >5 cm and neurovascular or bone invasion

TREATMENT

- Wide excision
- Postoperative XRT
- Postoperative chemotherapy if >5 cm (very sensitive to ifosfamide)
- To achieve better margin, consider preoperative chemotherapy if tumor encroaches on crucial structure

PROGNOSIS

- 60% 5-yr survival
- 30% 10-yr survival
- Better prognosis with re-excision
- Local recurrence does not correlate with mortality

References

Kawai A, et al. SYT-SSX gene fusion as a determinant of morphology and prognosis in synovial sarcoma. N Engl J Med 1998; 338:153–160.

Ladanyi M, et al. Impact of SYT-SSX fusion type on the clinical behavior of synovial sarcoma: a multi-institutional retrospective study of 243 patients. Cancer Res 2002; 62:135–140.

Lewis JJ, et al. Synovial sarcoma: a multivariate analysis of prognostic factors in 112 patients with primary localized tumors of the extremity. J Clin Oncol 2000; 18:2087–2094.

Tumoral Calcinosis

GENERAL

- Painless calcific masses around extensor surfaces of hips, elbows, shoulders, and gluteal areas
- Various genetic types
- Caused by a defect in phosphorus transport

HISTORY AND PHYSICAL EXAMINATION

- Seen in dialysis patients
- More common in African Americans
- 30% with positive family history

IMAGING

- Lobulated, calcified soft tissue mass adjacent to joints

PATHOLOGY

- Calcific deposits with focal mild mononuclear and, occasionally, multinucleated giant cell reaction

TREATMENT

- PhosLo in dialysis patients
- Surgical excision

Recommended Reading

Martinez S. Tumoral calcinosis: 12 years later. Semin Musculoskelet Radiol 2002; 6:331–339.

CHAPTER 7

Hand

Scott J. Ellis, Aaron Daluiski, Mark C. Drakos, Alison F. Kitay

Anatomy
 Abbreviation
Ossification of Carpal Bones
 Radial Artery
 Ulnar Artery
 Lateral Antebrachial Cutaneous Nerve
 Axillary Artery (Parts)
 Brachialis Innervation
 Triceps
Vascular Anatomy: Hand and Fingers
Anatomy: Palm Landmarks
Anatomy of the Median Nerve
 Innervation
 Martin-Gruber Anastomosis
 Variations of Palmar Cutaneous
  Nerve
 Variations of Motor Branch
Anatomy of the Radial Nerve
 Innervation
Anatomy of the Ulnar Nerve
 Innervation
Wrist Block
 Four Types of Injections (Using 2% Lidocaine
  without Epinephrine)
Dorsal Wrist Compartments
Approaches: Elbow/Forearm
 Kocher "J" Lateral Elbow
 Morrey Posterior Elbow Approach
 Volar Henry Approach to Radius
 Dorsal Thompson Approach to
  Radius
 Dorsal Approach
Physical Examination of Hand
 Intrinsic Minus (Claw)
 Intrinsic Plus
 Lumbrical Plus
 Retinacular Test
 Quadrigia Effect
Wrist Radiograph

Brachial Plexus
 Overview
 Preclavicular Branches
 Lateral Cord (C5-7)
 Posterior Cord (C5-T1)
 Medial Cord (C8, T1)
 Goals of Surgery (by Priority) in Brachial
  Plexus Injury
 Timing of Surgery
 Surgical Options
Nerve Injury
 Seddon Nerve Injury Classification
 Sequence of Nerve Function Failure
 Sequence of Nerve Function Recovery
 Recovery
 Common Nerve Injury Patterns
Anterior Interosseous Nerve Syndrome
 Symptoms
 Signs
 Six Possible Sites of Compression
 Differential Diagnosis
 Natural History
Carpal Tunnel Syndrome
 Diagnosis
 Carpal Tunnel Contents
 Transverse Carpal Ligament Attachments
 Predisposing Factors
 Diagnosis
 Treatment
 Endoscopic Carpal Tunnel Release
 Standard Carpal Tunnel Release
 Revision Carpal Tunnel Release
 Carpal Tunnel Release Technique
Cubital Tunnel Syndrome
 Diagnosis
 Treatment
 Subcutaneous Transposition
Radial Tunnel Syndrome
 Etiology

Radial Tunnel
Radial Tunnel versus Posterior Interosseous
    Nerve
Radial Tunnel Syndrome Treatment
Posterior Interosseous Nerve Syndrome
    Treatment
Pronator Syndrome
    Site of Impingement: Four Locations
    Treatment
Ulnar Tunnel Syndrome
    Guyon Canal Contents
    Guyon Canal Boundaries
    Etiology
    Treatment
Wartenberg Syndrome
    Etiology
    Diagnosis
    Treatment
Dorsal Wrist Ganglion
    Anatomy
    Presentation
    Natural History
    Treatment and Cure Rates
Mucous Cyst
Dupuytren Contracture
    Description
    Background
    Luck's Stages
    Structures Affected
    Structures Not Affected
    Cords Formed
    Non-surgical Management
    Indications for Surgery
    Surgeries
    Surgical Complications
    Operating Room Tips
Fracture of Hand: Open
    Classification and Treatment
**Flexor Tenosynovitis: Kanavel's Cardinal
    Signs**
Infection in Hand
    Fight Bite
Flexor Tendon Injury
    Fundamentals
    Functional Anatomy
    Phases of Tendon Healing
    Postoperative Protocols
Flexor Tendon Zones
Extensor Tendon Injury
    Anatomy
    Extension of Individual Joints
    General Principles of Treatment
    Extensor Zones
    Outcomes of Extensor Tendon Repair
    Intrinsic Tightness

Mallet Finger
    Definition
    Treatment
    Mallet Finger with Fracture
    Sequelae
**Flexor Digitorum Profundus Avulsion/Jersey
    Finger**
    Anatomy
    Classification
Traumatic Boutonniere Deformity
    Definition
    Cause
    Process
    Zone III Injury (Proximal Interphalangeal
        Joint)
**Ulnar Collateral Ligament: Gamekeeper's
    Thumb**
    Definition
    Associated Injuries
    Stener Lesion
    Diagnosis and Treatment
    Surgical Treatment
Sagittal Band Rupture
    Anatomy of Band
    Findings
    Treatment
Ring Avulsion Injuries
    Definition
    Urbaniak Classification
Replants
Chemical Burns
Flaps
Fracture: Metacarpal
    Fundamental Anatomy
    Metacarpal Head Fracture
    Metacarpal Neck Fracture
    Metacarpal Shaft Fracture
    Metacarpal Base Fracture
Fracture: Phalangeal
    Order of Most Commonly Fractured Bones
        in Hand
Pearls
    Fractures and Their Typical Angulation
    Treatment of Hand Fractures
Dislocations: Proximal Interphalangeal Joint
    Dorsal Dislocation
    Volar Dislocation
Swan Neck Deformity
    Description
    Rheumatoid Swan Neck Deformity
        Classification
Rheumatoid Arthritis Thumb Deformity Types
    Type I: Boutonniere Thumb
    Type II
    Type III

Type IV: "Gamekeeper's"
Type V
Rheumatoid Arthritis Boutonniere Deformity
Description
Stage I
Stage II
Stage III
Trigger Finger
Background
Finger Pulleys
Mechanics
History and Physical Examination
Steroid Injection
Operative Treatment
Basal Joint Osteoarthritis
Eaton Classification
Kirner Deformity
Description
Etiology
Epidemiology
Radiograph
Treatment
Clinodactyly
Description
Epidemiology
Treatment
Camptodactyly
Description
Etiology
Types
Epidemiology
Etiology
Treatment
Syndactyly
Description
Epidemiology
Types
Examination
Treatment
Thumb Hypoplasia
Background Anatomy
Blauth Classification of Thumb Hypoplasia
Ulnar Impaction
Ulnar Variance
Radiocarpal Ligaments
Volar Radiocarpal Ligaments
Dorsal Radiocarpal Ligaments
Intrinsic Ligaments of Wrist
Scapholunate Instability
Occult
Dynamic
Scapholunate Dissociation
Dorsal Intercalated Segment Instability (DISI)
Volar Intercalated Segment Instability (VISI)
Scapholunate Advanced Collapse

Triangular Fibrocartilage Complex and Distal Radioulnar Joint
Functional Anatomy
Components of Triangular Fibrocartilage Complex
Triangular Fibrocartilage Complex Tears
Radioulnar Synostosis
Description
Epidemiology
Surgery
Kienböck
Definition
Etiology
Epidemiology
Presentation
Radiographic Staging
Nonoperative Treatment
Operative Treatment

Anatomy

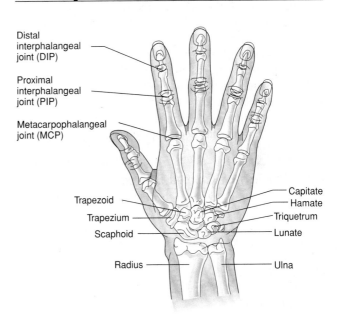

Bony structures of the wrist and hand. (From Bickley, Szilagyi P. Bates' Guide to Physical Examination and History Taking, 8th ed. Philadelphia: Lippincott Williams & Wilkins; 2003.)

ABBREVIATION

- AAROM: active-assisted range of motion
- AIN: anterior interosseous nerve
- APB: abductor pollicis brevis
- APL: abductor pollicis longus
- AROM: active range of motion
- BB: biceps brachii
- BR: brachioradialis

- CMC: carpal metacarpal
- DIP: distal interphalangeal
- DP: distal phalanx
- DRUJ: distal radial ulnar joint
- ECRB: extensor carpi radialis brevis
- ECRL: extensor carpi radialis longus
- ECU: extensor carpi ulnaris
- EDC: extensor digitorum communis
- EDQ: extensor digiti quinti
- EIP: extensor indicis proprius
- EPL: extensor pollicis longus
- EPB: extensor pollicis brevis
- FCR: flexor carpi radialis
- FCU: flexor carpi ulnaris
- FDP: flexor digitorum profundus
- FDS: flexor digitorum superficialis
- FPB: flexor pollicis brevis
- IO: interosseous
- MCP: metacarpal phalangeal
- MP: middle phalanx
- MN: median nerve
- ORL: oblique retinacular ligament
- PL: palmaris longus
- PT: pronator teres
- PQ: pronator quadratus
- PIN: posterior interosseous nerve
- PIP: proximal interphalangeal
- PP: proximal phalanx
- PROM: passive range of motion
- TFCC: triangular fibrocartilage complex

Ossification of Carpal Bones

- Capitate: 1
- Hamate: 1
- Triquetrum: 3
- Lunate: 5
- Trapezium: 5
- Scaphoid: 6
- Trapezoid: 8
- Pisiform: 12

RADIAL ARTERY

- Medial to biceps brachii (BB) tendon
- Courses anteriorly
- Lies volarly on supinator
- Courses just volar to insertion of pronator teres (PT) on radius
- Passes underneath brachioradialis (BR)
- Pierces first dorsal interosseous (IO) muscle
- Superficial branch travels between flexor pollicis brevis (FPB) heads and then under abductor pollicis brevis (APB)

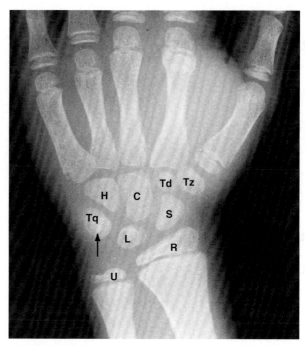

Posteroanterior view

Posteroanterior view of the inferior end of the forearm and hand of an 11-yo child. Ossification centers of all carpal bones are apparent. The *arrowhead* indicates the pisiform. Observe that the distal epiphysis of the ulna has ossified but that all epiphyseal plates (*lines*) "remain open" (i.e., they are still unossified). S, scaphoid; Td, trapezoid; Tz, trapezium. (From Moore KL, Dalley AF. Clinical Oriented Anatomy, 4th ed. Baltimore: Lippincott Williams & Wilkins; 1999. Courtesy of Dr. D. Armstrong, Associate Professor of Medical Imaging, University of Toronto, Toronto, Ontario, Canada.)

ULNAR ARTERY

- Disappears in cubital fossa deep to PT deep head
- Runs with ulnar nerve, but radial to it

LATERAL ANTEBRACHIAL CUTANEOUS NERVE

- Branches off musculocutaneous nerve
- Crosses arm volar to brachialis and exits laterally near lateral intermuscular septum
- Comes to lie on top of brachialis
- Landmark: in line connecting epicondyles, located 1 cm lateral to biceps tendon
- Medial antebrachial cutaneous (off medial cord, C8-T1) and brachial cutaneous (off medial cord, T1) nerves are more variable

AXILLARY ARTERY (PARTS)

- Parts determined by pectoralis minor
- Part I: proximal to pectoralis minor (one branch)

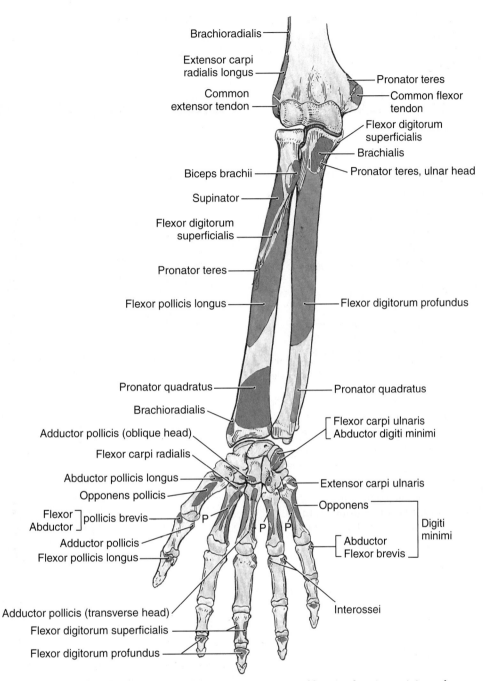

Brachioradialis
Extensor carpi radialis longus
Common extensor tendon
Biceps brachii
Supinator
Flexor digitorum superficialis
Pronator teres
Flexor pollicis longus
Pronator quadratus
Brachioradialis
Adductor pollicis (oblique head)
Flexor carpi radialis
Abductor pollicis longus
Opponens pollicis
Flexor ⎤ pollicis brevis
Abductor ⎦
Adductor pollicis
Flexor pollicis longus
Adductor pollicis (transverse head)
Flexor digitorum superficialis
Flexor digitorum profundus

Pronator teres
Common flexor tendon
Flexor digitorum superficialis
Brachialis
Pronator teres, ulnar head
Flexor digitorum profundus
Pronator quadratus
Flexor carpi ulnaris
Abductor digiti minimi
Extensor carpi ulnaris
Opponens
Abductor
Flexor brevis
Digiti minimi
Interossei
P P P

Muscles that move the forearm and wrist. Anterior view of bones showing origin and insertion of muscles. (From Agur MRA, Lee MJ. Grant's Atlas of Anatomy, 10th ed. Baltimore: Lippincott Williams and Wilkins; 1999.)

- Superior thoracic artery: to serratus anterior and pectoralis muscles
- Part II: directly beneath pectoralis minor (two branches)
  - Thoracoacromial artery:
    - Clavicular branch
    - Acromial branch
    - Deltoid branch: courses with basilic vein
  - Lateral thoracic branch: to serratus anterior (with long thoracic nerve)
- Part III: distal to pectoralis minor (three branches)
  - Subscapular
    - Circumflex scapular: seen posteriorly in triangular space
    - Thoracodorsal
  - Anterior circumflex

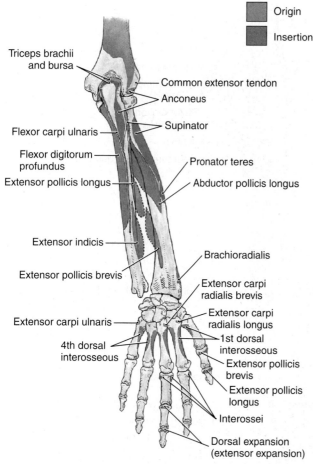

Origin
Insertion

Triceps brachii and bursa
Common extensor tendon
Anconeus
Flexor carpi ulnaris
Supinator
Flexor digitorum profundus
Extensor pollicis longus
Pronator teres
Abductor pollicis longus
Extensor indicis
Brachioradialis
Extensor pollicis brevis
Extensor carpi radialis brevis
Extensor carpi ulnaris
Extensor carpi radialis longus
4th dorsal interosseous
1st dorsal interosseous
Extensor pollicis brevis
Extensor pollicis longus
Interossei
Dorsal expansion (extensor expansion)

Muscles that move the forearm and wrist. Posterior view of bones showing origin and insertion of muscles. (From Agur MRA, Lee MJ. Grant's Atlas of Anatomy, 10th ed. Baltimore: Lippincott Williams and Wilkins; 1999.)

– Posterior circumflex: seen posteriorly in quadrangular space

BRACHIALIS INNERVATION

– Lateral part via radial n.
– Medial part via musculocutaneous n.
  – May be split longitudinally in anterior surgical approach

TRICEPS

– Long head (from scapula): nerve supply high in axilla
– Lateral head (from posterior humerus): nerve supply at spiral groove
  – Thus, these two heads can be split proximally without endangering radial n.

– Medial (deep) head has dual supply from radial n. and from some radial fibers "hitchhiking" with ulnar n.
  – Thus, medial head can be split longitudinally

Vascular Anatomy: Hand and Fingers

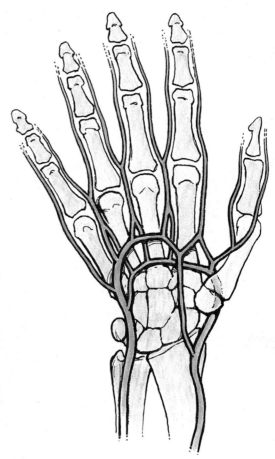

Anterior view of the palmar arterial arches of the hand. (Image from Grants Atlas of Anatomy.)

– Deep palmar arch arises from radial artery
– Superficial arch arises from ulnar artery: main supply to fingers
– Arteries volar to nerves in palm
– Nerves volar to arteries in fingers ("hurts before it bleeds")

Anatomy: Palm Landmarks

– Kaplan cardinal line: line along radial aspect of thumb web space toward pisiform (parallel to proximal transverse palmar crease)
  – Deep palmar arch found under this line

Surface Anatomy of the Hand. From Moore KL, Dalley AF II. Clinical Oriented Anatomy (4th ed.). Baltimore, Lippincott Williams & Wilkins 1999.

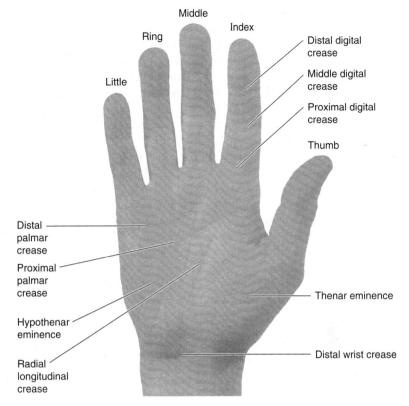

- Recurrent motor branch of median nerve located at intersection of Kaplan line and line drawn along ulnar aspect of long finger.
- Hook of hamate on line (tip of thumb rests on hook when thumb interphalangeal joint of opposite hand placed on pisiform)
- Superficial palmar arch: found below line connecting ulnar end of distal transverse palmar crease and radial end of proximal transverse palmar crease
- Palmar cutaneous branch of median branch of median nerve between flexor carpi radialis (FCR) and palmaris longus (PL)

Anatomy of the Median Nerve

- Median nerve (MN) is formed by the nerve roots of C5-T1 and the medial and lateral cords of the brachial plexus
- Runs in anterior compartment of forearm
- Follows the brachial artery on brachialis, medial to biceps
- Courses lateral to the artery in the upper arm and medial to it in the cubital fossa
- In medial midhumerus, MN is most anterior, brachial artery in the middle, and ulnar nerve most posterior
- There are no branches of MN in arm

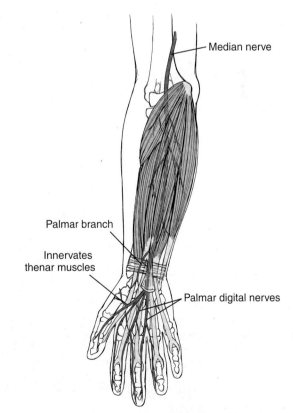

Course of the median nerve through the elbow, forearm, wrist, and hand.

- Under lacertus fibrosis, biceps tendon is most lateral, brachial artery in the middle, and MN most medial
- MN then runs between the two heads of PT: under the head with its origin on medial epicondyle and over the head with its origin on medial proximal ulna
- MN gives off anterior interosseous nerve (AIN) under origin of deep head of PT
- Both MN proper and AIN pass under fibrous arch origin of flexor digitorum superficialis (FDS)
- AIN trifurcates to innervate flexor pollicis longus (FPL), flexor digitorum profundus (FDP) of index/long finger, and pronator quadratus (PQ)
- MN proper continues on deep surface of FDS and innervates it
- MN is exposed in interval between FDS and FCR; it sends branches in ulnar direction in forearm, so dissect on its radial side
- Gives off palmar cutaneous branch 5 cm proximal to wrist, which runs between PL and FCR at level of wrist
- Courses through carpal tunnel deep to interval between FCR and PL

INNERVATION

- Motor branches of MN supply PT, FCR, PL, and FDS
- Motor branches of AIN division of MN include radial two digits of FDP (flexion of distal phalanx), flexor pollicis longus (FPL; flexion of distal phalanx), and PQ
- Motor branches of motor recurrent division of MN include APB, superficial head of FPB, and opponens pollicis (OP)
- MN also responsible for innervation of most radial two lumbricals
- Cutaneous distribution is via three terminal palmar digital branches that innervate skin of the radial two thirds of the palm: innervation includes the palmar aspect of the radial three and one-half digits and their dorsal aspects distal to the DIP joint

MARTIN-GRUBER ANASTOMOSIS

- Communication between median and ulnar nerves in forearm
- Occurs in 15%–30% of patients
- With such a communication, MN additionally supplies first dorsal IO muscle or other intrinsics
- Called Riche-Cannieu if in palm

VARIATIONS OF PALMAR CUTANEOUS NERVE

- Normally branches off 5 cm proximal to wrist and runs along ulnar side of FCR, then crosses retinaculum

- Divides separately into two branches and crosses retinaculum separately
- Arises from MN within carpal tunnel and then penetrates retinaculum
- If absent, may be replaced by branches of other nerves

VARIATIONS OF MOTOR BRANCH

- 50% are extraligamentous, recurrent branches
  - Arise from volar radial aspect of MN at distal radial end of carpal tunnel
  - Hook radially and proximally to enter thenar muscles between FPB and APB
- 30% are subligamentous, recurrent branches
  - Arise from anterior surface of MN within carpal tunnel and travel with MN through tunnel, and then hook back
- 20% are transligamentous
  - Arise from anterior surface of MN within tunnel and travel radially to pierce retinaculum, then enter thenar muscles
- Rare variations include those arising from ulnar side of MN, multiple motor branches, high proximal divisions, etc.

Anatomy of the Radial Nerve

- Radial nerve (RN) arises from C5-T1 and posterior cord of brachial plexus
- RN located on posterior wall of axilla, on top of subscapularis, teres major, and latissimus dorsi
- Then sends branch to the long head of triceps
- Runs in posterior compartment of arm
- RN approaches humerus 21 cm proximal to medial epicondyle
- Leaves humerus 14 cm proximal to lateral epicondyle
- Supplies lateral head of triceps in spiral groove of humerus
- At lateral aspect of humerus, RN trifurcates into branch for medial triceps head, inferior lateral brachial cutaneous nerve, posterior antebrachial cutaneous nerve, and rest of RN proper
- RN pierces intermuscular septum and enters anterior compartment
- Runs with deep brachial artery between brachioradialis and brachialis above elbow
- Supplies lateral part of brachialis, then brachioradialis, extensor carpi radialis longus (ECRL), anconeus, and extensor carpi radialis brevis (ECRB)
- Divides at radio-capitellar joint into superficial (sensory) and deep (motor) branches

- *Sensory branch* goes under brachioradialis and above supinator into lateral forearm along with radial artery
  - In midforearm, sensory branch is located under brachioradialis, with and lateral to radial artery
  - Sensory branch then courses between ECRL and FCR 5 cm from the radial styloid
  - In distal forearm, sensory branch overlies first dorsal compartment and comes to lie on extensor pollicis longus (EPL)
- *Motor branch* runs between two heads of supinator
  - Enters the supinator through arcade of Frohse and becomes posterior interosseous nerve (PIN)
  - ECRB, ECRL, and supinator are all supplied prior to arcade of Frohse
  - PIN exits on dorsal surface of distal supinator, travels over origin of abductor pollicis longus (APL), and then bifurcates 8 cm distal to elbow

INNERVATION

- RN supplies triceps brachii, anconeus, BR, and ECRL
- Deep radial nerve branch/PIN supplies ECRB, supinator, extensor digitorum communis (EDC), extensor carpi ulnaris (ECU), extensor digitorum minimi (EDM), APL, extensor pollicis brevis (EPB), EPL, and extensor indicis
- Ends in fourth compartment in wrist joint
- Cutaneous distribution is posterolateral aspect of arm and posterior aspect of forearm
- Superficial RN distribution supplies dorsal radial aspect of the first two and one-half digits proximal to most distal joint
- Extensor indicis proprius (EIP; last branch of PIN) is last to recover in PIN nerve palsy
- EDC (first branch of PIN) is first to recover
- ECRL recovers first in high radial nerve palsy

Anatomy of the Ulnar Nerve

- Ulnar nerve (UN) arises from nerve roots of C8-T1 and medial cord of brachial plexus
- Runs behind brachial artery in anterior compartment, then pierces intramuscular septum about two thirds along length of the humerus
- Traverses into the posterior compartment behind the medial epicondyle
- Courses along with ulnar collateral artery
- Like median nerve, UN has no branches in arm
- Its first branch is into elbow joint
- Its second branch is into the flexor carpi ulnaris (FCU)

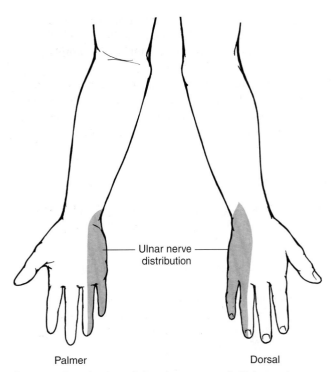

Ulnar nerve distribution

Palmer   Dorsal

Sensory distribution of the ulnar nerve. **A:** Palmar view. **B:** Dorsal view. (From Oatis CA. Kinesiology: The Mechanics and Pathomechanics of Human Movement. Baltimore: Lippincott Williams & Wilkins; 2004.)

- RN then runs between two heads of FCU and runs deep to both heads of PT
- Runs on surface of FDP and innervates half of it
- Runs deep and radial to FCU and ulnar to ulnar artery
- Gives off dorsal and volar sensory branches in distal forearm
- Dorsal branch eventually wraps around and dorsal to ECU at level of elbow joint but has significant variation
- Finally enters Guyon canal
- Just distal to the FCU insertion onto pisiform, UN divides into superficial and deep branches
- Superficial branch supplies ulnar aspect of skin of fingers
- Deep branch runs deep to all intrinsics except the index and long finger lumbricals by coursing between abductor digiti quinti (ADQ) and flexor digiti quinto brevis (FDQB)

INNERVATION

- UN supplies FCU and FDP of most ulnar two digits
- Deep ulnar nerve branch of UN supplies abductor digiti minimi (ADM), flexor digiti minimi brevis (FDMB), opponens digiti minimi (ODM), most ulnar two

lumbricals, palmar interossei, dorsal interossei, adductor pollicis, and deep head of FPB
- Superficial ulnar nerve branch of UN supplies palmaris brevis
- Its cutaneous distribution is the ulnar half of dorsum of hand up to last knuckle (supplied by dorsal cutaneous branch) and the ulnar one-third of the palm (supplied by the palmar cutaneous branch)

Wrist Block

FOUR TYPES OF INJECTIONS (USING 2% LIDOCAINE WITHOUT EPINEPHRINE)

- Median nerve:
  - Landmarks: through FCR sheath proximal to wrist flexion crease or just ulnar to PL to avoid hitting median nerve (eliciting paresthesias)
  - Remove and redirect with any paresthesias
  - Pop through antebrachial fascia
  - Aim 45 degrees distally, pointing slightly ulnar to avoid nerve
  - Inject 5 mL
  - Hold counterpressure just proximal to wrist crease to force solution into tunnel
- Ulnar nerve:
  - Landmarks: FCU
  - Inject 5 mL beneath FCU from either radial or ulnar side
  - Avoid entry into ulnar artery (palpate its pulse, aspirate before injecting)
- Dorsal sensory branch of radial nerve:
  - Landmark: radial styloid
  - Inject 5 mL subcutaneously over radial styloid
- Dorsal sensory ulnar nerve:
  - Landmark: ulnar styloid
  - Inject 5 mL over ulnar styloid

Dorsal Wrist Compartments

- APL, EPB
  - APL often consists of more than one strand
  - De Quervain: tenosynovitis of first dorsal compartment (assessed by Finkelstein test)
  - Septum between APL and EPB is found in one-third of individuals, needs to be released during surgical management of De Quervains
- ECRB, ECRL
  - Two tendons located radial to Lister tubercle
  - ECRB more ulnar: inserts metacarpal base of middle finger
  - ECRL more radial: inserts metacarpal base of index finger

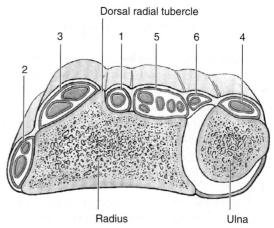

Transverse section of the distal end of the forearm showing the tendons in their synovial sheaths. 1: 3rd dorsal compartment with EPL, 2: 1st dorsal compartment with APL, EPB, 3: 2nd dorsal compartment with ECRL, ECRB, 4: 6th dorsal compartment with ECU, 5: 4th dorsal compartment with EDC, EIP, 6: 5th dorsal compartment with EDQ. (From Moore KL, Dalley AF. Clinical Oriented Anatomy, 4th ed. Baltimore: Lippincott Williams & Wilkins; 1999.)

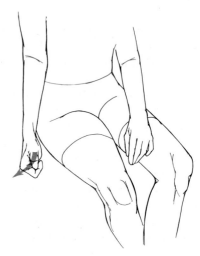

Finkelstein test, to rule out stenosing tenosynovitis of the extensor pollicis brevis and abductor pollicis longus.

- Intersection syndrome: between first and second dorsal compartments ("wet leather" crepitation)
- EPL
  - Tendon is located ulnar to Lister tubercle
  - Forms ulnar border of snuffbox
  - May rupture in distal radius fractures (more frequent in nondisplaced fractures)
- EDC, EIP
  - EIP is located ulnar to EDC to index finger
- Extensor digiti quinti (EDQ)
  - EDQ located ulnar to EDC to small finger

- EDQ and EDC small rupture most early in Vaughn-Jackson syndrome (RA)
- ECU

Approaches: Elbow/Forearm

KOCHER "J" LATERAL ELBOW

Incision
(Hoppenfeld & deBoer, 1994)
- Begins 5 cm proximal to elbow over supracondylar ridge and extends distally over and 5 cm beyond radial head
- Then curves in posteromedial direction to posterior ulnar ridge

Dissection
- Between triceps (radial n.) and ECRL/BR (radial n.) to expose lateral condyle and capsule over radial head
- Distal to radial head: separate anconeus from ECU (radial PIN)
- Anteriorly, reflect common origins of extensors off lateral epicondyle
- Incise capsule longitudinally (and collateral ligament)
- Dislocate elbow and inspect (Kanavel, 1974)

MORREY POSTERIOR ELBOW APPROACH

Incision
(Hoppenfeld & deBoer, 1994)
- Posteromedial

Dissection
- Protect and mobilize ulnar nerve
- Elevate triceps (radial n.) sharply off olecranon and go distally to also elevate anconeus (radial n.)
- Triceps can be reflected either in ulnar or radial direction

VOLAR HENRY APPROACH TO RADIUS

Incision
(Hoppenfeld, 1994)
- From anterior flexor crease of elbow (just lateral to biceps tendon) along course of FCR (median n.) to radial styloid

Dissection
- Proximally between BR (radial n.) and PT (median n.) and distally between BR and FCR (median n.)
- Distally, open volar compartment just ulnar to BR (radial n.) and bluntly develop plane between BR (radial n.) and FCR (median n.)
- Danger:
  - Distally: sensory branch of radial nerve beneath BR

- Proximally: PIN as it branches and passes through supinator
- Recurrent radial artery/vein can be ligated proximally to better expose supinator (PIN)
- Surgical pearls
  - Detach supinator in forearm supination to protect PIN
  - Origin of supinator can be found by staying lateral to biceps tendon and finding bursa between it and supinator
  - Pronate forearm to find PT and take it off middle one-third (in fracture)
- Volar approach poses less risk to PIN compared with dorsal Thompson

DORSAL THOMPSON APPROACH TO RADIUS

Incision
(Hoppenfeld, 1994)
- From lateral epicondyle to Lister tubercle (posterior wrist)

Dissection
- Between ECRB (radial n.) and EDC (PIN) distally, then work more proximally
- APL/EPB (radial n.) cross over radius at distal end of exposure with ECRL/ECRB (radial n.) going underneath them
- Supinator cloaks proximally one-third of radius and is elevated with forearm in supination (to move PIN out of danger)

DORSAL APPROACH

- Increased risk to sensory branch of radial nerve, but eases plate contouring.
- Indications: good for fractures of proximal one-third of radius

References
Hoppenfeld S, deBoer P. Surgical Exposures in Orthopaedics. The Anatomic Approach. New York: Lippincott Williams & Wilkins; 1994:604.
Kanavel AB. The classic. Infections of the hand. Clin Orthop Relat Res 1974; (104):3–8.

Physical Examination of Hand

- Intrinsic muscles of the hand: those that both take origin and have insertion within hand (i.e., dorsal and palmar interossei, lumbricals)
- Extrinsic muscles of the hand: have insertion in hand, but take origin proximal to hand

INTRINSIC MINUS (CLAW)

- Description: metacarpal phalangeal (MCP) hyperextension with interphalangeal (IP) joint flexion
- Causes:
  - Ulnar/median neuropathy
  - Volkmann contracture

INTRINSIC PLUS

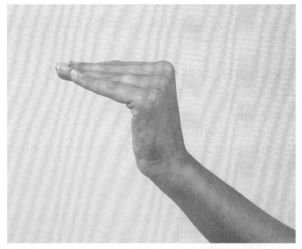

An intrinsic positive hand is positioned with the metacarpophalangeal (MCP) joints flexed and the interphalangeal (IP) joints extended. (From Oatis CA. Kinesiology: The Mechanics and Pathomechanics of Human Movement. Baltimore: Lippincott Williams & Wilkins; 2004.)

- Description: MCP joint flexion and IP joint extension
  - Bunnell test
    - Test flexion of IP joints with middle phalanx (MP) extended and then again with MP flexed
    - Less IP flexion with MP hyperextended indicates intrinsic tightness
    - Less IP flexion with MP flexion indicates extrinsic tightness

LUMBRICAL PLUS

Description
- Paradoxical extension of IP joints during attempted finger flexion

Anatomy
- Lumbricals take origin from flexor digitorum (FD), travel volar to transverse metacarpal ligaments, and insert radially on fingers into lateral bands

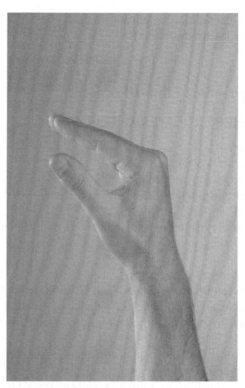

Lateral view of the wrist and hand of a white male, fingers extended, thumb partially abducted.

Etiology
- Retracted FDP tendon causes lumbrical origin tension and thus tensioned lumbrical origin
- Lumbrical becomes continuation of FDP

Treatment
- Surgically release radial lateral band (i.e., lumbrical insertion into extensor hood)

RETINACULAR TEST

- Oblique retinacular ligament (ORL) attaches at sides of proximal phalanx and proceeds distally to attach to portion of lateral bands
- ORL runs volar to proximal interphalangeal (PIP) and dorsal to distal interphalangeal (DIP)
- ORL tightens with PIP extension and DIP flexion

Description
- Assess DIP flexion with PIP in flexion and then again with PIP in extension
- Decreased DIP flexion is due to oblique retinacular ligament tightness if more DIP flexion occurs with PIP also flexed
- Vice versa: less DIP flexion occurs with PIP extended

QUADRIGIA EFFECT

Description
- Active flexion lag (i.e., inability to fully flex finger) in a digit adjacent to a digit with an injured FDP tendon

Etiology
- Tendons of FDP to individual fingers share a common muscle bell
- When one tendon comes to a flexion stop, all FDP tendons come to stop
- May also be caused if one FDP advances >1 cm

Wrist Radiograph
- True lateral
  - Scaphoid tubercle and pisiform overlap
  - Capitate in line with radius
- Ulnar variance
  - Taken with wrist in neutral, shoulder abducted to 90 degrees and elbow flexed at 90 degrees: view where ulnar styloid seen in best profile
- Pronation increases ulnar positive

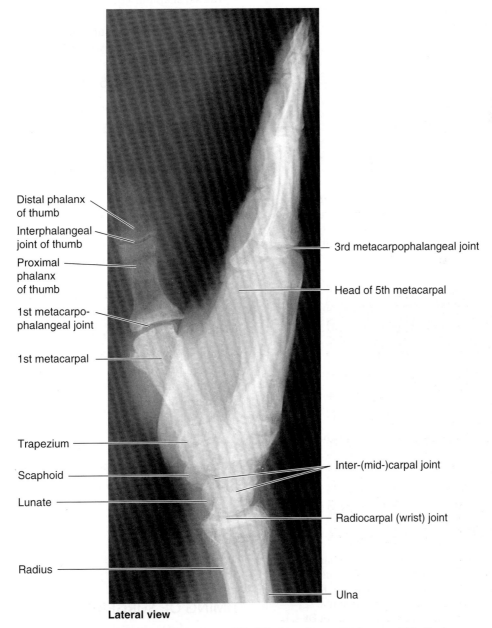

Lateral view

Lateral view of an adult hand. (Courtesy of Dr. E.L. Lansdown, Professor of Medical Imaging, University of Toronto, Toronto, Ontario, Canada.)

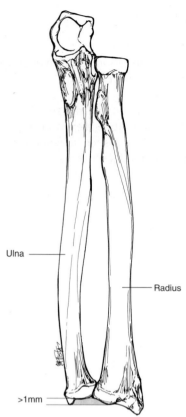

Ulna

Radius

>1mm

Ulnar variance. Ulnar variance is a >1.0-mm difference between the articular surfaces of the distal radius and distal ulna. (From Oatis CA. Kinesiology: The Mechanics and Pathomechanics of Human Movement. Baltimore: Lippincott Williams & Wilkins; 2004.)

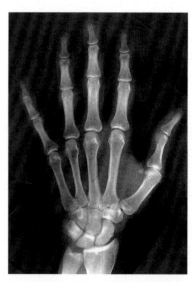

Anteroposterior radiograph of the wrist and hand. Notice the wide "joint space" at the distal end of the ulna because of the radiolucent articular disc. (From Moore KL, Agur A. Essential Clinical Anatomy, 2nd ed. Philadelphia: Lippincott Williams & Wilkins; 2002. Courtesy of Dr. E.L. Lansdown, Professor of Medical Imaging, University of Toronto, Toronto, Ontario, Canada.)

Brachial Plexus

OVERVIEW

- Roots: five (C5-T1)
- Trunks: three (superior, middle, inferior)
- Divisions: six (three anterior, three posterior)
- Cords: three (lateral, posterior, medial)
- Branches: five (musculocutaneous, axillary, radial, median, ulnar)

PRECLAVICULAR BRANCHES

- Long thoracic (C5-7 roots): serratus anterior
- Dorsal scapular (C5 root): rhomboids, levator scapulae
- Suprascapular n. (superior trunk): supraspinatus, infraspinatus, sensory to shoulder joint

LATERAL CORD (C5-7)

- Lateral pectoral n. (pectoralis major and minor)
- Musculocutaneous n.
- Median n.

POSTERIOR CORD (C5-T1)

- Mnemonic: ULTRA
  - *U*pper subscapular n. (upper portion subscapularis)
  - *L*ower subscapular n. (lower portion subscapularis and teres major)
  - *T*horacodorsal n. (latissimus dorsi)
  - *R*adial n.
  - *A*xillary n. (deltoid and teres minor)

MEDIAL CORD (C8, T1)

- Medial pectoral n. (pectoralis minor and major)
- Medial brachial cutaneous n. (sensation medial arm)
- Medial antebrachial cutaneous n. (sensation medial forearm)
- Ulnar n.
- Median n.

GOALS OF SURGERY (BY PRIORITY) IN BRACHIAL PLEXUS INJURY

- Elbow function
- Shoulder abduction
- Hand sensation
- Wrist extension
- Finger flexion

TIMING OF SURGERY

- Early (3 wk to 3 mo) in near-complete palsy
- Delayed (3–6 mo) in traction/low-energy injury

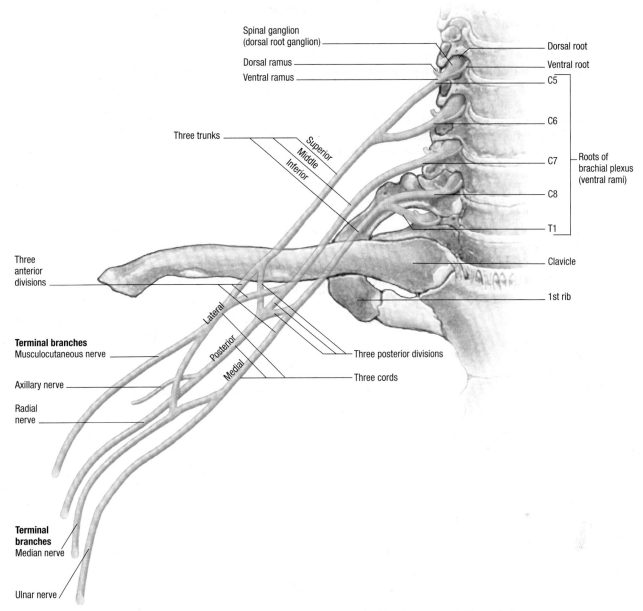

Spinal ganglion
(dorsal root ganglion)

Dorsal ramus

Ventral ramus

Dorsal root

Ventral root

C5

C6

C7

C8

T1

Roots of
brachial plexus
(ventral rami)

Three trunks

Superior
Middle
Inferior

Clavicle

1st rib

Three
anterior
divisions

Lateral

Posterior

Medial

Three posterior divisions

Three cords

Terminal branches
Musculocutaneous nerve

Axillary nerve

Radial
nerve

**Terminal
branches**
Median nerve

Ulnar nerve

Brachial plexus and branches. (Asset provided by Anatomical Chart Co.)

SURGICAL OPTIONS

- Direct repair
- Nerve transfer of expendable motor fascicles to denervated muscle
- Nerve grafting
- Direct muscle neurotization
- Muscle transfers

Nerve Injury

SEDDON NERVE INJURY CLASSIFICATION

(Leffert & Seddon, 1965)
- Neurapraxia
  - Local myelin damage

- Usually due to compression
- No distal degeneration
- No Tinel sign
- Axonotmesis
- Loss of axon continuity
- Some connective tissue intact
- Sunderland subclassification
  - Endoneurium, perineurium, epineurium all OK
  - Endoneurium disrupted
  - Endoneurium and perineurium disrupted
- Axons advance 1–2 mm/day with advancing Tinel sign along course
- Follow with electromyograms (EMGs)
- Fibrillations and possible sharp waves seen 2–5 wk after injury

- Neurotmesis
  - Complete physiologic disruption
  - Same EMG findings as axonotmesis
  - Treatment: primary repair within 1–3 wk
  - Gunshot wounds with nerve injury should have delayed repair when dead tissue declares itself: usually nerve is grafted
  - Epineurial repair is standard except for median and ulnar nerves at wrist where fascicular repair is better because fascicular function is segregated at that location
  - Results are affected by age (<40 yo better), tension, suture material/type, and nerve end condition
  - Graft is better than tension in repair because less blood flow
  - Motor fiber recovery is not as good

SEQUENCE OF NERVE FUNCTION FAILURE

- Motor
- Proprioception
- Touch
- Temperature
- Pain
- Sympathetic
- Recovery in reverse order

SEQUENCE OF NERVE FUNCTION RECOVERY

- Anesthesia
- Pressure
- Pain
- Moving touch
- Moving two-point discrimination
- Static two-point discrimination
- Threshold tests (monofilament, vibration)

RECOVERY

- Age is the single most important variable in predicting the outcome of nerve recovery
- Notable decline after age 30
- The level of injury is the second most important factor
- Motor fibers affected after sensory in compression
- After nerve cut, Wallerian degeneration leads to formation of bands of Büngner by Schwann cells
- Polyphasic motor units are sign of reinnervation
- Axons may grow at a rate of 1–2 mm/day

COMMON NERVE INJURY PATTERNS

- Radial nerve injury with humeral shaft fracture
- PIN injury with radial head or Monteggia-type fracture
- AIN injury with pediatric supracondylar fracture

Anterior Interosseous Nerve Syndrome

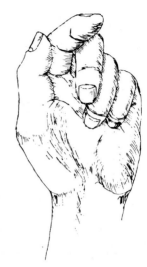

Median nerve palsy. (From Snell MD. Clinical Anatomy, 7th ed. Philadelphia: Lippincott Williams & Wilkins; 2003.)

SYMPTOMS

- Forearm pain 5 cm distal to elbow

SIGNS

- Decreased precise pinch (Kiloh-Nevin sign)
- Weak anterior interosseous muscles (FPL, FDL index and long finger, PQ)
  - PQ tested by resisted pronation of fully flexed elbow (thereby decreasing contribution of PT to pronation)
- No sensory deficit because AIN is a pure motor nerve

SIX POSSIBLE SITES OF COMPRESSION

- Deep head of PT
- Origin of FDS
- Origin of FCR
- Accessory muscle between FDS and FDP
- Gantzer muscle (accessory head of FPL)
- Thrombosis of ulnar collateral artery and aberrant radial artery

DIFFERENTIAL DIAGNOSIS

- Mannerfelt syndrome (attritional rupture of FPL)
- Bilateral AIN: seen in Parsonage-Turner syndrome (viral brachial neuritis)

NATURAL HISTORY

- Most resolved within 6 mo

Carpal Tunnel Syndrome

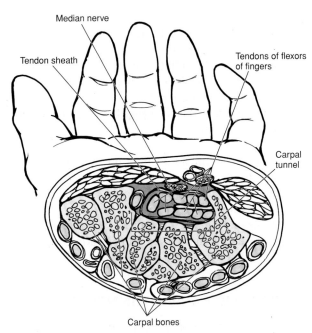

The carpal tunnel. (From Oatis CA. Kinesiology: The Mechanics and Pathomechanics of Human Movement. Baltimore: Lippincott Williams & Wilkins; 2003.)

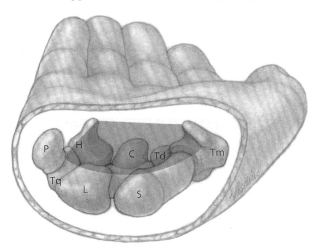

Open carpal tunnel release. The carpal tunnel is a fibroosseous canal. Associated bones that contribute to its boundaries include the hook process of the hamate (H), capitate (C), trapezoid (Td), pisiform (P), triquetrum (Tq), lunate (L), scaphoid (S), and trapezium (Tm). The roof is formed by the flexor retinaculum. (From Berger RA, et al. Wrist. In: Doyle JR, Botte MJ, eds. Surgical Anatomy of the Hand and Upper Extremity. Philadelphia: Lippincott Williams & Wilkins; 2003:486–531, with permission.)

- Impingement of median nerve by transverse carpal ligament
- Beware of double crush where compression in one place decreases threshold at another due to decreased axonal transport

- May also have concomitant C6 radiculopathy and carpal tunnel syndrome (CTS)
- May also have thoracic outlet syndrome and/or cubital tunnel syndrome
- Treat less morbid pathology first
- Pathogenesis: edema and fibrosis, not inflammatory

DIAGNOSIS

- Decreased sensation in median nerve distribution
- Weak thumb abduction: APB
- APB weakness also causes failure to pronate thumb: thus, thumb can't line up nails with fingers at 180 degrees; instead, is supinated and angled <100 degrees
- Palm spared
- Thenar atrophy occurs late in course
- No FPB atrophy because of innervation of deep head by ulnar nerve (FPB is main opposer)

CARPAL TUNNEL CONTENTS

- Median nerve is superficial and located just under transverse carpal ligament (TCL)
- FPL—most radial
- Four FDP
- Four FDS

TRANSVERSE CARPAL LIGAMENT ATTACHMENTS

- Pisiform and hamate hook medially
- Scaphoid tuberosity and ridge of trapezium laterally

PREDISPOSING FACTORS

- Diabetes mellitus (6%)
- Pregnancy
- Hypothyroid
- Collagen vascular disease
- EtOH
- Pyridoxine deficiency

DIAGNOSIS

- Katz diagram of symptoms—61% sensitivity, 71% specificity
- Nocturnal symptoms—variable sensitivity and specificity
- "Flick" sign of shaking hand to relieve symptoms—90% sensitivity and specificity in one study
- Phalen sign—flex at wrist for 60 sec; 40%–80% sensitivity/specificity
- Tinel—25%–60% sensitive, 70%–90% specific
- Durkin compression of 30 sec (most sensitive)

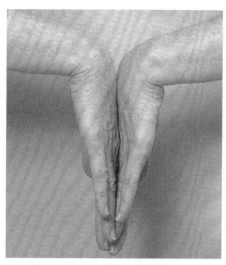

Phalen test. (From Bickley LS, Szilagyi P. Bates' Guide to Physical Examination and History Taking, 8th ed. Philadelphia: Lippincott Williams & Wilkins 2003.)

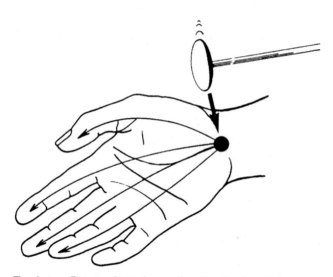

Tinel sign. Pain is elicited over the distribution of the median nerve by tapping over the volar carpal ligament. (MediClip image copyright © 2003 Lippincott Williams & Wilkins. All rights reserved.)

- Increase in two-point discrimination (>6 mm): occurs only late in course
- Monofilaments test threshold, thus useful in early disease
- Two-point discrimination tests only nerve-ending density
- Sensory latency >3.2 msec
- Motor latency >4.2 msec

TREATMENT

- Mild—rarely numb; may try injection
- Moderate—often numb; nonoperative versus surgical management

- Severe—numb all the time, atrophy or weakness; operative
- Splint
  - 80% of symptom relief within days
  - Reduces sensory latency
  - Best when wrist splint in neutral
- Nonsteroidal anti-inflammatory drugs (NSAIDs)
  - No proven symptom relief
  - Oral steroids—relieve symptoms but have questionable toxicity
- Steroid injections
  - Total 2 mL (1 mL lidocaine, 1 mL steroid) at crease ulnar to PL
  - 75% with symptom relief, recurs by 1 yr
  - 22% asymptomatic at 1 yr
  - 40% asymptomatic if symptoms <1 yr, normal two-point discrimination, no denervation, motor or sensor latency only 1–2 sec

ENDOSCOPIC CARPAL TUNNEL RELEASE

- Most common complication is incomplete TCL division
- 2-wk earlier return to work

STANDARD CARPAL TUNNEL RELEASE

- Pain relief within several days
- Pinch to preop at 6 wk
- Grip to preop at 3 mo

REVISION CARPAL TUNNEL RELEASE

- Only 25% complete relief
- No greater success if incomplete TCL release found
- Indications
  - Failed short incision or endoscopic technique
  - Night pain, relief with steroid injection
  - For severe late cases with atrophy and sensory changes, surgery less predictable due to endoneural fibrosis

CARPAL TUNNEL RELEASE TECHNIQUE

- Field block, then block incision
- Incision in line with flexed ring finger, not more distal than thumb web space and not more proximal than distal wrist crease
- Palmar cutaneous nerve is between FCR and PL
- Start proximally first, sweeping fat in ulnar direction; then make entrance hole in TCL
- Push Penfield into hole proximally to clear adhesion above and below TCL
- Divide proximal TCL with scissors

- Extend distally by sweeping TCL fibers in ulnar direction and cut deeper at same time
- End of TCL reached when fat is seen marking deep palmar arch (superficial arch is distal and fed by ulnar artery; deep arch is proximal and fed by radial artery)
- Close radial half of TCL to ulnar palmar fascia, which pushes some protective fat into the canal
- Splint 7–10 days
- Note: the TCL is continuous with antebrachial fascia

Cubital Tunnel Syndrome

- Most often due to compression of UN between the ulnar and humeral heads of FCU
- May also be due to compression at the arcade of Struthers (8 cm proximal to elbow at intramuscular septum), Osborne ligament, fibers within FCU, and anconeus muscle
- UN is large along the medial head of triceps and susceptible to compression

DIAGNOSIS

- Numbness, paresthesias in ring finger and small finger
- Clumsy or weak hand
- Beware of double crush with thoracic outlet syndrome, C7 impingement
- Weak intrinsics, wasting
- Weak FDP of ring and small finger (Pollock test)
- Weak FCU
- Froment sign (FPL compensates for weak adductor pollicis)
- EPL is secondary adductor of thumb in ulnar palsy
- Jeanne sign—compensatory thumb MP hyperextension
- Abducted small finger (Wartenberg sign); hidden if patient has Martin Gruber anastomosis where median nerve supplies some intrinsics such as first dorsal interossei
- Elbow flexion test
- Elbow Tinel

TREATMENT

- Elbow pads, extension brace
- Conservative treatment usually works
- Release FCU aponeurosis
- Anterior transposition
- Submuscular in severe neuropathy
- Medial epicondylectomy
- Intrinsic atrophy has poor prognosis
- Most common complication is injury to the medial antebrachial cutaneous nerve in all ulnar nerve anterior transpositions

SUBCUTANEOUS TRANSPOSITION

- 7 cm proximal to medial epicondyle and anterior to epicondyle, along nerve course
- Make skin flap anteriorly exposing flexor mass, taking care to preserve the medial brachial cutaneous nerve
- Free humeral attachment of FCU at epicondyle
- Dissect out branches to FCU, FDP
- Bring nerve anteriorly over flexor mass
- Take medial intermuscular septum all the way to arcade of Struthers where the nerve passes from anterior to posterior
- Suture subcutaneous tissue and fascia medial to nerve to keep it from sliding back

Radial Tunnel Syndrome

- Pain-only syndrome involving compression of PIN
- Radial tunnel is also known as PIN pain syndrome
- PIN syndrome is a similar disease involving the same nerve and same sites of compression, but different presentations, treatments, and outcomes

ETIOLOGY

- FLEAS
  - *F*ibrous bands at radiocapitellar joint
  - *L*eash of Henry—radial recurrents
  - *E*CRB
  - *A*rcade of Frohse (proximal aspect of supinator)
  - *S*upinator (distal edge)

RADIAL TUNNEL

- No motor or sensory deficits in radial tunnel, pain only
- Pain 5 cm distal to lateral epicondyle, anterior to mobile wad
- Pain with resisted supination of flexed elbow, resisted supination and wrist extension, resisted pronation and wrist flexion, and resisted middle finger extension

RADIAL TUNNEL VERSUS POSTERIOR INTEROSSEOUS NERVE

- Radial tunnel has normal nerve study, EMG/nerve conduction velocity (NCV) are not helpful in this condition
- PIN syndrome has motor deficit only, has abnormal nerve study, no pain or sensory component
- PIN has radial drift with wrist extension

RADIAL TUNNEL SYNDROME TREATMENT

- Usually conservative treatment for 6–12 mo
- Surgery only improves 50% of patients

POSTERIOR INTEROSSEOUS NERVE SYNDROME TREATMENT

- Decompress if symptoms >3 mo
- 85% get better with surgery
- Most direct approach is BR splitting
- Thompson (ECRB-EDC) gives best view of entire supinator
- Henry—anterolateral approach for elbow
- No surgery if polyphasics in EDC because nerve function will return

Pronator Syndrome

- Median nerve impingement at elbow
- Pain in volar forearm
- Palm affected
- Positive Tinel sign in forearm, - wrist, - Phalen
- Symptoms like CTS but no night pain
- Pain with resisted pronation
- Pain with resisted PIP flexion of long finger
- AIN spared

SITE OF IMPINGEMENT: FOUR LOCATIONS

- Supracondylar ligament of Struthers—third coracobrachialis head at medial epicondyle
- Lacertus fibrosus (bicipital aponeurosis)—resisted elbow flexion with supination
- PT—resisted pronation with extended elbow
- FDS proximal arch—resisted long finger PIP flexion

TREATMENT

- Splint 6 wk
- If conservative treatment fails attempt exploratory surgery

Ulnar Tunnel Syndrome

- Due to ulnar nerve compression in Guyon canal
- Traumatic or atraumatic causes
- Intrinsic muscle weakness
- Hypothenar atrophy
- Froment sign—adductor pollicis weak so thumb IP joint flexes
- Normal sensation on dorsum of hand
- Dorsal sensory branch of ulnar nerve branches proximal to wrist
- If patient has symptoms on dorsum of hand the problem is proximal to wrist, likely at elbow

GUYON CANAL CONTENTS

- Ulnar nerve
- Ulnar artery
- FCU tendon
- No synovium

GUYON CANAL BOUNDARIES

- Roof—volar carpal ligament
- Floor—TCL, pisohamate ligament
- Radial—hook of hamate
- Ulnar—pisiform, ADQ muscle

ETIOLOGY

- Magnetic resonance imaging (MRI) for ganglia—most common cause in atraumatic cases, 80%
- Computed tomography (CT) for hamate and pisiform fractures
- Ultrasound (US) for ulnar artery thrombosis
- Zone 1
  - Proximal to bifurcation and pisiform
  - Mixed motor and sensory branches
- Zone 2
  - Deep motor branch only
  - Located between ADQ and flexor digiti quint (FDQ)
  - Likely ganglia or hook of hamate fracture
- Zone 3
  - Superficial sensory branch only
  - Ulnar artery thrombosis, synovial inflammation

TREATMENT

- Conservative treatment—avoid aggravating activity, splint, NSAIDs
- Operative treatment includes decompression and possible volar carpal ligament and pisohamate ligament release

Wartenberg Syndrome

- Also known as Chiralgia paresthetica
- Compression of superficial radial nerve

ETIOLOGY

- Compression between BR and ECRL with forearm pronation
- Common causes include tight wrist watch, handcuffs, and ex-fix pins

DIAGNOSIS

- Paresthesias provoked with hyperpronation with clenched fist, wrist flexed, ulnar deviated
- No motor deficit
- Positive Tinel sign
- Use injection to differentiate from De Quervain tenosynovitis

TREATMENT

– Rest, NSAIDs, activity modification, wrist splints
– Surgical decompression after ~6 mo of conservative management and includes release of fascial band between brachioradialis and ECRL tendons

Dorsal Wrist Ganglion

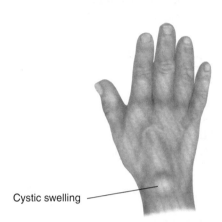

Cystic swelling

Ganglion. Ganglia are cystic, round, usually nontender swellings located along tendon sheaths or joint capsules. The dorsum of the wrist is a frequent site of involvement. Flexion of the wrist makes ganglia in this location more prominent; extension tends to obscure them. Ganglia may also develop elsewhere on the hands, wrists, ankles, and feet. (From Bickley LS, Szilagyi P. Bates' Guide to Physical Examination and History Taking, 8th ed. Philadelphia: Lippincott Williams & Wilkins; 2003.)

ANATOMY

– 75% connect with dorsal scapholunate ligament

PRESENTATION

– Pain from PIN compression

NATURAL HISTORY

– 50% spontaneous resolution
    – 80% resolution ≤1 yr in patient ≤10 yo

TREATMENT AND CURE RATES

– Closed rupture: 22%–66% cure rate
– Single puncture: 13% cure, 40% cure if splint worn for 3 wk
– Series of three aspirations: 85% cure
– Silk suture through skin (removed at 3 wk): 95% cure at 6 m; disadvantage: potential for infection
– Surgery:
    – 80% cure on average
    – Divide distal extensor retinaculum
    – Dissect to stalk on scapholunate ligament
    – 13% to 40% recur with cyst excision alone
    – 4% recur if cuff normal capsule also taken
– Steroids: no proven benefit
– Sclerosing agents: may cause damage

Synovial cyst of the wrist. (From Moore KL, Dalley AF. Clinical Oriented Anatomy, 4th ed. Baltimore: Lippincott Williams & Wilkins; 1999.)

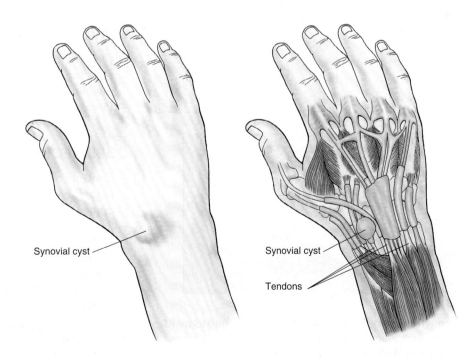

Synovial cyst

Synovial cyst

Tendons

Mucous Cyst

- Located at DIP joint
- Secondary to osteoarthritis (OA)
- Associated with dorsal ostephyte (must be taken to avoid recurrence)

Dupuytren Contracture

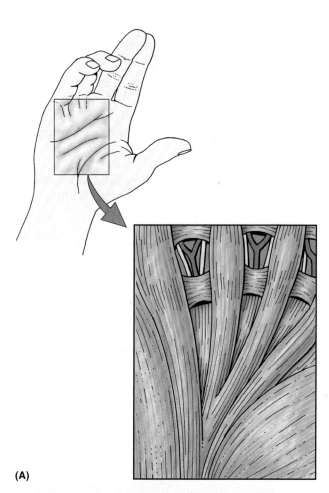

(A)

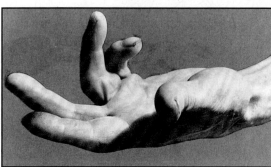

(B)

Dupuytren contracture of palmar fascia. (From Moore KL, Dalley AF. Clinical Oriented Anatomy, 4th ed. Baltimore: Lippincott Williams & Wilkins; 1999.)

DESCRIPTION

- Contracture of palmar and digital fascia leading to nodules, cords, and flexion contracture of fingers
- Most commonly affects ring and small fingers

BACKGROUND

- Rare before age 40, M > F (10:1)
- Autosomal dominant with variable penetrance

LUCK'S STAGES

(Luck, 1959)
- I—Proliferative: myofibroblasts
- II —Involutional: dense myofibroblast network, more collagen III than collagen I
- III—Residual, no myofibroblasts

STRUCTURES AFFECTED

- Pretendinous bands
- Spiral bands: continuation of pretendinous bands; enter digit deep to neurovascular structures and then become superficial to them
- Natatory ligaments
- Lateral digital sheet
- Grayson ligaments: a less distinct sheet than Cleland ligaments that goes from tendon sheath to lateral digital sheet, passing volar to the digital neurovascular structures

STRUCTURES NOT AFFECTED

- Cleland ligaments: dorsal to digital neurovascular structures and NOT involved; extends from side of phalanges to skin
- Palmar aponeurosis transverse fibers NOT involved

CORDS FORMED

- Central cord is continuation of pretendinous cord
- Lateral cord arises from lateral digital bands (which come off natatory ligaments)
- Spiral cord from:
  - Pretendinous band
  - Spiral band
  - Lateral digital sheet
  - Grayson ligaments
- Spiral cord displaces neurovascular bundle (NV) medially and superficially as it contracts
- Best predictor of central NV displacement is presence of PIP joint contracture

NON-SURGICAL MANAGEMENT

- Collagenase clostridium histolyticum injections into cord to lyse collagen
- Treated joint is manipulated day after injection to attempt cord rupture
- Night-time splint with no formal therapy required
- Most effective for MCP joint contracture: 77% reduction of contracture to within 5 degrees of full extension at MCP vs 40% reduction at PIP joint (ref: Hurst LC et al, Injectable collagenase clostridium histolyticum for Dupuytren's contracture. *NEJM* 2009; 361:968–979).
- Adverse effects include: ecchymosis, erythema, pain, and swelling related to injection/manipulation, potential for tendon rupture

INDICATIONS FOR SURGERY

- Functional limitation, which is usually at:
  - 30-degree MP joint contracture
  - Any PIP joint contracture
- MP joint contracture can usually be corrected regardless of severity
- PIP joint correction harder and cannot be completely corrected, thus need surgery at any amount of contracture

SURGERIES

- Fasciotomy—high recurrence
- Fasciectomy
  - Limited—high recurrence
  - Regional—remove only diseased tissue, good long-term results
- Total fasciectomy
  - Does not prevent recurrence
  - High complication rate
- Open palm technique: leave incision open to allow healing on own
  - Better in older patients with risk for stiffness since allows earlier motion
- Never perform concomitant carpal tunnel release because it increases complications and recurrence

SURGICAL COMPLICATIONS

- Stiffness
- Hematoma formation
- Neurovascular injury
- Infection
- Recurrence

OPERATING ROOM TIPS

- In proximal palm, subcutaneous layer present between fascia and skin

- Distally, fascia becomes closer to the skin; by distal palmar crease, fascia is just under skin
- Distal to middle crease of finger, there is subcutaneous layer between skin and fascia
- In palm, fascia and tendon sheath are close together
  - In proximal phalanx, areolar tissue separates sheath and fascia
  - Distal to PIP joint, fascia adheres to the tendon sheath: one must take care to avoid injuring sheath
- With significant contracture, neurovascular bundle may be easier to find proximally
- Neurovascular bundle is deep to natatory ligament in areolar tissue close to MP joint

Reference

Luck JV. Dupuytren's contracture; a new concept of the pathogenesis correlated with surgical management. J Bone Joint Surg Am 1959; 41-A(4):635–664.

Fracture of Hand: Open

CLASSIFICATION AND TREATMENT

(Swanson et al., 1991)
- Type I: clean, no delay, no systemic illness (diabetes mellitus [DM])—1.4% chance infection
- Type II: Grossly contaminated, delay in treatment ≥24 hr, or systemic illness (i.e., DM, RA)—14% chance of infection
- No increased infection with primary internal fixation or immediate wound closure

Reference

Swanson TV, et al. Open hand fractures: prognosis and classification. J Hand Surg [Am] 1991; 16(1):101–107.

Flexor Tenosynovitis: Kanavel's Cardinal Signs

(Kanavel, 1974)
- Presence of signs indicates purulent flexor tendon sheath infection
- Signs on physical exam:
  - Pain with passive extension (most important)
  - Flexed position
  - Symmetric enlargement ("fusiform swelling")
  - Tenderness along sheath

Infection in Hand

FIGHT BITE

Description

- Open wound to hand caused during fight when hand forced again mouth/teeth of other individual
- Wound may appear benign, but disastrous if not treated correctly

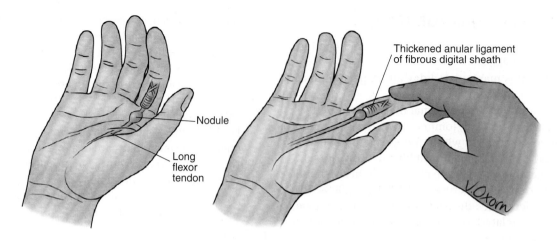

Digital tenovaginitis stenosans (Trigger finger)

Tenosynovitis. Injuries such as puncture of the palm by a rusty nail can cause infection of the synovial sheaths of the digits. When inflammation of the tendon and synovial sheath (tenosynovitis) occurs, the finger swells and movement becomes painful. Because the tendons of the second, third, and fourth digits nearly always have separate synovial sheaths, the infection usually is confined to the infected digit. In neglected infections, however, the proximal ends of these sheaths may rupture, allowing the infection to spread to the midpalmar space. Because the synovial sheath of the little finger is usually continuous with the common synovial sheath, tenosynovitis in this digit may spread to the common sheath and thus through the palm and carpal tunnel to the anterior forearm. Likewise, tenosynovitis in the thumb may spread through the continuous synovial sheath of the flexor pollicis longus (radial bursa). Just how far an infection spreads from the digits depends on variations in their connections with the common flexor sheath. Thickening of a fibrous sheath on the palmar aspect of the digit often results in stenosis (narrowing) of the osseofibrous tunnel of a finger. If the tendons of the flexor digitorum superficialis (FDS) and flexor digitorum profundus (FDP) enlarge (forming a nodule) proximal to the tunnel, the person is unable to extend the finger. When the finger is extended passively, a snap is audible. Flexion produces another snap as the thickened tendon moves. This condition is called digital tenovaginitis stenosans ("trigger finger" or "snapping finger"). (From Moore KL, Agur A. Essential Clinical Anatomy, 2nd ed. Philadelphia: Lippincott Williams & Wilkins, 2002.)

Treatment

- Must débride in emergency room (ER) or operating room (OR) and then IV antibiotics
- Most common pathogen is *Staphylococcus aureus* but *Eichenella corrodens* (a gram-negative anaerobe) is also common: treated with augmentin or second-generation cephalosporin
(Mennen & Howells, 1991)
- Cultures not useful: either negative or huge spectrum including anaerobes
- Treatment: early incision and drainage (I&D), hand baths, triple antibiotics, early rehab
- Antibiotics used: cloxacillin, gentamicin, metronidazole
- Complications:
  - 51% cellulitis
  - 18% amputations
  - 22% osteomyelitis
  - Delay to present associated with amputation and generally poor outcome

References

Kanavel AB. The classic. Infections of the hand. Clin Orthop Relat Res 1974; (104):3–8.

Mennen U, Howells CJ. Human fight-bite injuries of the hand. A study of 100 cases within 18 months. J Hand Surg [Br] 1991; 16(4):431–435.

Flexor Tendon Injury

FUNDAMENTALS

- Compared with ligaments, tendons have more collagen and are less viscoelastic
- FDP shares common muscle belly
- Fingers: nerves are volar to arteries in digit: "hurts before it bleeds"
- Palm: arteries volar to nerves

FUNCTIONAL ANATOMY

- MCP joint flexed by interosseous and lumbrical muscles

- PIP flexed by FDS, FDP
- DIP flexed by FDP only

PHASES OF TENDON HEALING

- Inflammation: days 0–5—invasion white blood cells, formation granulation tissue
- Fibroblastic/proliferation: days 5–28—fibroblast proliferation and matrix synthesis
- Remodeling: days >28—realignment of collagen
- Repair weakest between postoperative day (POD) 6–12
- Number of suture strands that pass repair site most important
- Epitendinous repair improves gliding and strength and lessens gap formation, which is initial event in repair failure

POSTOPERATIVE PROTOCOLS

- Kleinert: active extension, dynamic splint (rubberband) passive flexion
- Duran: passive extension, patient-assisted passive flexion

Flexor Tendon Zones

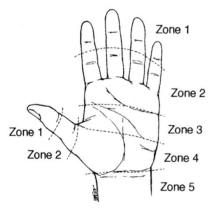

Zones used to describe flexor tendon lacerations. Zone I: midfinger pad to distal half of middle phalanx. Zone II: proximal half of middle phalanx to metacarpal phalangeal (MCP) joint, inclusive of the MCP. Zone III: distal palmar crease to midpalm. Zone IV: midpalm to wrist crease, carpus included. Zone V: wrist crease and proximal. (From Blackbourne LH. Advanced Surgical Recall, 2nd ed. Baltimore: Lippincott Williams & Wilkins, 2004.)

- Zone I: distal to FDS insertion; only FDP injured; "Jersey finger"
  - Avoid passive range of motion (PROM; Duran) after repair due to elongation
  - Dynamic splint PROM (Kleinert) better
- Zone II: "no man's land"—midphalanx to distal palmar crease (within flexor retinaculum); both FDP and FDS

injured; tendon and skin laceration may be at different levels

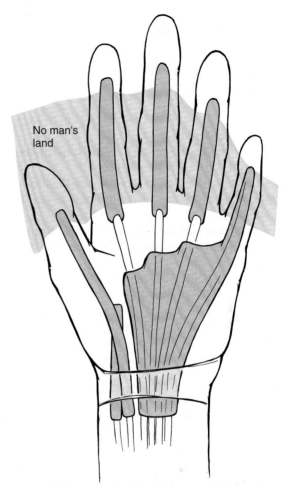

No man's land is the area where healing is most difficult for the fingers' flexor tendons. It encompasses much of the region where the digital tendons are in their synovial sheaths. (From Oatis CA. Kinesiology: The Mechanics and Pathomechanics of Human Movement. Baltimore: Lippincott Williams & Wilkins; 2004.)

- Early mobilization (Either Duran or Kleinert)
- Allowing wrist motion in dynamic splint allows 2 mm more tendon excursion
- Preserve A2 and A4 to prevent bowstringing
- Zone III: palm—concomitant neurovascular injuries common (median nerve, arterial arch); lumbricals located in this zone
  - Direct repair: good results (no retinacular structures, less scar)
- Zone IV: carpal tunnel
  - Surgical repair: postop adhesions common
  - Transverse ligament released/repaired
- Zone V: wrist and forearm
  - Primary end-to-end repair: good prognosis

- Thumb:
    - Primary end-to-end repair FPL
    - Avoid thenar muscles (i.e., recurrent motor branch median nerve)
    - Must preserve oblique pulley

Extensor Tendon Injury

ANATOMY

- Sagittal bands positioned over MCP joint to keep central band centered
- Extensor tendon trifurcates over proximal phalanx:
    - Central slip inserts into base of MP
    - Lateral bands go on to form terminal tendon
- Transverse retinacular ligament holds lateral bands in position
- Central slip is joined by separate lateral bands from interossei and lumbricals to insert into base of proximal phalanx
- Oblique retinacular ligament links PIP and DIP extension
    - ORL allows for Fowler tenotomy, whereby cutting extensor tendon still allows DIP extension through ORL
- Triangular ligament holds lateral bands together to form terminal tendon
- Juncturae tendinum can mask injury to EDC: these small tendinous bands connect EDC tendons of ring finger to EDC tendons of long and small fingers; may be able to extend a given digit through pull of adjacent digit through juncturae

EXTENSION OF INDIVIDUAL JOINTS

- MCP: sagittal bands of EDC
- PIP: lateral bands of lumbricals central slip of EDC
- DIP: terminal tendon, ORL

GENERAL PRINCIPLES OF TREATMENT

- Extensor is hood, thus hard to cut in entirety
- <50% laceration generally does not require surgery, treated with early range of motion (ROM) because sutures cause adhesions
- >50% generally requires repair

EXTENSOR ZONES

- Zones given odd number at joints, even number at shafts
- Treatment of extensor injury dictated by zone
- Zone I (DIP): mallet
- Zone II (middle phalanx): repair if >50%, treat like mallet
- Zone III (PIP joint): boutonniere
- Zone IV (proximal phalanx): usually cut <50%, thus treatment usually conservative
- Zone V (MCP joint): dynamic extension splint not shown to be helpful, therefore delayed mobilization acceptable; think "fight bight"
- Zone VI (metacarpal): management same as for zone V
- Zone VII (wrist: fibro-osseous sheath): delayed mobilization still acceptable
- Zone VIII: forearm, treatment with core suture, delayed mobilization

OUTCOMES OF EXTENSOR TENDON REPAIR

- Best results from repair obtained if no fracture present
- Most common problem is extension contracture (unable to make fist)
- Limited flexion can occur due to adhesion of extensor to bone
- Improved PIP flexion with MP extension

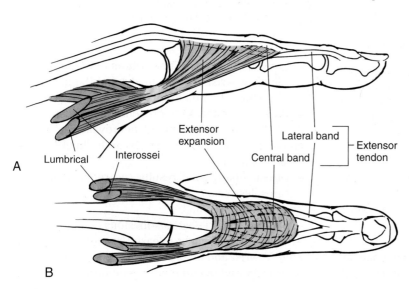

The extensor hood mechanism. The extensor hood mechanism consists of the central tendon (CT) and lateral bands (LB) of the extensor digitorum (ED) and the fibrous sheet that is an extension of the distal attachments of the lumbricals (L) and interossei (PI and DI). **A:** Lateral view. **B:** Dorsal view. (From Oatis CA. Kinesiology: The Mechanics and Pathomechanics of Human Movement. Baltimore: Lippincott Williams & Wilkins; 2004.)

INTRINSIC TIGHTNESS

- Results from intrinsic muscle tightness or crush injury
- Test for intrinsic tightness (see Physical Exam section)
- Treat with physical therapy or intrinsic tenolysis

Mallet Finger

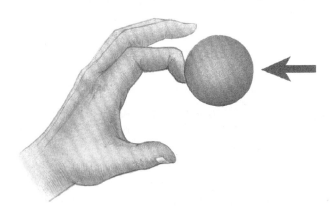

Hand and wrist. Tendon avulsion injury. (Asset provided by Anatomical Chart Co.)

DEFINITION

- Rupture of terminal tendon

TREATMENT

- 6–8 wk splinting (longer if lag still present)
- Can be splint many months after injury
- Surgery not often indicated

MALLET FINGER WITH FRACTURE

- Closed reduction if not subluxed
- If subluxed (>50%), reduce and pin; high associated complications with surgery

SEQUELAE

- Chronic mallets can develop swan neck deformity, which necessitates spiral oblique retinacular reconstructions (SORL)
  (Garberman et al., 1994)
- 40 patients with bony and soft tissue mallets treated within 2 wk (early) or after 4 wk (delayed) with continuous splinting
- <10-degree extension lag in 17/21 with early treatment and in 15/19 with late treatment
- Dorsal lip fracture of less than one-third of articular surface did not affect outcome
- Conclusion: splinting equally effective in restoring active extension in early and delayed group

Reference

Garberman SF, et al. Mallet finger: results of early versus delayed closed treatment. J Hand Surg [Am] 1994; 19(5):850–852.

Flexor Digitorum Profundus Avulsion/Jersey Finger

ANATOMY

- FDP inserts on volar aspect of base of distal phalanx
- Vincula: provide some connection of FDP to phalanges and provide conduit for blood supply to tendon
(Leddy & Packer, 1977)
- Jersey finger is a common sports injury, one player grabs another's jersey and a finger (most commonly the ring finger, 75%) gets caught and pulled
- Average age 16, athletes
- Delayed treatment in 75% due to delayed diagnosis
- Most common sport: football, rugby

CLASSIFICATION

(Leddy & Packer, 1977)
- Type I
  - FDP retracts into palm
  - Both vincula (longa and breve) ruptured
  - Must reinsert in 7–10 days before tendon becomes necrotic, contracted
  - If late, excise tendon and consider two-stage tendon graft
- Type II (most common)
  - FDP retracts to level of PIP joint
  - Long vincula intact (breve ruptured)
  - Often bony avulsion fragment at PIP joint seen on radiograph
  - Repair at up to 3 mo acceptable, but better to repair earlier
  - Can slip further and become type I
- Type III
  - FDP retracts to level of DIP joint
  - Large bony fragment trapped at A4 pulley
  - Early repair by open reduction and internal fixation (ORIF) of fragment
  - Late cases:
    - Late asymptomatic cases untreated
    - If DIP unstable in late cases, then fusion

Reference

Leddy JP, Packer JW. Avulsion of the profundus tendon insertion in athletes. J Hand Surg [Am] 1977; 2(1):66–69.

Traumatic Boutonniere Deformity

DEFINITION

- DIP hyperextension, PIP hyperflexion

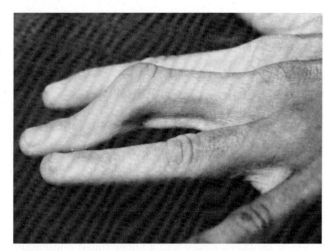

Boutonniere deformity. (From Bucholz RW, Heckman JD. Rockwood & Green's Fractures in Adults, 5th ed. Lippincott Williams & Wilkins, Philadelphia, PA; 2001.)

CAUSE

– Commonly by central slip rupture/avulsion/laceration

PROCESS

– May not become apparent until several weeks after injury
  – Triangular ligament attenuates
  – Lateral bands subluxate volar to PIP joint axis and become flexors of PIP joint
  – Intrinsic musculature to DIP joint tightens, causing DIP hyperextension
  – Leads to DIP and PIP capsular contractures over time

ZONE III INJURY (PROXIMAL INTERPHALANGEAL JOINT)

– Acute central slip rupture
– PIP joint extends with MP joint flexion/wrist flexion
– Elson test:
  – Performed with PIP bent 90 degrees over table
  – Resisted MP extension leads to DIP extension because all forces are sent to terminal tendon via intact lateral bands
  – DIP remains floppy if central slip is intact
  – Test key for early diagnosis

Treatment

– Acute: splint PIP in extension (leave DIP and MP free) for 6 wk
– Chronic, but passively correctable: splint
– Chronic, not correctable: surgery

Poor Prognosis
– Chronic deformity in patient >45 yo
– Fixed PIP contracture
– Associated fracture or surgery

Ulnar Collateral Ligament: Gamekeeper's Thumb

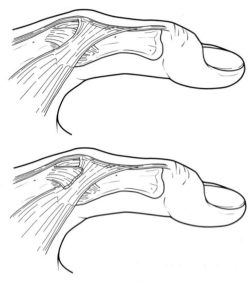

The Stener lesion occurs when the proximal portion of the torn proper collateral ligament on the ulnar side of the thumb middle phalanx (MP) joint comes to lie dorsal to the leading edge of the adductor aponeurosis. (From Bucholz RW, Heckman JD. Rockwood & Green's Fractures in Adults, 5th ed. Lippincott Williams & Wilkins; 2001.)

DEFINITION

– Injury of ulnar collateral ligament (UCL) of thumb MCP causing instability

ASSOCIATED INJURIES

– Dorsal capsule, volar plate, avulsion fracture of volar base of proximal phalanx

STENER LESION

– Aponeurosis of adductor pollicis interposes between distal avulsed fragment and its insertion in proximal phalanx
– Seen in complete ruptures only
– Prevents healing of UCL

DIAGNOSIS AND TREATMENT

- Apply radially directed force at MCP and full extension and at 30-degree flexion (compare to contralateral side)
  - If opens <30 degrees and has endpoint, incomplete rupture: treat with thumb spica
  - If opens <30 degrees and has no endpoint, block medial and radial nerves and repeat exam
  - If opens >30 degrees, complete rupture likely and needs open repair

SURGICAL TREATMENT

- Incision at border of dorsal and volar skin
- Find and protect superficial radial nerve
- Incise adductor pollicis aponeurosis 3 mm from EPL
- Expose enough to visualize volar plate (tears can extend toward it)
- Full inspection
  - Direct repairs of tears in middle two-thirds of ligament
  - Suture anchor in bony avulsion injury

Sagittal Band Rupture

ANATOMY OF BAND

- Covers extensor tendon and runs in palmar direction to attach to deep transverse metacarpal ligament
- May be seen with direct blow to MCP or forced flexion/extension of MCP joint; more common in RA
- Radial band more commonly torn
- Symptoms: popping MCP joint

FINDINGS

- MCP swelling and localized pain
- Ulnar deviation of digit (if radial band torn); radial deviation (if ulnar band torn)
- Extensor lag
- Extensor tendon subluxation or dislocation

TREATMENT

- Acute: splint MP joint in extension
- Chronic: repair or reconstruct, then hold MCP in extension for 4 wk

Ring Avulsion Injuries

DEFINITION

- Avulsion of tissue (skin, subcutaneous tissue, tendons) from digit without damage to bone or ligament
- Typically caused when ring avulsed from finger with force

URBANIAK CLASSIFICATION

(Urbaniak, 1981)
- I—circulation adequate: standard bone/soft tissue treatment
- II—circulation inadequate: vessel repair preserves viability
- III—complete degloving injury or amputation:
  - With proximal phalanx fracture or PIP joint injury, consider amputation
  - Complete amputations proximal to FDS treated with amputation

Reference

Urbaniak JR, et al. Microvascular management of ring avulsion injuries. J Hand Surg [Am] 1981; 6(1):25–30.

Replants

- Indications:
  - Thumb amputation
  - Multiple digit amputations
  - Metacarpal, wrist, or forearm amputation
  - Almost any body part in a child
  - Individual digit distal to FDS insertion
    - Single digit replantation proximal to FDS insertion results in significant functional impairment
- Sequence of replantation
  - Shorten and fix bone
  - Extensor tendon
  - Flexor tendon
  - Artery
  - Nerves
  - Veins
  - Wound
- Replant not recommended if:
  - Above-wrist amputation: Warm ischemia >6 hr, cold ischemia >12 hr
  - Digit amputation: warm ischemia >12 hr, cold ischemia >24 hr
- Most common complication after successful replantation: cold intolerance

Chemical Burns

- Hydrofluoric acid (rust remover)
  - Continues to burn until acid neutralized
  - Treatment: Calcium gluconate topically (SQ in severe burns)
- White phosphorus (fireworks)
  - Treatment: copper sulfate solution

Flaps

- Reconstructive ladder
  - Primary closure

- Secondary closure
- Skin graft
  - Full-thickness skin grafts (FTSGs): more fail, better cosmesis, more sensation
  - Thinner grafts contract more
  - FTSGs preferred for hand because they don't contract; nonmesh split-thickness skin grafts (STSGs) acceptable for dorsum
  - Grafts fail by shear, hematoma formation, infection
- Axial flaps have single arteriovenous (AV) pedicle
- Peninsular rotation is skin and pedicle
- Island rotation is pedicle only
- Random flaps are supported by microcirculation without pedicle
- Venous flaps have flow through venous system only when distal flap vein is hooked to donor artery and proximal flap vein is hooked to recipient vein
- Anastomoses should be out of zone of injury
- Flap blood supplies
  - Lateral arm: posterior collateral artery (off profunda brachii)
  - Scapular cutaneous: tiny branch of circumflex scapular artery
  - Latissimus dorsi musculocutaneous: thoracodorsal artery
  - Deltoid cutaneous: posterior circumflex humeral artery

Fracture: Metacarpal

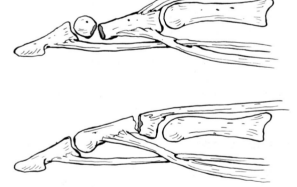

Fractures in the distal and proximal fourth of P2 may be deformed by the flexor digitorum superficialis (FDS) tendon. (From Bucholz RW, Heckman JD. Rockwood & Green's Fractures in Adults, 5th ed. Lippincott Williams & Wilkins; 2001.)

FUNDAMENTAL ANATOMY

- MCP joint is tight in flexion and loose in extension due to shape of metacarpal head

METACARPAL HEAD FRACTURE

- Rare and hard to see on radiograph
- Usually needs ORIF
- Rarely regains >45-degree motion after successful ORIF of intra-articular fracture

METACARPAL NECK FRACTURE

- Usually apex dorsal because of pull of volar intrinsics

Indications for Surgery

- >15-degree angulation second and third metacarpal (MC), >45-degree angulation of fourth and fifth MC

Surgical Technique

- Cross pins or two pins to fourth MC head

METACARPAL SHAFT FRACTURE

- Displacement limited by proximal and distal ligaments between metacarpals

Indications for Surgery

- Any rotational deformity, >10-degree dorsal angulation for second and third MC, >20-degree angulation for fourth and fifth MC

Surgical Technique

- Place pin axially through adjacent MC shaft
- Two interfragmentary screws acceptable only if fracture length is twice the diameter of the shaft
- Plating has high complication rate (stiffness)

METACARPAL BASE FRACTURE

Fingers

- Usually minimally displaced, associated with ligament avulsion
- Most can be treated with splinting, early ROM
- Reverse Bennett fracture dislocation: fifth MC base
  - Usually operative
  - 30-degree pronated view (60-degree supinated from neutral) shows subtle fifth carpal metacarpal (CMC) joint fracture/dislocation

Thumb

- Usually nonoperative if extra-articular because basal joint very forgiving and anatomic reduction not needed
- Bennett fracture: fracture/subluxation of metacarpal base
  - Volar-ulnar aspect of MC base remains reduced and held in place by anterior oblique ligament
  - MC shaft pulled proximally and dorsoradially by APL

- Distal MC adducted by adductor pollicis
- Reduction: abduct
- Surgical technique: pin axially into trapezium and across carpus
- Rolando fracture: T or Y fracture of MC base thumb with dorsal and volar lip fragments
  - Treatment operative: ORIF or external fixation

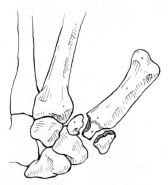

Rolando's (complete articular) fracture pattern that occur at the base of the thumb metacarpal. (From Bucholz RW, Heckman JD. Rockwood & Green's Fractures in Adults, 5th ed. Lippincott Williams & Wilkins; 2001.)

Fracture: Phalangeal

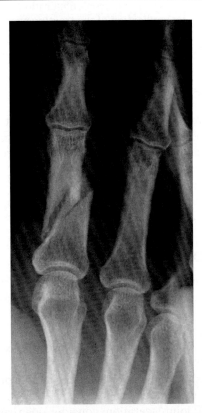

Long oblique and spiral fractures tend to instead shorten and rotate. (From Bucholz RW, MD and Heckman JD, MD. Rockwood & Green's Fractures in Adults, 5th ed. Lippincott, Williams & Wilkins, 2001.)

ORDER OF MOST COMMONLY FRACTURED BONES IN HAND

- Distal phalanx
- Metacarpal
- Proximal phalanx
- Middle phalanx

Pearls

- PIP joint is most unforgiving joint
- All digits should point at scaphoid tuberosity if properly aligned

FRACTURES AND THEIR TYPICAL ANGULATION

- Metacarpal: apex dorsal due to pull of interossei whose axis is more volar
- Proximal phalanx: apex volar due to fact that interossei flex proximal fragment; pull of extensor mechanism causes shortening
- Middle phalanx: angulation depends on location of fracture
  - Proximal one fourth: apex dorsal due to pull of central slip
  - Middle: variable
  - Distal one fourth: apex volar due to widely attached flexor digitorum (FD)

TREATMENT OF HAND FRACTURES

- For treatment of metacarpal fractures, see section on "Metacarpal Fractures"

Distal Phalanx
Extra-articular
- If closed, splint
- If open: I&D, reduce fracture and stabilize with longitudinal K wire, repair nail bed if lacerated

Intra-articular (Two Types)
- Dorsal lip (Mallet fracture)
  - Extension splint for 6–8 wk
  - ORIF if:
    - DIP joint subluxed
    - Fracture involves >30% articular surface
    - >2 mm displacement
- Volar lip fracture
  - Associated with FDP avulsion fracture
  - Common in football, most commonly ring finger
  - Primary repair especially if big fragment

Middle and Proximal Phalanges

- Nondisplaced phalangeal fracture: usually stable, immobilize for 3 wk, then active range of motion (AROM)
- Displaced phalangeal fracture:
  - Reduce
  - Don't accept any angulation >10 degree
  - Don't accept any rotation
  - AROM in 3–4 wk
  - ORIF: for unstable fracture, intra-articular displacement >1 mm, malalignment

Pearls

- Heals by 5–7 wk
- Radiographic lags clinical healing
- Consider Eaton volar plate arthroplasty if PIP joint heavily damaged

Phalangeal Condylar Fracture

- Usually unstable
- Get oblique radiograph for diagnosis and to define fracture (CT scan)
- Usually needs ORIF (various methods)

Middle Phalangeal Base Fracture

- Volar lip (dorsal fracture/dislocation)
  - Buddy tape if no history of dislocation and less than one-third of joint
  - Check for "V" sign
  - Fix if true dislocation and greater than one-third of joint
- Dorsal lip (volar fracture/dislocation)
  - Associated with central slip avulsion
  - Fix if >1 mm displaced or joint subluxated

Dislocations: Proximal Interphalangeal Joint

DORSAL DISLOCATION

Background

- One of most common articular injuries of hand
- Caused by hyperextension PIP

Radiograph

- Small avulsion fracture of middle phalanx indicates distal location of volar plate

Treatment

- Reduce with longitudinal traction, metacarpal block
- If reduction stable, early ROM with buddy taping for 3–6 wk
- If unstable, may need extension blocking splint to block at least 20 degrees of extension for approximately 3 wk

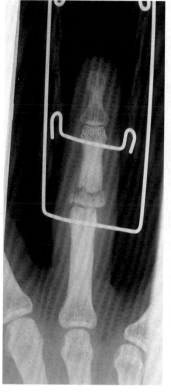
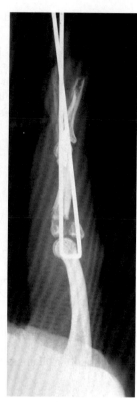

The Suzuki method of dynamic traction applied to a "pilon" fracture using a two-pin configuration reasonably well reduced by application of the traction system. (From Bucholz RW, Heckman JD. Rockwood & Green's Fractures in Adults, 5th ed. Lippincott Williams & Wilkins; 2001.)

- May need to operate if volar fracture fragment is >20% of volar surface
- Rotational deformity suggests entrapment of middle phalangeal condyle between lateral band and central slip: usually requires open reduction and repair

Complications

- Flexion contracture, pseudoboutonniere, hyperextension instability

VOLAR DISLOCATION

Background

- Can cause or be caused by rupture of central slip

Treatment

- Reduce with longitudinal traction and flexion of PIP and MCP joints
- Central slip competency tested by middle phalanx extension against resistance
- Volar PIP joint laceration: consider open dislocation, which needs I&D because of high incidence of amputation
- If slip intact, early ROM

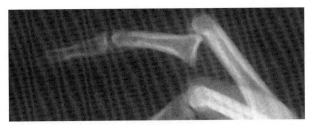

Three variants of proximal interphalangeal (PIP) joint dislocations are depicted. The most common is **(A)** dorsal, followed by **(B)** pure volar with central slip rupture, and least common is **(C)** rotatory subluxation often confused with pure volar dislocation. Note that rotatory P2 and P3 are seen in true lateral view, while P1 is seen as an oblique. (From Bucholz RW, Heckman JD. Rockwood & Green's Fractures in Adults, 5th ed. Lippincott Williams & Wilkins; 2001.)

– If slip torn, static extension splinting for 6 wk or open repair

Complications

– Extension contracture, PIP or DIP stiffness, progressive boutonniere if failure to treat central slip

Swan Neck Deformity

DESCRIPTION

– DIP flexion, PIP hyperextension

Etiology

– Can occur due to a variety of causes
  – Chronic mallet: avulsion extensor tendon distal phalanx
    – Volar plate laxity at PIP joint
    – FDS rupture or laceration at PIP joint
    – MCP subluxation
    – Intrinsic spasticity

A swan neck deformity in an individual with rheumatoid arthritis. A swan neck deformity in an individual with rheumatoid arthritis consists of hyperextension of the proximal interphalangeal (PIP) joint with flexion of the distal interphalangeal (DIP) joint. (Reprinted from the AHPA Teaching Slide Collection, 2nd ed., now known as the ARHP Assessment and Management of the Rheumatic Diseases: The Teaching Slide Collection for Clinicians and Educators. Copyright 1997. Used with permission of the American College of Rheumatology.)

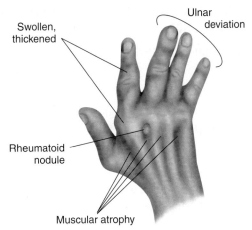

Chronic rheumatoid arthritis. As the arthritic process continues and worsens, chronic swelling and thickening of the metacarpophalangeal and proximal interphalangeal joints appear. Range of motion becomes limited and the fingers may deviate toward the ulnar side. The interosseous muscles atrophy. The fingers may show "swan neck" deformities (i.e., hyperextension of the proximal interphalangeal joints with fixed flexion of the distal interphalangeal joints). Less common is a boutonniere deformity (i.e., persistent flexion of the proximal interphalangeal joint with hyperextension of the distal interphalangeal joint). Rheumatoid nodules may accompany either the acute or the chronic stage. (From Bickley LS, Szilagyi P. Bates' Guide to Physical Examination and History Taking, 8th ed. Philadelphia: Lippincott Williams & Wilkins; 2003.)

Treatment

– Find cause and treat
  – Spiral oblique retinacular ligament reconstruction at DIP
  – Central slip tenotomy (proximal Fowler technique)
  – FDS tenodesis at PIP joint
  – Lateral band translocation at PIP joint (i.e., suture band to volar plate on one side)

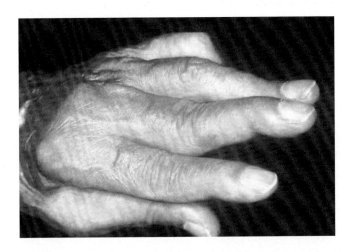

RHEUMATOID SWAN NECK DEFORMITY CLASSIFICATION

(Nalebuff & Millender, 1975)

Type I

- PIP flexible
- Treatment: FDS hemitenodesis
- Prevents hyperextension at PIP

Type II

- Intrinsic tightness
- PIP with decreased flex when MP extended
- Treatment: intrinsic release ± DIP fusion

Type III

- PIP flexion limited in all positions
- Radiograph shows normal PIP joint
- Treatment: free dorsally displaced lateral bands and allow them to reduce volarly; free flexor adhesions
- Dorsal skin left open distally
- Flexion therapy at 24–48 hr
- Extension block splint for 2–4 wk

Type IV

- Stiff PIP joint with poor radiographic findings
- PIP arthrodesis or arthroplasty
- Fuse index finger and long finger; index finger PIP fused at 25-degree flexion, middle finger PIP at slightly more flexion
- Replace ring finger, small finger: only if adjacent joints and soft tissues are intact.

Reference

Nalebuff EA, Millender LH. Surgical treatment of the boutonniere deformity in rheumatoid arthritis. Orthop Clin North Am 1975; 6(3):753–763.

Rheumatoid Arthritis Thumb Deformity Types

TYPE I: BOUTONNIERE THUMB

(Nalebuff, 1968)
- Description: MP flexed, IP hyperextension
- Treatment
  - If joints acceptably preserved, then perform synovectomy with rerouting EPL to MP joint capsule
- Usually, MP joint fused
- If IP needs fusion, then perform arthroplasty of MP joint; avoid fusing both joints

TYPE II

- Description: boutonniere with associated CMC joint involvement.
- Treat the same as I and III

TYPE III

- Description: swan neck deformity of thumb with CMC joint dislocation, MP joint hyperextended, and IP joint flexed
- Treatment
  - Hemitrapezial or complete trapezial resection
  - Volar capsulodesis or fusion for MP joint in hyperextension

TYPE IV: "GAMEKEEPER'S"

- Description: ulnar collateral ligament insufficiency with abduction deformity of MP joint, adduction contracture of metacarpal
- Treatment
  - If early, reconstruct
  - If late, fuse MP joint

TYPE V

- Description: MP hyperextension
- Volar capsulodesis vs. fusion

Reference

Nalebuff EA. Diagnosis, classification and management of rheumatoid thumb deformities. Bull Hosp Joint Dis 1968; 29(2):119–137.

Rheumatoid Arthritis Boutonniere Deformity

DESCRIPTION

(Nalebuff & Millender, 1975)
- PIP flexion, DIP hyperextension
  - Discontinuity of central slip and volar migration of lateral bands
  - Unable to flex DIP when making fist
  - Low surgical priority secondary to poorly predictable outcomes

STAGE I

- Mild extension lag, synovitis
- Treatment
  - Synovectomy, dorsal repositioning of lateral bands
  - ± Distal tenotomy

STAGE II

- 30- to 40-degree PIP flexion deformity
- Joint intact
- Treatment
  - Shorten central slip
  - Release lateral bands
  - Synovectomy

- Distal tenotomy
- Proximal phalanx (PP) K-wired in extension for 6 wk

STAGE III

- PIP stiff, no passive correction
- Treatment
    - Arthrodesis or arthroplasty
    - PIP fused in increasing flexion from 25 degrees at index finger to 50 degrees at small finger
    - In MF, arthroplasty may be preferred choice, coupled with reconstruction of central tendon in ring finger and small finger for grasping motion

Reference

Nalebuff EA, Millender LH. Surgical treatment of the boutonniere deformity in rheumatoid arthritis. Orthop Clin North Am 1975; 6(3):753–763.

Trigger Finger

BACKGROUND

- Idiopathic
- Usually affects patients >45 yo, more common in females
- Most commonly affected fingers: ring, long, and thumb

FINGER PULLEYS

- Thickened areas of flexor sheath
- Five annular (A1–A5): thicker than cruciate; odd-numbered located over joints (A1 over MP, A3 over PIP, A5 over DIP); prevent bowstringing of flexor tendons (A2 and A4 most important)
- Three cruciate pulleys (C1–C3); permit annular pulleys to pull together to allow flexion

MECHANICS

- Stenosing tenosynovitis (nodule in flexor tendon and thickening of sheath) causes size discrepancy between tendon and sheath.
- Tendon catches as it pulls through A1 pulley

HISTORY AND PHYSICAL EXAMINATION

- Tenderness of MCP head, but IP appears to trigger
- Symptoms worse in morning

STEROID INJECTION

- Use 0.5 mL of Celestone with 0.5 mL lidocaine without epinephrine
- Penetrate tendon to floor and withdraw needle while pushing plunger
- Loss of resistance indicates position in open sheath
- Palpate injection distal end of finger

OPERATIVE TREATMENT

- Local tourniquet
- Small 2-cm incision just distal to distal palmar crease (in thumb, just distal to MCP crease)

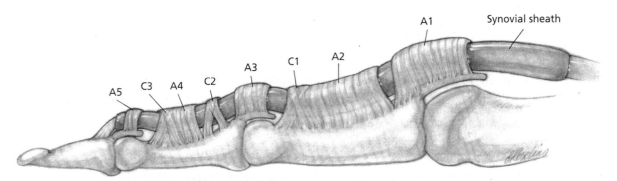

Trigger finger release. Digital flexor sheath. The digital flexor tendon sheath is composed of synovial (membranous) and retinacular (pulley) tissue components. The membranous portion is a synovial tube sealed at both ends. The retinacular (pulley) portion is a series of transverse (the palmar aponeurosis pulley), annular, and cruciform fibrous tissue condensations, which begin in the distal palm and end at the distal interphalangeal (DIP) joint. The floor or dorsal aspect of this tunnel is composed of the palmar plates of the metacarpophalangeal, proximal interphalangeal, and DIP joints and the palmar surfaces of the proximal and middle phalanges. (From Doyle JR. Hand. In: Doyle JR, Botte MJ, eds. Surgical Anatomy of the Hand and Upper Extremity. Philadelphia: Lippincott Williams & Wilkins; 2003:522–666, with permission.)

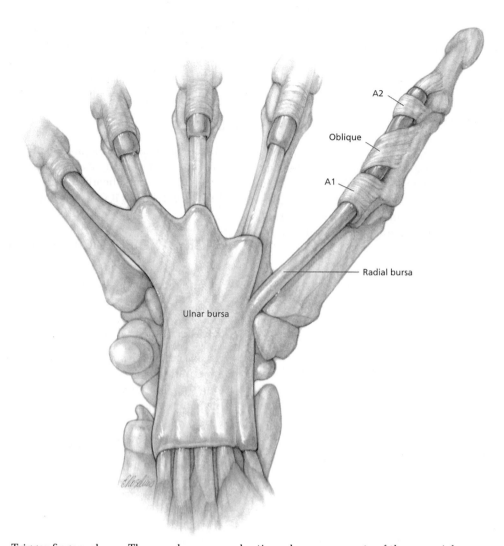

Trigger finger release. The membranous and retinacular components of the synovial sheaths in the proximal fingers, thumb, palm, and wrist. Note that the retinacular portion of the thumb flexor sheath is composed of only two annular and one oblique pulley. The radial bursa is a continuation of the flexor pollicis longus synovial sheath, which extends from the region of the interphalangeal joint of the thumb to 2.5 cm proximal to the wrist flexion crease. In the index, long, and ring fingers, the membranous portion of the sheath begins at the neck of the metacarpals and continues distally to end at the distal interphalangeal joint. In most instances, the membranous portion of the small finger synovial sheath continues proximally to the wrist. (From Doyle JR. Hand. In: Doyle JR, Botte MJ, eds. Surgical Anatomy of the Hand and Upper Extremity. Philadelphia: Lippincott Williams & Wilkins; 2003:522–666, with permission.)

- In thumb, digital nerve is more palmar and closer to flexor sheath, making radial digital nerve more vulnerable to injury
- Probe to find proximal edge of A1
- Slide edge of blunt-tip scissor across and under to cut A1
- Very important to conserve A2 and A4
- Confirm that symptoms (i.e., catching) resolved intraoperatively by asking patient to flex finger
- Apply pressure dressing

Basal Joint Osteoarthritis

EATON CLASSIFICATION

(Eaton et al., 1984)

Stage I
- Normal radiograph, basal joint may be wide due to synovitis
- Painful synovitis clinically
- Lax trapeziometacarpal joint on clinical examination

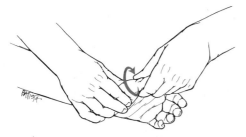

To assess the function of the first carpal metacarpal (CMC) joint, hold the joint between your thumb and index finger and gently circumduct the thumb.

- Initial treatment: splint, anti-inflammatory
- If conservative treatment fails, may perform volar ligament reconstruction with slip of FCR tendon

Stage II
- Radiographs: narrowing of trapeziometacarpal (TMC) joint, osteophytes, cysts, loose bodies <2 mm diameter, scaphotrapezial joint normal
- Treatment: conservative treatment first; if fails, then consider hemiresection interpositional arthroplasty (Eaton) or trapezial excision with ligament reconstruction/tendon interposition (LRTI; Burton)

Stage III
- Radiograph: severe narrowing of TMC joint
- Loose bodies >2 mm
- Scaphotrapezial joint normal
- Treatment: same as for stage II

Stage IV
- Radiograph: narrowing of TMC and scaphotrapezial joints
- Treatment: trapezial excision (LRTI)

Reference
Eaton RG, et al. Ligament reconstruction for the painful thumb carpometacarpal joint: a long-term assessment. J Hand Surg [Am] 1984; 9(5):692–699.

Kirner Deformity

DESCRIPTION
- Palmar and radial deformity (biplanar) of distal phalanx of short finger ("talon" or "parrot beak")

ETIOLOGY
- Unknown, but growth disturbance of distal phalangeal physis
- Insidious onset, painless swelling at DIP joint

EPIDEMIOLOGY
- F:M = 2:1
- Occurs in 1 in 400 children, onset prepubertal age (8–14 yo)
- Usually bilateral

RADIOGRAPH
- Widening distal phalanx (DP)
- Thinning of metaphysic
- Angulation (palmar and radial) of distal phalanx
- Radiolucent nidus at distal tuft

TREATMENT
- Usually no functional limitation, and surgery not necessary

Clinodactyly

DESCRIPTION
- Bent finger in the coronal (radial-ulnar) plane

EPIDEMIOLOGY
- Deformity usually at distal portion of middle phalanx
- Most commonly affects DIP joint of short finger
- Incidence: 1%–19% Caucasian population
- Usually bilateral
- Marked angulation associated with mental retardation (35%–79% incidence in patients with Down syndrome)
- Inheritance: autosomal dominant with variable penetration

TREATMENT
- Usually only cosmetic problem
- Splinting is not effective
- Consider closing wedge osteotomy in mature child with functional deficits

Camptodactyly

DESCRIPTION
- Flexion contracture of PIP joint (MCP joint hyperextended)

ETIOLOGY
- Anomalous insertion of lumbrical in abnormally proximal location into MCP capsule instead of radial lateral band

TYPES
- Infantile: <1 yo, M = F, most common
- Adolescent: F >> M, rare

EPIDEMIOLOGY

- Inheritance: usually sporadic
- Most common in short finger
- Two thirds of cases bilateral
- If unilateral, tends to affect right side

ETIOLOGY

- Multifactorial, unknown

TREATMENT

- Usually passively correctable, but progressive during growth spurts
- Treat early with splints
- Various surgeries available if hand dysfunction results, but usually give incomplete correction

Syndactyly

DESCRIPTION

- Webbing or fusion of two adjacent fingers

EPIDEMIOLOGY

- 1 in 2,000
- Most common congenital hand deformity
- May be isolated condition or occur as part of syndrome
- Often inherited
- Most common site: web space between ring finger and long finger

TYPES

- Simple: web contains only skin and SQ elements
- Complex: web contains skeletal elements
- Complete: soft tissue joined all the way to fingertip
- Incomplete: soft tissue joined only partially along length of finger

EXAMINATION

- Differential motion of individual digit indicates lack of bony involvement
- Confluence of nails (synonychia) suggests bony involvement
- Look for hidden polydactyly

TREATMENT

- Obtain preoperative Doppler (angiogram not necessary) to assess perfusion
- Early separation at 4–6 mo for complex syndactyly of ring finger–small finger connection
- Otherwise wait until 1 yo
- When symphalangism suspected, digit separation won't regain motion
- Most common technique: dorsal proximally based flap created and used to resurface commissure and insert onto palmar aspect of web; resultant defects along lateral walls of commissure covered with FTSG
- Always use FTSG because STSG contracts considerably
- Important to directly visualize all digital vessels

Thumb Hypoplasia

BACKGROUND ANATOMY

- APB: the most important muscle for thumb opposition
  - Insertions of APB
    - Radial proximal phalanx
    - Lateral MP joint capsule
    - Extensor apparatus
  - Function of APB: abducts and flexes thumb MC joint, flexes proximal phalanx, and extends IP joint to position thumb for function
- Opposition occurs mostly through CMC (TMC) joint, making it the most important joint

BLAUTH CLASSIFICATION OF THUMB HYPOPLASIA

(Blauth, 1967)

Type I (short)
- Most benign
- All parts of the digit present
- No surgery

Type II (Adducted)
- Tip doesn't reach index PIP (in length)
- Tight web space (adduction contracture)
- Deficient thenar muscles
- Instability at MCP joint
- Treatment
  - Web space release
  - Opponensplasty
  - MCP joint stabilization

Type III (Abducted)
- Muscle and bone deficiency
- Thenar muscle absence
- Web space deficiency
- Severe MCP joint instability
- Type IIIA—CMC joint stable, reconstruction as with type II or pollicization
- Type IIIB—CMC joint unstable, pollicization

Type IV (Pouce Flottant)

- Rudimentary thumb (short, unstable): positioned more distally and radially than on normal hand
- Connected to the hand by a slender pedicle, which contains a NV bundle
- Treatment: amputation with index pollicization at 6–12 mo

Type V (Absent)

- Complete absence of thumb
- Index pollicization
- Note: toe to thumb transfer for traumatic amputation, not for congenital hypoplasia

Reference

Blauth W. [The hypoplastic thumb]. Arch Orthop Unfallchir 1967; 62(3):225–246.

Ulnar Impaction

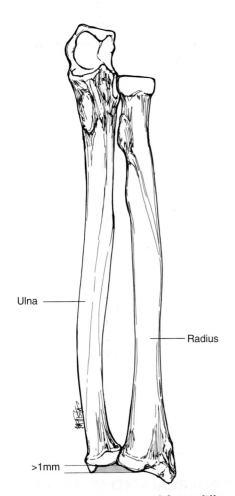

Ulnar variance. Ulnar variance is a >1.0-mm difference between the articular surfaces of the distal radius and distal ulna. (From Oatis CA. Kinesiology: The Mechanics and Pathomechanics of Human Movement. Baltimore: Lippincott Williams & Wilkins; 2004.)

ULNAR VARIANCE

- Description of relative heights of ulna and radius as seen on posteroanterior (PA) radiograph of wrist
  - Ulnar neutral: radius and ulna same length
  - Ulnar minus: ulna shorter than radius
  - Ulnar plus: ulna longer than radius

Ulnar Styloid Impaction

- Long ulnar styloid impacts triquetrum, causing chondromalacia, synovitis, and pain
- Maximum dorsiflexion and supination of wrist reproduces pain
- Supination causes recess of ulnar head relative to radius, thus would not reproduce pain caused by ulnocarpal impaction
- More common with neutral or negative ulnar variance
- Treatment: partial ulnar styloidectomy

Ulnocarpal Impaction

- More common with positive ulnar variance
- Supination and radial deviation increase minus variance
- Standard radiograph taken with shoulder abducted 90 degrees, elbow flexed 90 degrees, forearm neutral, wrist ulnar deviated
- Ulna impinges on lunate and triquetrum, causing wrist pain, restriction of motion, and cystic changes in carpal bones on plain radiograph

Radiocarpal Ligaments

VOLAR RADIOCARPAL LIGAMENTS

- Radioscaphocapitate ligament (RSCL)
  - Radial styloid to radial waist of scaphoid, around distal pole scaphoid
  - Interdigitates with fibers of triangular fibrocartilage complex (TFCC) just palmar to head of capitate
  - Minor insertion into body of capitate
- Long radiolunate ligament (LRL)
  - From just ulnar to RSCL to support interosseous scapholunate ligament
  - Inserts into radial half of palmar lunate
  - Separated from RSCL by interligamentous sulcus
- Radioscapholunate ligament (RSL) (Berger et al., 1991)
  - Also called ligament of Testut and Kuenz
  - Between LRL and short radiolunate ligament (SRL)
  - Neurovascular structure: surrounded by synovium; vascular origins from anterior interosseous artery and radial artery; neural origin from AIN
  - Travels to scapholunate (SL) interosseous ligament
- Short radiolunate ligament
  - Starts from just palmar to lunate facet of distal radius

– Attaches as a flat sheet to palmar lunate
– Ulnotriquetral ligament (UT)
  – Part of TFCC (see section on TFCC and distal radial ulnar joint [DRUJ])
– Ulnolunate ligament (UL)
  – Part of TFCC (see section on TFCC and DRUJ)

DORSAL RADIOCARPAL LIGAMENTS

– Dorsal intercarpal ligament (DIC)
  – Scaphoid to triquetrum
– Dorsal radiotriquetral ligament (DRTL)
  – Radius to triquetrum

INTRINSIC LIGAMENTS OF WRIST

– Scapholunate ligament
  – Only dorsal portion important
– Lunotriquetral ligament
  – Volar portion stronger

Reference

Berger RA, et al. Radioscapholunate ligament: a gross anatomic and histologic study of fetal and adult wrists. J Hand Surg [Am] 1991; 16(2):350–355.

Scapholunate Instability

OCCULT

– Partial scapholunate interosseous ligament (SLIL) injury
– Normal radiograph
– Normal stress radiograph
– Abnormal on fluoroscopy

Treatment

– Thumb spica if diagnosed acutely
– Arthroscopic and fluoroscopic confirmation with débridement of partial membranous SLIL injury
– If frank scaphoid subluxation on fluoroscopy, then Blatt dorsal capsulodesis (Blatt, 1987)

DYNAMIC

– Incompetent versus torn SLIL including critical dorsal portion
– Partial palmar extrinsics injury
– Normal radiograph
– Abnormal stress radiograph

Treatment

– Nonoperative treatment does not work even in acute setting
– Fluoroscopy, examination under anesthesia (EUA), arthroscopy
– If SLIL tear incomplete, dorsal capsulodesis will suffice

– Closed reduction with PP does not work universally, especially if not acute
– Direct open SLIL repair with supplemental dorsal capsulodesis if good tissue remains to repair

SCAPHOLUNATE DISSOCIATION

– Complete SLIL tear
– Volar or dorsal extrinsics torn
– Radiograph: SL gap >3 mm, SL angle >70 degrees
– Grossly abnormal stress radiograph

Treatment

– SLIL repair if acute and good tissue left for repair, scaphoid reducible, no degenerative changes
– Delayed repair controversial
– If no good tissue, Brunelli FCR tendon graft shows early promise
– Consider scaphocapitate (SC) or scaphotrapezio-trapezoid (STT) fusion with limited radial styloidectomy

DORSAL INTERCALATED SEGMENT INSTABILITY (DISI)

– With intact intercarpal ligaments (SL and LT), lunate remains balanced in neutral position by two counteracting forces from the scaphoid (which wants to volar flex) and the triquetrum (which tends to dorsally extend)
– With injury to the SL ligament, the lunate is no longer connected to the scaphoid and extends secondary to the unopposed pull from the triquetrum (DISI)
– Complete SLIL tear
– Volar extrinsics torn
– Secondary changes at most ligaments
– Radiograph:
  – SL angle >7 degrees
  – SL gap >3 mm
  – Radiolunate (RL) angle >15 degrees
  – Capitolunate (CL) angle <–15 degrees (flexed capitolunate joint >15 degrees)
– Nonoperative treatment only to stall salvage procedures
– Scaphocapitolunate (SCL) fusion if:
  – Scaphoid and lunate reducible
  – No degenerative joint disease (DJD)
– If scaphoid fixed in flexion, then proximal row carpectomy or partial or complete wrist fusion

VOLAR INTERCALATED SEGMENT INSTABILITY (VISI)

– volar flexion of lunate relative to longitudinal axis of radius and capitate
– secondary to LT ligament injury

- lunate flexes secondary to unopposed pull from scaphoid, loss of ulnar support from triquetrum
- SL angle <30

SCAPHOLUNATE ADVANCED COLLAPSE

- Same injury as in dorsal intercalated segment instability (DISI)

Classification
- I—styloid DJD
- II—radioscapholunate DJD
- III—CL DJD
- IV—pancarpal DJD

Treatment
- STT, SC, or SLC fusion if:
  - Mobile and reducible scaphoid
  - Proximal radiocarpal joint with no DJD
- Scaphoid excision with four-corner fusion (capitate-lunate-hamate-triquetrum) if:
  - Scaphoid fixed or proximal radiocarpal DJD present
  - Midcarpal DJD, but radiolunate normal
- Scaphoid excision with proximal row carpectomy (PRC) if:
  - Scaphoid fixed or proximal radiocarpal DJD present
  - Midcarpal joint normal

Reference
Blatt G. Capsulodesis in reconstructive hand surgery. Dorsal capsulodesis for the unstable scaphoid and volar capsulodesis following excision of the distal ulna. Hand Clin 1987; 3(1):81–102.

Triangular Fibrocartilage Complex and Distal Radioulnar Joint

FUNCTIONAL ANATOMY

- The different radius of the ulna and radius at the DRUJ permits rotation with translation
  - Pronation associated with palmar translation of radius
  - Supination associated with dorsal translation of radius
  - Radius migrates distally in supination
- There is debate over whether palmar or dorsal radioulnar ligaments tighten in pronation and supination
  - Primary stabilizer of DRUJ is TFCC
  - Dorsal and volar radioulnar ligaments are the main components of TFCC that stabilize DRUJ
  - Distal radioulnar ligament (DRUL) tight in pronation but volar radioulnar ligament (VRUL) prevents volar dislocation, and vice versa for supination
- Must anatomically reduce distal radius fractures to prevent DRUJ problems

- Ulnar styloid fractures can be pinned or excised/TFCC repair

COMPONENTS OF TRIANGULAR FIBROCARTILAGE COMPLEX

- Articular disc: acts as cushion
- Other structures that stabilize DRUJ
  - Dorsal and palmar radioulnar ligaments
  - ECU subsheath
  - Ulnolunate ligament
  - Ulnotriquetral ligament

TRIANGULAR FIBROCARTILAGE COMPLEX TEARS

- TFCC attaches to fovea and proximal one-third of ulnar styloid
- Large fragment can destabilize it
- Patient presents with limited pronation and supination and ulnar-sided wrist pain

Treatment
- Central portion is avascular: débridement
- Peripheral 40% is vascular: repair

Radioulnar Synostosis

DESCRIPTION

- Osseous fusion between ulnar and radius leading to fixed pronation deformity of forearm

EPIDEMIOLOGY

- 60% are bilateral
- One-third of cases associated with other congenital syndromes (i.e., Apert, Klinefelter)

SURGERY

- At age 5
- If unilateral, set in 10-degree pronation
- If bilateral, set dominant forearm in 10-degree pronation and nondominant forearm in 30-degree supination

Kienböck

DEFINITION

- Avascular necrosis of lunate (or lunatomalacia)

ETIOLOGY

- Unknown
- Associated with elevated intraosseous pressure and venous congestion

– Associated with negative ulnar variance
– Associated with lunate with single-nutrient vessel

EPIDEMIOLOGY

– Insidious onset of dominant wrist pain, no history of trauma
– Most common in third, fourth, and fifth decades

PRESENTATION

– Tender over dorsal lunate
– Decreased grip strength and range of motion
– Effusion, boggy synovitis

RADIOGRAPHIC STAGING

– Always obtain bilateral radiographs to rule out bilateral involvement
– Prognosis better for stage I and II disease
– Stage I—no radiographic changes, MRI shows early loss of marrow signal, bone scan abnormal
– Stage II—plain radiograph shows sclerosis of lunate
– Stage IIIA—plain radiograph shows lunate fragmentation/collapse without fixed scaphoid rotation
– Stage IIIB—lunate fragmentation/collapse with fixed scaphoid rotation
– Stage IV—degenerative changes in radiolunate and intercarpal joints

NONOPERATIVE TREATMENT

– Immobilize, NSAIDs
– May help with symptoms for many years
– Immobilization may lead to disuse osteoporosis, making sclerosis more pronounced

OPERATIVE TREATMENT

Revascularization
– Still controversial
– Dorsal pedicle distal radius graft (Sheetz et al., 1995)

Joint-leveling Procedures
– Indicated in patients without radiographic collapse
– Many types of procedures available
– Decreases load across lunate

– Weiss et al. (1991) showed that radial shortening led to decrease in pain in 87% patients at average follow-up 4 yr, also improved range of motion; radiographic appearance unchanged.
– Radial shortening
  – Less chance of nonunion than in ulnar lengthening
– Ulnar lengthening
  – More complicated because requires bone grafting
– Capitate shortening
  – Leads to greatest decrease in force across lunate
  – Decreases ROM because capsulotomy required
  – Load at scaphotrapezial joint increased

Lunate Resection Arthroplasty
– With silastic, titanium, coiled tendon
– Implant has been found to collapse, particulate debris may cause synovitis
– Currently has no role in treatment of Kienböck

Limited Intercarpal Fusion
– Good option in stage IIIB, especially if ulnar neutral or positive
– Addresses scaphoid rotatory subluxation at same time it unloads lunate
– Amount of decrease in lunate load similar to joint-leveling procedures
– STT performed
  – Some patients require later lunate excision
– SC easier, thus first choice

Wrist Denervation
– Buck-Gramcko (1993): PIN denervation alone led to 65% pain free at 6.5 yr

Salvage Procedure
– Indications: stage IV (wrist arthritis)
– Proximal row carpectomy
  – If lunate fossa of radius and capitate head are OK
– Wrist arthrodesis

References

Buck-Gramcko D. Wrist denervation procedures in the treatment of Kienbock's disease. Hand Clin 1993; 9(3):517–520.

Sheetz KK, et al. The arterial blood supply of the distal radius and ulna and its potential use in vascularized pedicled bone grafts. J Hand Surg [Am] 1995; 20(6):902–914.

Weiss AP, et al. Radial shortening for Kienbock disease. J Bone Joint Surg Am 1991; 73(3):384–391.

CHAPTER 8

Foot and Ankle

Tony S. Wanich, Matthew H. Griffith, John G. Kennedy, Padhraig F. O'Loughlin

General Topics
  Gait and Foot Biomechanics
  Tendons
  Tendon Disorders
  Plantar Fasciitis
  Arthroscopy
  Os Trigonum
  Os Peroneum
Forefoot Disorders
  Hallux Valgus—Adolescent
  Hallux Valgus—Adult
  Hallux Valgus—Distal Soft Tissue Procedure
  Hallux Valgus—Scarf Osteotomy
  Hallux Valgus—Treatments
  Hallux Rigidus
  Metatarsophalangeal Joint Dislocation
  Lesser Toe Deformities
  Bunionette
  Freiberg Infraction
  Sesamoids
Midfoot and Hindfoot Disorders
  Ankle Sprain and Instability
  Achilles Tendon Disorders
  Haglund Deformity
  Peroneal Tendon Dislocation
  Pes Planus
  Flatfoot in Adults
  Posterior Tibial Tendon Dysfunction
    (PTTD)
  Talus Osteochondritis Dissecans
Diabetes and Neurologic Disorders
  Charcot Arthropathy
  Diabetic Foot Ulcers and Infection
  Infection
  Amputations
  Foot Drop
  Morton Interdigital Neuroma
  Superficial Peroneal Nerve (SPN)
  Tarsal Tunnel Syndrome

Arthritis
  The Arthritides
  Arthrodesis of Ankle and Hindfoot
  Arthrodesis of Midfoot and Forefoot
  Ankle Arthroplasty

General Topics

GAIT AND FOOT BIOMECHANICS

Stance Phase
- About 62% of gait cycle
- Consists of:
  - Heel strike
  - Flat foot
  - Heel rise
  - Toe off
- Contralateral toe off soon after flat foot
- Contralateral heel strike soon after heel rise
- Divided into three periods: initial double support, single limb stance, second double support
- At heel strike, anterior compartment musculature contracts to dorsiflex; Gastrocnemius is relaxed
- Eversion through subtalar joint occurs after heel strike to unlock Chopart joint (talonavicular and calcaneocuboid joints)
- At heel rise, Gastrocnemius and Soleus (GS) fires and anterior compartment relaxes
- Posterior tibialis fires during heel rise to invert subtalar joint and lock Chopart joint

Swing Phase
- About 38% of gait cycle
- Lasts from toe off to heel strike
- Divided into two periods: early and late swing

Float Phase
- Period in running where both feet are off ground

Joint Motions
- Dorsiflexion/plantarflexion—ankle joint
- Inversion/eversion—subtalar joint
- Adduction/abduction—Chopart joint (talonavicular [TN] and calcaneocuboid [CC] joints)
- Supination—combination of dorsiflexion, eversion, and abduction
- Pronation—combination of plantarflexion, inversion, and adduction
- Ankle joint axis is oblique, parallel to malleolar tips, thus:
  - Inverts with plantarflexion
  - Everts with dorsiflexion
  - In coronal plane, axis is average of 82 degrees from anatomical axis of tibia
- Subtalar joint is oblique hinge
  - Axis is from medial talar head to lateral bottom of calcaneus
  - Acts almost like screw around that axis instead of hinge
  - With tibia internally rotated, hindfoot everts (heel strike)

- Extensor hallucis longus (EHL) and all extensor digitorum longus (EDL) should be repaired
- FHL must be repaired
- FDL of second toe does not need repair in case of puncture wound because results in no morbidity
- FHL is only posterior tendon with beef at heel

TENDON DISORDERS

Tibialis Anterior Tendon
Anatomy
- Origin—lateral tibia, intraosseous (IO) membrane
- Insert—medial cuneiform, base first metatarsal (MT)
- Innervation—deep peroneal nerve
- Function—control deceleration after heel strike, assist in toe clearance and ankle dorsiflexion after toe off, 80% of dorsiflexion power of ankle (Hintermann et al., 1994)

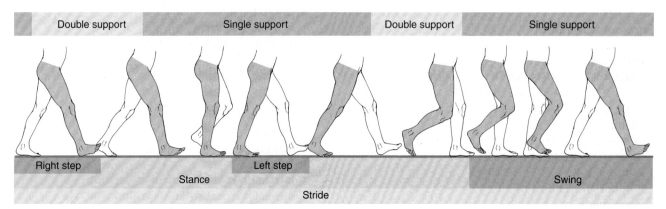

Gait cycle. (From Oatis CA. Kinesiology—The Mechanics and Pathomechanics of Human Movement. Baltimore: Lippincott Williams & Wilkins; 2004.)

- With tibia externally rotated, hindfoot inverts (toe off)

Recommended Readings
Chambers HG, Sutherland DH. A practical guide to gait analysis. J Am Acad Orthop Surg 2002; 10:222–231.
Mann RA, Coughlin MJ. Surgery of the Foot and Ankle, 7th ed. St. Louis: CV Mosby; 1999:2–35.

TENDONS

- Flexor hallucis longus (FHL) dorsal to flexor digitorum longus (FDL) at knot of Henry
- FHL runs right under sustentaculum
- Small toe has only one extensor, so must be repaired

Recommended Reading
Jones DC. Tendon disorders of the foot and ankle. J Am Acad Orthop Surg 1993; 1:87–94.

Reference
Hintermann B, et al. Foot movement and tendon excursion: an in vitro study. Foot Ankle Int 1994; 15(7):386–395.

Disorders
- Paratenonitis—indirectly runners/hikers training on downhill slopes or directly from irritation from ski boots during tucked position or hockey skates when crouched
- Tendinosis—rare because of course of tendon and minimal mechanical demands

- Discontinuity—younger patients due to laceration, older patients (>60 yo) due to rupture (traumatic, related to diabetes/gout/rheumatoid arthritis [RA], status post–steroid injection)

Findings
- Unable to heel walk, weak dorsiflexion, eversion during active dorsiflexion, altered contour during resisted dorsiflexion/inversion, palpable defect

Differential Diagnosis
- Peroneal nerve injury

Treatment
- Paratenonitis—padded tongues on footwear; rest, ice, compression, and elevation (R/I/C/E)
- Tendinosis—R/I/C/E
- Discontinuity
  - Conservative: functional bracing—controversial and only recommended in elderly population
  - Surgical: indicated in young, active patients; acute (<3 mo): end-to-end repair, no active plantarflexion until 6 wk; chronic or unable primary repair: sliding tendon graft or EHL transfer

Recommended Readings

Ouzounian TJ, et al. Anterior tibial tendon rupture. Foot Ankle Int 1995; 16:406–410.
Petersen W, et al. Blood supply of the tibialis anterior tendon. Arch Orthop Trauma Surg 1999; 119:371–375.

Flexor Hallucis Longus Tendon

Anatomy
- Origin—posterior fibula
- Insert—base of first distal phalanx
- Innervation—tibial nerve
- Function—plantarflex first interphalangeal (IP) joint, stabilize first metatarsophalangeal (MTP) joint

Disorders
- Frequently involved in athletes performing repetitive pushoff (ballet dancers)
- Tenosynovitis—aka "dancer's Achilles heel," most common injury of FHL; three sites: posterior ankle, behind flexor retinaculum, between sesamoids under distal hallucis tunnel
- Stenosing tenosynovitis—triggering of great toe resulting in hallux saltans; can occur in posterior talar tunnel, under flexor retinaculum, under intersesamoid tunnel
- Rupture—due to laceration, longitudinal tears, or tendinosis at tunnel behind talus, flexor retinaculum, intersesamoid tunnel, sustentaculum tali, knot of Henry

Findings
- Tenosynovitis—pain, swelling, tenderness in posterior ankle when moving from demi pointe to pointe
- Stenosing tenosynovitis—palpable nodule with tenderness
- Rupture—rupture proximal to interconnection with FDL: minimal pain and weakness, distal injury: greater functional loss

Differential Diagnosis
- Tenosynovitis—Achilles tendonitis, posterior tibial tendonitis, posterior impingement syndrome
- Stenosing tenosynovitis—hallux rigidus

Treatment
- Tenosynovitis—rest from aggravating activities, nonsteroidal anti-inflammatory drugs (NSAIDs), ice
- Stenosing tenosynovitis—conservative treatment (i.e., rest/ice/NSAIDs), steroid injection (risk rupture); surgical: tenolysis of tunnel with débridement
- Rupture—primary repair, ruptures distal to knot of Henry warrants FDL tenodesis, can use fascia lata/plantaris graft or FDL tenodesis for retracted tendon

Recommended Readings

Frenette JP, et al. Lacerations of the flexor hallucis longus in the young athlete. J Bone Joint Surg Am 1977; 59:673–676.
Sammarco GJ, et al. Flexor hallucis longus tendon injury in dancers and nondancers. Foot Ankle Int 1998; 19:356–362.

Flexor Digitorum Longus Tendon

Anatomy
- Origin—posteromedial tibia
- Insert—base of distal phalanges 2–5

Disorders
- Paratenonitis—less common than in FHL
- Lacerations

Treatment
- Paratenonitis—rest/ice/NSAIDs
- Laceration—primary repair if possible, reports of satisfactory outcome with conservative treatment but claw toe deformity

Peroneal Tendons

Anatomy
- Peroneus longus—upper two-thirds of lateral fibula insert inferior lateral surface of first MT and medial cuneiform
- Peroneus brevis—lateral two-thirds of fibula insert styloid process dorsolateral base of fifth MT

Disorders

- Paratenonitis with/without tendinosis—result of overuse
- Tendinosis
- Ruptures—typically, peroneus brevis develops longitudinal split that can develop into complete rupture
- Lacerations
- Subluxations—patients with flat or convex retromalleolar grooves may be predisposed
- Dislocations—commonly due to sports-related trauma
- Painful os peroneum—caused by fracture of ossicle, diastasis of multipartite os perineum, or attrition/rupture of peroneus longus

Findings

- Paratenonitis—pain/swelling/tenderness, worse with plantarflexion and inversion
- Dislocations—pain with resisted active eversion when ankle dorsiflexed
- Subluxation—sense of instability, painful snapping behind lateral malleolus, reproduce pain by pushing tendons out of retromalleolar groove
- Pain os peroneum—pain along peroneus longus distal to tip of fibula, pain with resisted eversion, plantarflexion of first ray

Differential Diagnosis

- Peroneal pathology
- Lateral ligament complex injuries
- Fractures of lateral malleolus, lateral process of talus, anterior process of calcaneus, cuboid, base of fifth MT, osteochondral fractures of talar dome

Treatment

- Paratenonitis—conservative: lateral heel wedge, rocker-bottom walking boot, or casting with non–weight bearing; surgical: tenolysis/débridement, decompression if evidence of impingement
- Tears—débridement and oversew with 6-0 nylon
- Subluxation/dislocation—conservative: NWB cast for 6 wk successful >50% cases, surgical: anatomical repair or placation of retinaculum; deepening retromalleolar groove; fibula osteotomy to create block; retinaculum reconstruction with soft tissue augmentation
- Painful os perineum—conservative: immobilization; surgical: symptoms >1 mo, excise os perineum, repair peroneus longus

Recommended Readings

Bruce WD, et al. Stenosing tenosynovitis and impingement of the peroneal tendons associated with hypertrophy of the peroneal tubercle. Foot Ankle Int 1999; 20:464–467.

Krause JO, et al. Peroneus brevis tendon tears: pathophysiology, surgical reconstruction, and clinical results. Foot Ankle Int 1998; 19(5):271–279.

Sobel M, et al. The dynamics of peroneus brevis tendon splits: a proposed mechanism, technique of diagnosis, and classification of injury. Foot Ankle Int 1992; 13:413–422.

PLANTAR FASCIITIS

Anatomy

- From medial plantar tubercle of calcaneus to plantar aspects of flexor sheaths and proximal phalanges
- Next dorsal layer is abductor hallucis, flexor digitorum brevis, abductor digitorum quinti, all originating from calcaneus
- Inferior calcaneal spur is at origin of flexor digitorum brevis (FDB; not plantar fascia) associated with heel pain in only 50%, but only 15% of asymptomatic patients have heel spurs
- Medial and lateral plantar nerves run dorsal to this level
- First branch of lateral plantar nerve is to abductor digitorum quinti (Baxter nerve), which can be compressed between deep fascia of abductor hallucis and medial head of quadratus plantae or by heel spur
- Medial calcaneal nerve can also be irritated

Differential Diagnosis of Plantar Heel Pain

- Herniated nucleus pulposus (HNP), spinal stenosis
- Stress fracture calcaneus
- Tarsal tunnel—pain inferior to medial malleolus
- Baxter nerve or medical calc nerve compression
- Heel pad atrophy—diagnosis of exclusion
- Worse in morning because sleep in plantarflexion and plantar fascia contracts, being stretched by first few steps
- Middle age
- 10% bilateral, rule out seronegative spondyloarthropathy
- Associated with Achilles tightness

Conservative

- Stretching program
- NSAIDs, heel pad or cup, short leg cast, night splint, physical therapy (PT), University of California Biomechanics Laboratory (UCBL) insert
- Silicone insert is best because absorbs most shock, custom-made polypropylene worst
- Steel shank with rocker-bottom heel
- 40% patients have 5 mo pain relief with one injection
- Shock wave therapy (3 × 1,000 impulses) effective and avoids surgery

- Surgery if fail conservative treatment × 1 yr
- Release medial one-third of fascia
- Most common complication is injury to medial calc nerve
- Complete release causes delayed flat arch, medial arch pain with weight bearing

Recommended Readings

Buchbinder R, et al. Ultrasound guided extracorporeal shock wave therapy for plantar fasciitis: a randomized controlled trial. JAMA 2002; 288:1364–1372.

Davies MS, et al. Plantar fasciitis: how successful is surgical intervention? Foot Ankle Int 1999; 20:803–807.

Furey JG. Plantar fasciitis: the painful heel syndrome. J Bone Joint Surg Am 1975; 57:672–673.

Sammarco GJ, et al. Surgical treatment of recalcitrant plantar fasciitis. Foot Ankle Int 1996; 17:520–526.

ARTHROSCOPY

- Indications include:
  - Osteoarthritis (OA)
  - Loose bodies
  - Synovectomy
  - Infection
  - Impingement
  - Instability
  - Osteochondral defect (OCD)

Distraction

- Invasive versus noninvasive
- Invasive using distractor with pins in tibia and calcaneus
- No more than 7–8 mm joint distraction, 90 N force, or 1.5 hr of invasive distraction is tolerated (injury to calcaneofibular ligament [CFL] if >90 N)
- Noninvasive safer, maximum 50 lb, no more than 1.5 hr

Setup

- Insufflate joint via anteromedial needle
  - Start just proximal and lateral to medial malleolus and aim cephalad
- Gravity inflow
- Mark out neurovascular structures

Portals

Anteromedial (AM)

- Just medial to tibialis anterior
- Incise skin, use clamp to spread down to capsule, and perform capsulotomy
- 9 mm lateral to greater saphenous vein
- 7.4 mm lateral to greater saphenous nerve

Anterolateral (AL)

- Just lateral to peroneus tertius tendon, distal to ankle joint between distal fibula and talus

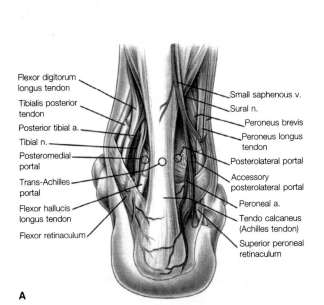 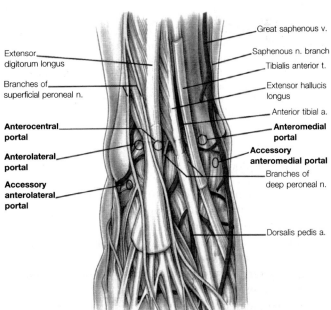

Portals for ankle arthroscopy. (From Ferkel RD. Arthroscopic Surgery: The Foot and Ankle. Philadelphia: Lippincott-Raven; 1996, with permission. Illustration by Susan Brust.)

- Transilluminate with camera through AM portal for incision to avoid neurovascular structures
- Incise skin, use clamp to spread down to capsule, and perform capsulotomy
- Traction and adduction of fourth toe may reveal intermediate dorsal cutaneous nerve (IDCN; branch of superficial peroneal nerve)
- 6.2 mm medial to IDCN (Most Commonly [MC] injured nerve)

Posterolateral
- Just lateral to Achilles, posterior to peroneal tendons, 1.5 cm proximal to tip of fibula
- Entry aided by distraction and direct arthroscopic visualization
- May be used for outflow with spinal needle
- Lesser saphenous vein and sural nerve in danger
- Sural nerve is always posterior to lesser saphenous vein, runs parallel, and is average of 3.5 mm apart

Not Recommended
- Posterocentral portal (through Achilles)
- Anterocentral portal
  - Between tendons of extensor digitorum communis (EDC)
  - Anterior tibial artery and deep peroneal nerve (DPN) at risk
- Posteromedial portal
- Posterior tibial artery and nerve, FHL, FDL, and calcaneal nerve at risk

Recommended Readings
Ferkel RD, Scranton PE Jr. Arthroscopy of the ankle and foot. J Bone Joint Surg Am 1993; 75:1233–1242.
Ferkel RD, et al. Neurological complications of ankle arthroscopy. Arthroscopy 1996;12:200–208.
Kitaoka HB. Master Techniques in Orthopaedic Surgery: The Foot and Ankle. Philadelphia: Lippincott Williams & Wilkins; 2002.

OS TRIGONUM
- Accessory bone found in up to 14% of normal feet
- Considered unfused lateral tubercle of talus
- Ossicle located posterior to talus
- Usually asymptomatic but may be involved in posterior impingement syndrome
  - Characterized by pain with plantarflexion ± limited plantarflexion
  - Higher incidence in ballet dancers
  - Can be caused by impingement of os trigonum between tibia and calcaneus with plantarflexion
  - Can confirm diagnosis with local anesthetic injection

Differential Diagnosis of Posterior Ankle Pain
- Fracture of lateral process of talus
- Tendonitis of Achilles, FHL, or peroneals
- Talar OCD
- Ankle sprain
- Haglund deformity
- Posterior impingement syndrome

Radiographic Evaluation
- Ankle series including 30 degrees oblique to assess lateral tubercle
- Some advocate bone scan to assess for symptomatic os trigonum or lateral process fracture; value is questionable
- Computed tomography (CT) scan may help

Treatment Options
Nonoperative Treatment
- Local steroid injection
- Immobilization
- Activity modification

Operative Treatment
- Excision of os trigonum often effective in relieving pain in refractory cases
- Beware of sural nerve injury when using posterolateral incision

OS PERONEUM
- Accessory bone in peroneus longus tendon in up to 26% of normal feet
- Found lateral to cuboid
- May be bipartite or multipartite
- Symptomatic os peroneum may be confused for cuboid fracture
- Injury to os peroneum may occur with inversion of ankle
  - May have associated peroneus longus tendon rupture

Radiographic Evaluation
- Foot series: anteroposterior (AP), lateral, oblique
- Bone scan advocated by some to assess for os stress fractures
- CT scan may help

Treatment Options
Nonoperative Treatment
- Immobilization with cast or CAM walker boot

Operative Treatment
- Excision of os peroneum with repair of peroneus longus tendon for refractory cases

Recommended Readings

Chao W. Os trigonum. Foot Ankle Clin 2004; 9(4):787–796, vii.

Myerson MS. Foot and Ankle Disorders, Vol. 2. Philadelphia: WB Saunders; 2000:965–967, 1501–1502.

Forefoot Disorders

HALLUX VALGUS—ADOLESCENT

- Almost always associated with increased intermetatarsal angle (IMA), metatarsus primus varus
- Normal IMA = 7 degrees, >9 degrees is pathological
- Associated with medial slope of first MT-cuneiform joint
- Associated with pes planus and ligamentous laxity
- Medial eminence less prominent
- Osteoarthritis usually not issue
- Associated with rounded MT head, increased distal metatarsal articular angle (DMAA) >15–20 degrees
- Congruent joints less likely to progress
- May have significant hallux valgus interphalangeus (>5 degrees valgus at IP joint), which must also be corrected to restore alignment
- Maternal transmission
- Mild: Hallux valgus angle (HVA) <25 degrees and IMA <13 degrees
- Moderate: HVA 30–34 degrees and IMA 13–15 degrees
- Severe: HVA >35 degrees and IMA >15 degrees

Nonoperative Treatment
- Shoe modification
- Splinting
- Often effective

Operative Treatment
- High failure rate with soft tissue procedures only
- Surgery usually bony and based on location of deformity
- Restore joint congruency and first ray alignment
- Medial sesamoid not removed because arthritic changes rare in this age
- Most common complication is recurrence (up to 50%)

Mild Deformity
- Chevron distal first MT osteotomy
  - Lateral translation of MT head
  - Can also correct DMAA if indicated by combining it with closing wedge

Moderate to Severe Deformity
- Proximal first MT osteotomy
  - Various techniques (crescentic, chevron, opening/closing wedge)

- Wait until physis closed
- Requires internal fixation
- Does not change MT length

Moderate to Severe Deformity With DMAA >20 degrees
- Double first MT osteotomy
  - Closing wedge distally
  - Opening wedge proximally (fill with wedge from distal osteotomy)
  - May add chevron distally for severe IMA to translate head laterally

Severe Deformity With Hypermobile First Ray in Pes Planus
- First cuneiform osteotomy
  - Opening wedge
  - Requires bone graft
  - May be used with open physis
- Coughlin triple osteotomy
  - First cuneiform osteotomy
  - Distal first MT osteotomy
  - Closing wedge osteotomy of proximal phalanx (Akin)

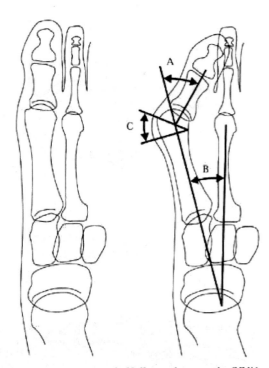

Radiographic measurements. **A:** Hallux valgus angle (HVA). **B:** Intermetatarsal angle (IMA). **C:** Distal metatarsal articular angle (DMAA). (From Chapman MW, et al. Chapman's Orthopaedic Surgery. Philadelphia: Lippincott Williams & Wilkins; 2001.)

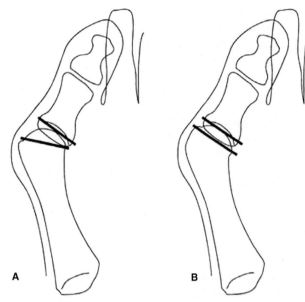

A

B

Distal metatarsal articular angle. **A:** Incongruent joint.
B: Congruent joint with increased distal metatarsal
articular angle (DMAA). (From Chapman MW, et al.
Chapman's Orthopaedic Surgery. Philadelphia: Lippincott
Williams & Wilkins; 2001.)

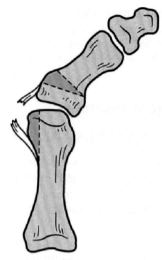

Akin osteotomy. (From Chapman MW, et al. Chapman's
Orthopaedic Surgery. Philadelphia: Lippincott Williams &
Wilkins; 2001.)

Chevron osteotomy. (From Chapman MW,
et al. Chapman's Orthopaedic Surgery.
Philadelphia: Lippincott Williams & Wilkins;
2001.)

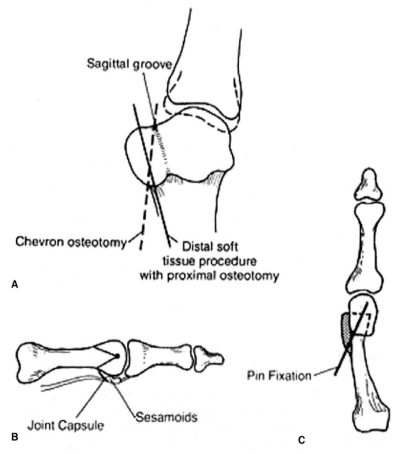

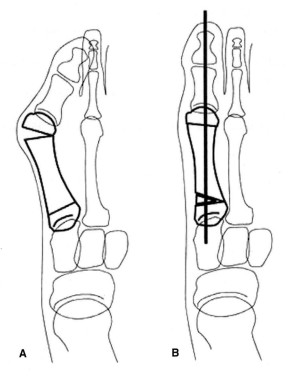

A   B

Double first metatarsal (MT) osteotomy. (From Chapman MW, et al. Chapman's Orthopaedic Surgery. Philadelphia: Lippincott Williams & Wilkins; 2001.)

Recommended Readings

Coughlin MJ, Carlson RE. Treatment of hallux valgus with an increased distal metatarsal articular angle: evaluation of double and triple first ray osteotomies. Foot Ankle Int 1999; 20(12):762–770.

Coughlin MJ, Mann RA. The pathophysiology of the juvenile bunion. Instr Course Lect 1987; 36:123–136.

Coughlin MJ, Roger A. Mann Award. Juvenile hallux valgus: etiology and treatment. Foot Ankle Int 1995; 16(11):682–697.

Myerson MS. Foot and Ankle Disorders, Vol. 2. Philadelphia: WB Saunders; 2000:213–288.

Thompson GH. Bunions and deformities of the toes in children and adolescents. Instr Course Lect 1996; 45:355–367.

Zimmer TJ, et al. Treatment of hallux valgus in adolescents by the chevron osteotomy. Foot Ankle 1989; 9(4):190–193.

HALLUX VALGUS—ADULT

- Lateral deviation of great toe, pronation of first MT
- Intrinsic and extrinsic causes
  - First ray hypermobility
  - Metatarsus primus varus
  - Abnormal MT length
  - Tight Achilles
  - Rheumatoid arthritis
  - Pronated foot
  - Lesser toe amputation (especially second) can cause bunion

Anatomy
- MT head has no muscle insertions
- Transverse MT ligament anchors sesamoids to second MT head; thus, sesamoids stay in place
- Four groups that encircle MTP joint
  - Dorsal: EHL, extensor hallucis brevis (EHB), thin capsule
  - Plantar: FHL, flexor hallucis brevis (FHB; sesamoids), plantar plate
  - Transverse and oblique heads of adductor hallucis insert on lateral sesamoid and lateral proximal phalanx
  - Abductor hallucis inserts on proximal phalanx medially

Physical Examination
- Check dorsiflexion while attempting to correct deformity
  - If dorsiflexion restricted with correction of hallux valgus, then expect this postop
- Hallux more pronated with more severe disease
- Should have no pain when barefoot unless degenerative joint disease (DJD) of MTP joint is already present
- Check stability of first MT-cuneiform joint (only 2%–3% of patients are hypermobile)
  - May present as callus under second MT head

Imaging (see figure p. 432)
- HVA normal <15 degrees
- IMA normal <9 degrees
- DMAA
  - Normal <10 degrees lateral deviation
  - Most patients with high DMAA are congruent
- Hallux valgus interphalangeus
  - Valgus angle at interphalangeal joint
- Angle between proximal articular surface of proximal phalanx and proximal phalangeal shaft (normal <10 degrees lateral)
- Obliquity of MT-cuneiform joint (normal <15 degrees medial)
- Sesamoid position
- Congruency of MTP joint (lateral subluxation of proximal phalanx on MT head)
- MTP joint arthrosis

Decision Making
- Restoration or preservation of MTP joint congruency most important
- If congruent, consider distal MT chevron sliding osteotomy or Akin proximal phalanx osteotomy with medial eminence excision
- If incongruent, classify further:
  - Normal: HVA <15 degrees, IMA <9 degrees
  - Mild: HVA 15–30 degrees, IMA 9–15 degrees

– Moderate: HVA 30–40 degrees, IMA 15–20 degrees
– Severe: HVA >40 degrees, IMA >20 degrees
- For mild: chevron or distal soft tissue procedure (DSTP) ± proximal osteotomy or Mitchell distal MT step-cut osteotomy
- For moderate: DSTP with proximal MT osteotomy or Mitchell
- For severe: DSTP with proximal MT osteotomy or MTP fusion

Special Considerations
- Fuse MTP if significant OA, severe deformity, RA, cerebral palsy (CP)
- Keller resection arthroplasty if minimal ambulatory, older, diabetic
- First MT-cuneiform fusion (Lapidus) with DSTP if hypermobile ± gastroc slide
- In general, 90% of patients satisfied, but 25% have residual pain

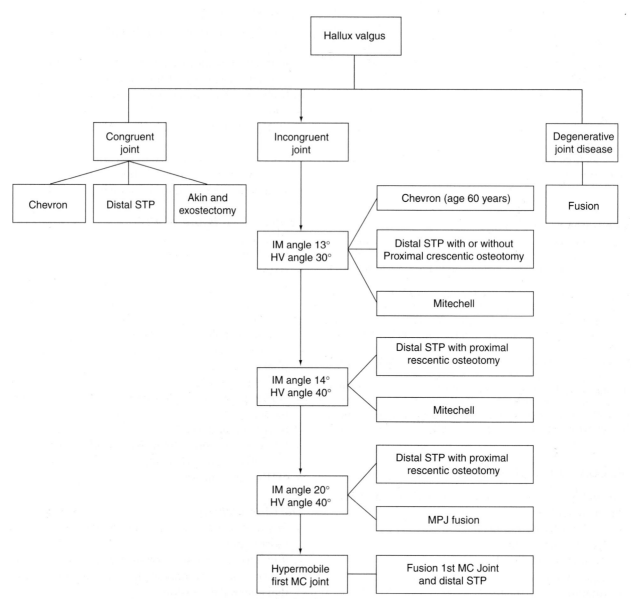

Treatment algorithm. (From Chapman MW, et al. Chapman's Orthopaedic Surgery. Philadelphia: Lippincott Williams & Wilkins; 2001.)

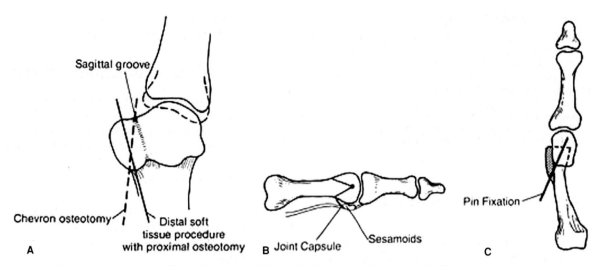

Chevron osteotomy. (From Chapman MW, et al. Chapman's Orthopaedic Surgery. Philadelphia: Lippincott Williams & Wilkins; 2001.)

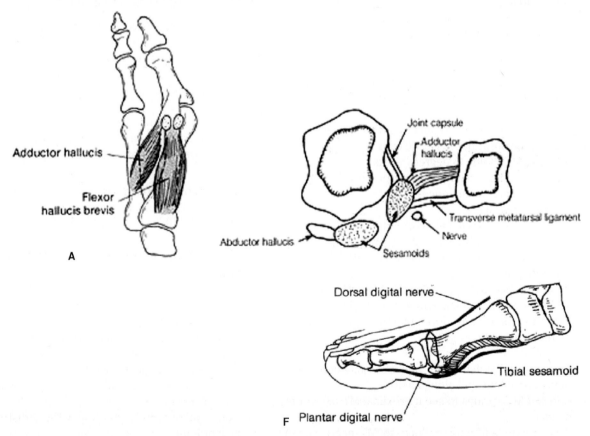

Distal soft tissue procedure. (From Chapman MW, et al. Chapman's Orthopaedic Surgery. Philadelphia: Lippincott Williams & Wilkins; 2001.)

Recommended Readings

Akin OF. The treatment of hallux valgus: a new operative procedure and its results. Med Sentinel 1925; 33:68.

Johnson KA, et al. Chevron osteotomy for hallux valgus. Clin Orthop 1979; (142):44–47.

Mann RA. Disorders of the first metatarsophalangeal joint. J Am Acad Orthop Surg 1995; 2:34–43.

Mann RA, Pfeffinger L. Hallux valgus repair. DuVries modified McBride procedure. Clin Orthop 1991; (272):213–218.

Myerson MS. Foot and Ankle Disorders, Vol. 2. Philadelphia: WB Saunders; 2000:213–288.

HALLUX VALGUS—DISTAL SOFT TISSUE PROCEDURE

- Incision in first web space centered on MT heads
- Stay in center to avoid deep peroneal nerves
- Weitlaner for exposure
- Find adductor hallucis along dorsal side of fibular sesamoid and lateral side of MT head
- Blade between MT head and fibular sesamoid through capsule, go distally until proximal phalanx hit, then cut adductor hallucis off proximal phalanx
- Then bring blade proximally to take capsule between sesamoid and MT
- Freer to inspect sesamoid by pushing it plantarly
- Weitlaner deeper and spread until intermetatarsal ligament stretched (between fibular sesamoid and second MT)
- Transect this intermetatarsal ligament, but avoid common digital nerve and vessels just underneath
- Freer under sesamoid to ensure no more adhesions
- Multiple perforations in lateral capsule and stretch by bringing MTP joint 15 degrees varus
- Medial midline incision from midproximal phalanx to 1 cm proximal to eminence
- Full-thickness flaps
- Watch out for dorsal and volar cutaneous nerves
- Vertical capsular incision 2 mm proximal to base of proximal phalanx and another parallel incision 4–8 mm more proximal
- Remove this flap, working inside out so tibial sesamoid protects plantar nerve from blade
- Extend capsulotomy dorsolongitudinally to expose medial eminence
- Inspect joint
- Find sagittal sulcus and remove eminence 2 mm medial to sulcus and along shaft
- Check if MT springs to see if proximal MT osteotomy needed
- If no, repair adductor hallucis to MT head capsule loosely
- Put MT phalangeal joint in neutral, allowing tibial sesamoid to be seen
- Repair medial capsulotomy, which should lead to neutral or slightly overcorrected MTP joint

HALLUX VALGUS—SCARF OSTEOTOMY

- Medial incision between junction of volar and dorsal skin
- 1.2-mm K-wires at corners of osteotomy
- Proximal pin 2 cm distal to MT-cuneiform joint
- Distal pin 5 mm proximal to dorsal cartilage surface
- Cuts parallel to long axis of foot, avoids shortening or lengthening
- Usually pure translation of distal fragment laterally
- Distal cut is dorsal
- Troughing occurs when distal fragment elevates MT head

Recommended Reading

Barouk LS. Scarf osteotomy for hallux valgus correction: local anatomy, surgical technique, and combination with other forefoot procedures. Foot Ankle Clin 2000; 5(3):525–558.

HALLUX VALGUS—TREATMENTS

Akin Proximal Phalanx Osteotomy
- Indications
  - Hallux valgus interphalangeus
  - Congruent joint, DMAA normal (<10 degrees)
  - As secondary procedure to chevron or distal soft tissue procedure
- Contraindications
  - Incongruent joint > worsens deformity
- Medial wedge removed 8 mm distal to joint

Recommended Reading

Frey C, et al. The Akin procedure: an analysis of results. Foot Ankle 1991; 12:1–6.

Chevron Distal Metatarsal Slide Osteotomy
- Indications—mild, congruent joint
- Contraindications—severe (HVA >35 degrees, IMA >15 degrees)
- Fixation harder if patient >50 yo
- 1 cm proximal to articular surface
- Head displaced 5 mm
- K-wire dorsomedial to plantar-lateral
- Add medial closing wedge if incongruent and DMAA >15 degrees
- Add Akin for more correction without disturbing congruent joint
- Nota Bene (NB): Transfer metatarsalgia if excessive shortening performed
- Limited correction of IMA

Recommended Reading

Trnka H-J, et al. The chevron osteotomy for correction of hallux valgus: comparison of findings after two and five years of follow up. J Bone Joint Surg Am 2000; 82:1373–1378.

Distal Soft Tissue Procedure (Modified McBride—leaves sesamoid)

- Indications—mild, congruent or incongruent joint
- Contraindications
  - Congruent with increased DMAA, severe arthrosis, cerebral palsy, connective tissue disorder
- Dorsal incision between first and second
- Metatarsal-sesamoid capsule cut
- (Adductor hallucis transferred to soft tissue near first MT neck)
- (Transverse MT ligament cut)
- Medial incision
- Excise eminence in line with MT shaft, just medial to sulcus
- Add MT osteotomy if IMA >15 degrees because IMA can be expected to correct 5 degrees by DSTP alone
- Complications—hallux varus if too much medial eminence or fibular sesamoid; hallux varus treated by extensor hallucis brevis or extensor hallucis longus static transfer to lateral MTP joint
- Can recur if done alone because soft tissues stretch out

Recommended Reading

Mann RA. Hallux valgus repair. DuVries modified McBride procedure. Clin Orthop 1991; (272):213–218.

Distal Soft Tissue Procedure Plus Proximal Metatarsal Osteotomy

- Indications—moderate
- Contraindications—congruent joint, arthrosis
- Crescent osteotomy with concavity to heel, over proximal one-third MT, halfway between being perpendicular to first MT and perpendicular to bottom of foot (this 120-degree cut avoids excess dorsiflexion)
- Corrects IMA but avoids excess lateralization of MT head, which will cause varus
- Closing wedges not done because ends up short, dorsiflexed with resulting transfer metatarsalgia
- Longer recovery—4 mo to normal shoes

Recommended Reading

Mann RA, et al. Repair of the hallux valgus with a distal soft tissue procedure and proximal MT osteotomy. J Bone Joint Surg Am 1992; 74-A:124–129.

Mitchell Distal Metatarsal Step-Cut Osteotomy

- Indications—moderate
- Contraindications—severe, congruent, short MT
- Complications—transfer metatarsalgia due to dorsiflexion of MT head
- More technically demanding—complex biplane double step-cut

Recommended Reading

Glynn MK, et al. The Mitchell distal metatarsal osteotomy for hallux valgus. J Bone Joint Surg Br 1980; 62-B(2):188–191.

Distal Soft Tissue Procedure With Metatarsal-Cuneiform Fusion

- Indications—hypermobile first ray, severe
- Contraindications—congruent joint, athlete
- Usually takes 4–6 mo for union
- Fuse in slight plantarflexion, lateral deviation to prevent transfer metatarsalgia

Recommended Reading

Sangeorzan BJ, et al. Modified Lapidus procedure for hallux valgus. Foot Ankle 1989; 9:262–266.

Metatarsal-Phalanx Fusion

- For severe, OA, CP, short first MT
- Contraindications if OA of IP or MT-cuneiform joints
- Do not do concomitant osteotomy because IMA will correct if fusion takes
- Fuse with proximal phalanx in 15-degree valgus, 15 degrees dorsiflexed from plantar surface of foot

Recommended Reading

Mann RA, et al. Arthrodesis of the first metatarsophalangeal joint for hallux valgus in rheumatoid arthritis. J Bone Joint Surg Am 1984; 66(5):687–692.

Keller

- Resect base of proximal phalanx
- Removal of medial eminence
- Loss of toe pushoff strength > only for minimal ambulators
- Achieves great pain relief for hallux rigidus

Recommended Reading

Richardson EG. Keller resection arthroplasty. Orthopedics 1990; 13:1049–1053.

HALLUX RIGIDUS

- Loss of range of motion (ROM; especially dorsiflexion) of first MTP joint due to DJD
- Characteristic dorsal exostosis on MT head, extends medially and laterally
- Present in 1 of 45 people >50 yo

- Ratio of women to men is 2:1
- If in child, think OCD lesion
- Etiology may include:
  - OA
  - Trauma
  - Inflammatory arthritis (RA, seronegative)
  - Metabolic disorder (gout)
  - Congenital abnormality (long first ray, irregular ball-and-socket MTP joint)
  - Acquired causes (obesity, footwear)

History and Physical Examination

- Decreased ROM (normal 30 degrees plantarflexion [PF], 90 degrees dorsiflexion [DF])
- 60-degree extension needed for activities of daily living (ADLs)
- Localized swelling, tenderness
- Gait (painful push-off): shifts weight to lateral border, may externally rotate hip to clear floor, may toe off using lesser toes
- Dorsal medial cutaneous nerve sensitive (Tinel sign, paresthesias)
- Pain with forced dorsiflexion
- May have mechanical block from osteophytes on MT head > proximal phalanx
- Palpable dorsal bony protuberance

Imaging

- Standing AP, lateral, oblique radiograph (XR) of foot
- Dorsal osteophyte on MT head and proximal phalanx, which may fracture
- Staging (Hattrup & Johnson, 1988)
  - Stage I—minimum narrowing, dorsal osteophyte
  - Stage II—only plantar joint is preserved
  - Stage III—complete joint narrowing

Nonoperative Treatment

- Stiff sole shoe
- Orthotic with Morton extension
- Full-length rigid orthosis that limits dorsiflexion at MTP joint
- Office manipulation under ankle block

Operative Treatment

Cheilectomy
- Indicated for early stages
- Dorsal incision, medial to EHL
- DPN is lateral; saphenous nerve is medial
- Remove dorsal bone until 60–80 degrees dorsiflexion
- Remove at least dorsal one-third, starting just above where cartilage has been lost
- Take lateral osteophyte in line with shaft
- Take dorsal one-third of proximal phalanx
- Average postop increase in dorsiflexion is 25 degrees

- Relieves impingement but may still have pain
- Maximum improvement by 4 mo

Moberg Osteotomy
- Indicated in young active patient with good joint space but inadequate dorsiflexion
- Medial incision
- Dorsal closing wedge at proximal aspect of proximal phalanx
- Exchanges plantarflexion for dorsiflexion
- Done alone in child without exostosis
- Stable internal fixation necessary because cheilectomy requires early motion

Metatarsophalangeal Arthrodesis
- Indicated in an active patient with no residual joint space
- Fuse at 15–25 degrees dorsiflexion, 15–25 degrees valgus to MT shaft
- Fixation with crossed screws, dorsal plate, or K-wires
- Eliminates pain
- Return to most activities
- Heel height, running limited
- Reliable functional results, especially in young

Modified Keller Interpositional Arthroplasty
- Indicated for elderly with severe involvement
- Maintains motion
- Resect proximal half of proximal phalanx
- Interpose space with EHB and capsule
- Complications include transfer metatarsalgia, shortening, weak push-off

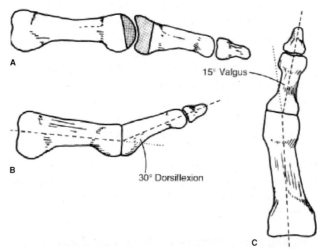

First metatarsophalangeal (MTP) joint arthrodesis. (From Chapman MW, et al. Chapman's Orthopaedic Surgery. Philadelphia: Lippincott Williams & Wilkins; 2001.)

Recommended Readings

Hamilton WG, Hubbard CE. Hallux rigidus: excisional arthroplasty. Foot Ankle Clin 2000; 5(3):663–671.

Mann RA. Disorders of the first metatarsophalangeal joint. J Am Acad Orthop Surg 1995; 2:34–43.

Shereff MJ, Baumhauer JF. Current concepts review—hallux rigidus and osteoarthrosis of the first metatarsophalangeal joint. J Bone Joint Surg Am 1998; 80:898–908.

Reference

Hattrup SJ, Johnson KA. Subjective results of hallux rigidus following treatment with cheilectomy. Clin Orthop Relat Res 1988; (226):182–191.

METATARSOPHALANGEAL JOINT DISLOCATION

– Almost always dorsal

Jahss Type I

– Disruption of sesamoid-plantar plate through weak proximal attachment to first MT
– No injury to intersesamoid ligament
– Sesamoids stuck in joint, not reducible
– Requires open reduction

Jahss Type II

– Sesamoid complex disrupted
– IIA:
  – Intersesamoid ligament torn
  – Intermetatarsal space wide
  – MT head dislocates through split between two sesamoids
  – Closed reduction okay
– IIB:
  – Intersesamoid ligament okay
  – Transverse fracture through one or both sesamoids
  – Proximal half of sesamoid stays in place; distal half becomes loose body
  – Requires open reduction as well

Recommended Reading

Jahss MH. Traumatic dislocations of the first metatarsophalangeal joint. Foot Ankle 1980; 1:15–21.

LESSER TOE DEFORMITIES

– All caused by narrow toe box
– Flexible ones passively correct with standing

Anatomy

– 37% distal phalanx (DP) fused to middle phalanx (MP) in fifth toes
– Terminal extensor tendon and FDL insert on DP
– Extensor digitorum longus central slip and flexor digitorum brevis insert on MP

– Extensor mechanism gets contribution from EDL and from extensor digitorum brevis (EDB) laterally
– No fifth EDB
– FDB from calcaneus inserts on MP, causing flexion of proximal interphalangeal (PIP)
– FDL inserts base of DP, causing flexion of distal interphalangeal (DIP)
– Lumbricals start from long flexor tendons and insert on medial toes and extensor mechanism
– Plantar plate is primary stabilizer of MTP joint

Hammer Toe

– MTP/DIP joint extended, PIP joint flexion deformity, callus over PIP joint
– Fixed or flexible
– If flexible, can be reduced by ankle plantarflexion or dorsal pressure over plantar surface of MT head
– Caused by long ray, small toe box, neuromuscular disorder
– If flexible:
  – Percutaneous FDL tenotomy
  – Girdlestone-Taylor flexor-to-extensor transfer
– If fixed:
  – DuVries distal proximal phalangeal (PP) condylectomy
  – ± FDL tenotomy through plantar capsule

Recommended Readings

Coughlin MJ, et al. Operative repair of the fixed hammer-toe deformity. Foot Ankle Int 2000; 21:94–104.

Myerson M, et al. The pathologic anatomy of claw and hammertoes. J Bone Joint Surg Am 1989; 71:45–49.

Padanilam TG. The flexible hammer toe: flexor to extensor transfer. Foot Ankle Clin 1998; 3:259–268.

Claw Toe

– MTP hyperextension, PIP/DIP flexion
– Metatarsalgia, plantar ulceration
– Cause diabetes mellitus (DM), RA, compartment, cavus
– Same treatment as hammer toe, except address MTP also with EDL/EDB tenotomies/lengthenings

Recommended Readings

Feeney MS, et al. Selective lengthening of the proximal flexor tendon in the management of acquired claw toes. J Bone Joint Surg Br 2001; 83:335–338.

Sans AK, et al. Idiopathic clawed toes. Foot Ankle Clin 1998; 3:245–258.

Mallet Toe

– DP flexed on MP
– Caused by OA
– Distal MP condylectomy if rigid, flexor tenotomy if flexible

Recommended Reading

Murphy GA. Mallet toe deformity. Foot Ankle Clin 1998; 3:279–292.

Intractable Plantar Keratosis

- Proliferations of hyperkeratotic tissue on plantar area usually MT heads
- Surgical if conservative fails—modified DuVries or dorsiflexion osteotomy

Recommended Readings

Marks RM. Anatomy and pathophysiology of lesser toe deformities. Foot Ankle Clin 1998; 3:199–214.
Richardson EG. Lesser toe deformities: an overview. Foot Ankle Clin 1998; 3:195–198.

BUNIONETTE

- Prominent fifth MT head
- Causes include:
  - Extrinsic pressure (tight footwear)
  - Congenital (fifth MT shaft bowing, fourth MT brachymetatarsia, primary hypertrophy of fifth MT head, abnormal transverse MT ligament insertion)
  - Iatrogenic (failed surgery on adjacent MT, forefoot varus after correction of hindfoot deformity)
  - Inflammatory (rheumatoid nodules), trauma

History and Physical Examination

- Pain, swelling, and decreased ROM in fifth MTP joint
- Adduction deformity of fifth MTP
- Hyperkeratotic skin changes
- Antalgic gait
- Splayfoot: hallux valgus with metatarsus primus varus plus bunionette

Imaging

- Weight-bearing AP, lateral, and oblique radiographs
- Fifth MT-proximal phalangeal angle (normal 16 degrees)
- Fourth to fifth IMA (normal 7 degrees)
- Lateral deviation angle—reflects MT bowing by measuring angle between proximal and distal portions of MT shaft
- Evaluate MT head shape, osteophytes

Radiographic Staging

- Type I: fifth MT head enlarged or pronated (lateral plantar condyle rotated more laterally)
- Type II: lateral bowing of fifth MT
- Type III: wide 4–5 IMA

Treatment Options

Nonoperative Treatment
- Callus shaving
- MT pad
- Wide-toe box shoe
- NSAIDs

Operative Treatment
- Surgery indicated for symptomatic bunionette refractory to conservative treatment

Lateral Condylectomy and Capsulorrhaphy

- Primary treatment for type I (no correction of IMA)
- Also can be adjuvant to other procedures

Distal Osteotomy
- Crescentic, chevron, or oblique
- Shifts head medially 33%–40%, little change in IMA (1 degree per 1 mm translation)
- Fixation with screws, K-wires, or bioabsorbable pins
- Treatment for types I and III

Midshaft Osteotomy
- Oblique or closing wedge
- Allows correction of IMA
- Less risk of transfer lesion
- Fixation with screws

Proximal Osteotomy
- Closing or opening wedge, chevron
- Allows large correction of IMA
- Contraindicated in high degrees of bowing (therefore, little correction possible)
- Risk of disrupting blood supply, destabilizing tarsometatarsal (TMT) joint

Metatarsal Head Resection
- Salvage procedure
- Risk of transfer lesion to fourth MT

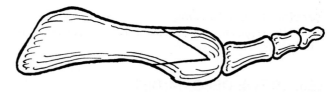

Crescentic osteotomy. (From Chapman MW, et al. Chapman's Orthopaedic Surgery. Philadelphia: Lippincott Williams & Wilkins; 2001.)

Recommended Readings

Moran MM, Claridge RJ. Chevron osteotomy for bunionette. Foot Ankle Int 1994; 15(12):684–688.
Myerson MS. Foot and Ankle Disorders, Vol. 2. Philadelphia: WB Saunders; 2000:335–358.

FREIBERG INFRACTION

- Primary articular osteochondrosis of lesser MT heads
- Proposed etiologies include trauma, vascular abnormalities, and repetitive stress leading to avascular necrosis (AVN)
- Female-to-male ratio: 11:1, 11–17 yo
- Second MTP joint in up to 80%, bilateral 6%
  - Long second ray may increase stresses on MT head

History and Physical Examination

- Forefoot pain (metatarsalgia), worse with activity
- Limited motion in MTP joint
- May be asymptomatic until adulthood when arthrosis develops
- Swelling, thickened soft tissues, warmth (signs of synovitis)
- Antalgic gait
- May develop palpable dorsal osteophyte

Imaging

- Initial radiographs may be normal or show fragmented head and joint space narrowing
- Early stage has subchondral bone collapse dorsocentrally with intact cartilage
- Middle stage with central collapse progressing peripherally
- Advanced stage with loose bodies, frank DJD

Staging

- I—Fissure fracture in epiphysis
- II—Bone resorption and resultant central head depression
- III—Head collapse with intact plantar cartilage
- IV—Plantar piece breaks free as loose body
- V—End-stage arthritis, deformity

Nonoperative Treatment

- Activity modification
- MT pad
- Shoe modification
- Cast immobilization
- Steroid injection
- Period of non–weight bearing
- Physical therapy

Operative Treatment

- Joint débridement with cheilectomy good for early stages
- Dorsiflexion osteotomy will unload affected joint and shift normal plantar cartilage into center of joint
  - Perform proximally to minimize shortening and maximize elevation and distal fragment size

- Extra-articular MT shortening (4 mm)
- DuVries-type MTP arthroplasty
  - Dorsal incision through skin, extensor mechanism, and capsule
  - Resect 3–4 mm of MT head perpendicular to shaft using sagittal saw
  - Reshape MT head with burr until it is round
  - Interpose capsule or EDB
  - Fix with 0.062-in. retrograde K-wire at 0–10 degrees MTP dorsiflexion, ankle neutral
  - Protect weight bearing for 6 wk, then remove K-wire; buddy tape for 6 wk
  - Pin with 0.045-in. K-wire, protect weight bearing, and remove at 4 wk
- Joint replacement with silicon implant has high risk of complications and is controversial

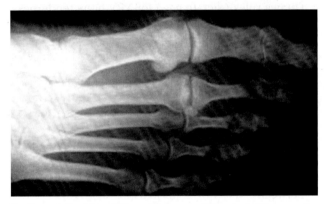

Freiberg infraction. (From Chapman MW, et al. Chapman's Orthopaedic Surgery. Philadelphia: Lippincott Williams & Wilkins; 2001.)

Recommended Readings

DuVries HL. Surgery of the Foot. St. Louis: Mosby–Year Book; 1959:359–360.
Myerson MS. Foot and Ankle Disorders, Vol. 2. Philadelphia: WB Saunders; 2000:785–799.

SESAMOIDS

- Encased within FHB tendon to increase mechanical advantage and to weight bear under MT head
- Most constant is sesamoids beneath first MT
- 80% of bipartite sesamoids involve tibial one
- 25% of patients have bilateral bipartite tibial sesamoids

Turf Toe

- Volar plate avulses off MT head
- Hallux rigidus can result
- Avoid complete excision of both sesamoids because of hallux cock-up deformity
- Two-thirds of either sesamoid can be removed safely

Recommended Reading

Rodeo SA, et al. Turf-toe: an analysis of metatarsophalangeal joint sprains in professional football players. Am J Sports Med 1990; 18(3):280–285.

Midfoot and Hindfoot Disorders

ANKLE SPRAIN AND INSTABILITY

Ankle Sprain

- Twisting injury with subsequent swelling, ecchymosis, tenderness, and painful ROM
- Most commonly, anterior talofibular ligament (ATFL) injury
- Grade I—microtear
- Grade II—partial tear
- Grade III—complete rupture
- Ottawa rules (dictate need for XR): bony tenderness to palpation (TTP) in distal fibula, tibia, navicular, or base of fifth MT and inability to bear weight
- Early mobilization with weight bearing in brace is most effective treatment of sprain
- Expect normal activity in 4–8 wk

Ankle Instability

History
- Present with repeated episodes of ankle giving way, with pain and swelling and asymptomatic periods in between
- Soccer player with ankle injury is two to three times more likely to get another injury
- Recurrent sprains in 80% of high school varsity basketball players
- Functional instability is diagnosed by history of feeling of ankle giving way, and difficulty walking on uneven ground

Physical Examination
- May see limited dorsiflexion, tight Achilles
- Mechanical instability is:
  - Anterior drawer: >10 mm anterior translation or >3 mm difference compared with other side
  - Talar tilt: >9 degree or >3 degree difference compared with other side

Treatment
- Can try period of physical therapy and/or bracing
- Surgery is indicated when both mechanical and functional instability are present
- Repeated episodes of giving way do not predispose to OA, so operative indication is patient's unwillingness to accept episodes of instability
- Anatomical and nonanatomical repairs described:

- Nonanatomical: Chrisman-Snook reconstruction uses half of peroneus brevis (PB) to reconstruct ATFL and CFL through drill hole in fibula
  - 84% good/excellent results
  - 100% restricted inversion
  - 20% restricted dorsiflexion
  - Ligaments not isometric, abnormal biomechanics
- Anatomical: Broström shortens, imbricates, and reimplants ATFL into bone
  - Gould modification uses extensor retinaculum to reinforce repair and uses lateral talocalcaneal ligament to reinforce CFL repair
  - Motion and weight bearing in 2 wk
  - Full activity in 12 wk
  - 93% good/excellent results
  - Poor outcome if:
    - >10 yr of instability
    - Associated OA
    - Generalized hypermobility

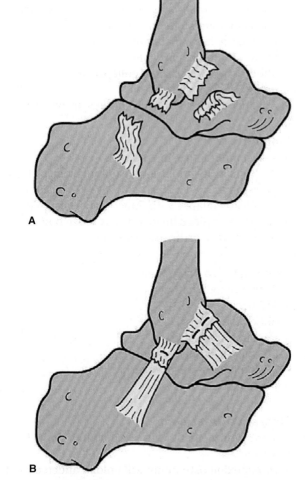

Modified Broström repair. (From Chapman MW, et al. Chapman's Orthopaedic Surgery. Philadelphia: Lippincott Williams & Wilkins; 2001.)

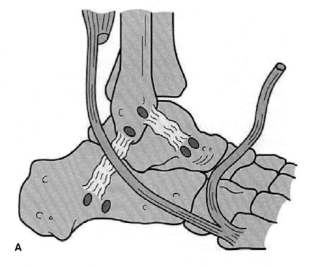

A

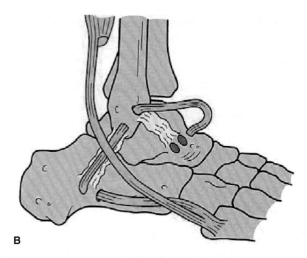

B

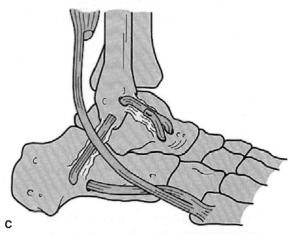

C

Chrisman-Snook reconstruction. (From Chapman MW, et al. Chapman's Orthopaedic Surgery. Philadelphia: Lippincott Williams & Wilkins; 2001.)

Subtalar Sprain
- Occurs in combination with lateral injury
- Present in 10% patients with lateral instability
- Subtalar arthrography aids in diagnosis

Syndesmosis Injury
- 10% of all ankle ligament injuries include partial tear of anterior syndesmosis
- Mechanism of injury: internal rotation of tibia on fixed everted foot
- Usually unable to bear weight
- Squeeze test: compressing tibia-fibula at midcalf causes pain at distal syndesmosis
- External rotation of foot causes pain
- Cotton test: side-to-side motion of talus in mortise indicates syndesmotic instability
- Fibular drawer: increased distal fibular translation anteriorly and/or posteriorly and elicits pain
- Check external rotation stress XRs in plantarflexion and dorsiflexion (may require sedation)
- Bone scan or magnetic resonance imaging (MRI) if too painful for stress XR
- Treat in non–weight-bearing cast
- Recovery significantly longer than with ankle sprain only
- Failed conservative treatment can be managed surgically with one to two screws across syndesmosis

Midfoot Sprain
- TMT, intertarsal, or midtarsal joints
- Stiff-soled shoe helpful for mild sprains
- Beware of Lisfranc sprain or fracture: perform weight-bearing and/or abduction stress XRs (may require sedation) if suspected
    - CT scan may show bony injury, displacement, or avulsion fracture at insertion of Lisfranc ligament
    - MRI can aid in assessment of suspected ligamentous injury
- Stable, nondisplaced midfoot sprain treated with cast, non–weight bearing for 6 wk
- Lisfranc fracture or unstable ligamentous injury treated with open reduction and internal fixation (ORIF) of unstable joints
- Some surgeons advocate immediate fusion of unstable joints after Lisfranc injury

Sinus Tarsi Syndrome
- Pain and tenderness over sinus tarsi
- Interosseous talocalcaneal ligament, which is in sinus tarsi, can be injured with lateral ankle sprain (ATFL/CFL)
- Treat like ankle sprain
- Repeated local injections can be helpful

Recommended Readings

Brodsky AR, et al. An analysis of outcome measures following the Broström-Gould procedure for chronic lateral ankle instability. Foot Ankle Int 2005; 26(10):816–819.

Broström L. Sprained ankles VI: surgical treatment of "chronic" ligament ruptures. Acta Chir Scand 1966; 132:551–565.

Chrisman OD, Snook GA. Reconstruction of lateral ligament tears of the ankle: an experimental study and clinical evaluation of seven patients treated by a new modification of the Elmslie procedure. J Bone Joint Surg Am 1969; 51:904–912.

Gould N. Repair of lateral ligament of ankle. Foot Ankle 1987; 8:55–58.

Hamilton WG, et al. The modified Broström procedure for lateral ankle instability. Foot Ankle 1993; 14:1–7.

Myerson MS. Foot and Ankle Disorders, Vol. 2. Philadelphia: WB Saunders; 2000:1399–1419.

Richardson EG. Orthopaedic Knowledge Update: Foot and Ankle 3. Rosemont, IL: American Academy of Orthopaedic Surgeons; 2003:103–111.

Snook GA, et al. Long-term results of the Chrisman-Snook operation for reconstruction of the lateral ligaments of the ankle. J Bone Joint Surg Am 1985; 67:1–7.

Thompson MC, Mormino MA. Injury to tarsometatarsal joint complex. J Am Acad Orthop Surg 2003; 11:260–267.

ACHILLES TENDON DISORDERS

– Includes paratenonitis, tendinosis, and rupture
– 15% ruptures with prior tendinosis
– 75% in sports (running MC) in age 30–40 yo
– Male-to-female ratio: 5:1
– Most common site 4 cm proximal to insertion (low vascularity, watershed area)

History

– Increase in training intensity often present
– Rupture may or may not be preceded by tendonitis/pain
– Often hear pop and experience acute posterior ankle pain with tendon rupture

Physical Examination

– Paratenonitis is characterized by swelling, pain, warmth, and tenderness
– Tendinosis is tendon degeneration and can be painless
  – May coexist with paratenonitis
  – May have palpable nodules
– Acute onset of pain with palpable nodule may represent partial tear
– Weakness of dorsiflexion, inability to heel rise
– Thompson squeeze test positive
– Palpable defect, swelling, and tenderness

Imaging

– Radiographs may be negative
– May see avulsion fracture of calcaneus or incongruity of tendon shadow on lateral view with tendon rupture
– Loss of Kager triangle on lateral XR highly suggestive of Achilles tear
  – Normally, well-defined triangle formed by posterior tibia, Achilles tendon, and calcaneus
– Ultrasound is inexpensive, allows dynamic testing, and is valuable in evaluating tendon thickness and gap size
– MRI aids in evaluating partial tears and chronic degeneration

Treatment

Paratenonitis

– Mainstay is nonoperative treatment:
  – Immobilization (23 hr/day for 10 days in CAM walker boot)
  – Ice
  – NSAIDs
  – Heel lift, cushioned shoes, or orthotics may help after period of immobilization
  – Stretching and PT for tight heel cord
  – Steroid injections not recommended
  – May inject local anesthetic to free adhesions (brisement)
– Surgery is indicated only for resistant cases
  – Medial longitudinal incision used
  – Thickened paratenon is débrided, taking care to preserve blood supply to tendon

Tendinosis

– Mainstay is nonoperative treatment
– Treated similar to paratenonitis
– For resistant cases, can perform débridement of thickened paratenon and diseased tendon
  – Tendon is split longitudinally; degenerative areas are débrided
  – Tendon is repaired with nonabsorbable sutures
  – Weight bearing allowed in postop boot, which is used for 2–4 wk
  – Early ROM is important

Tendon Rupture

– Nonoperative treatment
  – Cast or boot with elevated heel that is slowly lowered to neutral over 6–8 wk, at which time ROM is begun
  – Indicated for older, sedentary patients
  – Rerupture rates 8%–39% (therefore, surgical treatment is often preferred, with rerupture of 0%–2%)
– Operative treatment
  – Indicated if tendon ends not apposed at 20 degrees of plantarflexion on ultrasound
  – Relative indication in younger active patients

- Medial longitudinal incision used over defect
- Tendon ends are repaired with modified Bunnell technique or Krakow (stronger)
- Immobilize in cast or boot for 6–8 wk; elite athletes may start ROM earlier
- Resistance exercises started at 8–10 wk, running at 4–6 mo
- Most common complication of surgical repair is wound breakdown
- Percutaneous repair is weaker and risks injury to adjacent neurovascular structures
- V-Y lengthening for 2- to 3-cm gap between ends
- Turned-down tendon flap or FDL/FHL tendon augment for chronic rupture with gap >3 cm

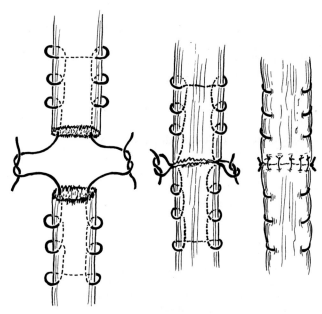

Repair of an acute Achilles tendon rupture. (From Hansen ST. Functional Reconstruction of the Foot and Ankle. Philadelphia: Lippincott Williams & Wilkins; 2000.)

Recommended Readings

Jarvinen TA, et al. Achilles tendon disorders: etiology and epidemiology. Foot Ankle Clin 2005; 10:293–308.

Khan RJ, et al. Treatment of acute Achilles tendon ruptures: a meta-analysis of randomized, controlled trials. J Bone Joint Surg Am 2005; 87:2202–2210.

Myerson MS. Achilles tendon ruptures. Instr Course Lect 1999; 48:219–230.

Myerson MS. Foot and Ankle Disorders, Vol. 2. Philadelphia: WB Saunders; 2000:1367–1398.

Myerson MS, McGarvey WC. Disorders of the Achilles tendon insertion and Achilles tendonitis. Instr Course Lect 1999; 48:211–218.

Richardson EG. Orthopaedic Knowledge Update: Foot and Ankle 3. Rosemont, IL: American Academy of Orthopaedic Surgeons; 2003:91–102.

Therman H. Treatment of Achilles tendon ruptures. Foot Ankle Clin 1999; 4:773–787.

HAGLUND DEFORMITY

- Bony prominence on superolateral aspect of posterior calcaneal tuberosity
- Most common in women 15–30 yo
- May coincide with retrocalcaneal bursitis
- Etiology is posterior heel inflammation caused by mechanical irritation from shoe wear; less common is trauma to apophysis during childhood

History and Physical Examination

- Diagnosis is clinical
- Posterior heel pain with activity
- Worse with running up hill or push-off
- Tenderness, erythema, and swelling over Achilles tendon insertion
- May have palpable bony prominence
- Differential diagnosis includes retrocalcaneal bursitis and Achilles tendonitis and is difficult to differentiate

Imaging

- AP, lateral, and oblique radiographs of foot and ankle
- May reveal long calcaneus or posterior "beak" near Achilles insertion
- Many radiographic measurements described to evaluate posterior calcaneus, but none has been shown to aid in diagnosis of Haglund deformity
  - Philip-Fowler angle is angle between line drawn from anterior tubercle to medial process of plantar tuberosity and line along posterosuperior prominence at Achilles insertion; value >75 degrees is diagnostic

Nonoperative Treatment

- Treat same as retrocalcaneal bursitis or Achilles tendonitis
- Ice, NSAIDs
- Shoe modification (heel lift, open-backed shoe)
- Physical therapy not helpful
- Steroid injections contraindicated

Operative Treatment

- Indication for surgery is continued pain refractory to conservative measures
- Results of surgery are mixed; reserve for severe refractory cases
- Complications include continued pain, stiffness, and nerve injury

Ostectomy

- Short vertical, lateral incision between Achilles tendon and sural nerve
- Excise bony prominence (large resection not necessary)
- May excise bursa if indicated

Calcaneal Osteotomy
- Indicated for abnormal calcaneal shape (long calcaneus, high angle of calcaneal inclination)

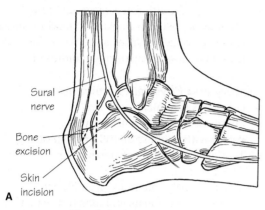

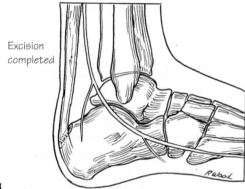

Lateral radiograph demonstrating Haglund deformity. (From Hansen ST. Functional Reconstruction of the Foot and Ankle. Philadelphia: Lippincott Williams & Wilkins; 2000.)

Recommended Readings
Myerson MS. Foot and Ankle Disorders, Vol. 2. Philadelphia: WB Saunders; 2000:1368–1398.
Myerson MS, McGarvey W. Disorders of the insertion of the Achilles tendon and Achilles tendonitis. J Bone Joint Surg Am 1998; 80:1814–1824.

PERONEAL TENDON DISLOCATION

- PB has more muscle distally and more anterior at lateral malleolus (shorter one has more muscle and faces hard rock)
- Peroneus longs (PL) is more lateral
- They share one sheath
- Peroneus quartus—anomalous muscle with muscle most distally
- Os peroneum in PL in 5% of people
- Sudden forceful dorsiflexion of inverted foot with reflex contracture of peroneals
- Most commonly caused by skiing injury

- Tender behind fibula
- Active dorsiflexion of plantarflexed and everted foot > subluxation
- I—"Bankart," where superior retinaculum is intact but tendons slide over cartilage ridge "labrum" and into false pouch between lateral fibula and retinaculum
- II—anterior tear of retinaculum
- III—avulsion fracture off posterior fib
- IV—posterior tear of retinaculum

Treatment
- Find and fix all pathoanatomical features, including débridement and repair of longitudinal tendon tears
- Difficult to tell what pathology is preop

Acute
- Avulsion of periosteal attachment of sheath and superior retinaculum
- Repair avulsion directly
- If seen acutely, short leg cast 6 wk with tendons reduced

Chronic
- Associated with longitudinal tears of PB
- May require:
  - Deepening fibular groove
  - Fascia to create new retinaculum
  - Fibular bone block
  - Rerouting tendons through fibula

Recommended Readings
Kollias SL. Fibular grooving for recurrent peroneal tendon subluxation. Am J Sports Med 1997; 25:329–335.
Oden RR. Tendon injuries about the ankle resulting from skiing. Clin Orthop 1987; (216):63–69.

PES PLANUS

Incidence/Natural History
- Flatfoot standard in infants and children, normal biological variant
- Typically flexible, asymptomatic
- Natural history usually asymptomatic in adulthood
- Incidence 8.6% in children with footwear versus 2.8% in children without

Pathoanatomy
- Major component calcaneus valgus, superior articular surface tilted medially with talus rotated medially and plantar
- Talar head prominent medially
- Subluxation between talus and navicular; navicular and cuneiform
- Stretching of medial ligamentous complex of talonavicular joint

Etiology
- Congenital vertical talus, tarsal coalition, skewfoot, accessory navicular

Clinical History
- Most children flexible, nonpainful flatfoot
- Note age of walking, family history, sports limitations
- Shoe wear patterns
- History of ankle sprains

Physical Examination
- Examine arch sitting and standing
- Rule out Achilles contracture
- Forefoot mobility/deformity
- Tiptoe may reconstitute arch—posterior tibialis
- Pattern of shoe wear

Radiography
- Unnecessary for asymptomatic flatfoot
- AP/lateral weight-bearing feet
- Standing AP ankle if foot in extreme valgus
- AP talocalcaneal angle >35 degrees—heel valgus

Treatment
- No proven benefit of orthotics or custom shoes
- Accessory navicular—excise if symptomatic and not responsive to conservative measures
- Surgical treatment of flexible flatfoot rare, only when medial foot pain despite conservative care
- Soft tissue procedures—Achilles lengthening, Durham procedure: transfer posterior tibialis with elevation of long ligamentous and capsular flap
- Bony procedures—calcaneal osteotomy for extreme calcaneal valgus, Evans procedure for calcaneal lengthening, medial cuneiform opening wedge osteotomy to correct forefoot adductus, talar neck osteotomy for severe structural deformities
- Arthrodesis—indicated in rigid flatfeet, patients with neuromuscular conditions

Recommended Readings
Caldwell GD. Surgical correction of relaxed flatfoot by the Durham flatfoot plasty. Clin Orthop 1953; 2:221–226.
Gould N. Evaluation of hyperpronation and pes planus in adults. Clin Orthop 1983; (181):37–45.
Rao UB, et al. The influence of footwear on the prevalence of flat foot: a survey of 2300 children. J Bone Joint Surg Br 1992; 74(4):525–527.

FLATFOOT IN ADULTS

Introduction
- 10%–25% incidence in general population, generally asymptomatic
- Congenital or acquired
- Lack requirements for normal arch dynamics

Anatomy
- Major medial longitudinal arch—calcaneus, talus, navicular; medial, middle, and lateral cuneiforms; first, second, and third MTs
- Spring ligament complex—important static component of medial longitudinal arch stability
    - Superomedial calcaneonavicular ligament
    - Inferior calcaneonavicular ligament
    - Tibioligamentous portion of superficial deltoid
- Plantar fascia—originates from plantar calcaneus and inserts on plantar forefoot
    - "Windlass effect" creates arch in gait
    - Medial, lateral, central components
    - Central component most important in arch pathology
- Long plantar ligament—anterior tuberosity of inferior calcaneus and inserts onto bases of second and third MTs
- Dynamics structures
    - Posterior tibial tendon—inserts on navicular tuberosity, across cuneiform and cuboid, medial MT bases; most powerful inverter of foot
    - Tibialis anterior, peroneus longus and brevis, gastrocsoleus muscles—antagonists to tibialis posterior
    - Intrinsic musculature of foot
- Theory of arch maintenance
    - Truss theory
    - Curved beam theory

Pathology
- Theory of primary static element failure followed by dynamic elements
- Failure of plantar fascia or other key soft tissue component leading to flattening of medial longitudinal arch
- Disruption or laxity of soft tissue restraints leads to uncoupling of tarsal bones
- Dynamic imbalance leading to posterior tibialis insufficiency as talocalcaneonavicular complex loses stiffness
- Peroneus brevis becomes deforming force along with Achilles tendon leading to hindfoot valgus and late findings of chronically subluxed joints of hindfoot and midfoot

Etiology
- Posterior tibial tendon insufficiency—most common, females 45–65 yo
- Long-standing idiopathic flatfeet

- Rigid flatfeet as result of tarsal coalition, congenital vertical talus, subtalar disease
- Degenerative/inflammatory arthritides
- Posttraumatic
- Soft tissue injuries
- Neuropathic—diabetic, spinal cord injuries, Hansen disease

Differential Diagnosis
- Subfibulare impingement
- Sinus tarsi syndrome

Physical Examination
- Forefoot abduction
- Hindfoot valgus
- Medial navicular sag
- Prominent medial malleolus
- "Too many toes sign"—from behind, see more lateral toes on involved side
- Difficulty with repetitive heel rise
- Tenderness over posterior tibial tendon (most commonly, just distal to medial malleolus), sinus tarsi, deltoid ligament, spring ligament
- Achilles tightness, contracture

Radiographs
- Weight-bearing AP/lateral views
- Perialar lateral subluxation
- Loss of talus/first MT alignment
- Sag talonavicular joint and/or naviculocuneiform joint
- Decreased calcaneal pitch
- Tibiotalar subluxation (must rule out)
- MRI—degeneration of posttibial tendon

Posttibial Tendon Insufficiency Clinical Staging
- Stage 1—tenosynovitis or tendonitis, no loss of single limb heel rise strength; normal radiographs; MRI: possible edema, intrasubstance degeneration
- Stage 2—tendon elongation, flexible planovalgus posture; radiographs increased lateral talocalcaneal angle, decreased calcaneal pitch, uncovered talar head; MRI: tendon degeneration/discontinuity, spring ligament changes
- Stage 3—fixed deformity; radiographs perialar subluxation, plantarflexed talus, secondary degenerative changes subtalar and transverse tarsal joints
- Stage 4—fixed deformity with valgus angulation of talus

Treatment
- Stage 1—nonoperative usually successful, short leg walking cast, arch support with medial heel wedge, ankle stirrup brace, NSAIDs; surgical intervention if symptoms persist or recur within 3 mo: tendon decompression and débridement, tenolysis, possible tendon augmentation with FDL or FHL
- Stage 2—nonoperative for poor surgical candidates: shoe modification with arch support, high-top shoe, offset medial sole, reinforced medial counter, medial heel wedge, UCBL orthosis; surgical options:
  - Tendon débridement and shortening—only if limited area of degeneration and attenuation without frank rupture
  - Jahss/Shereff—excision of degenerated tendon, augmentation with FDL
  - FDL transfer with spring ligament repair—most common soft tissue procedure, FDL transfer to navicular, spring ligament repair pants over vest technique
  - FDL transfer with medial displacement calcaneal osteotomy—indicated in patient where there's concern for loss of correction with soft tissue reconstruction alone
  - Lateral column lengthening with soft tissue reconstruction—indicated in patients with lateral perialar subluxation, hindfoot valgus, and subfibulare impingement and laterally based hindfoot pain; FDL transfer, spring ligament repair, lateral wedge into calcaneocuboid joint
  - Spring ligament reconstruction
    - Rerouting peroneus longus
    - Cobb procedure—reroute half of distal anterior tibial tendon
- Stage 3—nonoperative: custom ankle-foot orthotic (AFO); operative: triple arthrodesis
- Stage 4—nonoperative: AFO; operative: pantalar arthrodesis

Recommended Readings

Deland JT. The adult acquired flatfoot and spring ligament complex: pathology and implications for treatment. Foot Ankle Clin 2001; 6(1):129–135.

Evans D. Calcaneo-valgus deformity. J Bone Joint Surg Br 1975; 57(3):270–278.

Gazdag AR. Rupture of the posterior tibial tendon: evaluation of injury of the spring ligament and clinical assessment of tendon transfer and ligament repair. J Bone Joint Surg Am 1997; 79(5):675–681.

Helal B. Cobb repair for tibialis posterior tendon rupture. J Foot Surg 1990; 29(4):349–352.

Jahss MH. Spontaneous rupture of the tibialis posterior tendon: clinical findings, tenographic studies, and a new technique of repair. Foot Ankle 1982; 3(3):158–166.

Kitaoka HB. Stability of the arch of the foot. Foot Ankle Int 1997; 18(10):644–648.

Mann R. Phasic activity of intrinsics muscles of foot. J Bone Joint Surg Am 1964; 46:469–481.

Mann RA. Rupture of the posterior tibial tendon causing flat foot: surgical treatment. J Bone Joint Surg Am 1985; 67(4):556–561.

POSTERIOR TIBIAL TENDON DYSFUNCTION (PTTD)

- Most common form causes adult acquired flatfoot
- Degenerative tendinosis in middle-age female
- Longitudinal tears 14 mm proximal to insertion where it is less vascular
- Posterior tibial tendon has only 1 cm excursion
- Unable to be repaired because degenerative
- Can be associated with avulsion fracture off accessory navicular
- Associated with obese, pes planus, women

Anatomy

- Posterior tendon arises from tibia, fibula, and IO membrane
- Comes around groove on medial malleolus and inserts into navicular
- Sends bands to cuneiforms, MT 2–4, and sustentaculum tali
- Initiates hindfoot inversion during midstance gait, bringing hindfoot to neutral and allowing lateral Achilles tendon best mechanical advantage to plantarflex
- Controls transverse tarsal joints and thus flexibility
- Deformity due to unopposed peroneus brevis
- Talonavicular joint capsule, calcaneal-navicular spring ligament, and deltoid ligaments are also involved in arch loss

Diagnosis

- Usually clinical
- Medial pain along tendon, shoeing problem
- Lateral impingement between calcaneus and fibula
- "Too many toes" from abduction of midfoot
- Hindfoot excess valgus, medial arch collapse
- Unable to single heel rise
- May vault with Achilles to compensate in tiptoeing
- Test inversion strength of everted, plantarflexed foot (to eliminate tibialis anterior)
- Hindfoot equinus usually due to gastrocnemius muscle only and not entire gastrocsoleus complex

Radiography

- Weight-bearing AP and lateral of foot and ankle
- Hindfoot short from subtalar joint collapse
- Talus plantarflexed, collapse of talonavicular joint
- Talo—first MT should be 0 degrees in AP and lateral
- Compare inferior portion of medial cuneiform to inferior base of fifth MT to assess arch collapse
- Navicular subluxed laterally with midfoot abduction
- Talar head uncovered

PTTD Staging

Stage I

(Johnson & Strom, 1989)

- No deformity
- Pain along tendon
- Gastrocnemius may be contracted
- Immobilization, NSAIDs, brace × 3 mo
- Débridement, tenosynovectomy relieves pain
- Consider FDL transfer if tendon degenerated

Stage II

- Dynamic flexible deformity
- Tendon torn, elongated
- Limb weak, unable to tiptoe in single stance
- Heel valgus
- Midfoot pronates
- Forefoot abducts
- Subtalar joint flexible
- Shoe modification—medial arch
- UCBL, articulated corrective custom molded AFO, Arizona
- Posterior tibial tendon reconstruction with FDL transfer and medializing calcaneal osteotomy or lateral column lengthening, ± spring (calc-navic) ligament imbrication
- Tendon transfer alone relieves pain but does not correct deformity

Stage III

- Fixed hindfoot deformity
  - Talonavicular joint unreducible
- Fixed forefoot pronation deformity
- Arthrosis evident
- ± Lateral pain
- Isolated talonavicular fusion, subtalar fusion ± FDL transfer, double, or triple arthrodesis with heel cord lengthening
- Isolated talonavicular fusion insufficient if lateral impingement pain
- Custom molded AFO if low demand

Stage IV

- Ankle involvement—valgus tilt
- Tibiocalcaneal or pantalar fusion

Recommended Readings

Deland JT. Posterior Tibial Tendon Dysfunction in Clinical Orthopedics. Philadelphia: Lippincott Williams & Wilkins; 1999:883–890.

Shereff MJ. Treatment of ruptured posterior tibial tendon with direct repair and FDL tenodesis. Foot Ankle Clin 1997; 2:281–296.

Reference

Johnson KA, Strom DE. Tibialis posterior tendon dysfunction. Clin Orthop 1989; (239):196–206.

TALUS OSTEOCHONDRITIS DISSECANS

- Most commonly due to trauma; other differential diagnoses: DJD, AVN, endocrine
- 10% bilateral without trauma
- Medial more common than lateral
- Medial usually nondisplaced, cup shaped, deeper, posterior (possible inversion plantarflexion external rotation mechanism)
- Lateral usually traumatic as cause (inversion dorsiflexion force can create this in cadavers), wafer shaped, displaced, anterior
- Radiographs often normal or subtle
  - Mortise in plantarflexion to view posterior
  - Mortise in dorsiflexion to view anterior
- MRI if diagnosis unknown
  - MRI can predict fragment stability
- CT if diagnosis known, defines bone better
  - Scan in coronal and axial, no reconstructions

Berndt and Harty Classification System

(Berndt and Hard, 1959)
- I—Small compression fractures
- II—Incomplete avulsion
- III—Complete avulsion without displacement
- IV—Complete avulsion, displaced
- Plain x-ray findings do not correlate with findings on scope, so treatment should be based on actual findings

CT-Based Classification System

(Ferkel & Sgaglione, 1993–1994)
- I—Cystic lesion within dome, intact cartilage; may be able to graft from below
- IIA—Cyst communicates with dome surface
- IIB—Open lesion with overlying nondisplaced fragment
- III—Nondisplaced lesion with lucency, similar to IIB
- IV—Displaced fragment
- I, II—Conservative first (short leg cast, PWB 6 wk)
- Steroid injection shown not to help
- Delay in surgery for up to 1 yr does not compromise surgical results
- III, IV—Surgery, except in children (they get conservative therapy first)
  - Scope
  - Drilling of intact lesions
  - Débride detached lesions
  - Fix if bony attachment, acute, young
  - Bone grafting if necessary
- OCD with lateral instability
  - In acute, OCD treated surgically, instability treated conservatively
- In chronic, OCD treated first because requires postop motion; lateral reconstruction done later if needed because requires immobilization

Recommended Reading

Loomer R, et al. Osteochondral lesions of the talus. Am J Sports Med 1993; 21:13–19.

References

Berndt AL, Harty M. Transchondral fractures (osteochondritis dissecans) of the talus. J Bone Joint Surg Am 1959; 41-A:988–1020.

Ferkel RD, Sgaglione NA. Arthroscopic treatment of osteochondral lesions of the talus: long term results. Orthop Trans 1993–1994; 17:1011.

Diabetes and Neurologic Disorders

CHARCOT ARTHROPATHY

Etiology

- Most common cause is leprosy worldwide
- Most common cause is DM in United States
- Tabes dorsalis (70% lower extremity [LE], 20% lumbosacral [LS] spine)
- Syringomyelia—most common cause of upper extremity (UE) neuropathic joint
  - Order C-spine MRI if UE involvement
  - Syrinx disrupts decussating pain and temperature fibers of spinothalamic tract
- Myelomeningocele
- Occurs as result of repetitive loading of neuropathic joint (no protective sensation)

History and Physical Examination

- Present with painless, swollen, red, warm joint ± deformity
- With elevation for 2 hr, erythema and swelling should resolve (differentiates from infection)
- Consider ligament disruption or fracture-dislocation
- Absence of fever, high white blood cell (WBC) count, high erythrocyte sedimentation rate (ESR), and presence of normal glucose rule out infection
- Semmes-Weinstein monofilament is most accurate test for sensation
  - Protective sensation is present if patient can feel 5.07 Semmes-Weinstein
- Most have good perfusion with ankle-brachial index (ABI) >0.6

Imaging

- Atrophic or hypertrophic pattern
- Bony fragmentation, fracture, dislocation

- Both osteomyelitis and Charcot have bone edema on MRI
- Simultaneous indium and technetium polyphosphate scan can diagnose infection

Staging
(Eichenholtz, 1966)
- Based on clinical and XR findings

I—Acute/Dissolution
- Inflammation, edema, erythema
- Bony fragmentation
- Treatment: elevation, rest × 6–8 wk; then total contact cast for weight bearing when swelling and warmth decreased

II—Subacute/Coalescence
- Reparative process begins
- Decreasing inflammation
- Coalescence and resorption of bony fragments
- Stabilize with removable boot or short leg cast
- Avoid surgery during this fragmented stage due to tenuous fixation

III—Chronic/Resolution
- Inflammation resolved
- Bone consolidated
- Distribute force evenly with custom orthoses or brace (AFO)

Treatment
- Gold standard for majority of Charcot fractures, dislocations, and ulcers is total contact casting followed by bracing/orthoses
- Operative indications include chronic recurrent ulcers, joint instability, fracture-dislocations compromising soft tissues, and chronic pain (rare)
- Can treat in acute stage with ORIF
- Reconstructive surgery in subacute or chronic stage indicated only in unstable deformed foot when cast, brace, or orthosis has failed to prevent recurrent ulcerations
- Reconstruction involves open realignment and fusion
- Success of surgery depends on:
  - Minimal soft tissue swelling
  - Bone that can support hardware
  - Adequate vascularity
  - Absence of infection
- Stable pseudoarthrosis is acceptable result
- Patients with fused ankles and/or hindfoot should be protected with AFOs/rocker bottoms to prevent tibial stress fractures

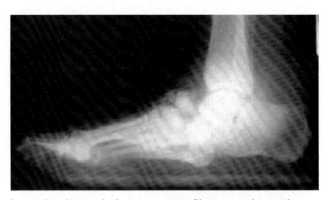

Lateral radiograph demonstrating Charcot arthropathy. (From Chapman MW, et al. Chapman's Orthopaedic Surgery. Philadelphia: Lippincott Williams & Wilkins; 2001.)

Recommended Readings
Brodsky JW. Management of Charcot joints of the foot and ankle in diabetes. Semin Arthroplasty 1992; 3:58.
Johnson JE. Operative treatment of neuropathic arthropathy of the foot and ankle. J Bone Joint Surg Am 1998; 80:1700–1709.

Reference
Eichenholtz SN. Charcot Joints. Springfield, IL: Charles C Thomas; 1966.

DIABETIC FOOT ULCERS AND INFECTION
- 15% people >65 yo have DM
- Foot infections affect 20% of diabetics
- Risk of amputation increases with age, duration, history of proteinuria or retinopathy, and smoking, and in males
- Up to 15% diabetics require some amputation
- Neuropathy in 5%–60% diabetics

Etiology
- Retina, kidneys, and nerves do not require insulin transport pump
- In nerves, excess glucose converted to sorbitol, which slows axonal transport
- Nerve damaged by sorbitol buildup, not from microvascular disease
- Ulcer occurs in neuropathy with abnormal or repetitive loading on insensate foot
- Neuropathy can be sensory, motor, and/or autonomic
- Occurs distal > proximal (stocking glove)
- Loss of protective sensation enables abnormal or repetitive stresses to injury tissues
  - 5.07 Semmes-Weinstein monofilament threshold for protective sensation

- Motor neuropathy leads to intrinsic dysfunction, claw, or hammer toe deformities and resultant abnormal contact pressures
  - Claw/hammer toe has MTP hyperextension with high pressures on plantar surface
  - PIP flexion contracture may lead to dorsal ulceration
- Autonomic dysfunction leads to decreased sweat and dry splitting and fissuring
- Other deformity, such as bunion, bunionette, Charcot arthropathy, or even callosities/corns, can lead to abnormal contact pressures
- Tight heel cord increases pressure on forefoot
- Vasculopathy (low O_2 tension) usually not cause of diabetic ulcers but prevents subsequent healing
- Toe pressure >45 mm associated with 85% healing, <40 mm with 0% healing
- Transcutaneous pO_2 <20 predicts poor wound healing

Classification
- Brodsky's depth-ischemia system (number for depth and letter for ischemia)
  - Depth grading
    - Grade 0: at risk
    - Grade 1: superficial ulcer, no infection
    - Grade 2: deep ulcer with exposed tendon or joint, with or without infection
    - Grade 3: extensive ulceration with exposed bone or deep infection
  - Ischaemia grading
    - Grade A: no ischemia
    - Grade B: ischemia, no gangrene
    - Grade C: partial gangrene
    - Grade D: complete foot gangrene

Nonoperative Treatment
- Débridement
  - Must débride callus, eschar, and necrotic tissue down to clean base
  - Often can be done in office without anesthesia
  - Can augment with wet-to-dry dressings or enzymatic agents
- After débridement, nonoperative treatment will usually achieve wound healing
- Strict non–weight bearing with dressing changes
- Shoe modifications
- Total contact casting takes pressure off area and prevents shear around ulcer
  - For superficial ulcer without infection
  - More success with forefoot ulcer than heel ulcers
  - Apply well-molded cast with little padding, ankle at 5 degrees dorsiflexion, knee at 90 degrees
  - 90% healing of low-grade ulcers

- Topical adjunctive agents: dimethyl sulfoxide, Dakin solution (sodium hypochlorite), acetic acid, hydrogen peroxide, insulin, and Betadine
- Some advocate hyperbaric oxygen

Surgical Treatment
- Indicated for refractory or recurrent ulcers
- Correct deformity and abnormal pressures
- Tendon releases and/or soft tissue procedures can be used to correct toe deformities
- Metatarsal condylectomy, head resection, or dorsiflexion osteotomy can treat plantar ulcer under MT heads
- Joint arthroplasty/resections for ulcers about PIP joints of lesser toes or IP of hallux
- Heel cord lengthening can decrease forefoot pressures
- Arthrodesis of ankle, hindfoot, or midfoot can be used to correct severe deformity
- Ostectomy can be used to remove prominent portion of bone; best done after ulcer heals to decrease risk of infection
- Skin coverage with split-thickness skin graft (STSG) or rotational flap has high failure rate and is rarely indicated

INFECTION
- Diabetics have increased risk for infection
  - High serum glucose is nutrition for bacteria
  - Abnormal polymorphonuclear leukocyte (PMN) chemotaxis and phagocytosis
  - Often have poor blood flow to area
- Usually polymicrobial: *Clostridium perfringens*, *Staphylococcus epidermidis*, anaerobes, gram-negative rods

Diagnosis
- Usually evident on examination: drainage, erythema, pus, foul odor
- Some advocate bone scan and/or indium-labeled white cell scan to diagnose osteomyelitis and to differentiate from soft tissue infection
- Include Charcot neuroarthropathy in differential
  - Usually can differentiate between them by brief period of elevation; in Charcot joint, erythema subsides with elevation, unlike infection

Nonoperative Treatment
- Broad-spectrum antibiotics
- Indicated only for minor cellulitis with no systemic effects
- Contraindicated in osteomyelitis, abscess, fasciitis, or systemic infection

Operative Treatment

- Surgical irrigation and débridement of necrotic tissue
- Open and débride sinus tracts and infected tendon sheaths
- Wounds usually left open to heal by secondary intention
- Broad-spectrum antibiotics for 6 wk in osteomyelitis
- Amputation may be necessary
  - In hallux, try to preserve base of proximal phalanx to maintain windlass mechanism
  - Preserve base of lesser toe proximal phalanges to prevent toe migration
  - Remove infected sesamoids
  - If more than two MT heads must be removed, resect all
  - Transmetatarsal amputation when first MT head is involved with two others
  - Lengthen tight heel cord with any of these amputations
  - Midfoot osteomyelitis (OM) treated with débridement versus Chopart's amputation (transverse tarsal joint) with heel cord lengthening
  - Calcaneal OM can be treated with débridement versus total calcanectomy
  - Consider below-knee amputation (BKA) or above-knee amputation (AKA) for nonambulatory or ill patient or after failure of lesser amputations
- See Amputations section for more information

Recommended Readings

Guyton GP, Saltzman CL. The diabetic foot: basic mechanisms of disease. J Bone Joint Surg Am 2001; 83:1083–1096.
Myerson MS. Foot and Ankle Disorders, Vol. 2. Philadelphia: WB Saunders; 2000:411–435.

AMPUTATIONS

Indications

- Overall, 80% done for vascular insufficiency
- Also performed for trauma, malignancy, congenital defect, or infection
- In trauma, Mangled Extremity Severity Score (MESS) can aid in deciding amputation versus limb salvage
  - Score based on four groups:
    1. Skeletal/soft tissue injury
       - Low energy (1 point)
       - Medium (2)
       - High (3)
       - Massive crush (4)
    2. Shock
       - Normotensive (0)
       - Transiently hypotensive (1)
       - Prolonged hypotension (2)
    3. Ischemia
       - None (1)
       - Mild (2)
       - Moderate (3)
       - Advanced (4)
    4. Age
       - <30 (0)
       - 31–50 (1)
       - >50 (2)
- Score of ≥7 shown to have 100% predictive value of amputation

Determination of Level

- Biological amputation level is most distal amputation with high probability of wound healing
- Ischemic index: ratio of Doppler pressure at level of amputation to brachial pressure
  - >0.5 predicts healing
  - ABI: ischemic index at ankle
- Transcutaneous partial pressure of oxygen ($TcpO_2$) is gold standard
  - Reflects oxygen delivery to area
  - >40 mm Hg predicts high rate of healing
  - <20 mm Hg predicts poor healing
- In malignancy, level is selected based on achieving adequate margins

Surgical Considerations

- Strip periosteum at level of bone cut to prevent bony overgrowth
- Attach muscles to bone end and not antagonistic muscles to optimize function
- Bury nerve end in ample soft tissue to avoid irritation
- Do not close soft tissues under tension

Toe Disarticulations

- Distal phalanx of great toe
  - FHL is shortened and its associated sesamoid is removed
  - Better function than first MP amputation
- Great toe MP disarticulation
  - Remove both sesamoids to avoid proximal displacement
  - Trim prominent crista on plantar surface of MT head
- Second MP disarticulation
  - Removes lateral support to first toe and can perpetuate bunion
  - Better to perform amputation through proximal metaphysis of MT (ray amputation) and approximate first and third rays
- Third and fourth MP disarticulation tolerated
- With fifth MP disarticulation, trim prominent lateral condyle if present

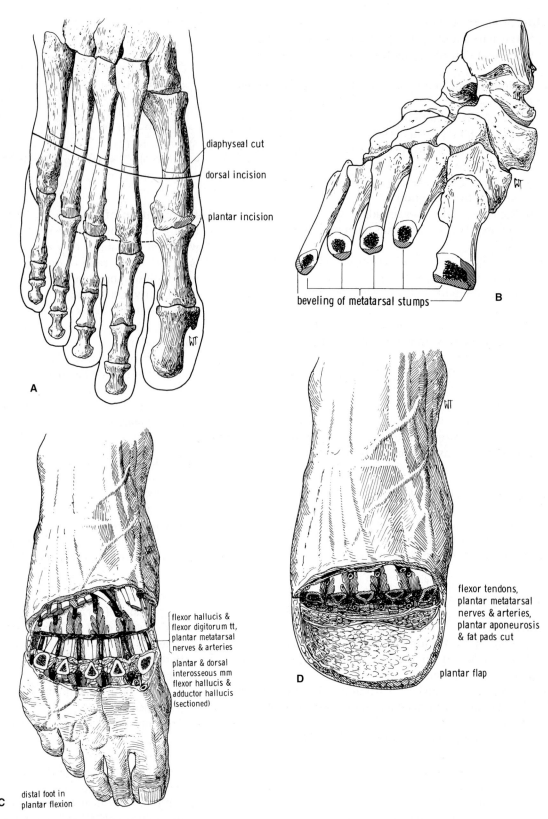

A

diaphyseal cut

dorsal incision

plantar incision

B

beveling of metatarsal stumps

C

flexor hallucis & flexor digitorum tt, plantar metatarsal nerves & arteries

plantar & dorsal interosseous mm flexor hallucis & adductor hallucis (sectioned)

distal foot in plantar flexion

D

flexor tendons, plantar metatarsal nerves & arteries, plantar aponeurosis & fat pads cut

plantar flap

Transmetatarsal amputation. (From Chapman MW, et al. Chapman's Orthopaedic Surgery. Philadelphia: Lippincott Williams & Wilkins; 2001.)

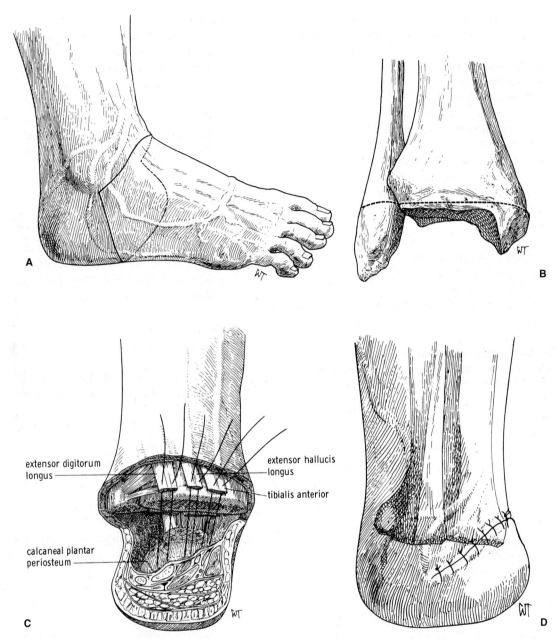

extensor digitorum
longus

extensor hallucis
longus

tibialis anterior

calcaneal plantar
periosteum

Syme amputation. (From Chapman MW, et al. Chapman's Orthopaedic Surgery.
Philadelphia: Lippincott Williams & Wilkins; 2001.)

- All five toes can be disarticulated at MP joint
- Remove cartilage and volar plate with disarticulation

Ray Amputation
- First ray:
  - Leave as much MT length as possible
  - Poor function because medial column of foot is lost
- Second to fifth rays: amputate ray at proximal metaphysis of MT

- With multiple ray amputations, cascade ray lengths so they are progressively shorter laterally to improve foot rollover with gait

Transmetatarsal Amputation
- Is an amputation across all MT diaphyses
- Consider when most of first MT or multiple lesser rays must be removed
- Bevel plantar bone ends to decrease pressure
- Angle lengths from medial to lateral to create 15-degree cascade
- Close flap dorsally

Lisfranc (Tarsometatarsal) Disarticulation
– To prevent equinus contracture, preserve insertions of:
  – Tibialis anterior
  – Peroneus longus
  – Peroneus brevis
– Leave bases of second and fifth MTs
– May lengthen gastrocnemius if tight

Chopart (Midtarsal) Disarticulation
– Through talonavicular and calcaneocuboid joints
– Transfer tibialis anterior to navicular
– Excise 2–3 cm Achilles tendon to prevent equinus contracture

Syme Ankle Disarticulation
– Through ankle joint
– Retains heel pad
– Must have posterior tibial artery to perfuse heel pad

Recommended Readings

Helfet DL, et al. Limb salvage versus amputation: preliminary results of the Mangled Extremity Severity Score. Clin Orthop 1990; 256:80–86.

Myerson MS. Foot and Ankle Disorders, Vol. 2. Philadelphia: WB Saunders; 2000:466–503.

Oishi CS, et al. The role of non-invasive vascular studies in determining levels of amputation. J Bone Joint Surg Am 1988; 70:1520–1530.

FOOT DROP

– Causes of weakness in dorsiflexion:
  – Muscle injury
  – Nerve injury
  – Lower motor neuron (LMN) disorders

Evaluation
– Assess range of motion of ankle, subtalar, and foot joints and any deformity
– Assess motor strength of all muscle groups and look for contractures or spasticity
– Consider cause of foot drop and determine if muscle strength could improve, stay same, or worsen
– Slap foot gait—cannot clear foot during swing phase and forefoot strikes ground first
  – Compensate by flexing hip and knee

Nonoperative Treatment
– Orthosis (AFO) for passively correctable foot drop
  – Can improve function and prevent tight heel cord
  – Indicated for flaccid paralysis of foot (all dorsiflexors and plantarflexors flaccid) or for patients passively correctable to neutral where improvement in weakness is expected

Operative Treatment
– Includes combination of tenodesis, tendon transfer, tendon release, osteotomy, or arthrodesis that is customized to each patient

Tenodesis
– Can be primary treatment for patients with flaccid paralysis of both dorsiflexors and plantarflexors
– Extensor tendons secured to tibia to hold foot in neutral
– Ankle is dorsiflexed to 10 degrees above neutral and MTP joints are held in neutral; if ankle dorsiflexion is limited, perform percutaneous Achilles tenotomy
– Attach tibialis anterior, EHL, and EDL to anterior tibia by scoring tibia to cause scarring between bone and tendon and secure with staples or suture anchors
– May stretch out with time requiring shortening of tendons

Tendon Transfer
– Ideally, transfer muscle that fires in phase with muscle that is being replaced
– Tendon transferred should be in line with direction of muscle pull to optimize function (no angulation of tendon)
– Posterior tibialis is most commonly used, although FHL, FDL, EHL, PL, and peroneus tertius can be used alone or in combination
– Excursion of posterior tibialis is about 2 cm compared to about 4 cm for dorsiflexors, so proper tension at transfer is essential to maximize function
– Posterior tibialis can be passed through IO membrane into anterior compartment and secured into tunnel in lateral cuneiform, as described by Hsu and Hoffer (1978)
– Determine proper tension by noting resting length and maximum length tendon can be stretched, and secure at halfway point
– Secure tendon with ankle dorsiflexed at 20 degrees (if dorsiflexion limited, lengthen Achilles)
– Deformity should be corrected by calcaneal osteotomy or, if severe, triple arthrodesis (wait 3–6 mo after fusion to transfer tendon to allow early ROM)

Arthrodesis
– Triple or pantalar arthrodesis can be used as primary treatment of foot drop
– Can be augmented with tendon transfer for muscle balancing
– Results in stiff foot with risk of arthritis in adjacent joints
– Development of deformity over time can occur, especially in patients with spasticity or muscle imbalance

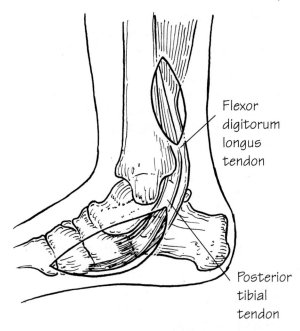

Flexor digitorum longus tendon

Posterior tibial tendon

Posterior tibial tendon transfer through intraosseous (IO) membrane to dorsum of foot. (From Hansen ST. Functional Reconstruction of the Foot and Ankle. Philadelphia: Lippincott Williams & Wilkins; 2000.)

Recommended Reading
Myerson MS. Foot and Ankle Disorders, Vol. 2. Philadelphia: WB Saunders; 2000:883–899.

Reference
Hsu JD, Hoffer MM. Posterior tibial tendon transfer anteriorly through the interosseous membrane: a modification of the technique. Clin Orthop 1978; (131):202–204.

MORTON INTERDIGITAL NEUROMA

- Not true neuroma but entrapment neuropathy with nerve perineural fibrosis and degeneration
- More common in between third and fourth because of increased thickness receiving supply from medial and lateral plantar nerves
- Increased motion between third and fourth space because first, second, and third MTs are fixed to MT-cuneiform joints and fourth and fifth MTs are fixed to more mobile cuboid
- More common in females because their shoes hyperextend MTP joint, causing excess plantarflexion of MT, which exposes nerve to increased trauma, especially if partially tethered to transverse MT ligament
- 15% bilateral
- Burning pain, radiates to digits
- Worse with high heels
- Reproducibility with palpation of intermetatarsal space

- Mulder sign—clicking with reproduction of pain with medial lateral pressure across MTs
- Radiograph with close apposition of MT heads
- Lidocaine/steroid injection for diagnosis and treatment
- Wide soft shoe, pad behind MT heads, injections help but usually not enough to wear heels

Surgery
- Dorsal incision in web space extending 3 cm proximal to level of MT heads
- Self-retainers
- Take intermetatarsal ligament
- Take nerve with neuroma proximal to MT head and distal to bifurcation
- If stump neuroma occurs after primary neurectomy, revision to shorter stump produces good results

Recommended Readings
Coughlin MJ, et al. Operative treatment of interdigital neuroma: a long term follow up study. J Bone Joint Surg Am 2001; 83:1321–1328.
Weinfeld SB, et al. Interdigital neuritis: diagnosis and treatment. J Am Acad Orthop Surg 1996; 4:328–335.

SUPERFICIAL PERONEAL NERVE (SPN)

- SPN pierces fascia at 9 cm from distal fibula
- SPN divides into medial dorsal cutaneous nerve (MDCN) and IDCN 6.5 cm proximal to tip of distal fib
- IDCN passes over retinaculum, anterior to common extensor tendon of fourth and fifth toes, then runs toward web between third and fourth toes
- MDCN passes over retinaculum, runs parallel and just lateral to EHL tendon, and divides just distal to inferior retinaculum into dorsal digital branches, ending up distally over dorsomedial aspect of hallux MTP joint

Study of the Superficial Peroneal Nerve by Blair and Botte (1994)
- 25 cadaver lower limbs
- Loupe magnification
- Three distinct branching pattern types were noted as follows.

Type A (72%)
- SPN penetrates crural fascia at 12 cm proximal to ankle joint
- Divides at 4 cm proximal to ankle joint into large medial dorsal cutaneous nerve and intermediate dorsal cutaneous nerve
- (Lateral dorsal cutaneous nerve comes form sural nerve)

Type B (16%)
- MDCN and IDCN penetrate fascia independently
- MDCN travels like SPN (penetrates 12 cm above joint)
- IDCN penetrates fascia posterior to fibula at 5.5 cm above joint, then crosses lateral to fibula at 4.5 cm above joint

Type C (12%)
- MDCN and IDCN arise separately
- MDCN travels like SPN
- IDCN penetrates fascia anterior to fibula at 5 cm above joint and courses closely to anterior border of fibula
- Note:
    - In all three branching types, MDCN was about one-half of distance from tip of lateral malleolus to medial malleolus. IDCN was one-third of that distance. If these nerves are not at these locations, look for MDCN more medially and IDCN more laterally because this tends to occur in types B and C

Reference
Blair JM, Botte MJ. Surgical anatomy of the superficial peroneal nerve in the ankle and foot. Clin Orthop 1994; (305):229–238.

TARSAL TUNNEL SYNDROME

- Canal created by flexor retinaculum
- Posterior tibial nerve runs anterior to FHL
- Just distal to medial malleolus and proximal to abductor hallucis, it divides into medial plantar, lateral plantar, and medial calcaneal nerves
- Medial and lateral plantar nerves arise from under retinaculum in 93% of people
- Medial plantar nerve runs under abductor hallucis fascia, under knot of Henry (FDL crossing plantar to FHL), gives rise to nerve between first and second and between second and third
- Lateral plantar nerve runs under abductor hallucis fascia, crosses foot superficial to quadratus plantae, and goes to web between fourth and fifth
- Nerve between third and fourth arise from medial and lateral plantar nerve
- Common digital nerve passes plantar to transverse MT ligaments before bifurcating in web spaces
- DM, hypothyroidism, pregnancy, flexor tendon synovitis, excess pronation, os trigonum
- Ganglion of tendon sheath, lipoma, exostosis, fracture fragment, enlarged venous plexus
- Diffuse plantar radicular pain
- Percussion sign
- Sensory and motor usually normal
- Diagnosis made by history, examination
- MRI to evaluate for mass effect

- Electromyography (EMG)/nerve conduction velocity (NCV) do not correlate with surgical outcome
- Best surgical response when both MRI and EMG/NCV are positive
- Arch support avoids excess pronation
- Steroid injections
- Release retinaculum distally to medial and lateral plantar nerve by releasing deep fascia of abductor hallucis

Recommended Readings
Bailie DS. Tarsal tunnel syndrome: diagnosis, surgical technique, and functional outcome. Foot Ankle Int 1998; 19: 65–72.
Sammarco GJ, et al. Outcome of surgical treatment of tarsal tunnel syndrome. Foot Ankle Int 2003; 24(2):125–131.

Arthritis

THE ARTHRITIDES

Rheumatoid Arthritis
- Affects up to 0.5%–1.5% of population
- Women 2 to 10 times more common
- Complain of morning stiffness and symmetric joint involvement, especially of small joints of hands and feet
- About half of RA patients have active foot/ankle disease
- Juvenile rheumatoid arthritis (JRA) can be monarticular, pauciarticular, or polyarticular, but foot/ankle involvement rarely disabling
- With new disease-modifying agents, severe disease is much less common
- Synovitis leads to periarticular erosions and arthrosis
    - Decreases as disease progresses, but joint destruction continues
- Can also get tenosynovitis, rheumatoid nodules, vasculitis, mononeuritis multiplex, and systemic illness
- Subtalar and midtarsal involvement leads to planovalgus foot
- Forefoot involvement includes hallux rigidus, valgus, or varus and hammer toes
- Ankle affected in up to 50%

Radiographs
- Early: periarticular osteopenia and erosions
- Late: osteophytes from secondary OA, spontaneous fusion (midfoot/hindfoot ankylosis more common than forefoot)

Nonoperative Treatment
- NSAIDs, disease-modifying drugs (DMDs)
- Physical therapy for strengthening and stretching

- Shoe modification
- Orthotics for hindfoot valgus or flatfoot
- AFO or UCBL orthosis for ankle/hindfoot deformity or instability
- Steroid injections

Operative Treatment

Ankle
- Involved in 50%
- Clinical symptoms usually greater than XR findings
- Synovitis, tenosynovitis, arthritis, and fibular stress fractures possible
- Synovitis may be treated with arthroscopic or open synovectomy
- End-stage DJD: arthrodesis versus arthroplasty

Hindfoot
- Commonly affected
- Valgus deformity from joint inflammation and subsequent ligamentous laxity
- Arthrodesis of affected joints—subtalar, talonavicular, or triple arthrodesis
- Options for treating ankle and hindfoot DJD:
  - Talectomy and tibiocalcaneal fusion
  - Ankle and subtalar fusion
  - Pantalar arthrodesis (poor functional results)

Forefoot
- Involvement common and difficult to treat effectively nonoperatively
- Wide range of possible forefoot presentations, and each case must be tailored to patient's deformity
- Standard rheumatoid foot reconstruction:
  - First MTP fusion with screws
  - Manual arthrolysis to correct lesser toe deformity
  - Lesser MTP joint resections with retrograde pinning
  - Extensor tenotomies to prevent deformity recurrence

Seronegative Spondyloarthropathy
- Includes:
  - Ankylosing spondylitis
  - Psoriatic arthritis
  - Reiter syndrome
  - Arthritis of inflammatory bowel disease
- HLA-B27 positive in 50%–90% of cases
- Possibly also an infectious etiology implicated in some cases:
  - *Salmonella* species
  - *Shigella*
  - *Yersinia*
  - *Chlamydia* species

- Musculoskeletal manifestations may include:
  - Inflammatory synovitis
  - Enthesitis (patellar, posterior tendon, Achilles, FHL, FDL)
  - Heterotopic bone formation
  - Ankylosis
  - Periostitis
  - Joint destruction and osteolysis (leads to pencil-in-cup deformity)
- Skin lesions seen with Reiter syndrome or psoriasis
- Gastrointestinal (GI) and genitourinary (GU) inflammatory disease may be present

Ankylosing Spondylitis
- Clinical manifestations include:
  - Back/neck pain
  - Stiffness and ankylosis
  - Arthritis
  - Uveitis
  - Iridocyclitis
  - Cardiovascular and renal involvement
- Foot and ankle involvement includes enthesitis and arthritis
- Treatment is largely nonoperative with NSAIDs, DMDs, and physical therapy

Psoriatic Arthritis
- Foot and ankle manifestations include:
  - Digital swelling (dactylitis)
  - Onycholysis
  - Arthritis mutilans (bony resorption leads to telescoping digits)
- Nonoperative treatment includes NSAIDs, DMDs, orthotics, and PT
- Operative treatment is usually resection arthroplasty for forefoot arthritis mutilans
  - Arthrodesis has high failure rate in these patients

Reiter Syndrome
- Triad (only present in one-third of patients with Reiter syndrome):
  - Uveitis
  - Urethritis
  - Arthritis
- Foot and ankle involvement includes bony proliferation, periostitis, and possibly spontaneous fusion
- Nonoperative treatment includes:
  - NSAIDs
  - DMDs
  - Possibly antibiotics (reactive arthritis may be secondary to bacterial infection in another location)
  - PT for stretching and ROM
  - Orthotics
- Operative treatment rarely required

Gout
- Monosodium urate crystal deposits
- Usually from high purine intake with decreased urate excretion
- Acute phase:
    - Includes severe pain, swelling, and redness
    - First MTP in 90%, can also affect subtalar joint, ankle, or tendon insertion
    - Lasts days to weeks
- Interval phase is asymptomatic
- Chronic gout is chronic arthritis secondary to crystal deposits and DJD
    - May have significant deformity
    - Tophi may occur in soft tissues and erupt through skin, causing draining ulcer
    - Hallux valgus common
- Clinical diagnosis confirmed by joint fluid analysis: needle shaped, yellow, negatively birefringent in polarized light
    - Fluid is inflammatory: high WBC count (may be >50,000) with left shift
- Serum uric acid level >7 mg/dL in men and 6 in women
- Nonoperative treatment (mainstay)
    - NSAIDs (Indocin) and colchicine for acute attack
    - Increase excretion with probenecid
    - Inhibit production with allopurinol (xanthine oxidase inhibitor)
    - Change medications that increase serum uric acid (thiazide diuretics)
- Operative treatment
    - Rarely needed, especially in acute gout
    - Arthritis and deformity can be treated with resection arthroplasty or fusion
    - Symptomatic tophi are treated with debulking

Recommended Readings

Myerson MS. Foot and Ankle Disorders, Vol. 2. Philadelphia: WB Saunders; 2000:1189–1222.

Richardson EG. Orthopaedic Knowledge Update: Foot and Ankle 3. Rosemont, IL: American Academy of Orthopaedic Surgeons; 2003:155–175.

ARTHRODESIS OF ANKLE AND HINDFOOT

- Primary indication is osteoarthrosis (cartilage degradation and subchondral bone hypertrophy) refractory to more conservative means
- Osteoarthrosis can be primary or secondary to trauma, RA, neuroarthropathy, talar avascular necrosis, or infection

Preoperative Considerations

- Assess hip and ankle for arthritis, deformity, or contracture; more proximal joints should usually be corrected first
- Assess ligamentous stability
- Assess leg lengths
- Assess contractures and muscle strength, especially in neuropathic patients; simultaneous tendon lengthening or transfer may be required
- Consider bone quality in regard to optimal fixation
- Assess all joints of foot and ankle clinically and radiographically, and select most appropriate procedure
    - Selective joint injection with lidocaine aids in assessment of their contribution to pain

Nonoperative Treatment

- NSAIDs
- Steroid injections
- Orthotics—stiff-soled or rocker-bottom shoe, wedges, AFO, or hinged ankle orthosis

Surgical Options

- Depends on patient characteristics and joints affected
- Arthroscopy
- Excision of anterior osteophytes (cheilectomy)
- Supramalleolar osteotomy
- Distraction arthroplasty
- Total ankle replacement (TAR)
- Arthrodesis of affected joints
- Contraindications to ankle/hindfoot arthrodesis:
    - Severe vasculopathy
    - Active infection

Ankle Arthrodesis
- Indications: painful, debilitating DJD of tibiotalar joint with or without deformity that is refractory to conservative treatment
- May be performed arthroscopically or through miniarthrotomy when no correction of deformity is desired; benefit is minimal soft tissue injury and high rate of fusion
- Open transfibular approach enables deformity correction, and resected fibula can be used as bone graft
- Correct position for ankle arthrodesis
    - Neutral plantarflexion
    - Valgus 0–5 degrees
    - External rotation 0–10 degrees (balance to other side)
    - Tibial crest should align with second ray
- Fixation using two to three 6.5- to 7.0-mm compression screws that are crossed in coronal and sagittal planes
- Non–weight bearing in cast for 6–8 wk

Subtalar Arthrodesis
- Indications:
    - Posttraumatic OA (often following calcaneus fracture)
    - Irreparable calcaneus fracture
    - Subtalar instability or deformity
- Use lateral incision over sinus tarsi

- Fuse joint in 5–7 degrees of valgus
  - May require bone graft laterally when correcting valgus deformity
  - May require lateral closing wedge osteotomy when correcting varus deformity
- Fixation using one to two 6.5- to 7.0-mm cannulated screws in compression, starting at calcaneal tuberosity posteriorly and aiming into talar neck

Tibiocalcaneal Arthrodesis
- Indications:
  - Severe deformity
  - Significant talar bone loss or destruction
  - Failed TAR
  - Revision after failed ankle fusion

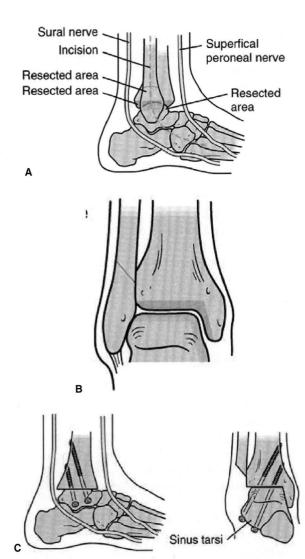

Ankle arthrodesis. (From Chapman MW, et al. Chapman's Orthopaedic Surgery. Philadelphia: Lippincott Williams & Wilkins; 2001.)

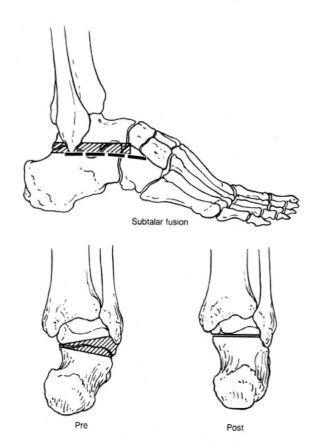

Subtalar arthrodesis. (From Chapman MW, et al. Chapman's Orthopaedic Surgery. Philadelphia: Lippincott Williams & Wilkins; 2001.)

- Anterolateral incision for joint preparation
- Fibular osteotomy can aid in correction of large deformity and provides bone graft
- Fixation with IM nail (load sharing)

Triple Arthrodesis
- Involves fusion of subtalar, TN, and CC joints
- Indications: correction of deformity or instability
- Use two incisions
  - Lateral incision accesses subtalar and calcaneocuboid joints
  - Medial incision accesses talonavicular joint
- Decorticate joints, remove bone as necessary to correct any deformity
- Correct hindfoot to 5 degrees of valgus and fix as described for subtalar fusion
- Correct transverse tarsal joint and forefoot to neutral/plantigrade

Pantalar Arthrodesis
- Indications:
  - End-stage DJD of ankle, subtalar, and Chopart joint
  - Significant instability of these joints

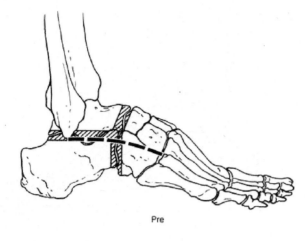

Pre

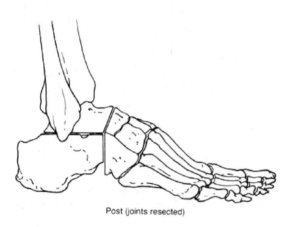

Post (joints resected)

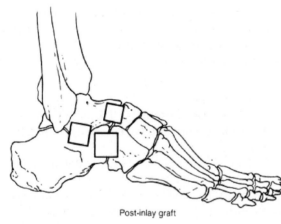

Post-inlay graft

Triple arthrodesis. (From Chapman MW, et al. Chapman's Orthopaedic Surgery. Philadelphia: Lippincott Williams & Wilkins; 2001.)

- Pantalar fusion has significant functional impairment and higher energy expenditure with gait than BKA (avoid if possible)
- Complications: include tibial stress fracture and arthritis of midfoot and forefoot joints

Recommended Readings

Myerson MS. Foot and Ankle Disorders, Vol. 2. Philadelphia: WB Saunders; 2000:1049–1058.

Richardson EG. Orthopaedic Knowledge Update: Foot and Ankle 3. Rosemont, IL: American Academy of Orthopaedic Surgeons; 2003:155–175.

ARTHRODESIS OF MIDFOOT AND FOREFOOT

First Metatarsophalangeal Joint Arthrodesis

- Indicated for hallux rigidus and salvage treatment of hallux valgus and varus
- Other surgical options include resection or interpositional arthroplasty, joint replacement, osteotomy, or débridement

Surgical Considerations

- Shape of bone cuts depends on surgeon's preference (flat, cup and cone, etc.)
- Release FHB and allow sesamoids to retract proximally or excise sesamoids to prevent painful compression under MT head
- Shoe wear preference dictates angle of dorsiflexion
- Key is balanced forefoot without abnormally high or low contact pressure on first IP joint
- Place foot on flat surface intraoperatively to find optimal MTP sagittal alignment for fusion
- Fuse in neutral supination/pronation—balance by aligning nails of toes
- Fuse in 10 degrees of valgus (never varus)
- Fixation with one to two screws, K-wires, or plate
- Simultaneous correction of metatarsus primus varus not indicated; after fusion, deforming forces are neutralized, and it should self-correct
- Heel weight bearing in postop shoe or splint
- Fusion rate 85%–100%

Complications

- Nonunion 0%–15% (depends on patient)
- Malunion with resulting pain or instability

First Interphalangeal Joint

Indications

- Instability
- Dorsal instability occurs secondary to stiff MTP joint
- IP volar plate and FHL stretch out with increased dorsiflexion through this joint
- Volar plate advancement is alternative to fusion
- Trauma
- Deformity correction (claw toe)
- As part of correction of hallux varus

Surgical Considerations

- Dorsal incision
- Incise extensor hood, retract EHL laterally

- Make cuts perpendicular to shaft, taking minimal bone
- Fuse in neutral alignment in all planes and do not supinate or pronate
- Fixation with single retrograde lag screw or multiple threaded K-wires

Complications
- Nonunion rate is higher than MTP fusion
- Malunion: hyperextension causes difficulties with shoe wear; rotation causes painful pressure areas

Lisfranc Arthrodesis (Tarsometatarsal)
- Most common indication is posttraumatic OA, also primary OA
- Advocated by some as primary treatment for Lisfranc injury instead of ORIF; similar results reported

Surgical Considerations
- Assess affected joints and any deformity
- Radiography of unaffected foot to guide correction
- Usually two dorsal longitudinal incisions used (one medial and one lateral)
- Protect neurovascular (NV) bundle, which lies near EHL
- Identify and protect superficial cutaneus nerves, which are very sensitive and susceptible to neurapraxias
- Débride, decorticate, and mobilize joints to be fused
  - Usually TMT joints 1–3 are enough
  - With severe fracture-dislocations, fourth and fifth TMT joints may need to be pinned (remove at 6 wk); occasionally, one must fuse between cuneiforms
  - Avoid fusing cuboid to lateral cuneiform to leave medial and lateral arches free

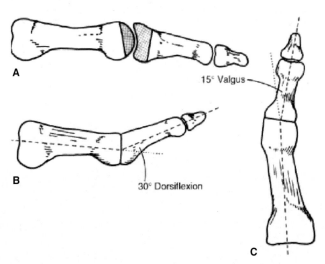

First metatarsophalangeal (MTP) joint arthrodesis. (From Chapman MW, et al. Chapman's Orthopaedic Surgery. Philadelphia: Lippincott Williams & Wilkins; 2001.)

- Secure first TMT joint provisionally in similar alignment as unaffected foot, then assess remaining joints
- Fix first TMT joint with crossed 4-0 cortical screws, one from MT to cuneiform and one from cuneiform to MT
- Reduce second TMT joint and fix with 4-0 cortical screw from distal-lateral to proximal-medial
- Transverse screw can then be used to fuse medial and middle cuneiforms if indicated
- Finally, fuse third TMT joint with screw from distal-lateral to proximal-medial
- Sangeorzan et al. (1990) reported good/excellent results in 69% after Lisfranc arthrodesis, although only 25% returned to full preinjury activities
  - Nonunion rate of 19%

Recommended Readings
Myerson MS. Foot and Ankle Disorders, Vol. 2. Philadelphia: WB Saunders; 2000:972–998.
Richardson EG. Orthopaedic Knowledge Update: Foot and Ankle 3. Rosemont, IL: American Academy of Orthopaedic Surgeons; 2003:155–175.

Reference
Sangeorzan BJ, et al. Salvage of Lisfranc's tarsometatarsal joint by arthrodesis. Foot Ankle 1990; 10:193–200.

ANKLE ARTHROPLASTY
- Indication is severe ankle arthritis with pain-limiting activities of daily living that is refractory to nonoperative modalities
- May be secondary to:
  - Posttraumatic OA (most common)
  - Primary OA
  - Inflammatory arthritis
  - Talar dome AVN
- Patient selection important; should be:
  - >50 yo
  - <250 lb
  - No expectations to return to vigorous sport or manual labor
- Absolute contraindications include:
  - AVN of talar body
  - Infection
  - Varus or valgus deformity >20 degrees
  - Neuropathy
  - Poor leg muscle function
  - Previous ankle fusion with removal of malleoli
- Relative contraindications include:
  - Ankle ROM <20 degrees
  - Young active patients
  - Obesity
  - Poor soft tissues
  - Vascular compromise

- Ankle instability
- Severe osteoporosis
- Segmental bone loss
- Alternative treatment options:
  - First try NSAIDs, weight loss, steroid injections, ice/heat
  - AFO with rocker-bottom shoe
  - Leather lace-up brace
  - Arthrodesis is good option for obese, young, or active patients

Preoperative Considerations

- Tibial deformity >10 degrees may be treated with osteotomy before TAR
- CT scan may aid in assessing bone quality and evaluating deformity
- Subtalar varus or valgus deformity that is large and not passively correctable should be treated with osteotomy
- If THR or TKR is needed, they should be performed before TAR in staged fashion
- Subtalar or talonavicular fusions can be performed at time of TAR if significant arthritis is present
- Tight heel cord should be lengthened
- Lax lateral ligaments should be reconstructed

Surgical Procedure

- Supine with bump under ipsilateral buttock
- Tourniquet high on thigh
- External fixator pins placed (EBI system uses one in talus and calcaneus, two in tibia)
- Use fixator to hold ankle in neutral with deformity corrected
- Anterior incision between tibialis anterior and EHL; beware of SPN superficially and anterior tibial artery and deep peroneal nerve deep to EHL
- Lateral incision over fibula with 5-cm skin bridge from anterior incision; preserve branches of SPN

- Expose tibia, fibula, and talus; excise syndesmotic ligaments; and mobilize
- Place alignment jig parallel to tibial spine, secure cutting guide to tibia using two pins, check with fluoroscopy
- Remove enough distal tibia and talus using oscillating/reciprocating saw to have bleeding bone
- Remove small amount of articular side of medial malleolus and one-third of medial fibula
  - If too far medial, may fracture medial malleolus
  - If too far lateral, talus is translated laterally and deltoid is overtightened
- Cut slot for tibial fin, taking care not to violate posterior cortex
- Insert tibial trial and check cuts
- Align talar fin cutting jig with second ray, centered on talar dome
  - Make cut about 5 mm deep; do not violate posterior cortex
- Check trial components (should fit loosely)
- Remove ex-fix and insert final components
- Balance soft tissues (often must release posterior one-half deltoid ligament)
- Should have 5-degree ankle dorsiflexion with knee extended; if not, perform gastroc recession or take more bone
- Fuse syndesmosis with bone from bone cuts and 3.5-mm screws
- Layered closure (repair capsule to cover hardware and repair extensor retinaculum)
- ROM started at 2 wk, protect weight bearing for 6 wk

Recommended Readings

Easley ME, et al. Total ankle arthroplasty. J Am Acad Orthop Surg 2002; 10:157–167.

Kitaoka HB. Master Techniques in Orthopaedic Surgery: The Foot and Ankle. Philadelphia: Lippincott Williams & Wilkins; 2002.

CHAPTER 9

Spine

Christopher R. Good, Wakenda K. Tyler, Russel C. Huang

Anatomy of Cervical Spine
   Cervical Lateral Masses
   Vertebral Artery
Anatomy of Lumbar Spine
   Lumbar Pedicles
   Axial Plane Levels
   Sagittal Plane Levels
Anatomy of Thoracic Spine
   Thoracic Pedicles
   Radicular Artery of Adamkiewicz
Atlantoaxial Rotatory Displacement
   Grisel Syndrome
   Traumatic
   Transverse Ligament Injury
Cervical Spine: ACDF
   Advantages of C-spine ACDF
   Landmarks
   Surgical Approach
   Corpectomy
   Bone Graft
   Complications of C-spine ACDF
   C-spine—ACDF: Plates
C-spine—Disc Disease
   Pathology of Spondylosis
   Risk Factors for Spondylosis
   Surgery Indications
C-spine—Myelopathy
   Causes
   Spondylotic Myelopathy
   Pathology
   Natural History
   Presentation
   Diagnosis
   C-spine—Myelopathy—Treatment
C-spine—Rheumatoid Arthritis
   Atlantoaxial Subluxation
   Subaxial Subluxation
   Atlantoaxial Impaction (Cranial Settling, Basilar
      Invagination)

Radiographic Parameters
Combinations
Ranawat's Clinical Grades
Natural History
Complications
C-spine—Radiculopathy
   Causes
   Epidemiology
   Anatomy
   Natural History
   Presentation
   Differential Diagnosis
   C-spine—Radiculopathy—Treatment
Cauda Equina Syndrome
Disc Calcification Syndrome
ICBG
   Posterior
   Anterior
Infection—Postop
Infection—Spondylodiscitis/Osteomyelitis (OM)
Infections—Tuberculosis
   Differential Diagnosis
   Pathology
   Surgery
Klippel-Feil Syndrome
Kyphoplasty
   Complications
Kyphosis—Adult
   Etiology
Kyphosis—Scheuermann
   Differential Diagnosis
   Natural History
   Treatment
LS-spine—Low Back Pain
   General
LS-spine—Degenerative Scoliosis
   Cause
   Natural History
   Presentation

Imaging
Nonsurgical Treatment
Surgical Treatment
LS-spine—Disc Herniation/Radiculopathy
Red Flags
Physical Examination
Imaging
Anatomy
Nonoperative Treatment
Prognosis for Nonoperative
 Treatment
Indications
Surgical Candidate
Surgical Results
Complications
LS-spine—Pedicle Screws
Roles of Internal Fixation
Historical Perspective
Pedicle Screws
Biomechanics
Potential Problems
LS-spine—Spinal Stenosis
Classification
Pathophysiology
Stenosis Locations
Differential Diagnosis
Diagnosis
Differential Diagnosis
Natural History
LS-spine—Stenosis: MRI Findings
LS-spine—Stenosis: Treatment
MRI
Sagittal Cuts
Axial Cuts
Contrast
Normal Disc
Abnormal Nucleus
Abnormal Annulus
Disc Morphology
Facets
Spinous Processes
Intraosseous Herniated Nucleus
 Pulposis
MRI—Postoperative
Scar vs. Disc
Arachnoiditis
Neurologic Exam
Upper Motor Neuron Signs
Lower Motor Neuron Signs
Cervical and Peripheral Nerves
Lower Extremity
Neurologic Exam—Quick
ASIA Scale Motor Source
Neurologic Injury
Causes

Os Odontoideum
Cause
Ossiculum Terminale
Scoliosis—Adolescent
Anatomy
Evaluation—Radiographic
Natural History
Curve Progression
Adolescent Scoliosis—Classification
Scoliosis—Adolescent—Treatment
Scoliosis—Adult
Natural History
Indications
Complications (Common and Severe)
Scoliosis—Congenital
Scoliosis—Congenital—Treatment
**Scoliosis—History and Physical
Examination**
Scoliosis—Infantile
Treatment
Scoliosis—Juvenile
Treatment
Scoliosis—King-Moe Classification
Scoliosis—Lenke Classification
Scoliosis—Neuromuscular
SRS classification
Risk Factors for Progression
Pelvic Obliquity
Fusion Level
Instrumentation
Correction
Complications
**Scoliosis—Selection of Fusion
Level**
Upper
Lower
Scoliosis—Selective Fusion
Indications
Spondylolisthesis—Adult, Isthmic
Diagnosis
**Spondylolysis, Spondylolisthesis—
Pediatric**
Natural History
Spondylolysis
Spondylolisthesis
T-spine—Disc Disease
Indications for Surgery
LS-spine Total Disc Replacement
Indications
Requirements
Contraindications
Advantages
Results
Trauma—Atlanto-occipital Dissociation
Traynelis Classification

Diagnosis
Treatment
Trauma—C-spine Radiographs
Lateral view
AP View
Open-mouth View
C-spine Flexion/Extension Views
MRI
Trauma—C1 Fracture
Treatment
Jefferson Burst Fracture
Trauma—C2—Odontoid Fracture
Anterior Odontoid Screw
Trauma—C2 Fracture (Hangman's)
Overall
Trauma—Cervical—Pediatric
Pseudosubluxation
Spinal Cord Injury without Radiographic
   Abnormality
Trauma—Cervical Body Fracture
Trauma—Cervical Facet Dislocation
Unilateral
Bilateral
MRI
Treatment
Trauma—Cervical Stability List
Trauma—Cervical Subaxial Fractures
Compression Flexion (20%)
Vertical Compression (15%)
Distractive Flexion (10%)
Compression Extension
Distractive Extension (22%)
Lateral Flexion (20%)
Trauma—Halo, Tongs
Halo
Gardner-Wells Tongs
Trauma—Occipital Condyle Fracture
Trauma—Sacrum Fracture
Vertical Fracture
Transverse Fracture
H-shaped Fracture
Trauma—Spinal Cord Injury
ASIA Scale Motor Source
Frankel/ASIA Classification
Motor Index Score
Treatment
Complications
Trauma—Spinal Cord Syndromes
Trauma—Steroids
Protocol
Contraindications
Trauma—Thoracolumbar Fracture
Stability
Trauma—TL Burst Fracture
Trauma—TL Compression Fracture
Treatment
Benign vs. Malignant Fracture
Trauma—TL Flexion Distraction
   (Seat Belt)
Trauma—TL Fracture-Dislocation
Trauma—Gun Shot Wound

Anatomy of Cervical Spine

- C1
  - Posterior arch fuses at 3 years old (yo)
  - Anterior arch fuses in two sites at 7 yo
- C2
  - Alar ligaments stabilize dens to occiput
  - Synchondrosis between dens and body of C2 fuses at 6 yo
  - Space available for the Cord is greatest at C1-2, thus low incidence of spinal cord injury with fractures at this level
- Power's ratio
  - Ratio of basion to posterior arch over opisthion to anterior arch
  - Ratio >1 = occipitoatlantal dislocation
- C3-6
  - Space available for the cord (SAC) decreases at C3-6 as cord enlarges for upper extremity (UE) motor neurons
  - C2-6 are bifid
  - Vertebral foramen C1-6
  - Carotid tubercle of C6
- C7
  - Tapered, not bifid, most prominent
  - Lateral masses are between articular processes
  - Transverse process has anterior and posterior tubercles and vertebral artery foramen
- Posterior longitudinal ligament attached to annulus
- Anterior longitudinal ligament is stronger
- Lordosis due to intervertebral disc shape
- Ligamentum flavum runs from superior margin of lower lamina to inferior half of anterior surface of upper lamina
- Posterior atlanto-occipital membrane is flavum of occiput C1
- Steel's rule of thirds (C1/2 articulation)
  - 1—dens
  - 2—cord
  - 3—meninges, epid fat, veins, cerebrospinal fluid (CSF)
- Spinal canal is triangular with rounded angles, width greater than depth

CERVICAL LATERAL MASSES

- Cephalad and caudad roots are equidistant from midpoint of lateral mass

– Pedicle screw is possible at C7 instead of lateral mass screw because lateral mass thinner and pedicle wider

VERTEBRAL ARTERY

– Vertebral artery enters C6 transverse foramen and goes up, then around lateral masses of C1 to perforate posterior atlanto-occipital membrane, then into foramen magnum
– Anterior spinal artery in cervical-spine arises from vertebral arteries
– Anterior spinal artery runs in anterior median fissure
– Two posterior spinal arteries
– Distance between the vertebral arteries increases from C3 to C6
– Vertebral veins are medial to artery, thus more likely to get injured in ACDF

Recommended Readings

Bono CM, Garfin SR, eds. Spine. Philadelphia: Lippincott Williams & Wilkins; 2004.

Fardon D, Garfin S, eds. Orthopaedic Knowledge Update: Spine 2, 2nd ed. Rosemont, IL: American Academy of Orhopaedic Surgeons; 2002.

Anatomy of Lumbar Spine

– Normal lordosis 40–80 degrees

LUMBAR PEDICLES

– Average distance of pedicle to superior root is 5 mm, inferior root is 1.5 mm, lateral dural edge
– L3 pedicle is usually perpendicular to floor in sagittal plane, but check on x-ray
– Depth is around 50 mm
– Pars marks medial extent of pedicle at L2-4

AXIAL PLANE LEVELS

– Pedicular
– Infrapedicular
– Discal
– Pedicle and transverse processes are only posterior structures seen in only one level

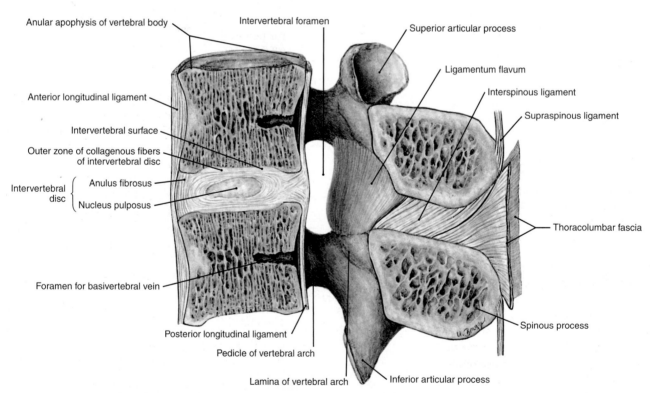

Median Sagittal Section through two lumbar vertebrae and an intervertebral disk. Note (1) The anterior and posterior longitudinal ligaments ventral and dorsal to the bodies of the lumbar vertebrae. (2) The ligamentum flavum forms an important ligamentous connection between the laminae of adjacent vertebral arches on the dorsal aspect of the vertebral canal. (From Clemente CD, Anatomy: A Regional Atlas of the Human Body 5th ed. Philadelphia: Lippincott Williams & Wilkins 2007 with permission.)

- Superior articular facet is mainly in pedicular level but also in discal level
- Superior facet of inferior level is more anterior and more lateral

SAGITTAL PLANE LEVELS

- Zones: central, lateral, foraminal, extraforaminal

Central Zone
- Contains thecal sac
- Underneath lamina
- Medial to medial aspect of inferior facet

Lateral Recess (Subarticular Zone)
- Contains traversing nerve root
- Pedicle is lateral
- Vertebral body is anterior

Foramen (Pedicular Zone)
- Contains dorsal root ganglion
- Cephalad pedicle is superior
- Caudad pedicle is inferior
- Posterior is pars of cephalad vertebra and superior facet of caudad vertebra
- Body and disc are anterior

Pars
- Is the concave lateral part of lamina
- Landmark for nerve root anteriorly and posterior branch of lumbar radicular artery laterally
- Laminar overlap decreases from L1 to S1; less bone resection needed for L5-S1 discectomy vs. more cephalad level

Recommended Readings
Ebraheim NA, et al. Are anatomic landmarks reliable in determination of fusion level in posterolateral lumbar fusion? Spine 1999; 24(10):973–974.
Wiltse LL, et al. A system for reporting the size and location of lesions in the spine. Spine 1997;22(13):1534–1537.

Anatomy of Thoracic Spine

- Normal kyphosis 20–50 degrees

THORACIC PEDICLES

- T4—10 mm high, 4.5 mm wide
- T12—14 mm high, 7.8 mm wide
- T1 medial angulation 30 degrees
- T2 medial angulation 26 degrees
- T4 anteromedial inclination 13.9 degrees
- T12 anteromedial inclination 0.3 degrees
- Medial pedicle wall two times thicker

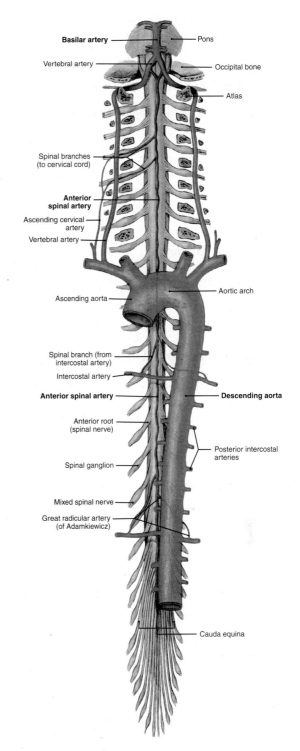

Anterior Spinal Artery. Note: The anterior spinal artery is formed by vessels from the vertebral arteries. It receives anastomotic branches from certain cervical, thoracic and lumbar segmental arteries along the spinal roots. An especially large branch (artery of Adamkiewicz) arises in the lower thoracic or upper lumbar region. (From Clemente CD, Anatomy: A Regional Atlas of the Human Body 5th ed. Philadelphia: Lippincott Williams & Wilkins 2007 with permission.)

- From T9 to L5, horizontal diameter increases from 7 mm to 15 mm; vertical diameter is 1.5 cm

RADICULAR ARTERY OF ADAMKIEWICZ

- Major supply to anterior spinal artery to lower spinal cord
- From the left side in 80%
- Usually with ventral root of T9, T10, or T11, but can be anywhere from T5 to L5
- Comes off segmental artery at the level of costotransverse junction, then enters intervertebral foramen

Recommended Reading
Fardon D, Garfin S, eds. Orthopaedic Knowledge Update: Spine 2, 2nd ed. Rosemont, IL: American Academy of Orhopaedic Surgeons; 2002.

Atlantoaxial Rotatory Displacement

- C1-2 bilateral dislocation occurs at 65 degrees' rotation in cadaver studies
- With ruptured transverse ligament, unilateral dislocation occurs at 45 degrees' rotation

GRISEL SYNDROME

- Common cause of acquired childhood torticollis
- Occurs after colds in children—due to inflammation and spasm
- Possibly due to synovial impingement
- Cock-robin deformity (head tilted, long sternocleidomastoid muscle [SCM] in spasm on opposite side to bring it back) vs. congenital muscular torticollis (head tilted toward and turned away from side of short fibrotic SCM)
- Neurologic injury rare

Diagnosis
- Anteroposterior (AP): dens open-mouth view with one lateral mass appears wider and closer to midline because rotated forward
- Lateral: anterior wedge-shaped lateral mass seen and posterior arches superimposed, suggesting fusion
- Plain radiographs are not useful except to rule out tumor
- Check temperature to rule out infection
- Dynamic rotation computed tomography (CT) (with head turned maximally to one side, then the other) needed

Classification
Type A
- Rotation without translation
- Atlantodens Interval <3 mm

Type B (II)
- Unilateral facet subluxation
- ADI 3–5 mm
- A and B probably have normal range of motion

Type C (III)
- Unilateral facet subluxation
- Translation >5 mm

Type D
- Very rare
- C1-2 facet dislocation
- Posterior displacement of C1

Treatment
- Based on duration of symptoms
- <1 wk: soft collar immobilization, non-sterioidal anti-inflammatory drugs, and rest
- 1 wk to 1 mo: cervical traction ± halo, immobilization for 6 wk if reducible, muscle relaxants
- >1 mo: cervical traction with halo for <3 wk
- Recurrence common if symptoms last >1 mo

Surgical Indications
- Neurologic involvement
- Anterior displacement
- Failure to achieve and/or maintain reduction
- Deformity present >3 mo because closed reduction rarely works and fusion needed for pain relief
- Recurrence of deformity

Surgery (C1-2 Fusion)
- Gallie's fusion doesn't work well because wires near spinous process don't get good rotational control
- Brook's fusion works better

Recommended Reading
Fielding JW, Hawkins RJ. Atlanto-axial rotatory fixation (fixed rotatory subluxation of the atlanto-axial joint). J Bone Joint Surg Am 1977;59(1):37–44.

TRAUMATIC
Type I (ADI <3 mm)
- Acute traumatic type I treated with 3–5 lb traction or hard collar and if no reduction in 1–2 wk, then skeletal traction to reduce, then maintain 1–2 wk, then halo vest
- Adults tend to need skeletal traction and halo more so than children

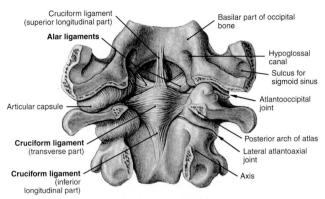

Cruciform ligament (superior longitudinal part)

Alar ligaments

Articular capsule

Cruciform ligament (transverse part)

Cruciform ligament (inferior longitudinal part)

Basilar part of occipital bone

Hypoglossal canal

Sulcus for sigmoid sinus

Atlantooccipital joint

Posterior arch of atlas

Lateral atlantoaxial joint

Axis

Atlantooccipital and Atlantoaxial joints showing the cruciform ligament (posterior view). Note: The posterior arches to the atlas and axis have been removed and the cruciform ligament is seen from this posterior view. It consist of the transverse ligament and the longitudinal fascicles that extend superiorly and inferiorly. (From Clemente CD, Anatomy: A Regional Atlas of the Human Body 5th ed. Philadelphia: Lippincott Williams & Wilkins 2007 with permission.)

- If not reduced by skeletal traction, then open to reduce and fuse C1-2

Type II, III (ADI 3–5 mm or >5 mm)
- Considered unstable
- Initially halo vest if in child with normal neurology
- In adult, C1-2 fusion
- Consider direct transoral reduction with anterior C1-2 plate

TRANSVERSE LIGAMENT INJURY

Classification
- I—midsubstance tear—surgery
- II—avulsion—nonoperative, 75% heal with immobilization alone
- **ADI <3 mm,** normal
- **ADI >5 mm,** complete tear
- ADI >7 mm indicates tear of alar ligaments and tectorial membrane (PLL)
- In children, <5 mm is normal, >10 mm is tear

Treatment
- Collar for ADI <5 mm
- Halo for ADI >5 mm if bony avulsion only
- C1-2 fusion for ADI >5 mm if not avulsion

Recommended Readings
Dickman CA, Sonntag VK. Injuries involving the transverse atlantal ligament: classification and treatment guidelines based upon experience with 39 injuries. Neurosurgery 1997;40(4): 886–887.

Fielding JW, Hawkins RJ. Atlanto-axial rotatory fixation (fixed rotatory subluxation of the atlanto-axial joint). J Bone Joint Surg Am 1977;59(1):37–44.

Cervical Spine: ACDF

ADVANTAGES OF C-SPINE ACDF
- Indirect decompression of canal and foramen by distraction of disc space
- Minimized manipulation of cord

LANDMARKS
- C1—angle of mandible
- C3—hyoid bone
- C4—thyroid cartilage
- C6—cricoid cartilage (marks two most common sites of disc disease)
- C6—carotid tubercle

SURGICAL APPROACH
- Left-sided approach because consistent recurrent laryngeal nerve on left
- Can access C3 to T1
- Interscapular roll on bed
- Horizontal incision unless more than two levels, then oblique in line with SCM
- Take platysma in line with skin
- Superficial layer of deep cervical fascia taken to expose sternocleidomastoid muscle
- Midlayer of deep cervical fascia taken and carotid sheath palpated laterally
- Deeper dissection bluntly with peanut
- Elevate longus colli but stop laterally when body curves posteriorly to avoid vertical artery and sympathetic chain
- More lateral dissection safer at more cephalad part of body because vertical a. protected by transverse process there
- Helps to remove anterior osteophytes before placing retractors under longus colli
- Disc incised and removed with curettes and pituitary rongeurs
- Remove disc to posterior longitudinal ligament and until uncovert junctions are visualized
- 3-0 angled curetted used to permit placement of 1–2-mm punch Kerrison posterior to body to remove phytes
- PLL taken only if soft disc behind it or PLL is part of compressive lesion

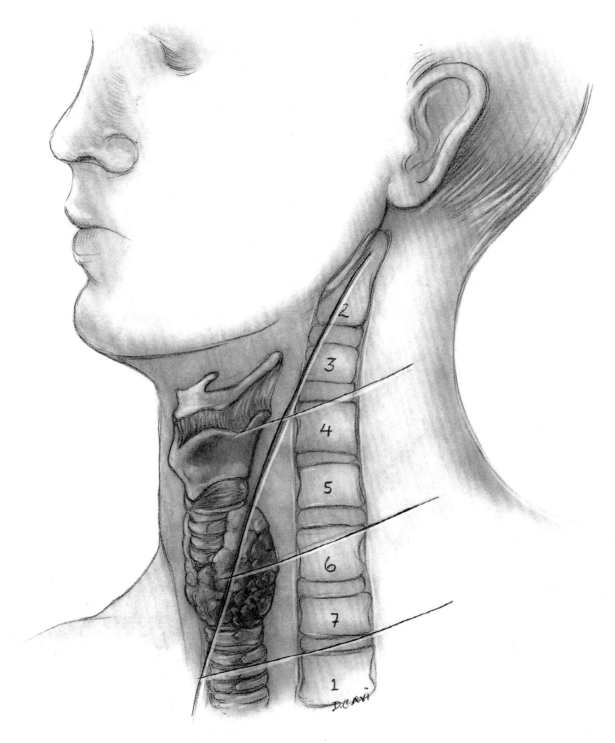

Superficial landmarks are helpful in placing the skin incision. The hyoid bone is at the level of C3, the thyroid cartilage is at the C4-C5 level, and the cricoid lies at the C6 level. (From Bradford DS, Master Techniques in Orthopeadic Surgery: The Spine 2nd ed. Philadelphia: Lippincott Williams & Wilkins 2004 with permission.)

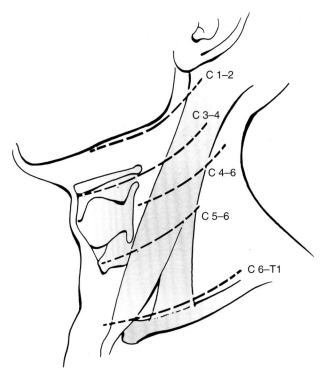

Landmarks for the incision of the Smith-Robinson approach for anterior cervical discectomy and fusion. C1-2 is at the level of the mandible. C3 is at the level of the hyoid. C4-5 is at the level of the superior and inferior borders of the thyroid cartilage. C6 is at the level of the cricoid cartilage. C7-T1 exposure is just above the clavicle. (From Fischgrund J, Herkowitz H. In: Bradford DS, ed. Master techniques in orthopaedic surgery: spine. Philadelphia: JB Lippincott, 1997 with permission.)

CORPECTOMY

- Anterior half removed with Leksell
- High-speed drill for remaining cancellous bone
- Burr to thin posterior cortex
- Remaining cortex removed with curette or punch
- Decompression carried laterally to uncinate junctions
- Should go no more lateral than palpated pedicle to protect vertical a.
- Maximum width is 18–20 mm
- If vertebrectomy not needed to remove retrovertebral material, multilevel graft may be better to maintain alignment than strut even though more surfaces need to fuse

BONE GRAFT

- Autograft increases union more than allograft in more than one level
- Plate lowers pseudo rate in allograft
- Multiple techniques—Smith Robinson horseshoe, Cloward bicortical dowel, "keystone," trapezoid

- More cancellous increases fusion but not as structural as cortical
- Increased fusion with more aggressive decortication of end plates (Emery with only 4% pseudo in single level vs. 12% in Robinson's without decortication)
- Should be recessed behind anterior margin of superior and inferior end plates
- Harvest with saw instead of osteotome
- For iliac crest bone graft, stay at least 2 cm from ASIS to avoid LFCN
- Complications of ICGB—5% hematoma, 1% infection, 10% lateral femoral cutaneous nerve damage, 15% persistent pain

Reference
Robinson R, Smith G. Anterolateral cervical disc removal and interbody fusion for cervical disc syndrome. Bull Johns Hopkins Hosp 1955;96(223).

Recommended Readings
Albert TJ, Murrell SE. Surgical management of cervical radiculopathy. J Am Acad Orthop Surg 1999;7(6):368–376.
Clements DH, O'Leary PF. Anterior cervical discectomy and fusion. Spine 1990;15(10):1023–1025.
Williams JL, et al. Late results of cervical discectomy and interbody fusion: some factors influencing the results. J Bone Joint Surg Am 1968;50(2):277–286.

COMPLICATIONS OF C-SPINE ACDF

- 5% persistent neurologic symptoms due to inadequate phyte removal
- Recurrent laryngeal traction
  - Refer if hoarseness not better by 6 wk
  - Cloward—8% transient, 2% permanent
- Chylothorax from left-sided laceration to thoracic duct
  - Avoid by staying medial to carotid sheath
- Esophageal injury
  - Detected by indigo carmine extravasation, must repair and give IV antibiotics and total parenteral nutrition (TPN) until it heals
- Graft dislodgement
  - Associated with
    - More bodies removed
    - Longer graft
    - Corpectomies with fusion ending at C7
- Horner's from sympathetic chain
- Superior laryngeal n. (at C3-4)
  - Gives sensation, thus leads to difficult swallowing
  - Affects high notes (singers)
- Pseudarthrosis
  - 15% overall nonsmokers, without plate
  - 10% pseudarthrosis one level
  - 44% pseudarthrosis three levels
  - Observe if painless because

– Fusion does not correlate with outcome
– PSF alone if no radiculopathy
– 20% adjacent segment degeneration due to fusion or just natural history?
- Respiratory compromise
  – 6% airway complications in anterior cervicals
  – Associated with
    – >3 vertebral body exposure
    – EBL >300 mL
    – Exposure above and including C4
    – Operative time >5 hr

Recommended Readings

Sagi HC, et al. Airway complications associated with surgery on the anterior cervical spine. Spine 2002;27(9):949–953.

Wang JC, et al. Graft migration or displacement after multilevel cervical corpectomy and strut grafting. Spine 2003;28(10): 1016–1021; discussion 1021–1022.

C-SPINE—ACDF: PLATES

Biomechanics

- Tension band in extension
- Buttress plate during flexion

Advantages

- Increases fusion rate in multilevel ACDF and/or when allograft used
- Decreases graft dislodgement
- Provides stability when stabilized structures lost
- Decreases rate of graft collapse
- Reduces segmental kyphosis

Disadvantages

- Increases cost, surgical time
- Plate-related complications

Multilevel Corpectomies

- High stresses at graft–vertebrae junction
  - Anterior plating of multilevel corpectomies
  - 9% of grafts dislodge in two-level
  - 50% of grafts dislodge in three-level
  - Recommended posterior fixation

Recommended Readings

Connolly PJ, et al. Anterior cervical fusion: outcome analysis of patients fused with and without anterior cervical plates. J Spinal Disord 1996;9(3):202–206.

Vaccaro AR, et al. Early failure of long segment anterior cervical plate fixation. J Spinal Disord 1998;11(5):410–415.

C-spine—Disc Disease

- Incidence parallels decade of life for 30s–50s, then up to 70%–80% after that

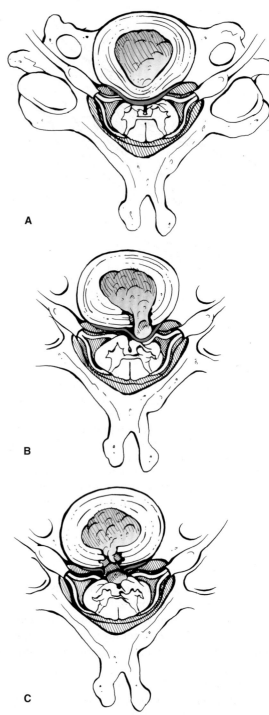

A

B

C

Three common types of cervical disc herniation. **(A)** Central protrusion, with the outer anulus remaining intact. **(B)** Posterolateral extrusion, with the anulus having a tear and the nucleus being restrained by fibers of the posterior longitudinal ligament. **(C)** Central sequestered fragment, lying posterior to the posterior longitudinal ligament. (From Jenis L, An H. Cervical disc disease. In: Chapman MW, ed. Chapman's orthopaedic surgery, 3rd ed. Philadelphia: Lippincott Williams & Wilkins 2001 with permission.)

- Male greater than Female
- Rule out shoulder pathology, Pancoast tumor

PATHOLOGY OF SPONDYLOSIS

- First disc desiccation, then narrowing, bulging; kyphosis (natural lordosis due to discs) narrows foramen
- Uncinate spurring, facet arthrosis
- Most common disc disease at C5-6 because greatest motion there, then C4-5 or C6-7

RISK FACTORS FOR SPONDYLOSIS

- Smoking, lifting, driving
- Three patterns, progression
  - Discogenic mechanical neck pain
  - Radiculopathy
    - Hard disc (ophyte)
    - Soft disc (Herniated Nucleus Pulposus, usually posterior–lateral)
    - Affects caudad-exiting root
    - In Lumbar spine, affects caudad-traversing root
  - Myelopathy (usually with radiculopathy)
- Three types of disc herniations
  - Intraforaminal—most common, motor and sensory changes, dermatomal
  - Posterolateral—usually motor only
  - Midline—myelopathy
- Plain xr—nonspecific
  - Use to rule out tumor, signs of infection
  - 70% of those >70 yo have + xr
- Magnetic resonance imaging (MRI)—false positives
  - 14% asymptomatic HNP or stenosis in those <40 yo
  - 28% in those >40 yo
- Nonsteroidal anti-inflammatory drugs (NSAIDs), collar, moist heat
- Physical therapy (PT), traction, injections, pain clinic

SURGERY INDICATIONS

- Painful radiculopathy >6 wk
- Progressive significant weakness
- Myelopathy (except in extreme elderly)
- Confirmatory imaging (MR, CT myelogram) and for surgical planning
- See treatment for cervical radiculopathy and ACDF

Recommended Reading

Miller M, ed. Review of Orthopaedics, 4th ed. Philadelphia, PA: Saunders; 2004.

C-spine—Myelopathy

CAUSES

- Usually spondylosis
- Instability (compensatory subluxation at segments adjacent to stiff spondylosis)

- Cervical kyphosis
- Congenital stenosis (13 mm)
- Ossification of posterior longitudinal ligament

SPONDYLOTIC MYELOPATHY

- Disc degeneration with hypertrophic osseous and ligamentous changes, annular bulging
- Chondro-osseous spurs at annular insertion into end plates
- Uncovertebral junction hypertrophy, which may lead to foraminal stenosis
- Facet junction hypertrophy, which can cause foraminal narrowing
- Loss of lordosis contributes
- Ligamentum flavum thickens

PATHOLOGY

- Combination of ischemia and direct mechanical effects
- Mild to moderate associated with degeneration of lateral white matter tracts
- Severe associated with necrosis of central gray matter (occurs when ratio of anterior-posterior diameter to medial–lateral diameter is <1:5)
- Anterior white columns resistant to infarction even in severe compression

NATURAL HISTORY

- Very slow progression, episodic stepwise deterioration with long periods of plateau
- Deterioration associated with trauma
- Many with asymptomatic compression
- Prognosis poor after moderate signs and symptoms develop
- Lees and Turner (1963)
- Clarke and Robinson (1956)

PRESENTATION

- Wide spectrum
- Mild symptoms with neck pain only
- 15% with moderate/severe myelopathy have no neck pain
- Radicular arm pain alone
- Paresthesias common, typically nondermatomal global in upper extremity
- **Changes in gait (shuffling) early**
- Unilateral or bilateral upper extremity weakness, **clumsiness,** fine motor loss—change in writing, difficulty with buttons, zippers, coins
- Weakness in proximal lower extremities (LEs) manifest as difficulty getting out of chair or stairing

(proximal muscle groups more involved as opposed to lumbar stenosis, where distal groups more involved)—thus, presentation with foot drop is rare
- Bowel, bladder (urgency) rare
- Neck extension decreases canal diameter (asymptomatic cervical stenosis with central cord syndrome from hyperextension injury), thus limited or painful
- Finger escape sign—when asked to extend and adduct fingers, small and ring finger abduct and flex in less than a minute because of weak intrinsics
- Grip and release test—should be able to do 20 times in 10 sec
- Gross atrophy—myelopathy of the hand
- Shoulder girdle atrophy and fasciculations in C4-5, C5-6 loss of anterior horn cells
- Hyperreflexia in UEs and LEs unless concomitant root compression
- Upper motor neuron (UMN) long tract signs—Hoffman, inverted radial reflex, clonus, Babinski
- Ulnar drift of ring and small finger with active elevation of upper extremity
- Cranial nerve abnormalities or hyperactive jaw jerk indicates cranial or brainstem lesion—neurologic consult, image brain
- Heel walk, toe walk, toe-to-heel tightrope gait picks up subtle disease

DIAGNOSIS

- By history and physical examination
- XRs
  - Xr changes of spondylosis age related and occur in most people >50 yo
  - Flexion–extensions for instability
  - Pavlov/Torg ratio (<0.8 is abnormal) less useful
  - Better is sagittal diameter <13 mm (normal 17 mm) on plain xr
- MRI
  - If clinical myelopathy, MR indicated to see soft tissue and cord
  - Stenosis
  - Signal changes (edema vs. myelomalacia)
    - T2 signal changes don't correlate with preoperative deficits
  - Cord flattening (compressive ratio >30%)
- CT myelogram
  - Study of choice when MRI is contra-indicated
- Electrodiagnostics
  - To differentiate cervical radiculopathy from carpal tunnel syndrome (CTS), cubital tunnel, or thoracic outlet syndrome
  - To differentiate from amyotrophic lateral sclerosis (ALS), multiple sclerosis (MS), and severe peripheral neuropathy

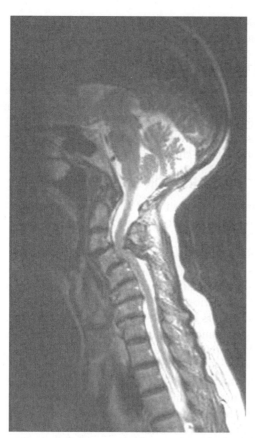

Sagittal T2-weighted MRI in a myelopathic patient. Note the decreased room available for the cord and loss of lordosis resulting from severe spondylosis. (From Bono C, Garfin SR, Orthopaedic Surgery Essentials: Spine Philadelphia: Lippincott Williams & Wilkins 2004 with permission.)

References
Clarke E, Robinson PK. Cervical myelopathy: a complication of cervical spondylosis. Brain 1956;79(3):483–510.
Lees F, Turner JW. Natural history and prognosis of cervical spondylosis. Br Med J 1963;5373:1607–1610.

Recommended Readings
Emery SE. Cervical spondylotic myelopathy: diagnosis and treatment. J Am Acad Orthop Surg 2001;9(6):376–388.
Miller M, ed. Review of Orthopaedics, 4th ed. Philadelphia, PA: Saunders; 2004.

C-SPINE—MYELOPATHY—TREATMENT

- Nonoperative treatment debatable
- Surgical indications
  - Gait changes
  - Progressive dysfunction
  - Hand involvement
  - Age? (ability of 80 yo to get better?)

Nonoperative
- Observe if no signs/symptoms of myelopathy
- Exception is severe compression that could cause cord injury from mild trauma
- If mild with only slight gait change and mild hyperreflexia and no functional loss, individual pattern of deterioration or plateauing checked q6–12mo

Surgical Approach
- Mostly anterior decompression likely involving corpectomies and strut
- Aggressive anterior cervical discectomy and fusion may be alternative if disease mainly around disc
- Kyphosis is contraindicated for posterior approach
- Anterior for one to two levels and posterior for three or more levels involved
- Approach does not affect neurologic improvement

Posterior
- For diffuse canal stenosis or dorsal compression from buckled ligamentum flavum
- Since most spondylosis is predominantly anterior, posterior cervical decompression and fusion is an indirect technique that requires posterior shifting of cord, which requires lordotic C-spine
- Multilevel lami without fusion almost never indicated because late subluxation and kyphosis

Laminoplasty
- Posterior canal expansion via trap door while preserving posterior elements
- Indicated in myelopathy with multilevel stenosis
- Never in kyphosis, patient must be neutral or lordotic
- Prevents progressive kyphosis seen with laminectomy
- Associated with failure to relieve axial neck pain, loss of 40% range of motion, postoperative radiculopathy (C5)

Indications for AP Cervical Fusion
- Severe osteoporosis
- Preexisting kyphosis
- Prior laminectomy
- In greater than three-level corpectomy
- Anterior decompression with posterolateral fusion and lateral mass plating in postlami kyphosis

Results of Surgery
- 80% pain relief
- 90% neurologic improvement

Prognosis
- **Degree of severity of myelopathy is most important**
- Cord compression, age
- Single better chronicity than multiple levels

- Poorer postoperative neurologic recovery if preoperative cord cross-sectional area <30 mm^2

Complications
- Graft related in anterior struts
- Strut revision if no bony contact, esophagus threatened, or significant kyphosis
- Recurrent laryngeal stretch and hoarseness 2% in anterior
- 1%–2% neurologic injury
- Steroids in high-risk patients
- If significant cord signal changes, then trauma dose methyprednisone
- Motor C5 palsy 5–8% due to short root and maximal lordosis at that level; slow but progressive recovery in most; can occur after anterior
- Dural leaks in OPLL from long-standing erosions
- Adjacent segment degeneration cause of relapse years later

Recommended Readings
Bono CM, Garfin SR, eds. Spine. Philadelphia: Lippincott Williams & Wilkins; 2004.
Emery SE. Cervical spondylotic myelopathy: diagnosis and treatment. J Am Acad Orthop Surg 2001;9(6):376–388.

C-spine—Rheumatoid Arthritis

- In 25%–85% of rheumatoid arthritis (RA), associated with severity markers, long-standing disease
- C-spine had 32 synovial articulations; upper C-spine depends largely on soft tissue constraints

ATLANTOAXIAL SUBLUXATION

- Most common, usually anterior subluxation
- Direct damage of transverse, apical, and alar ligaments and pannus extension into junction
- atlantodens interval >3.5 mm is abnormal
- Disruption of transverse ligament occurs at ADI of 3–5 mm
- Worsens with duration
  - Reducible, then fixed, then invaginates
  - Invagination can make AAS look better
- Space available for the spinal cord <14 mm predicts neurologic impairment

Surgery Indications
- *SAC <14 mm even if neurologic exam normal
- Concomitant atlantoaxial impaction
- Ranawat IIIA
- ? for pain, Ranawat II, IIIB
- Halo needed if PSF/wire
- Halo avoided if Magerl transarticular screws or Harm's technique

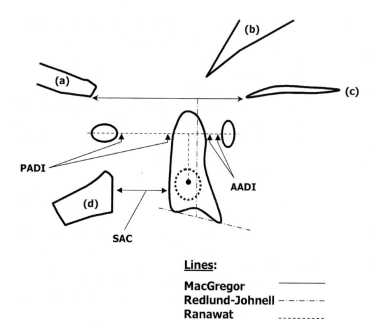

Radiographic parameters of cervical rheumatoid arthritis: (a) occiput, (b) clivus, (c) hard palate, (d) C2 arch. (From Bono C, Garfin SR, Orthopaedic Surgery Essentials: Spine Philadelphia: Lippincott Williams & Wilkins 2004 with permission.)

Lines:

MacGregor ————
Redlund-Johnell – – – – –
Ranawat - - - - - - - -

SUBAXIAL SUBLUXATION

- Second most common, due to wide involvement
- Neural canal is narrower in the subaxial region, thus myelopathy with lesser subluxation
- Anterior subluxation, usually at C2-3, at C3-4, or caudal to a previous fusion
- White and Panjabi—3.5 mm translation or 11 degrees angular instability
- Sagittal diameter <14 mm is indicated for operation (posterior spinal fusion)
- Extend across entire segment if upper C-spine needs fusion also

ATLANTOAXIAL IMPACTION (CRANIAL SETTLING, BASILAR INVAGINATION)

- Least common, most dangerous
- Vertical translation of dens and settling of occiput leading to cord compression by dens in foramen magnum
- Almost always preceded by atlantoaxial subluxation
- Can decrease ADI, giving false impression of improvement
- Sudden death—compression of medulla, vertebral artery thrombosis
- Vertebrobasilar insufficiency—dizzy, diplopia, dysesthesias, dysphagia
- Dysphagia—pressure on nucleus of glossopharyngeal nerve
- Hydrocephalus from cerebrospinal fluid flow occlusion

RADIOGRAPHIC PARAMETERS

- McRae line (across foramen magnum—0 mm), Chamberlain line (hard palate to back of foramen magnum—3 mm), McGregor line (hard palate to back of occiput—4.5 mm)
  - Bony landmarks difficult to identify
- Ranawat index—<13 mm abnormal (15 mm for males, 13 mm for females)
- Surgery indications
  - Dens in foramen magnum, Ranawat <13 mm
  - Cord compression
  - Cervicomedullary angle <135 degrees on MR
  - Fuse to occiput, odontoidectomy rarely needed because pannus resolves

COMBINATIONS

- C1-2 with basilar invagination is highly associated with paralysis
- *Flexion/extension radiographs a must
- MRI, flexion/extension MRI
- Somatosensory evoked potentials

RANAWAT'S CLINICAL GRADES

- I—Neck pain, no neural deficit
- II—Subjective weakness with hyperreflexia and dysesthesia
- IIIA—Objective weakness and long-tract signs, ambulatory
- IIIB—Objective weakness and long-tract signs, nonambulatory
  - **IIIB—25% 6-mo mortality even with surgery**

NATURAL HISTORY

- One-third stay the same
- One-third progress neurologically
- One-third progress by xr but neurologic stable

COMPLICATIONS

- Wound dehiscence
- Swallowing difficulties in flexed position (put in halo first in good position)

Recommended Readings
Boden SD, et al. Rheumatoid arthritis of the cervical spine. A long-term analysis with predictors of paralysis and recovery. J Bone Joint Surg Am 1993;75(9):1282–1297.
Fielding JW, et al. Tears of the transverse ligament of the atlas. A clinical and biomechanical study. J Bone Joint Surg Am 1974;56(8):1683–1691.
Ranawat CS, et al. Cervical spine fusion in rheumatoid arthritis. J Bone Joint Surg Am 1979;61(7):1003–1010.

C-spine—Radiculopathy

CAUSES

- Disc (20%)—usually acute symptoms
- Spondylosis ± disc (70%)
  - Facet junction hypertrophy and/or
  - Neurocentral junction hypertrophy
  - Usually insidious onset
- Instability, listhesis
- Chemical irritation

EPIDEMIOLOGY

- Peak age 50–55 yo
- Most common C7, then C6
- Over 5-yr follow-up one-third still had symptom recurrence, 25% underwent surgery, 90% of nonsurgical cases treated were asymptomatic

ANATOMY

- Facets 30–50 degrees to transverse plane
- Foramen 45 degrees to sagittal plane
- Each level composed of five joints
- Root exits above named pedicle
- C4 comes out at C3-4
- Ventral motor n. root is anteroinferior and lies next to uncovert junction
- Dorsal sensory n. root lies next to superior articular process
- In normal cases, root takes up one-third of foramen
- Foraminal size decreases with extension

NATURAL HISTORY

- Lees and Turner—cervical radiculopathy rarely progressed to myelopathy
- Long-term follow-up of nonoperative treatment with two-thirds having recurrent symptoms
- One-quarter with persistent pain unable to return to original work

PRESENTATION

- Most with radicular and trapezial periscapular pain
- Exacerbation with extension and tilting to affected extremity
- Shoulder abduction relief sign specific for soft disc herniation
- Breast pain, cervical angina
- Sensory changes don't follow strict dermatomal pattern
- Half of patients with root compression have strict radicular pattern
- Motor deficits in two-thirds
- Reflex changes in two-thirds
- C2, C3—jaw pain, occiput headache
- C4—neck and trapezial pain, numb at base of neck to scapular area, diaphragm weakness not described
- C5—epaulet pattern; deltoid, supraspinatus, infraspinatus, biceps weak; biceps reflex inconsistent
- C6—neck to lateral aspect of forearm to hand dorsum between thumb and index fingers to tips; brachioradialis reflex depressed, wrist extension weak; infraspinatus, serratus anterior, triceps, supinator, EPL may be affected
- C7—posterior arm and forearm to middle finger; absent triceps common, triceps weakness almost always; wrist flexors, pronators, finger extensors, and lateral dorsi
- C8, T1—rare; least likely to be associated with pain; sensory changes below wrist; motor changes involve interossei, all ulnar n. muscles, thenars, anterior interosseus nerve muscles

DIFFERENTIAL DIAGNOSIS

- Myelopathy
- Entrapment syndromes
  - C6-7 with CTS
  - C7 with radial n. entrapment
  - C8-T1 with cubital tunnel, AIN
- Thoracic outlet syndrome
  - Thenar—interosseous (IO) wasting
- Tumors—Pancoast, schwannoma
- XR
  - By 50 yo, 25% of asymptomatic patients have xr degenerative changes

- By 75 yo, 75% asymptomatic patients have xr degenerative changes
- Cervical plain xr myelogram
  - injection at C1-2 or lumbar
  - 21% filling defects in asymptomatic patients
  - CT myelography much better
- MR
  - As good as CT myelography
  - Foraminal stenosis seen better on CT than MR
  - More problems with motion artifact compared to MR of LS spine
- Electrodiagnostics
  - Only if clinical doubt
  - Compression that leads to cervical radiopathy usually occurs proximal to sensory dorsal root ganglion, thus sensory action potentials usually normal
  - Thus, nerve conduction velocity and latency changes typically not found in cervical radiopathy
  - electromyogram is modality of choice for differentiated radiopathy from peripheral compression syndromes and correlates better clinically than xr's
  - Cervical root stimulation may be better than EMG

Reference
Lees F, Turner JW. Natural history and prognosis of cervical spondylosis. Br Med J 1963;5373:1607–1610.

Recommended Reading
Albert TJ, Murrell SE. Surgical management of cervical radiculopathy. J Am Acad Orthop Surg 1999;7(6):368–376.

C-SPINE—RADICULOPATHY—TREATMENT

Nonoperative
- In hard or soft discs, always nonoperative to start unless progressive or disabling deficit
- Soft collar for <2 wk, isometric paraspinal strengthening, gentle stretching during weaning; more aggressive strengthening in 6 wk if no pain
- Short course of bedrest; inverted V pillow, which flexes neck and internally rotates shoulders
- Home traction controversial
- Oral steroid not recommended

Surgical Indications
- Recalcitrant radiopathy >6 wk
- Progressive or disabling deficit such as deltoid palsy, wrist drop
- Static deficit with pain
- Instability with radiopathy

Choice of Approach
- ACDF
  - Generally preferred if

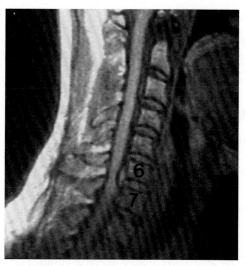

T2-weighted MRI reveals soft disc herniations at C4-5, C5-6, and C6-7. (From Bono C, Garfin SR, Orthopaedic Surgery Essentials: Spine Philadelphia: Lippincott Williams & Wilkins 2004 with permission.)

  - Axial neck pain
  - Central disease
  - Any segmental kyphosis
  - Bilateral symptoms, multisegments
- Less risk to neural elements
- Access to central and lateral lesion
- Hard to get to C7-T1 in burly patients
- Posterior laminoforaminotomy
  - Generally preferred if
    - Soft disc with mainly arm pain
    - Caudal lesion in large, short neck
    - Unilateral, one level
- No need for fusion, no immobilization
- Ideal in young athletic male smoker unilateral without hard disc disease

ACDF

Anterior Discectomy, No Fusion
- Advocated by some because no pseudo, no graft or graft site problems, and similar short-term results to ACDF
- Requires removal of PLL to avoid buckling
- Need long-term results

Posterior Laminoforaminotomy
- Direct visualization of compressed root with decompression without fusion
- Keyhole foraminotomy with removal of lamina and facet over root
- Midline incision, preserve interspinal ligaments
- High-speed burr or 3-0 angled curette with 2-mm Kerrison punch to take medial one-third to one-half of facet, one-half of superior lamina, one-third of inferior lamina, lateral ligamentum flavum
- Will destabilize if too aggressive

- Root unroofed posterior, superior, and inferior
- If HNP present, lift root superiorly and follow inferior aspect of pedicle by palpation to axilla of root
- 93%–96% G/E at about 2 yr
- Transient worsening <1 wk in 8%
- 2% prolonged postsurgical paresis
- Avoid venous air emboli by prone position
- 1%–2% wound infections

Cauda Equina Syndrome

- 50% of compressions of thecal sac lead to dysfunction
- LBP with radiation down posterior thighs
- Weak toe flexors bilaterally
- Difficulty in initiating micturition
- Urinary retention is the most important symptom. Without urinary retention, the chance of true cauda equina syndrome is 1/10,000
- Saddle (perianal) anesthesia
- Obtain confirmatory imaging
- Emergent surgical treatment
- Don't do microdiscectomy

Disc Calcification Syndrome

- Children
- Usually affects C-spine
- Pain
- Decreased ROM
- Low-grade fevers
- High erythrocyte sedimentation rate
- Xr with disc calcification in annulus without erosion
- Self-limiting
- Conservative treatment

ICBG

POSTERIOR

- Superior gluteal a. and v. enter sciatic notch above piriformis
- Sup cluneal n.'s come from dorsal rami of L1-3, then go distally over posterior iliac crest
- Posterior superior iliac spine to superior cluneal n. is 69 mm
- PSIS to sup glut a. is 63 mm
- So make incision parallel to cluneal n.'s and stay within 7 cm from PSIS

ANTERIOR

- Variations of lateral femoral cutaneous nerve
  - 58% cross under inguinal ligament
  - 29% cross at anterior superior iliac spine

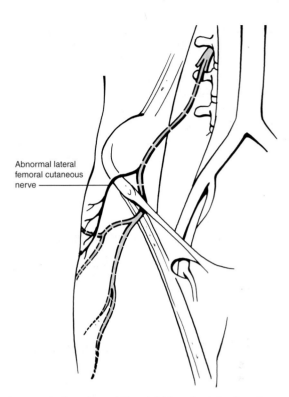

Anteroposterior view of the right hemipelvis showing an anomalous course of the lateral femoral cutaneous nerve, which may be 2 cm lateral to the anterior superior iliac spine. (From Garfin SR. Complications of spine surgery. Baltimore: Williams & Wilkins, 1989.)

- 11% cross within 2 cm posterior to ASIS
- Only 2% cross more than 2 cm posterior to ASIS
- Maintain 2-cm working distance to ASIS and dissect on outer table

Recommended Reading
Murata Y, et al. The anatomy of the lateral femoral cutaneous nerve, with special reference to the harvesting of iliac bone graft. J Bone Joint Surg Am 2000;82(5):746–747.

Infection—Postop

- Lumbar discectomy—<1%
- Lumbar fusion—2%
- Lumbar instrumentation—5%–6%
- Cervical—0.1%–0.3%
- Increasing pain and spasms postoperatively or continued longer than expected
- Fever and local signs, WBC count unreliable indicators of infection
- ESR and c-reactive protein useful
- ESR
  - Peaks postoperative day (POD) 4–5
    - Average in discectomy—75
    - Average in lumbar fusion—102

- Downward trend and normal at days 21–42
- Can be normal with infection if on steroids
- CRP
  - Peaks POD 2–3
  - Normal in 5–14 days
- Most common bug is *Staphylococcus*
- Gram negatives from direct contamination or septicemia
- Most common source of septicemia causing infection is pre- or postoperative urinary tract infection (UTI)

Recommended Readings

Bono CM, Garfin SR, eds. Spine. Philadelphia: Lippincott Williams & Wilkins; 2004.

Fardon D, Garfin S, eds. Orthopaedic Knowledge Update: Spine 2, 2nd ed. Rosemont, IL: American Academy of Orhopaedic Surgeons; 2002.

Infection—Spondylodiscitis/Osteomyelitis (OM)

- Usually hematogenous, seeds body
- Venous and arteriolar theory
- End plate erosion leads to disc destruction, epidural or paraspinal abscess, late deformity
- In C-spine, penetration of prevertebral fascia can lead to mediastinum
- In children, vascular channels cross cartilage growth plate and end within nucleus to inoculate bugs; thus, infection in children can start in disc. In adults, no such channels; thus, bugs get to disc by direct extension from vertical body
- In elderly and immunocompromised
- H/o preceding infection (upper respiratory infection, UTI, skin, IV site, dental)
- Risk factors for neurologic compromise include diabetes mellitus (DM), RA, old age, steroids, cephalad level, and *Staphylococcus*
- Presentation depends on location, bug virulence, and immune status
- Severe nonmechanical pain at rest and paraspinal spasm
- 50% with fevers
- 10% radicular pain, neurologic changes
- Weight loss
- Psoas abscess causes pain with extension
- Dysphagia, torticollis in C-spine
- Meningitis if it extends into epidural space
- ESR, white blood cell, CRP
- Xr—end plate destruction (late)
  - Usually nondiagnostic in 2–3 wk: differential diagnosis—destructive spondyloarthropathy from long-term hemodialysis

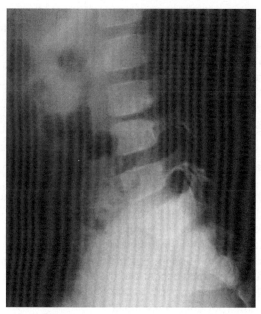

Plain radiograph of discitis in a child. Note the classic disc space narrowing at L3-4 and the more subtle loss of lordosis. (From Bono C, Garfin SR, Orthopaedic Surgery Essentials: Spine Philadelphia: Lippincott Williams & Wilkins 2004 with permission.)

- **Don't use indium scan in spine because only 17% sensitive; use technetium/gallium combination scan**
  - 90% sensitive, 85% accurate
  - Gallium 67 citrate is an analog of ferritin and is secreted by WBCs at sites of infection
  - Technetium 99m alone depends on local blood flow and can cause false negative in area of relative ischemia in children and elderly
- MRI
  - 95% sensitivity/specificity, 94% accurate
    - Gold standard, must use gadolinium
  - **Disc involved on MRI with pyogenic infection, uninvolved with tuberculosis (TB)**
  - Triad—T1 with decreased signal in bone marrow, contrast enhancement of marrow on T1, T2 with increased signal in disc ± bone
  - Phlegmon with high signal intensity (SI) on T2 and enhances on contrast T1
  - Abscess with low SI on T1, high SI on T2, peripheral rim enhancement on contrast T1
  - 80% of patients with epidural abscess have spondylodiscitis at time of imaging
- Myelogram contraindicated in setting of suspected infection
- Culture all potential sources—urine
- Blood cultures (gets bug in 50%)
- CT biopsy (gets bug in 70%)

- >50% from *Staphylococcus aureus* in children and adults
- Gram-negative *Escherichia coli, Pseudomonas,* and *Proteus* after genitourinary (GU) infection/procedure
- *Pseudomonas* in intravenous drug abuser, *Salmonella* from gastrointestinal (GI) source in sickle cell
- Low virulence coagulase-negative *Staphylococcus* and *Streptococcus viridans* cause indolent infection
- Bedrest, brace, IV antibiotics for 12 wk
- Antibiotics
  - Delay antibiotics until cultures taken
  - CRP used to time switch to po's
- Surgery if
  - Unable to confirm organism
    - Open biopsy gets diagnosis in >80%
  - Destruction leading to deformity
  - Epidural or paraspinal abscess
  - Failed antibiotics
  - ANY neurologic sign at any time during presentation
    - Higher levels (cervical) more worrisome
    - Seen in RA, diabetes mellitus, elderly
    - Operate even if seen late
- Indications for nonoperative treatment of epidural abscess
  - Medically unstable
  - Length of abscess prohibits surgery
  - No neurologic deficits
  - Complete paralysis >3 days
- Approach
  - Usually anterior decompression
  - Autologous strut graft because of infection
  - Vascular rib graft
  - Titanium cage filled with autograft
  - Posterior fixation usually not needed
  - Avoid lami if anterior column infected
  - If needed, stage posterior
  - Hyperalimentation
- Consider posterolateral approach in fragile patient
- Consider costotransversectomy if only culture, biopsy, or abscess drainage needed

Infections—Tuberculosis

- Worldwide most common cause of painful spine deformity in children
- Most common infection of pediatric spine
- <10% of TB involves bone but half of those are in spine
- Most common extrapulmonary location is spine
- With primary lung infection or later
- Indolent, present with mild back pain
- Three patterns—peridiscal (most common), central (in body), anterior (under ALL)

- Most common in thoracic spine, then lumbar, then cervical
- Starts in body metaph (earliest xr finding is lucency there) and spreads under anterior longitudinal ligament to cause skip lesions
- Paraspinal abscess common, may calcify (Ghon complex)
- Cutaneous sinus in severe cases
- **Disc spared,** distinguishing it from pyogenic infection
- Posterior elements spared
- 90% have two or more levels involved
- 15% involve skip lesions

DIFFERENTIAL DIAGNOSIS

- Non-TB spondylitis
  - Can't tell radiographically
- *Actinomyces, Nocardia, Brucella,* atypical mycobacteria, fungals
- Sarcoidosis
- Neoplasm (spares disc, usually one level)
- histocytosis X
- Technetium and gallium scans have high false-negative rates for TB (30%, 70%, respectively)

PATHOLOGY

- Granulomas, chronic inflammation
- Giant cell with "C"-formation nuclei
- Caseating necrosis
- acid fast bacilla
- CXR to rule out active pulmonary disease
- Ambulatory chemotherapy for 9 mo if no neurologic deficit or deformity
- Four-drug treatment——isoniazid, rifampin, ethambutol, pyrazinamide
- 10%–20% recurrence

SURGERY

- Modified Hong Kong
  - Anterior debr, + strut
- 9 months of chemotherapy
- Best neurologic recovery with anterior decompression compared with medications only and laminectomy

Klippel-Feil Syndrome

- Failure of segmentation or formation at 3–8 wk of gestation
- Triad present in only 50%
  - Low posterior hairline
  - Short webbed neck
  - Limited cervical ROM

- Rotation worse than flexion/extension because other levels compensate
- Associated with
  - Congenital scoliosis (60%)
  - Renal aplasia (33%)
  - Synkinesis (mirrorlike movements)
    - Incomplete pyramidal decussation
    - Improves with age
  - Sprengel shoulder (one-third)
    - Failure of scapular/clavicle descent
  - Congenital heart disease
  - Brainstem abnormalities
  - Congenital cervical stenosis
- Natural history unknown
- Workup
  - Spine flexion/extension xr's
  - Ear exam for deafness
  - Renal ultrasound (US), cardiac echo
- High-risk patterns for instability
  - C2-3 fused with O-C1 synostosis
  - Long fusion with abnormal O-C1 junction
  - Single open interspace between two fused segments
- Conservative therapy if asymptomatic
- Presents in second or third decade when unfused segments become hypermobile and degenerate
- Surgery for pain, instability, myelopathy

Recommended Readings

Herman MJ, Pizzutillo PD. Cervical spine disorders in children. Orthop Clin North Am 1999;30(3):457–466, ix.

Tracy MR, et al. Klippel-Feil syndrome: clinical features and current understanding of etiology. Clin Orthop Relat Res 2004;(424):183–190.

Kyphoplasty

- Aka vertebroplasty if no balloons
- Vertebroplasty first in France to treat C2 hemangioma for pain relief
- Began in United States in 1993
- 85%–90% pain relief and back to activities of daily living (ADLs)
- Recent RCT's of vertebroplasty show no superior outcome compared to sham surgery.
  - Buchbinder NEJM 2009

COMPLICATIONS

- Related to extrusion
- 1% in osteoporosis
- 5% in tumors
- Always polymethylmethacrylate, fat, bone emboli but clinically silent

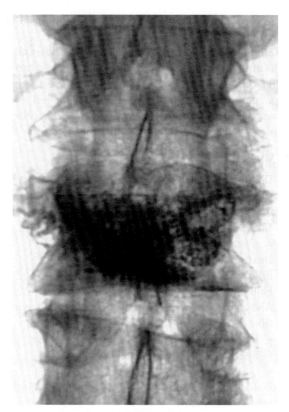

Postoperative radiograph after a midlumbar vertebroplasty performed through a unipedicular approach with a curved needle. (From Bono C, Garfin SR, Orthopaedic Surgery Essentials: Spine Philadelphia: Lippincott Williams & Wilkins 2004 with permission.)

Reference

Buschbinder R, Osborne RH, et al. A randomized trial of vertebroplasty for painful osteoporotic vertebral fractures. N Engl J med 2009;361(6):557–568.

Recommended Readings

Lane JM, et al. Minimally invasive options for the treatment of osteoporotic vertebral compression fractures. Orthop Clin North Am 2002;33(2):431–438, viii.

Lin J, Lane JM. The osteoporotic spine. Eura Medicophys 2004;40(3):233–237.

Kyphosis—Adult

ETIOLOGY

- Fractures, osteoporosis, or Scheuerman
- Osteoporosis
  - Rarely need biopsy
  - Nonoperative management is a must
  - Indications for surgery
  - Burst fracture with deformity or neurologic symptoms
  - Extended segmental fixation
  - Anterior column reconstruction

- Posttraumatic
  - Likely unrecognized ruptured posterior tension band
  - Anterior decompression if neurologic
  - anterior/posterior spinal fusion for deformity >55 degrees
  - Pedicle subtraction osteotomy corrects about 30 degrees, avoids anterior surgery

Recommended Readings

Bridwell KH, et al. Pedicle subtraction osteotomy for the treatment of fixed sagittal imbalance. J Bone Joint Surg Am 2003;85-A(3):454–463.

Cho KJ, et al. Comparison of Smith-Petersen versus pedicle subtraction osteotomy for the correction of fixed sagittal imbalance. Spine 2005;30(18):2030–2037; discussion 2038.

Kyphosis—Scheuermann

- Thoracic kyphosis >45 degrees
- >5-degree anterior wedging of three sequential vertebrae
- Normal kyphosis is 20–45 degrees from T3-12
- Normal kyphosis increases with age
  - 20 degrees in children
  - 25 degrees in adolescents
  - 40 degrees in adults
- Normal kyphosis apex at T7-8, lordosis apex at L3
- 1%–8% of population
- Adolescent males
- Possibly due to juvenile osteoporosis, defective end plates, or mechanical factors
- Autosomal dominant with high penetrance, variable expressivity
- Kyphosis not flexible
- Tight hamstrings
- 50% have thoracic pain in adolescence but decreases to 25% after skeletal maturity
- Heavy labor associated with T-L or L kyphosis
- Can't diagnose by xr in those <10 yo because ring apophysis has not ossified

DIFFERENTIAL DIAGNOSIS

- Infectious spondylitis
- Morquio Syndrome
- Tumor, trauma, neuromuscular disease
- Congenital kyphosis, postlami kyphosis
- Other xr findings
  - Disc narrowing
  - End plate irregularities
  - Spondylolysis (30%–50%)
  - Scoliosis (33%)
  - Schmorl nodes

NATURAL HISTORY

- Very controversial
- Problematic in old age due to osteoporotic fractures
- Risk of progression unknown
- Murray and Weinstein, 1993
  - 67 patients with prior diagnosis from 1920 to 1986 based on three consecutive wedged vertebrae
  - Average current kyphosis 71 degrees
  - Average follow-up 32 yr, consistent with controls
  - A little more back pain (64%) but no interference on ADLs
  - Normal pulmonary function tests if curve <100 degrees
  - Restrictive lung disease if curve >100 degrees and apex high (between T1-8)
  - Warned against many complications of surgery in setting of little future disability

TREATMENT

- Observe if <50 degrees
- No proven benefit of physical therapy, hamstring stretching
- Modified Milwaukee for progressive curve >50 degrees in patients with **>1 yr growth remaining (Risser 3)**
- Brace >18 mo, until wedging becomes 5 degrees or less
  - Considered effective
  - Brace fails if curve >74 degrees (Sachs et al., 1987)
- Surgery for mature patients, curve >75 degrees, pain, failed brace
- PSF with segmental compression
  - If flexible
  - Luque rods avoided because passing sublaminar wires at ends of curve disrupts posterior ligaments and can lead to kyphosis at the ends of the fusion
  - **Late loss of correction**
- A/PSF
  - If no correction to <50 degrees on extension xr
  - For large curves
  - Anterior release, interbody fusion
  - Do thoracotomy at two ribs above apex
  - Isola, two rods, three claws proximally, three claws distally
  - **Proximally, include end vertebra on curve, usually T2**
  - **Distally, through first lordotic disc**
  - Consider limiting correction to 50%
- Postural roundback
  - Kyphosis is flexible
  - No vertebral body changes
  - Treatment with extension exercises
  - Surgery is rarely indicated

References
Murray PM, et al. The natural history and long-term follow-up of Scheuermann kyphosis. J Bone Joint Surg Am 1993;75(2):236–248.
Sachs B, et al. Scheuermann kyphosis. follow-up of Milwaukee-brace treatment. J Bone Joint Surg Am 1987;69(1):50–57.

LS-spine—Low Back Pain

– Non specific, without identifiable cause

GENERAL

– Complex bio-psycho-social problem
– 80% lifetime prevalence
– 5% of patients with LBP disability account for 7% of the cost
– In 85% of patients, pain cannot be reliably attributed to a specific disease or specific spinal abnormality (Non-specific Low Back Pain)

Natural History of Acute Non-Specific LBP
– 80% improved by 6 weeks
– 10% become chronic

Risk Factors for Chronic Disabling LBP
– Depression
– Poor social support
– Job dis-satisfaction
– Poor coping skills

History and Physical Exam
– Used to screen patients for serious specific causes of low back pain
– Patients with risk factors ("red flags") require further work-up
– Patients without risk factors do not require imaging initially

Risk Factors of Serious Causes of Low Back Pain
– Cancer
    – History of cancer with new LBP
    – Unexplained weight loss
    – Age >50 at first onset of LBP
    – Failure to improve after 1 month
– Infection
    – Fever. IV Drug use, recent infection
– Cauda Equina Syndrome
    – Urinary retention
– Vertebral Compression Fracture
    – Osteoporosis, steroids, older age, focal tenderness
– Inflammatory Spondyloarthropathy
    – Younger age, morning stiffness, better with exercise, awakening due to LBP
– Lumbar Radiculopathy
    – Nerve root tension signs, motor/sensory/reflex changes

Lumbar Spinal Stenosis
– >6 years old, relieved with sitting

Treatment of Non-Specific Low Back Pain
Treatment of Acute Non-Specific Low Back Pain
– Reassurance
– Continued activities as tolerated
– Heat
– Medium firm mattress
– Spinal manipulation during acute severe symptoms
– Exercise therapy when acute severe symptoms improved
– Over-the-counter pain medications
– Judicious use of muscle relaxants, benzodiazepines, and narcotics

Treatment of Chronic Low Back Pain
– Bio-Psycho-Social therapy
– Screen for Depression
– Education, physical fitness, stress management
– Exercise therapy with addition of psychologic therapy

Surgical Treatment of Low Back Pain
– Results not predictable
– Over half of patients who undergo surgery for low back pain do not achieve good/excellent outcome
– Surgery results equivalent to physical therapy with cognitive intervention (Brox Spine 2003)

References
Brox JI, et al. Randomized clinical trial of lumbar instrumented fusion and cognitive intervention and exercises in patients with chronic low back pain and disc degeneration. Spine (Phila PA 1976). 2003;28(17):1913–1921.
Chou R, et al. Diagnosis and treatment of low back pain: a joint clinical practice guideline from the America College of Physician and the American pain Society. Ann Intern med 2007;147(7):478–491.

LS-spine—Degenerative Scoliosis

– Minimal structural abnormalities
– Advanced degenerative changes
– Mostly lower lumbar curves

CAUSE

– Unknown, osteoporosis, degenerative disc disease, osteoarthritic changes, compression fracture, facet tropism, lateral listhesis

NATURAL HISTORY

(Pritchett & Bortel, 1993)
– 68% convex left

- Of those who had xr's over 10 yr, 73% progressed at 3 degrees/yr
- Progression associated with
  - Cobb angle >30 degrees
  - Apical rotation > grade II
  - Lateral listhesis >6 mm
  - Intercrest line at or below L4-5 disc
- Larger curves in older people progressed more
- More severe pain, shorter pain-free intervals with larger deformity

PRESENTATION

- Wide range from asymptomatic to debilitating back and leg pain with imbalance
- Sagittal and coronal balance usually OK
- Most symptoms c/w spinal stenosis except symptoms did not get better with sitting
- Unilateral radicular symptoms most common on concavity side
- Bilateral or unilateral leg pain on convex side due to stenosis in the primary curve or the lower lumbar compensatory curve
- In patients with degenerative scoliosis and only back pain, hard to establish deformity as cause of axial pain
- Axial pain can be on convexity or concavity but most common on convexity
- Can have rib cage impingement, flat-back fatigue, loss of waistline
- In degenerative scoliosis, 85% have stenosis symptoms and 16% have stenosis and mechanical symptoms; in adult idiopathic scoliosis, 85% have only mechanical symptoms, 7% have stenosis symptoms, and 7% have both

IMAGING

- Myelography with contrast column compression greatest on apex of curve concavity
- MR gantry aligned with deformity
- Discograms useful in idiopathic scoliosis but not in degenerative scoliosis since patients present with neurogenic claudication instead of mechanical back pain, DDD is ubiquitous, and pain is not reliably provoked
- Hip dual-energy S-ray Absorptiometry scan for bone minderal density

NONSURGICAL TREATMENT

- Brace for pain relief but causes truncal deconditioning, thus use if patient's function better in brace; usually LSO but TLSO if rib impingement
- In progressive curve with minimal pain and OK balance, observe

SURGICAL TREATMENT

- Consider patient population who are elderly, osteoporotic, variable life expectancy, comorbidities
- Vaccaro and Ball (2000)—decompression alone leads to further collapse, instability, increased back and nerve pain
- 85% relief of pain and walking with decompression and fusion
- Must fuse if signs of instability such as lateral listhesis >5 mm, anterolisthesis, residual disc space height instead of more stable complete collapse, sagittal or coronal imbalance
- Fusion to sacrum rarely indicated
- Three-column osteotomy (posterior pedicle subtraction) can correct 30 degrees per level vs. Smith-Peterson (posterior column only) osteotomy, which corrects 8–10 degrees per level
- 20%–40% complication rates

References

Pritchett JW, Bortel DT. Degenerative symptomatic lumbar scoliosis. Spine 1993;18(6):700–703.
Vaccaro AR, Ball ST. Indications for instrumentation in degenerative lumbar spinal disorders. Orthopedics 2000;23(3): 260–271; quiz 272–273.

Recommended Reading

Tribus CB. Degenerative lumbar scoliosis: evaluation and management. J Am Acad Orthop Surg 2003;11(3):174–183.

LS-spine—Disc Herniation/Radiculopathy

- Lumbar MRI abnormal in asymptomatic patients
- Age 20–39
  - 21% HNP
  - 56% bulge, 34% degeneration
- Age 40–59
  - 22% HNP
  - 50% bulge, 59% degeneration
- Age 60–79
  - 36% HNP
  - 21% stenosis
  - 79% bulge, 93% degeneration
- 50%–80% lifetime incidence acute LBP
- Disc pressure least with supine laying < standing straight < sitting straight < standing and leaning forward < sitting and leaning forward
- Back pain from annular degeneration precedes leg pain, then lessens as leg pain predominates
- Symptoms increase with sitting, flexion episodes

RED FLAGS

- H/o tumor, infection, trauma, elderly, bowel/bladder
- Bilateral LE numb and weak, rectal pain, sensory change in perineum, paralysis of sphincter, sudden

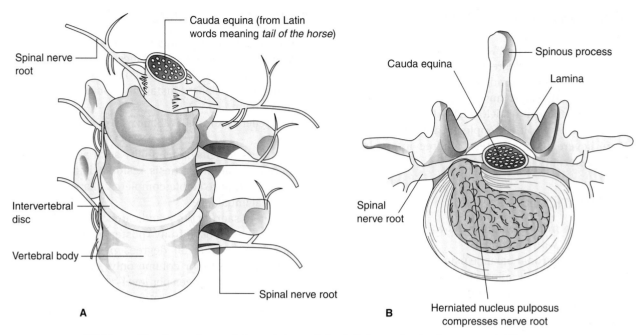

(A) Normal lumbar spine vertebrae, intervertebral disks, and spinal nerve root. **(B)** Ruptured vertebral disk. (From Smeltzer SC, Bare BG. Textbook of Medical-Surgical Nursing, 9th Ed. Philadelphia: Lippincott Williams & Wilkins, 2000.)

loss of bowel/bladder control should alert to cauda equina syndrome

PHYSICAL EXAMINATION

- **Positive tension sign** (straight leg raise) is an absolute prerequisite to take to operating room
  - Only for L5 or S1 roots
  - Pain/paresthesia at 30–70 degrees (first 15–30 degrees causes no root movement at foramen, greatest movement at 60–80 degrees and at L5 root)
  - Positive only if neurologic leg pain re-created below knee (not back pain)
  - Crossed SLR most specific
- Lasègue maneuver—ankle dorsi worsens symptoms on SLR
- Bowstring sign—flex hip and knee, then extend knee while putting thumb in popliteal fossa over tibial n.; positive only if dermatomal pain re-created either retro- or antegrade
- Femoral nerve stretch for L3, L4 roots done by extending hip with flexed knee

IMAGING

- Pursue red flags, failed nonoperative techniques >1 mo
- Get plain xr for LBP >6 wk
- EMG/NCV for patients with confounding neuropathy

- MRI very sensitive and specific but only confirmatory, for preoperative plan

ANATOMY

- Water increases closer to center of nucleus
- Proteoglycan increases in center
- Collagen II increases in center (nucleus)
- Total collagen decreases in center
- Collagen I decreases in center (in annulus)
- Biochemical changes of aging disc
  - With age, total prostaglandins and water content decrease and shift to more keratan sulfate
  - Loss of clear transition between nucleus and annulus
  - Increases in total collagen content
  - Loss of negatively charged PGs (which normally attract water)
- L5 and S1 roots slide 1 cm during flexion/extension
- Cord and roots stretch with flexion
- Canal and foramen enlarge with flexion
- L4-5 or L5-S1 are most common HNPs
- Strong genetic predisposition (twin study)
- HNP differentiated from lumbar spondylosis
- Posterolateral herniation
  - Most common by far
  - Affects lower level traversing root
- Foraminal far lateral herniation
  - Affects upper level exiting root

NONOPERATIVE TREATMENT

- NSAIDs
- Oral steroids
- Antidepressants, antiepileptics
- Epidural steroids with short-term improvement in leg pain and sensory deficit but no long-term effects
- Selective nerve root injections allow 2/3's of patients to avoid surgery
- Formal PT vs. home exercises, aerobic conditioning
- McKenzie extension program can decrease radicular pain and centralize pain pattern
- Williams flexion program better in mechanical LBP without radicular symptoms
- Best prognosis in young patients, those not pursuing lawsuits, and those with symptoms lasting <6 mo

PROGNOSIS FOR NONOPERATIVE TREATMENT

- 80% sciatica improve without surgery

INDICATIONS

- Cauda equina (emergent)
- Rapidly progressive motor deficit
- **Persistent disabling pain**

SURGICAL CANDIDATE

- Persistent deficit or sciatica/radiculopathy (not back pain) despite 6 wk of conservative therapy and
- Tension sign and
- Confirmatory MRI

SURGICAL RESULTS

- 90% relief of leg pain
- 15%–30% still with persistent back pain
- 50% patients complete motor recovery, less for sensory recovery
- <25% of patients recover reflexes
- Four-year results of Sport trials show that patients who underwent discectomy surgery achieved greater improvement than non-operatively treated patients (when as-treated analysis was used, Weinstein Spine 2007)

COMPLICATIONS

- 5% dural tears
- 5%–8% recurrent herniation over lifetime
- 1% discitis (fine immediately postoperatively but then 2–3 wk later, present with progressive back pain; must get MR with gadolinium to rule out discitis; usually treat with IV antibiotics even if needle biopsy negative; treat for *Staphylococcus*)

Reference
Weinstein JN, et al. Surgical versus nonoperative treatment for lumbar disc herniation: four-year results for the Spine Patient Outcomes Research Trial (SPORT). Spine (Phila PA 1976) 2008;33(25):2789–2800.

Recommended Readings
Atlas SJ, et al. The Maine lumbar spine study, part II. 1-year outcomes of surgical and nonsurgical management of sciatica. Spine 1996;21(15):1777–1786.
Saal JA, et al. The natural history of lumbar intervertebral disc extrusions treated nonoperatively. Spine 1990;15(7):683–686.
Weber H. Lumbar disc herniation. A controlled, prospective study with ten years of observation. Spine 1983;8(2):131–140.

LS-spine—Pedicle Screws

ROLES OF INTERNAL FIXATION

- Corrects deformity
- Provides early stabilization
- Increases rate and rapidity of fusion

HISTORICAL PERSPECTIVE

- Harrington –
  - Showed decreased pseudo rates from 40% to 1%–15%
  - 15% hook disengagement
  - Rod fracture at smooth-ratcheted junction
  - No rotational correction of deformity
  - Caused new lumbar flat-back deformity
- Luque
  - Introduced concept of segmental fixation
  - Dural tears and neurologic injury from sublamina wires
  - Limited ability to resist axial loads
- Cotrel-Dubousset
  - Used multiple hooks to avoid sublamina wires
  - Required intact laminae and facets
  - Hard to place over multiple adjacent segments

PEDICLE SCREWS

- Can be used in short- or long-segment fusions
- Do not require intact posterior elements
- Improve fusion by increasing stability

BIOMECHANICS

- Stronger in flexion, compression, torsion
- Primary mode of failure is bending fatigue
- The larger the inner diameter, the greater the bending rigidity
- Pull-out strength related to difference between inner and outer diameter (important in osteoporosis)
- Smaller thread pitch provides slightly stronger pull-out

- Anterior cortex violation gives increased pull-out strength but has 25% but risk of vascular injury
- Zdeblick (1993)
  - Prospective randomization of 124 patients, fused
  - No internal fixation—64% fusion, 71% good/excellent
  - Semirigid—77% fusion, 87% gd/ex
  - Rigid fixation—95% fusion, 95% gd/ex
- Lorenz et al. (1991)
  - Prospective randomization
  - Fusion for DDD ± instrumentation
  - Low back pain (LBP)—100% fusion, 80% of patients had decreased pain
  - No internal fixation—20% pseudo, 50% of patients had decreased pain

POTENTIAL PROBLEMS

- 5% radiculitis from misplacement
- 0%–12% neurologic injury (3.2% from SRS)
- Infection
  - 1% in decompression
  - 2% in decompression with fusion
  - 7% in decompression, fusion, with instrumentation
  - Related to operative time, use of fluoro
- Soft tissue irritation from bulkiness
- Impingement on unfused superior facet
- Increases degeneration from rigid subadjacent segment
- Difficult XR, CT, MRI evaluation of fusion
- Screw breakage (6%–30%)
- Increases blood loss?

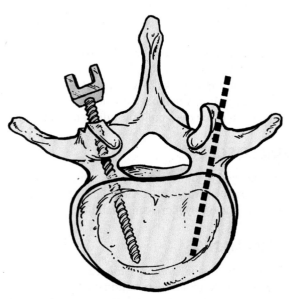

Lumbar fusion. Insertion of pedicle screw medially and inferiorly close to the anterior cortex without penetrating it. (From Koval KJ, MD and Zuckerman, JD, MD. Atlas of Orthopaedic Surgery: A Multimeidal Reference. Philadelphia: Lippincott Williams & Wilkins, 2004.)

- Tamponade effects of paraspinals against decorticated posterior elements lost with bulky screws
- Decreased space for bone graft

References
Lorenz M, et al. A comparison of single-level fusions with and without hardware. Spine 1991;16(8 Suppl):S455–458.
Zdeblick TA. A prospective, randomized study of lumbar fusion. preliminary results. Spine 1993;18(8):983–991.

Recommended Readings
Vaccaro AR, Garfin SR. Internal fixation (pedicle screw fixation) for fusions of the lumbar spine. Spine 1995;20(24 Suppl): 157S–165S.
Vaccaro AR, Garfin SR. Pedicle-screw fixation in the lumbar spine. J Am Acad Orthop Surg 1995;3(5):263–274.

LS-spine—Spinal Stenosis

- Combination of degenerative and developmental narrowing
- Soft tissue (flavum, disc) contributes 40% to narrowing
- M > F; late middle age
- Stenosis due to degenerative listhesis four times more common in females (L4-5)

CLASSIFICATION

- More common in females, DM, sacralized L5, more sagittal-oriented facets
- Developmental
  - Short pedicles, medial facets
  - Trefoil canal (vs. oval or round)
  - Achondroplasia
- Acquired—spondylosis
- Combined
  - Spondylolisthesis/instability
  - Dynamic stenosis
- Degenerative spondylolisthesis

PATHOPHYSIOLOGY

- Anterior posterior diameter of foramen decreased by bulging annulus anteriorly, hypertrophic facets posteriorly
- Foraminal height decreased by loss of disc height and associated facet subluxation
- Cortical evoked potentials highly sensitive to compression and affected by clinical symptoms
- Venous congestion, arterial constriction, block of axoplasmic flow, demyelination, wallerian degeneration
- Sensory fibers more sensitive than motor to compression and slower to recover
- Mechanism of pain unknown

STENOSIS LOCATIONS

Central Canal Stenosis
- Central sac or traversing root (L5 or lower) vs. inferior facet, flavum
- Central thecal sac compression causes nonspecific severe back pain and severe limitation in ambulation

Lateral Recess Stenosis
- Lateral dura near take-off of root
- Divided into three zones
  - Entrance zone
  - Midzone
  - Exit zone

Symptoms
- Back pain (from spondylosis or central stenosis), stiffness
- Worse in extension, positive shopping cart sign (patient leans forward over cart)
- Cycling is OK, treadmill painful
- "Simian" posture with shoulders anterior to pelvis

- Buttock pain extending to lateral thigh (proximal to distal)
- Neurogenic claudication (pain extending to legs, relieved by sitting down or leaning forward) in only 50% of patients
- 70% have equal back and leg pain
- Most common radicular pain is L5 then S1; half have more than one root involved
- Neurologic exam normal in >50%, typically some diminished reflexes only
- Postexercise exam may bring out motor weakness, most common in L5
- SLR and tension signs rarely positive
- Painless motor claudication rare
- Gait disturbance from poor proprioception rare
- Bowel/bladder—some urgency and frequency but frank incontinence rare

DIFFERENTIAL DIAGNOSIS

- If gait disturbance with positive Romberg, consider cervical myelopathy or intracranial d/o

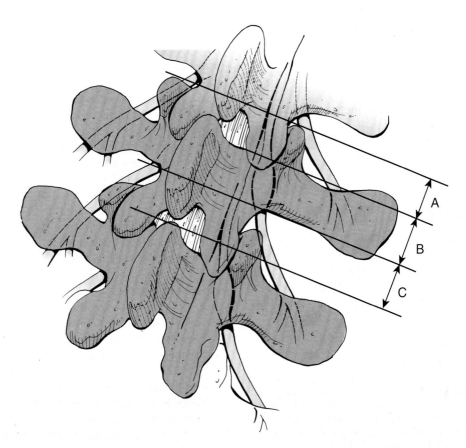

The lateral spinal canal in the lumbar spine showing the different zones. **(A)** Entrance zone. **(B)** Mid zone. **(C)** Exit zone. (Redrawn with modification from Lee CK, Rauschning W, Glenn W. Lateral lumbar spinal canal stenosis: classification, pathologic anatomy and surgical decompression. Spine 1988;13:313–320.)

- Peripheral vascular disease with symptom onset at consistent level of exercise, cramping in large muscle groups, pain distal to proximal
- Abdominal aortic aneurysm can cause back pain
- Hip osteoarthiritis can cause buttocks pain
- DM peripheral neuropathy can be ruled out with EMG-NCV

DIAGNOSIS

- By history and physical examination because xr findings ubiquitous
- Xr—medially placed facets, degenerative spondylolisthesis, scoliosis
- Dynamic laterals with >3-mm motion = instability
- 3-ft-long standing xr's in all revision surgeries to look for any malalignment
- MRI or CT myelography
  - Thecal sac <100 mm^2 = central stenosis
  - Can see lateral and foraminal compression
  - Used to determine operative level
  - Myelography shows cut-off of contrast
  - 21% of patients 60–80 yo have MR evidence of stenosis
- Plain myelography defines roots better in scoliotics

DIFFERENTIAL DIAGNOSIS

- Hip OA, peripheral neuropathy, metastatic disease
- Vascular
  - Pain distal to proximal
  - Relief with standing, stopping

NATURAL HISTORY

- Mild stenosis (no functional limitation) does well for many years
  - Waiting does not affect later surgery
- Severe stenosis (limits activity, walking) does better with earlier operation; waiting 1–2 yr sacrifices operative results

Recommended Readings

Atlas SJ, et al. Long-term outcomes of surgical and nonsurgical management of lumbar spinal stenosis: 8 to 10 year results from the Maine lumbar spine study. Spine 2005;30(8):936–943.

Atlas SJ, et al. The Maine lumbar spine study, part III. 1-year outcomes of surgical and nonsurgical management of lumbar spinal stenosis. Spine 1996;21(15):1787–1794; discussion 1794–1795.

Lee CK, et al. Lateral lumbar spinal canal stenosis: classification, pathologic anatomy and surgical decompression. Spine 1988;13(3):313–320.

LS-SPINE—STENOSIS: MRI FINDINGS

Central
- Normal canal and thecal sac is plump oval
- Flat ovals or triangles indicate stenosis
- No universally accepted grading

Lateral Recess
- Located on medial side of pedicles
- Roots lie in these recesses after leaving thecal sac before exiting through foramen
- There is foramen on top and bottom of each lateral recess
- Stenosis if shape of recess is deformed and root is compressed

Foraminal
- Should have vertical oval appearance on sagittal with root (dorsal root ganglion) in the upper half of oval
- Stenosis from disc abnormalities narrows the lower part of the foramen to cause a keyhole appearance
- Although DRG looks free with fat around it, as the nerve goes laterally and inferiorly, disc or other material can compress on spinal nerve or dorsal and ventral rami at any point in foramen

LS-SPINE—STENOSIS: TREATMENT

Nonoperative
- NSAIDs, avoid narcotics
- Williams flexion exercises
- Bracing only short term to prevent truncal deconditioning
- Epidural steroids effective in lumbar radicular syndromes but few studies for degenerative stenosis; can be used to help PT
- Trans-foraminal/selective root injections

Surgical Indications
- Persistent pain, limitations in ADLs
- Progressive weakness (rare indication)

Decompression
- Lami and partial facetectomy of all moderate and severe levels seen (vs. only symptomatic levels)
- Preserve 50% of facets when undercutting
- Preserve 1 cm of dorsal pars surface
- #4 Penfield to mobilize compressed root to assess decompression
- Probe neural foramen with dural elevator
- Foraminotomy usually needed in severe level
  - Part of superior facet of caudad level
  - Part of pars
  - Annulus
  - Pedicle of cephalad level
- Fusion ± Internal Fixation

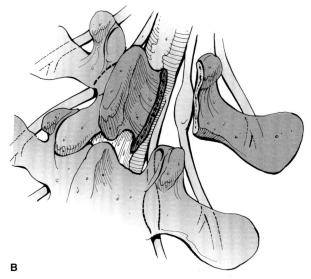

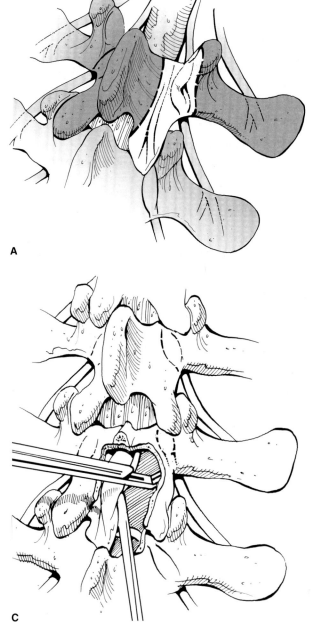

The extent of decompression for mid zone stenosis. **(A** and **B)** Total laminectomy and total removal of the inferior articular facet ensure adequate decompression but may lead to a significant amount of instability of a motion segment. The osteophytes and hypertrophic ligamentum flavum under the pars interarticularis can be excised and curettaged without sacrificing the facet joint or an entire lamina. Careful undercutting of the facet and removal of the bone from the undersurface of the lamina overlying the root canal can be performed with a Kerrison rongeur **(C)**. This can achieve neural decompression, while minimizing destabilization of the spine. (Redrawn with modification from Lee CK, Rauschning W, Glenn W. Lateral lumbar spinal canal stenosis: classification, pathologic anatomy and surgical decompression. Spine 1988;13:313–320.)

- – If degenerative spondylolisthesis or degenerative scoliosis because better results (Herkowitz & Kurz, 1991)
- – If unstable from taking total of more than one facet
- – If >3 mm motion on dynamic laterals, then fusion; if >5 mm and local mechanical symptoms, then internal fixation
- – NOT indicated in just spondylosis
- – Internal fixation increases fusion but does not improve patient outcome (Herkowitz & Kurz, 1991)
- – Most accurate way to diagnose pseudo is surgical exploration

- – Four-year results of SPORT trial for spinal stenosis and degenerative spondylolisthesis show that patients who underwent decompression/instrumented fusion surgery maintained substantially greater pain relief and improvement in function (when as-treated analysis was used, Weinstein JBJS 2009)

Results
- – Severe stenosis = better outcome
- – Generally 80%–85% successful
- – Katz et al. (1991)
  - – Only 57% patients with successful surgery

- Unsuccessful surgery associated with single-level decompression, multiple medical problems
- 5%/yr degeneration at adjacent levels to decompression area
- Predominant back pain associated with worse outcome (Katz et al., 1995)

Complications

- By 5–10 yr, good results wear off from return of stenosis
- 2%–3% infection rate, 0.4% nerve root injury from bad pedicle screw
- 14% dural tears

Revision

- Better outcome if pain-free interval after index procedure, if presentation occurs >18 mo after index procedure
- Worse outcome with periroot fibrosis

References

Herkowitz HN, Kurz LT. Degenerative lumbar spondylolisthesis with spinal stenosis. A prospective study comparing decompression with decompression and intertransverse process arthrodesis. J Bone Joint Surg Am 1991;73(6):802–808.

Katz JN, et al. Clinical correlates of patient satisfaction after laminectomy for degenerative lumbar spinal stenosis. Spine 1995;20(10):1155–1160.

Katz JN, et al. The outcome of decompressive laminectomy for degenerative lumbar stenosis. J Bone Joint Surg Am 1991; 73(6):809–816.

Weinstein, et al. Surgical compared with nonoperative treatment for lumbar degenerative spondylolisthesis. Four-year results in the Spine Patient Outcomes Research Trial (SPORT) randomized and observational cohorts. J Bone Joint Surg Am 2009;91(6):1295–1304.

MRI

SAGITTAL CUTS

- Cord, central canal
- Disc signal, height
- Bodies, spinous processes
- Roots, foramen
- Ligaments
- Epidural space

AXIAL CUTS

- Roots
- Cord
- Disc contour
- Bodies
- Central canal
- Lateral recess
- Ligaments
- Epidural space
- Facet junctions

CONTRAST

- Usually only postoperatively or if concern for tumor, infection

NORMAL DISC

- Medium signal like muscle on T1
- Homogenous high-signal-intensity disc with low signal of annulus on T2

ABNORMAL NUCLEUS

- On T2, low SI line that cuts disc in half on sagittal view is intranuclear cleft, very early sign of degeneration

ABNORMAL ANNULUS

- Radial tears of annulus seen as focal areas of high SI on posterior annulus on T2 or contrasted T1 called high intensity zones (HIZs)
- Painful as vascular and neoneural granulation tissue grows into tear
- High intensity zone shown to be in 56% of asymptomatic patients at the average age of 40
- Anterior annulus is thicker than posterior

DISC MORPHOLOGY

- Compare axial cut through vertical body vs. cut through disc
- Bulge—circumferential, symmetric
- Protrusion—focal asymmetric; AP size < medial–lateral size on axial
- Extrusion—more protrusion
  - AP size > medial–lateral size on axial
  - On sagittal, goes above ± below
  - Spontaneous reduction in size of extrusions and protrusions with nonoperative therapy well documented
  - **Only 1% of asymptomatic patients have extrsns** (Jensen et al., 1995)
- Sequestered—disc material loses attachment to parent disc
  - Sequestered fragment is higher signal than parent on T2 due to inflammation
  - Cause of failed surgery
- Focal disc locations—central, paracentral, foraminal, extraforaminal
  - 90% central and paracentral
  - 90% at L4-5 or L5-S1
- In C-spine osteophytes usually accompany disc and are hard to differentiate one from other

- In older patients, herniations tend to include end plates and annulus instead of only nucleus
- Small epidural hematomas associated with HNP with intermediate SI on T1 and high SI on T2 hard to distinguish from sequestered fragment
- Vacuum discs are cracks in desiccated nucleus that fill up with N2 and seen as horizontal signal void on all sequences; the finding can be confused with infection; N2 pockets can fill up with high SI fluid on positional change
- Calcified discs seen as heterogeneous high SI on T1, but as more Ca^{2+} builds up, becomes low SI
- Modic changes to vertical body from degenerated disc
  - Focal or diffuse bands parallel to end plates
  - Type I—low SI T1, high SI T2 (inflammation)
  - Type II—high SI T1, same as fat T2
  - Type III—Low SI T1 and T2 (sclerosis)
- Modic vs. infection—infection has high SI on T2, which would be unusual in degenerative disc adjacent to Modic changes

FACETS

- Can get Modic changes in pedicles adjacent to degenerative facet junction
- Synovial cysts with low SI on T1 and high SI on T2 can arise from facets
- Ligamentum flavum covers laminae and facets

SPINOUS PROCESSES

- Baastrup disease (kissing spine)—degenerative hyperlordosis causes spinous processes (SPs) to touch and form pseudo-joints; seen as high-SI bursal fluid between SPs on T2

INTRAOSSEOUS HERNIATED NUCLEUS PULPOSIS

- Aka Schmorl nodes
- Inflammatory reaction may occur with vascularization of disc material and marrow edema
- Schmorl node can rim enhance and appear "aggressive"

MRI—Postoperative

- Not possible to tell meningocele from pseudomeningocele (dural defect with leak of CSF) on MRI
- Marrow in body adjacent to operated disc appears same postoperatively as preoperatively
- Epidural scars light up with contrast most prominently during the first year after surgery but enhancement may last years

- Contrast enhancement of intrathecal nerve roots is common up to 6 months after surgery
- Disc contrast enhancement may last for years, usually posteriorly by annulus and rarely in center of disc; shouldn't be confused with infection because adjacent bodies should appear normal

SCAR VS. DISC

- Scar tissue over 6 mo old enhances diffusely and early after gadolinium given
- Scar has irregular margins and is not continuous with disc
- Scar causes retraction of dural sac rather than causing mass effect
- Disc does not enhance until late if at all and only enhances peripherally
- Difficult to distinguish in first 6 mo postoperatively

ARACHNOIDITIS

- Caused by injection into subarachnoid space
- From infection or bleeds
- Inflammation and subsequent adhesions
- On MR T2, nerves of cauda equina are clumped, wavy, angled, and irregular on sagittal cuts vs. normal gentle curves
- Nerves may adhere to dura, giving appearance of empty dural sac on axial cuts
- Contrast does not help

Recommended Readings

Bono CM, Garfin SR, eds. Spine. Philadelphia: Lippincott Williams & Wilkins; 2004.

Fardon D, Garfin S, eds. Orthopaedic Knowledge Update: Spine 2, 2nd ed. Rosemont, IL: American Academy of Orhopaedic Surgeons; 2002.

Jensen MC, et al. Magnetic resonance imaging of the lumbar spine in people without back pain. N Engl J Med 1994;331(2): 69–73.

Neurologic Exam

- Heel walk
- Toe walk
- Toe-to-heel tightrope gait
- Romberg sign—loss of balance with arm forward and eyes closed is sign of posterior column dysfunction

UPPER MOTOR NEURON SIGNS

- Spasticity, hyperreflexia
- Clonus
- Babinski—big toe dorsiflexes, others flare (normal is plantarflexion of all toes)

- Hoffman—thumb and IF IP junctions contract with flicking of middle finger DIPJ or sudden extension of distal interphalangeal joint
- Inverted radial—biceps or brachioradialis reflex that is suppressed but generalizes to finger flexors; normal is to extend wrist; indicates cord compression at C6
- Gait disturbances
- Finger escape sign—ulnar digits abduct when patient is asked to keep fingers in full extension
- Jaw jerk—hyperreflexia upon tapping masseter and temporalis of cranial nerve V indicates upper motor neuron lesion at brainstem
- Lhermitte—rapid flexion causes electric shock down back, may be a sign of myelopathy
- Crossed adductor sign—tapping of VMO causes hip adduction

LOWER MOTOR NEURON SIGNS

- Fasciculation with atrophy
- Areflexia
- Spurling—extension and lateral bend exacerbate radicular symptoms
  - Some describe Spurling as lateral bend and rotation to symptom side with loading
- Distraction/compression of C-spine relieves/worsens radicular symptoms
- Shoulder abduction relieves radicular pain in arm

CERVICAL AND PERIPHERAL NERVES

Sensory Exam
- C5 and axillary—lateral deltoid
- C6 and median—tip of thumb
- C7—tip of long finger
- C8 and ulnar—tip of little finger; radial: dorsal thumb web
- T1—medial forearm
- Musculocutaneous—lateral forearm

Reflexes
- C5—biceps
- C6—brachioradialis
- C7—triceps

Motor
- C5 and axillary—shoulder abduction
- C6 and musculocutaneous—elbow flexion
- C6 and radial—wrist extension (not posterior interoseus nerve)
- C7 and radial—elbow, finger extension (PIN)
- C7 and median—wrist flexion
- C8 and median—finger flexion
- Median, C8, T1—thumb intrinsics
- Ulnar, C8, T1—hand intrinsics

- C5—deltoid, supraspinatus, infraspinatus, biceps
- C6—brachioradialis, wrist extension weak; infraspinatus, serratus anterior, triceps, supinator, EPB
- C7—triceps, wrist flexion, pronators, finger extensors, EPL, and lateral dorsi
- C8-T1—all ulnar n. innervated mm., hypothenar, dorsal and volar interossei, all lumbricals, plus thenar, flexor policis longus, FDS, all FDPs

LOWER EXTREMITY

Sensory Exam
- L1—inguinal ligament area
- L4 and femoral—medial leg to ankle
- L5 and peroneal—dorsum foot
  - Deep peroneal = first webspace
- S1 and posterior tibial—sole of foot

Reflexes
- T7-T10—supraumbilical abduction reflexion
- T11-L1—infraumbilical abduction reflexion
- T12-L1—cremasteric reflexion
- L4—quads
- S1—Achilles
- S2-4—anal wink
- S3-4—bulbocavernosus

Motor
- L1, L2, L3—iliopsoas
- L3, L4—hip adductors
- L4 and femoral—quadriceps
- L4 and DPN—tibial anterior
- L5 and DPN—exensor hallucis longus
- L5—gluteus medius
- L5 and S1—medial and lateral hamstrings
- S1 and posterior tibial—plantarflexion
- S1 and superficial peroneal nerve—peroneals
- S1—gluteus maximus

Neurologic Exam—Quick

- Breathing, shrug—C4
- Deltoid—C5
- Biceps—C5
- (Sh IR—C5)
- (Sh ER—C6)
- Wrist extension—C6
- Triceps, wrist flexion—C7
- Finger flexion—C8
- Intrinsics, interossei—T1
- Iliopsoas—L1-2
- Quadriceps—L3
- Tibial anterior—L4
- EHL—L5
- Gastrocnemius—S1

Sensory dermatomes

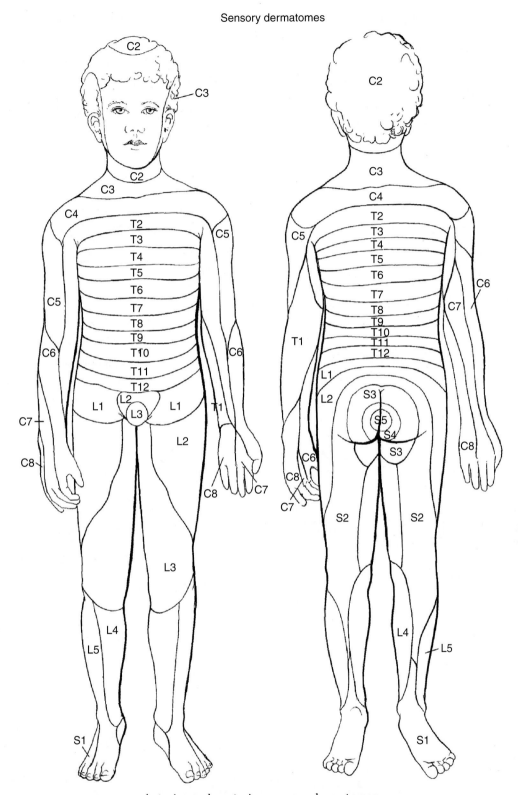

Anterior and posterior sensory dermatomes.

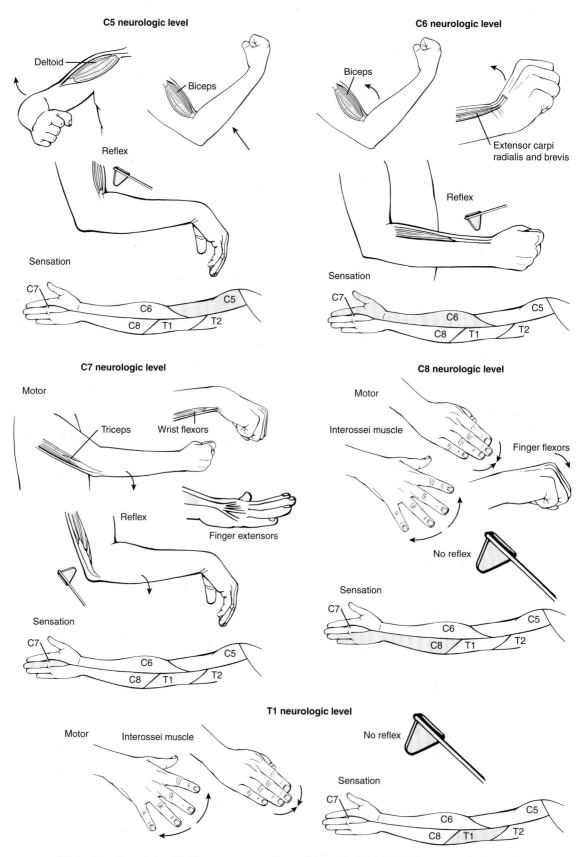

Clinical testing of the C5-T1 nerve roots. (From Klein JD, Garfin SR: History and physical examination. In Weinstein JN, Rydevik BL, Sonntag VKG, eds. Essentials of the spine. New York: Raven Press, 1995:71–95.)

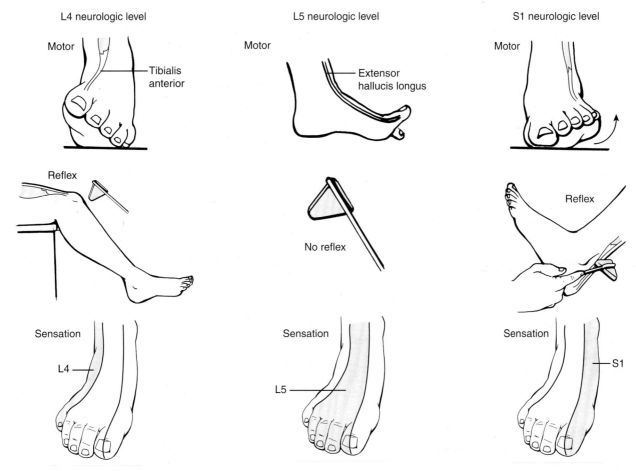

Clinical testing of the L4-S1 nerve roots. (From Klein JD, Garfin SR: History and physical examination. In Weinstein JN, Rydevik BL, Sonntag VKG, eds. Essentials of the spine. New York: Raven Press, 1995:71–95.)

- Bladder sphincter—S2
- Anal sphincter—S3
- Upper outer arm—C5
- Thumb—C6
- Middle finger—C7
- Small finger—C8
- Medial forearm—T1
- Nipples—T4
- Umbilicus—T10
- Groin—L1
- Anterior thigh—L2
- Knee—L3
- Medial malleolus—L4
- Small toe—S1
- Posterior thigh—S2
- Anal—S3-5

ASIA SCALE MOTOR SOURCE

- C5—elbow flexors
- C6—wrist extensors
- C7—elbow extensors
- C8—finger flexors
- T1—small finger abductor
- L2—hip flexors
- L3—knee extensors
- L4—ankle dorsiflexors
- L5—hallux extensors
- S1—ankle plantarflexors

Recommended Reading

Bono CM, Garfin SR, eds. Spine. Philadelphia: Lippincott Williams & Wilkins; 2004.

Neurologic Injury

CAUSES

- Acute cord contusion
- Subacute cord compression by
  - Instruments
  - Instrumentation
  - Hematoma

- Stretching of cord
  - From deformity correction
- Vascular insult
  - Deformity correction
  - Compression
  - Sacrificing segmentals
- Postoperative—delayed onset (24–48 hr)
  - Caused by epidural hematoma or vascular insult
- Requires immediate operation for removal of instrumentation (ROI), hematoma decompression, and steroids (30 mg/kg initial dose, then 5.4 mg/kg/hr for 23 hr)
  - Maintain adequate blood pressure
  - Imaging and consults delay treatment

Os Odontoideum

- Smooth corticated round/oval ossicle separated from axis
- Blood supply to dens
  - Paired anterior and posterior ascending arteries off vertebral
  - Cleft perforators from carotid

CAUSE

- Failure of fusion of os
  - Fusion at 3–6 yo but fusion line may remain for many years
- Probably traumatic—unrecognized fracture, nonunion
- Usually dens is three times length of C3 body
- Most asymptomatic, incidental diagnosis
- Neurologic symptom from os into cord in extension or odontoid into cord in flexion
- C1-2 instability can also cause vertebral artery insufficiency with seizure, vertigo, syncope, visual disturbances
- Surgery if neurologic symptoms, instability
  - >5 mm on flexion/extension xr
  - Atlanto-Dens interval >10 mm
  - Space available for the Cord <13 mm
  - Translation >40%, >20 degrees angulation
- Avoid contact sports
- Prophylactic fusion controversial
  - No contact sports after fusion

Recommended Reading

Schiff DC, Parke WW. The arterial supply of the odontoid process. J Bone Joint Surg Am 1973;55(7):1450–1456.

Ossiculum Terminale

- Tip of dens
- Appears at age 3

- Fuses to dens at 12 yo
- Much smaller than os odontoideum
- No clinical significance

Scoliosis—Adolescent

- Structural lateral curve that occurs near onset of puberty without known cause
- 7 degrees of angle of trunk rotation is criterion for referral
- Must be >10 degrees for diagnosis
- Curve >10 degrees in 2%–3% of those <16 yo
- Curve >20 degrees in 1 of 2,500
- M = F if ~10 degrees but F > M in treatment
- Most curves are right thoracic, left lumbar
- Cause (?)—pineal gland/melatonin, platelet calmodulin, osteopenia, equilibrium system

ANATOMY

- Normal kyphosis is 25–50 degrees, apex T6-T8
- Apex of lordosis at L3-4
- Normally lordosis is two times kyphosis

EVALUATION—RADIOGRAPHIC

- Nash-Moe method
  - To assess rotation
  - 1—concave side pedicle disappearing
  - 2—concave side pedicle disappeared
  - 3—convex pedicle at center of body
  - 4—convex pedicle past midline
- Cobb method
  - Interobserver variability 7.2 degrees and intraobserver 4.9 degrees without preselected endpoints
  - 10-degree measurement difference needed to be 95% confident that a true change occurred
- Structural curves have the following (mnemonic DWARF):
  - Displacement of apex
  - Wedging of body or disc space
  - Angulation
  - Rotation
  - Flexibility (lack of)
- Nonstructural curves have no rotation and correct with bending
- When to do MRI
  - Most common findings in scoliosis are Arnold-Chiari and hydromelia
  - Structurally abnormal
  - Excessive kyphosis
  - <11 yo
  - Rapid progression
  - Neurologic signs/symptoms

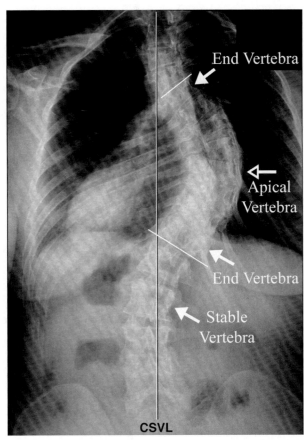

Radiograph showing the central sacral vertical line (CSVL), apical vertebra, stable vertebra, and end vertebrae. The stable vertebra is the most proximal lower thoracic or lumbar vertebra that is bisected most closely by the CSVL. (From Bono C, Garfin SR, Orthopaedic Surgery Essentials: Spine Philadelphia: Lippincott Williams & Wilkins, 2004, with permission.)

- Associated syndromes
- Left curves
- Do et al., 2001
  - 327 patients with operative scoliosis of average 57 degrees
  - Prospective study with preoperative MRIs
  - Two with syrinx, four with Chiari I, one with fatty infiltration of T10
  - None required neurosurgery or more workup
- Bone scan if pain associated with scoliosis
- Risser
  - Starts from lateral to medial and divided into 4, with 5 being complete ossification
  - Risser 1–4 takes 1.4 yr
  - Risser 4–5 takes 2 yr
  - When iliac apophysis starts to ossify, females have 3–5 cm and males have 5–8 cm of growth of sitting height (spine growth)
- Tanner

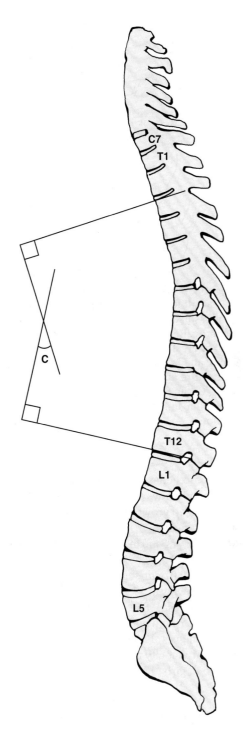

Sagittal alignment of the spine showing the Cobb method of quantifying spinal deformities. (From Bono C, Garfin SR, Orthopaedic Surgery Essentials: Spine Philadelphia: Lippincott Williams & Wilkins 2004 with permission.)

- Growth spurt coincides with onset of pubic hair in both sexes and breast budding in girls
- Peak growth velocity (time of maximum rate of curve progression) precedes menarche by 6 mo, also closure of triradiate cartilage

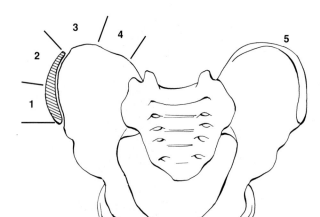

Risser sign—progressive ossification of the iliac apophyses is a soft indicator of skeletal maturity. Risser 1 (beginning of ossification) usually is visualized around the time of menarche. Risser 4 (entire apophysis visualized but not fused to crest) signifies the patient is past peak height velocity and is nearing the end of spinal growth. Risser 5—the entire apophysis has fused to the crest. (From Bono C, Garfin SR, Orthopaedic Surgery Essentials: Spine Philadelphia: Lippincott Williams & Wilkins 2004 with permission.)

- Menarche precedes Risser 1 by 6 mo
- Axillary hair in boys and menarche in girls coincide with decreased growth phase—at this point, 18 mo of growth remain
- Menarche 12 yr/8 mo in whites, 12 yr/3 mo in blacks (range 9–16 yo)
- Spine grows at 0.07 cm/segment/yr
- Spine stops growing at 17 yo in females, 19 yo in males
- Tanner and Davies, 1985
  - Adolescent growth spurt begins
    - 10.5 yo in girls, 12.5 yo in boys
  - Peak height velocity at
    - 11.5 yo in girls, 13.5 yo in boys

NATURAL HISTORY

(Weinstein et al., 2003)
- Back pain similar to background (60%)
- Decreased pulmonary function (forced vital capacity) only seen in thoracic curve >100 in nonsmokers
- Direct correlation between thoracic curve magnitude and vital capacity and forced expiratory volume in the first second
- Hypokyphosis contributes to decreased pulmonary function
- No increases in mortality with curve <100 degrees

- All curves <30 degrees at maturity don't progress
  - 68% of curves >50 degrees at maturity progress
- T curves >50 degrees at maturity progress at 1 degrees/yr
- L curves >30 degrees likely to progress and shift
  - Don't progress if L5 below intercrest line
- Mild/moderate scoliosis has no effect on pregnancy, delivery

CURVE PROGRESSION

(Lonstein & Carlson, 1984)
- In untreated

	5–19 degrees	20–29 degrees
Risser 0, 1	22%	68%
Risser 2, 3, 4	1.6%	23%

- Factors associated with progression (>6-degree change is significant)
  - Young age at diagnosis, Risser 0–1, premenarchal
  - Magnitude of curve
  - Thoracic curve because they present earlier
  - Double curves
  - Females 10 times more likely than males of same curvature

ADOLESCENT SCOLIOSIS—CLASSIFICATION

Curve Patterns as Described by King and Moe

Location	Type	Description
Thoracic	I	Principal lumbar, secondary thoracic curve
	II	Principal thoracic, secondary lumbar curve
	III	Thoracic curve only (apex ≥ T10)
	IV	Long thoracic curve (extends to L4)
	V	Double thoracic curve
Double major		Equally structural thoracic & lumbar curves
Lumbar		Apex in lumbar spine
Thoracolumbar		Apex at thoracolumbar junction

From: Bono CM, Garfin SR, eds. Othropaedic Surgery Essentials: Spine Philadelphia: Lippincott William & Wilkins, 2004.
Adapted from King HA, Moe JH, Bradford DS, et al. The selection of fusion levels in thoracic idiopathic scoliosis. J Bone Joint Surg, 1983;65A:1302.

Curve Patterns as Described by Lenke et al.

Type	Proximal Thoracic	Main Thoracic	Thoracolumbar/Lumbar	Curve Type
1	Nonstructural	Structural (major*)	Nonstructural	Main thoracic
2	Structural	Structural (major*)	Nonstructural	Double thoracic
3	Nonstructural	Structural (major*)	Structural	Double major
4	Structural	Structural (major*)	Structural	Triple major
5	Nonstructural	Nonstructural	Structural (major*)	Thoracolumbar/lumbar
6	Nonstructural	Structural	Structural (major*)	Thoracolumbar/lumbar; main thoracic

		Modifiers		
Lumbar Spine Modifier	*Location of Central Sacral Vertical Line at Lumbar Apex*		*Thoracic Sagittal Modifier*	*Sagittal Profile T5-12*
A	Between pedicles		–	Hypokyphotic <10°
B	Touches apical body		N	Normal 20–40°
C	Lateral to body		+	Hyperkyphotic >40°

From Lenke LG, Betz RR, Harms J, et al. Adolescent idiopathic scoliosis: a new classification to determine extent of spinal arthrodesis. J Bone Joint Surg, 2001;83A(8):1169.

References

Do T, et al. Clinical value of routine preoperative magnetic resonance imaging in adolescent idiopathic scoliosis. A prospective study of three hundred and twenty-seven patients. J Bone Joint Surg Am 2001;83-A(4):577–579.

Lonstein JE, Carlson JM. The prediction of curve progression in untreated idiopathic scoliosis during growth. J Bone Joint Surg Am 1984;66(7):1061–1071.

Tanner JM, Davies PS. Clinical longitudinal standards for height and height velocity for North American children. J Pediatr 1985;107(3):317–329.

Weinstein SL, et al. Health and function of patients with untreated idiopathic scoliosis: a 50-year natural history study. JAMA 2003;289(5):559–567.

SCOLIOSIS—ADOLESCENT—TREATMENT

Treatment Guidelines

Bracing
- Indications for bracing
  - 30–40 degrees in growing child
  - 25–29 degrees with known progress, Risser 0–1
- Prerequisites for bracing
  - Growth—Risser 0, 1, 2
  - Braceable curve (cervical–thoracic isn't)
  - Compliant patient (impossible to measure)
- Contraindications for bracing
  - Completed growth
  - Growing child with >45 degrees
  - Curve <25 degrees without progression
  - Thoracic lordosis
    - Brace pushes on rib of apical body
    - This makes brace lordogenic
    - Decreased pulmonary function if kyphosis <10 degrees
  - Noncompliant patient, obesity
- Prescription for brace
  - Need level pelvis as foundation

General Treatment Algorithm for Adolescent Idiopathic Scoliosis

(From Bono C, Garfin SR, Orthopaedic Surgery Essentials: Spine Philadelphia: Lippincott Williams & Wilkins 2004 with permission.)

- Three-point fixation with localizer pad at rib of apex or lower (lower because ribs pointed down and pad will provide upward force), at posterior axillary line
  - For double curve, push on transverse processes of lumbar curve
  - Decrease lordosis to "unlock" spine
  - Milwaukee for apex above T7
  - Boston for apex below T8 (Boston = below)
- Expect 75% success rate for brace
- More success if correction >50% in brace
- Goal is to prevent progression
- Full-time wear (23 hr) is standard
  - Wean on and off
  - Full time for 2 yr
  - Until past peak velocity
    - Marked by menarche or
    - Documented growth curve
  - Part-time wear (16 hr) is better than nothing
  - Less than part-time wear (8 hr) is not better than wearing no brace
  - At 5 yr follow-up, curve is equal to beginning

Surgery
- Indications of skeletal immaturity
  - Premenarchal Risser 0–2
  - Curve >40 degrees
  - Curve progresses in appropriate brace
- Indications of skeletal maturity
  - Thoracic curve >50 degrees
  - Thoracolumbar, lumbar curve >40 degrees with marked apical rotation/translation
  - Double major curve >50 degrees
  - Significant imbalance
- Posterior spinal fusion is gold standard for most
  - Get coronal correction by connecting precontoured concave rod and rotating 90 degrees into sagittal plane
  - Left rod placed first
  - Pulling the left pedicle screw or left hooks to left rod derotates and brings down right-sided posterior hump
  - Most distal hook is one level proximal to stable vertebra
  - Distraction of left concave rod increases and restores thoracic kyphosis and decreases right-sided curve
  - Compression of same left rod in lumbar spine corrects scoliosis and restores lumbar lordosis
- Most predictable balance with fusion to stable vertebra
  - Center sacral line is perpendicular to ilium and bisects midline of sacrum
  - Stable vertical line is most closely bisected by this line

- Indications for anterior release/fusion
  - If >45 degrees or <50% correction on bend xr's
  - In thoracolumbar, and high left curves to save levels
  - Incision on convex side
  - Incision along rib of upper fused level
  - Above T10—thoracotx alone
  - T11-L1—thoractx and retroperitoneal with diaphragmatic detachment (thoracoabdominal approach)
  - L1-5—retroperitoneal alone
  - Release posterolateral corner of disc to allow derotation and lordotization
  - Compression on convex side
  - No anterior instrument distal to L4 for fear of common iliac vessels
  - Contraindicated in
  - Kyphosis above proposed level
  - Compensatory curve >20 degrees in bending
- Harrington—fuse to one above and two below end vertebrae in stable zone
  - His distraction and compression rods led to good coronal correction but distraction led to lumbar hypolordosis "flat-back" deformity

Scoliosis—Adult

- Untreated adolescent scoliosis or
- De novo degenerative scoliosis (>40 yo)
  - Usually lumbar, lesser magnitude
  - Associated with rotatory subluxation
  - Associated with lateral listhesis
  - Associated with stenosis on concavity
  - Patients also get symptoms on convexity-side leg from fractional curve at lower roots

NATURAL HISTORY
- Adult scoliosis' association with pain controversial (most notable in large lumbar or T-L curves)
- Progression rare if <30 degrees
- If >50 degrees (especially right thoracic), progresses at 1 degree/yr
- Degenerative scoliosis progresses at 3.3 degrees/yr
- Respiratory failure rare
- Life expectancy unaffected
- Pregnancy unaffected
- Pain usually in concavity of curve but try not to attribute pain to scoliosis

INDICATIONS
- Curve progression
- Intractable concave pain, **not LBP**
- Intractable stenosis symptoms

- Cardiopulmonary compromise (rare)
- Cosmesis?
- PSF + instrumentation is standard
  - Smaller flexible thoracic curves
- ASF alone rare because adults usually rigid
- A/PSF for >70 degrees; rigid, lumbar component of double major curve; or if you fuse to sacrum.
- A/PSF improves correction and fusion

COMPLICATIONS (COMMON AND SEVERE)

- 15%–20% pseudo in L, TL curves
  - Decreased if A/PSF
  - If asymptomatic, observe
  - Gold standard for diagnosis is reexploration
- Implant failure
- Loss of correction

- Inadequate pain relief
  - 30%–70% relief of pain only

Recommended Reading
Weinstein SL, Ponseti IV. Curve progression in idiopathic scoliosis. J Bone Joint Surg Am 1983;65(4):447–455.

Scoliosis—Congenital

- I—failure of formation
  - Unilateral hemivertebrae
  - Bilateral hemivertebrae = butterfly
- II—failure of segmentation
  - Unilateral—bar
  - Bilateral—block
- III—mixed

Diagrammatic representation of classification system of congenital scoliosis. (Modified from McMaster MJ. Congenital scoliosis. In: Weinstein SL, ed. The pediatric spine: principles and practice, 2nd ed. Lippincott Williams and Wilkins, Philadelphia, 2001.)

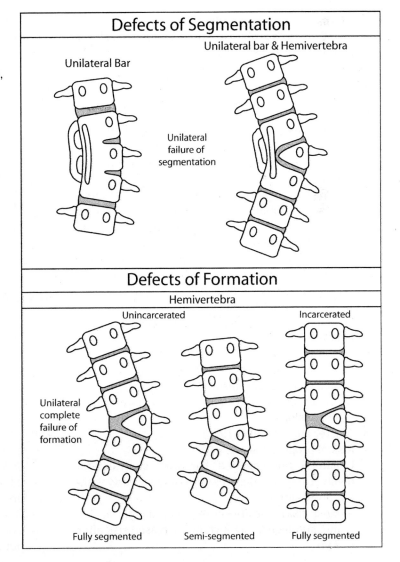

- Hemimetameric shift—"musical chairs" of components as they come from lateral and fuse in midline, worse when shifted hemivertebrae are farther apart
- Diastematomyelia—congenital longitudinal split of cord into two hemi-cords with fibrous tissue or bony spur in between, causes 5% of congenital scoliosis; this becomes tether in scoliosis correction; may split into one or two dural tubes
- Diplomyelia is split into two full cords with bilateral roots from each cord; true cord duplication; one dural tube; ? different manifestation of same disorder as diastematomyelia
- Multiple anomalies are often hereditary
  - Jarcho-Levin thoracodysplasia in Puerto Ricans is AD, variable penetrance
- Family history rare in isolated single anomaly
- Other systems
  - Cord (12%–40%), cardiac (10%)
  - GU most common (25%)—get US
  - VACTERLS
  - Sprengel
- Females progress more than males
- T-L curve progresses most, upper thoracic least; L-S curves don't progress much
- Most common neurologic defect is cranial nerve palsy, then bowel/bladder, lower motor neuron
- Paraplegia common in congenital kyphosis
- XR
  - Supine cone-down views allow better evaluation by eliminating natural kyphosis and lordosis
  - If you find one hemivertebra, look at entire spine to find other half
  - Loder et al. (1995)—with preselected levels intraobserver variability is ± 10 degrees, interobserver variability is 12 degrees; suggested 23-degree increase to ensure progression
  - Facanha-Filho et al. (2001)—similar study as Loder but interobserver variability 3.4 degrees, intraobserver variability 2.8 degrees
- CT with 3D reconstruction
- Indications for MRI in congenital scoliosis
  - If patient having surgery
  - Abnormal neurologic exam
  - Cavovarus, equinus, hemihypertrophy, i.e., suspected spinal dysraphism
  - No increased risk of cord abnormality in worse congenital lesions
- McMaster and Ohtsuka (1982)
  - Risk of progression
  - Unilateral unsegmented bar with contralateral hemivertebra (10 degrees/yr)—surgery early without observation
    - Most risky anesthesia 0–3 mo, anemic at 3–6 mo, still high 6 mo–2 yr; no increased risk after 2 yo

- Unilateral unsegmented bar (6–9 degrees/yr)—surgery without observation
- Segmented hemivertebra (1–2.5 degrees/yr)
  - Disc above and below
  - ASF or
  - A and P excision and fusion (Boach)
  - **Hemiepiphysiodesis (for those <5 yo with lots of growth left, moderate curve, no kyphosis)**
  - Excision if <4 yo
  - Double hemivertebra—two times progression
- Partially segmented hemivertebra
  - Observe or
  - Excision and fusion
- Incarcerated hemivertebra—observe
  - Normal hemidisc on contralateral side
  - Hemivertebra pedicle in line with others
  - No growth potential
  - Curves usually <20 degrees
  - Minimal to no progression
  - Nonsegmented hemivertebra—observe
    - No disc space above and below
  - Block or wedge (<1 degree/yr)—observe
- Unsegmented bar is always worse than hemivertebra
- Treatment of congenital lordosis is purely surgical, correction vs. stabilization
- Treatment of congenital kyphosis is also surgical
- All sharp short curves, rigid curves, and kyphotic and lordotic curves are contraindications to bracing

References

Facanha-Filho FA, et al. Measurement accuracy in congenital scoliosis. J Bone Joint Surg Am 2001;83-A(1):42–45.

Loder RT, et al. Variability in Cobb angle measurements in children with congenital scoliosis. J Bone Joint Surg Br 1995;77(5):768–770.

McMaster MJ, Ohtsuka K. The natural history of congenital scoliosis. A study of two hundred and fifty-one patients. J Bone Joint Surg Am 1982;64(8):1128–1147.

SCOLIOSIS—CONGENITAL—TREATMENT

- Treatment goal
  - Short straight spine
- Bracing
  - No role in congenital except maybe to control compensatory curve
- Surgery if
  - >10 degrees of progression
- PSF alone
  - In those <5 yo—two-thirds fail
  - In 5–10 yo—one-third fail
  - If triradiate closure used to time surgery—? % failure
  - Fusion rates don't increase with instrumentation
  - Correction not much better with instrumentation but increases neurologic injury

- ASF
  - Increases risk of cord ischemia from anterior approach, increased in congenital scoliosis
- Convex hemiepiphysiodesis
  - Winter et al. (1988)—13 patients, half of growth plate taken anteriorly, unilateral concave fusion posteriorly, cast 6 mo; seven got true epiphysis effect (curve corrects over time), five got fusion effect, one failed
  - Mixed results
  - Most useful before 5 yo
  - For progressive curve <50 degrees
  - Contraindicated in kyphosis and/or posterolateral quarter vertebra because anterior fusion may make it worse
- Hemivertebra excision
  - Lazar and Hall (1999)—11 patients, average 18 mo old, A and P, two laminar hooks for two levels, great correction, no complications
  - Bradford and Boachie-Adjei (1990)
    - Acutely corrects deformity and stabilizes
    - Highest neurologic risk
    - Clearest role in lumbosacral hemivertebra because safer and greatest impact on balance

References

Bradford DS, Boachie-Adjei O. One-stage anterior and posterior hemivertebral resection and arthrodesis for congenital scoliosis. J Bone Joint Surg Am 1990;72(4):536–540.

Winter RB, et al. Convex growth arrest for progressive congenital scoliosis due to hemivertebrae. J Pediatr Orthop 1988;8(6):633–638.

Scoliosis—History and Physical Examination

- Onset, progression?
- Menstruation?
- Gait
  - Pelvic obliquity
  - Wide or circumductive gait
- Symmetry
  - Shoulder
  - Scapulae
  - Pelvis
- Skin—cafe-au-lait, hairy patches
- Adams forward-bending test
  - Paravertebral prominences
  - Scoliometer
    - ATR (angle of trunk rotation)
    - 5 degrees ATR = 11-degree curve
    - 7 degrees ATR = 20-degree curve
  - Right thoracic prominence in right thoracic curve because rotation is into the concavity
  - Left lumbar curve has left prominence

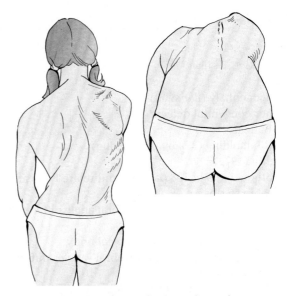

Abnormal Spinal Curvatures Scoliosis Lateral curvature of the spine with an increase in convexity on the side that is curved is seen in scoliosis. (From Weber J RN, EdD and Kelley J RN, PhD. Health Assessment in Nursing, 2nd edition. Philadelphia: Lippincott Williams & Wilkins, 2003.)

- Plumb line
  - Sagittal balance is C2 or C7 body to L5-S1 disc
- Neurologic exam
  - Abdominal reflex—early spinal cord pathology
  - Clonus? Babinski
- Tone, spasticity, foot deformities
- Leg length
- Tanner stage
  - I—prepubertal
  - II—straight fine pubic hair
    - Testes larger
    - Small raised breast buds
  - V—full maturity

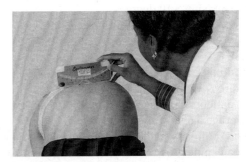

Scoliosis Idiopathic scoliosis occurs most often in adolescent girls. The rotation of the spine usually results in a right-sided prominence. (From Bickley, LS and Szilagyi, P. Bates' Guide to Physical Examination and History Taking, 8th Ed. Philadelphia: Lippincott Williams & Wilkins 2003.)

Scoliosis—Infantile

- 2 mo–3 yr
- Left-sided T curve
- M > F
- Plagiocephaly (flat skull)
- Other congenital defects
  - Bat ear
  - Rib molding (? baby positioning)
- Mehta (1972)
  - Studied xr's of 138 patients and related apical vertebra to ribs
  - Defined phase and rib vertebral angle difference
- Phase I
  - No overlap of rib head to apical body
  - 80% progress if rib vertebral angle difference >20 degrees
  - 20% progress if RVAD <20 degrees
- Phase II—overlap
  - All will progress

TREATMENT

- Rule out congenital and neuromuscular causes
- Observe for
  - Curve <25 degrees
  - RVAD of Mehta <20 degrees
  - These will likely resolve
- Brace for
  - Curve 25–35 degrees
  - Progression ~10 degrees
  - RVAD 20–25 degrees
  - Don't use total contact because will mold baby
  - Use localizer pads in brace
  - 100% progress despite brace
  - Hope for brace to control curve until before adolescent spurt around age 10 or 11; then they usually require A/PSF
- Surgery for
  - Curve >35 degrees
  - Progression >10 degrees
  - Preoperative MRI rule out cord lesion
  - SQ rodding (no fusion) or
  - **ASF & PSF**
- SQ rodding
  (Mineiro & Weinstein, 2002)
  - 11 patients early scoliosis, multiple causes
  - Average 5.6 yr at rod placement
  - 8 of 11 already had A/PSF by 5-yr follow-up
  - Mean spine growth at 5 yr follow-up 2 cm
  - Multiple distraction procedures

References

Mehta MH. The rib-vertebra angle in the early diagnosis between resolving and progressive infantile scoliosis. J Bone Joint Surg Br 1972;54(2):230–243.

Mineiro J, Weinstein SL. Subcutaneous rodding for progressive spinal curvatures: early results. J Pediatr Orthop 2002;22(3): 290–295.

Scoliosis—Juvenile

- 4–10 yo
- Mix of juvenile and adolescent forms
- <6 yo, M > F; >6 yo, F > M
- High risk of progression
  - 70% required treatment
  - Half of those were braced
  - Other half needed surgery
- Robinson and McMaster (1996)
  - 109 patients with juvenile scoliosis
  - 104 of 109 progressed
  - 70 of 104 required fusion
  - 67 of 84 had major T curves fused
  - 3 of 20 had TL or L curves fused
  - Pattern of final curve not apparent at early stage
  - Thoracolumbar and lumbar curves progress less than major thoracic curves
  - In brace, average progression 1–3 degrees/yr before 10 yo, then 4–11 degrees/yr after 10 yo

TREATMENT

- <25 degrees
  - Observe with checks q6mo
- >25 degrees, 3–6 yo
  - Treat like infantile scoliosis
- >25 degrees or progression, >6 yo
  - Full-time brace for 2 yr
  - If curve <20 degrees after 2 yr, brace, then can wear part time, then wean
- Delay fusion until onset of adolescent growth spurt unless curve >50 degrees
- ASF and PSF to prevent crankshaft
- Anterior and posterior fusion for
  - Severe deformity >80 degrees
  - Kyphotic element >50 degrees
  - Curves requiring anterior release
  - Females <10 yo, males <13 yo
    - Risser <1
    - Open triradiate
    - Tanner I or II
    - At or before peak height velocity
    - Vertical body apophysis open
  - Crankshaft
    - Increases rotation after good PSF
    - Due to continued anterior growth
    - Increases Cobb by 10 degrees or increases apical rotation

Reference

Robinson CM, McMaster MJ. Juvenile idiopathic scoliosis. curve patterns and prognosis in one hundred and nine patients. J Bone Joint Surg Am 1996;78(8):1140–1148.

Scoliosis—King-Moe Classification

(King et al., 1983)
- For thoracic curves
- Clarified that most lumbar curves were compensatory and usually did not require fusion
- Type I—13%
  - Reverse "S" shaped
  - L curve > T curve
  - T curve more flexible
  - Fuse T and L (usually to L3 or L4)
    - To L3 if minimal rotation and levels above pelvis on bending xr
  - Consider selective anterior left fusion
- Type II—33%
- Reverse "S" shaped
- T curve > L curve
- L curve more flexible
- Fuse T, and L if L curve >50 degrees
  - IIA—L curve <35 degrees, >70% flexible
    - Apical L body touches center sacral line
    - L-S fractional curve <12 degrees
    - OK for selective T fusion
  - IIB—opposite of IIA
    - Not OK for selective T fusion
    - Can't adapt to thoracic correction
    - Becomes unbalanced
- Selective T fusion should not end just above junctional kyphosis
- If lumbar curve >45–50 degrees in select T fusion, avoid vigorous correction of thoracic curve beyond lumbar flexibility; this will lead to truncal decompensation to left
- Type III—33%
  - T curve only
  - L vertebrae don't cross midline
  - Selective T fusion to L1 or L2
- Type IV—9%
  - Long thoracic curve apex T10 where L4 tilts toward the thoracic curve
  - Must fuse through L4
  - Fuse to L3 with pedicle screw if L3 neutral and reverses wedge on bends
- Type V—12%
  - Double thoracic "S"-shaped curve
  - Left shoulder elevated
    - Vs. isolated right thoracic curve, where right shoulder elevated
  - T1 tilts into the concavity of the upper curve
  - Left upper T curve usually rigid, thus must fuse to T1 or T2
  - If upper T curve not treated, will lead to worsening of left shoulder elevation
  - Fuse lower T curve alone if shoulders level and upper T flexible (corrects to <20 degrees)
- Triple curve

- Left upper thorax, right thorax, left lumbrical/T-L
- Lower right thoracic curve is usually dominant and usually requires treatment
- The other two curves treated according to criteria of double curves

Reference
King HA, et al. The selection of fusion levels in thoracic idiopathic scoliosis. J Bone Joint Surg Am 1983;65(9):1302–1313.

Scoliosis—Lenke Classification

(Lenke et al., 2001)
- Curve type (1–6)
- Lumbar spine modifier (A–C)
- Thorax sagittal modifier (–, N, +)
- Curve type
  - Main thoracic—51%
  - Double thoracic (prox T, T major)—20%
  - Double major (T major, TL/L)—11%
  - Triple major (proximal T, T major, TL/L)
  - TL/L—12%
  - TL/L, main thoracic (T, TL/L major)
- Major—largest Cobb measurement, always structural
- Minor—all other structural curves
- Structural criteria
  - Proximal T
    - Side bend >25 degrees
    - T2–T5 kyphosis >20 degrees
  - Main T
    - Side bend >25 degrees
    - T10-L2 kyphosis >20 degrees
  - TL/L (thoracolumbar, lumbar)
    - T10-L2 kyphosis >20 degrees
- Location of apex (SRS)
  - Thoracic—T2 to T11/12 disc
  - Thoracolumbar—upper end plate of T12 to lower end plate of L1
  - Lumbar—L1/2 disc to L4
- Lumbar modifiers
  - Based on relationship of center sacral vertical line to apex of lumbar spine
  - Center sacral vertical line should bisect sacrum and be parallel to lateral edge of film
  - Pelvic oblique of 2 cm OK but if more, use shoelift to even pelvis
    - A—CSVL between pedicles
    - B—CSVL touches apical body
    - C—CSVL completely medial
- Thoracic sagittal modifier
  - Based on kyphosis from T5 to T12
  - (–)—hypo <10 degrees
  - (N)—normal (10–40 degrees)
  - (+)—hyper (>40 degrees)

- The major curve (with largest Cobb) distinguishes between 3 and 6
- Lumbar A and B are only for types 1–4
- Types 5 and 6 are always lumbar C
- In 1–4, main thorax is major
- in 5–6, TL/L is major with main thorax structural in 6 and nonstructural in 5
- In operated series, most common overall are 5CN, 3CN, 1BN, 1AN, 2AN, and 1CN
- Type 1 is most common curve type
- Most common lumbar is C
- Most common kyphosis modifier is N
- Fusion
  - 90% predictive of fusion of appropriate structural curves
  - Fuse only major curve (largest) and structural minor curves
  - Don't fuse lumbar A and B unless there's TL kyphosis >20 degrees
  - Lumbar C should be fused unless it's 1C or 2C and balance of lumbar curve can be maintained

Reference

Lenke LG, et al. Multisurgeon assessment of surgical decision-making in adolescent idiopathic scoliosis: curve classification, operative approach, and fusion levels. Spine 2001; 26(21):2347–2353.

Scoliosis—Neuromuscular

SRS CLASSIFICATION

Neuropathic

- Upper motor neuron—cerebral palsy, Charcot-Marie-tooth, Friedrich ataxia, trauma-spinal cord injury, tumor
- Lower motor neuron—polio, spinal muscular atrophy, dysautonomia

Myopathic

- Duchenne, Becker, arthrogryposis
- See CP, Myelomeningocele, Duchenne
- 20% in CP, 60% in myelomeningocele
- 90% in males with demyelinating disease
- 100% in those <10 yo with high paralysis above T12
- Deformity due to
  - Poor trunk balance
  - Muscle asymmetry
  - Spasticity
- Curves usually flexible
- Early onset
- Rapid progression during growth
- Continued progression after maturity
- Deformity interferes with function
- Other factors
  - Nutrition (increases risk with albumin <3.5)
  - Poor bone stock, seizure medications
  - Respiratory function (FVC = volume of first second of exposure)
  - Low-grade urosepsis

RISK FACTORS FOR PROGRESSION

- Early onset
- High-level paralysis
- Asymmetric paralysis

PELVIC OBLIQUITY

- Rotational deformity at lumbosacral junction
- Caused by contraction of spino-femoral, pelvic-femoral, or spino-pelvic muscles
- Hips/lower extremity may be cause
  - Pelvis higher on dislocated side
  - If hips are causing obliquity, there is usually lower lumbar fractional curve
  - If spine is causing obliquity, lower lumbar bodies are parallel to pelvis
  - Examine prone with hips over the end of table; if pelvic obliquity goes away with abduction/adduction of hips, then pelvic-femoral m. are cause and should be released
  - Instead of plumb line, extend center sacral line up toward head to determine balance
- Observe
  - If curve <25 degrees
  - If large curve in severe MR
- Brace/nonoperative treatment
  - For moderate flexible curve
  - During growing period
  - Only when upright, not full time
  - Don't correct in brace but rather molded to just hold patient up
  - Open in back
  - Doesn't work to control curve progression
  - Wheelchair custom molds, head band
  - Watch out for skin breakdown, gastrointestinal, pulmonary function
- Surgery indicated for
  - Loss of sitting balance due to scoliosis and pelvic obliquity with decrease in function
- Indications for anterior release, anterior spine fusion
  - Unable to correct to <50 degrees on bends
  - Inadequate post elements for fusion
  - Postlami kyphosis, myelomeningocele

FUSION LEVEL

- Usually fusion to T2 of T3 to prevent kyphosis at proximal end of instrumentation

- Most need fusion to pelvis, especially if no ambulatory potential
- In ambulatory patients, lower lumbar motion should be saved but lowest fused level must be horizontal; i.e., there must be no pelvic oblique or oblique takeoff of L5 on S1
- Lower lumbar motion needed to elevate hemipelvis in swing
- Fusion to pelvis usually not needed in Duchenne because curves milder and usually no pelvic oblique

INSTRUMENTATION

- Luque-Galveston most common in North America
- Devised by Allen and Ferguson
- Two contoured cross-linked (rectangular) rods with sublami wires
- Multiplanar rod gives triangulation fixation
- Potential sacro-iliac junction pain
- Lucency devices at tip of rod in pelvis but resolves as fusion matures

CORRECTION

- PSF instrumentation alone 39%
- PSF segmental instrumentation 48%
- A/PSF instrumentation 59%
- A/PSF segmental instrumentation 58%
- Isola-Galveston PSF 66%
- Pelvic oblique corrected 31% in PSF, 66% in A/PSF
- Isola-Galveston PSF 81% pelvic oblique correction
- **Postoperative improvement in function directly relates to truncal balance**
- With curve correction, moment arms reduced, convex tension forces reduced, lower pseudarthrosis
- Improved trunk height improves diaphragmatic efficiency and appetite
- Upper extremity function may decrease because rigid spine removes compensatory skills to accommodate for proximal limb weakness
- Curve should be corrected to <35 degrees to prevent progression

COMPLICATIONS

- 25% complications, 10% mortality
- Pseudarthrosis 7% in PSF segmental
- Pseudarthrosis 24% in MMC, 17% in CP
- Instrumentation failure 20% in myelomeingocele, 12% in CP
- 8% wound infection (15% MMC, 6% CP)
  - Most common due to mixed gram negative and positive
- Pulmonary distress most common in FVC <50%

Recommended Readings

Banta JV, et al. The treatment of neuromuscular scoliosis. Instr Course Lect 1999;48:551–562.
Berven S, Bradford DS. Neuromuscular scoliosis: causes of deformity and principles for evaluation and management. Semin Neurol 2002;22(2):167–178.
Larsson EL, et al. Long-term follow-up of functioning after spinal surgery in patients with neuromuscular scoliosis. Spine 2005;30(19):2145–2152.

Scoliosis—Selection of Fusion Level

UPPER

- End Cobb vertebra
- Stable, neutral
- No cephalad kyphosis on lateral
- Upper level is midway between sides of rib cage
- Normal sagittal and transverse plane angular
- Usually one to two levels above upper end vertical for major thoracic curves
- Is upper end vertical for double thoracic and compensatory thoracic curves
- In sagittal plane it is the first vertical above a normal intersegmental alignment

LOWER

- End Cobb vertebra
- Neutral or nearly neutral
- No caudal kyphosis on lateral
- Rarely below L4 in idiopathic scoliosis
- Disc opens both ways during bending (indicates flexibility beyond fused body)
- Becomes stable and horizontal during bending
- For single and double thoracic curves, it is usually one below lower end vertical
- May be end vertical in double thoracic
- May be two below end vertical in single thorax
- Transverse plane angulation <10 degrees
- Should be the stable vertical after instrumentation

Scoliosis—Selective Fusion

INDICATIONS

- Primary TL or L curve <60 degrees
  - Similar to King-Moe type I
- T curve must be <40 degrees, flexion to <20 degrees
  - Nonsurgical curve that can be braced
  - Dr. Hall's criteria
- No TL kyphosis
  - Dwyer and Zeilke's anterior spine fusion were kyphogenic due to inadequate stiffness of rods
- Contraindicated in double T curve
- Limited anterior fusion of apical three to four levels

- Fuse to one vertical above and one below apex body; if apex at disc, fuse to two above and two below disc
- Apex body's lateral border is most vertical and farthest lateral
- Include levels with wider disc space on convex side on bending xr's
- Distal unfused disc must open both ways on bending or be normal on MRI
- Emphasis on overcorrection
- ASF limited to L4 distally due to vessels

Recommended Reading

Cassella MC, Hall JE. Current treatment approaches in the nonoperative and operative management of adolescent idiopathic scoliosis. Phys Ther 1991;71(12):897–909.

Spondylolisthesis—Adult, Isthmic

DIAGNOSIS

- Pain on extension
- Asymptomatic as child but disc space narrows, leads to foraminal narrowing, presents in middle age
- Lysis or grade I slippage is not associated with increased risk for back pain
- 80% of lysis seen in plain xr's; add a few more percent with obliques
- L5-S1 rarely moves on flexion-extension xr, especially in adult due to iliolumbar ligaments
- L4-L5 lysis usually moves on flexion-extension and tends to be more symptomatic

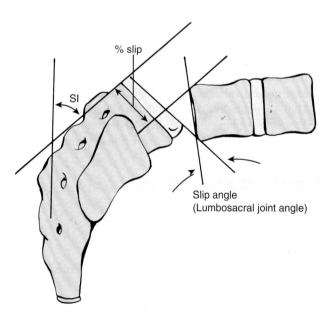

Calculation of the slip angle as a measure of kyphosis and of the percent slip of one vertebral body on the other. (From Bono C, Garfin SR, Orthopaedic Surgery Essentials: Spine Philadelphia: Lippincott Williams & Wilkins 2004 with permission.)

- MRI for radicular symptoms
- SPECT scan or CT to see lysis
- Sagittal MR
  - L5-S1 isthmic listhesis compresses L5 root
  - L4-5 degenerative listhesis compresses L5 root
  - L4-5 isthmic listhesis affects L4
  - Usually no central stenosis
  - Foraminal stenosis
- Encourage flexion exercises instead of extension
- Indications for surgery
  - Leg pain below knee of 6 mo
  - Neurologic deficit
- Better outcome in low grade slips with interbody fusion (Kwon JSDT 2005)
- If >50% slip at L5-S1, consider fusion L4 to S1
- If high grade slip, consider trans-sacral fibular allograft (Speed's procedure)
- 25% incidence of neurologic injury with reduction of high grade slip

Recommended Readings

Meyerding HW. Spondylolisthesis; surgical fusion of lumbosacral portion of spinal column and interarticular facets; use of autogenous bone grafts for relief of disabling backache. J Int Coll Surg 1956;26(5 Part 1):566–591.

Wiltse LL, Jackson DW. Treatment of spondylolisthesis and spondylolysis in children. Clin Orthop Relat Res 1976;(117): 92–100.

Spondylolysis, Spondylolisthesis—Pediatric

- In children, lysis most common at L5, which leads to L5-S1 listhesis, which will compress L5 root if neurologic symptoms
- Wiltse and Jackson (1976) on listhesis
  - I—congenital abnormal L5-S1 facet
  - II—isthmic (most common in kids)
    - A—lytic pars stress fracture
    - B—elongated intact pars
    - C—acute pars fracture
  - III—degenerative (most common L4 on L5)
  - IV—traumatic
  - V—pathologic
  - VI—postsurgical
- Lysis incidence 4% in 6 yo, 6% in 14 yo
  - 75% seen by age 6 already
  - 75% present with some slippage
- Most common in boys, whites, gymnasts, lineman, weight lifters—repetitive extension
- 25%–50% in Alaskan Eskimos
- Associated with spina bifida occulta and Scheuermann
- 20% unilateral
- Most common symptom is pain
- **Dull back ache during growth spurt**

- Flat heart-shaped buttocks
- Lumbar lordosis, hip/knee flexed
- Waddling gait—Phalen-Dickson sign
- Restricted forward bend
- Tight hamstrings
- Upside down napoleon's hat
- Trapezoidal L5, rounded S1 body
- Slip percentage (Meyerding)
  - Sacrum is divided into 4s
- Slip angle
  - Perpendicular to tangent to posterior sacrum
  - Vs. inferior end plate of L5
- **SPECT scan most sensitive**
- Bone scan to differentiate acute from chronic
  - Hot indications healing potential
  - Contralateral pars may be hot from stress transfer
- CT with 1-mm cuts can help make other diagnosis; best seen at cut through mid-VB at inferior aspect of pedicle where a complete ring of bone without "defects" from facets should be normally seen
- Hard to make diagnosis on MRI

NATURAL HISTORY

- 90% of slippage has already occurred at initial presentation (Seitsalo, 1991)
- Most have slippage of <30%–50%
- **5% progress after diagnosis, likely related to disc degeneration**
- Risk factors for slippage
  - Dysplastic
  - Girls
  - Young, preadolescent
  - >50% initial slippage, slippage angle >40 degrees
  - Dome S1, trapezoid L5 predictive?

SPONDYLOLYSIS

- Observe if painless, ? xr until mature
- Activity modification if chronic, cold scan
- Brace if pain, acute fracture on bone scan
  - Early bracing better than activity modification
  - Antilordotic thoraco-lumbar-sacral othosis
  - Boston overlap brace
    - Xiphoid to pubis
    - Bottom of scapula to buttocks apex
  - Healing takes 3–4 mo
  - Pain and HS tightness should improve
  - 25% heal with brace only
  - 80% feel better, despite failure to heal
- Fix if nonoperative treatment fails, cold bone scan
  - For L3 or L4 usually
  - Wire transverse processes to spinous process, iliac crest bone graft
  - Pedicle screw to rod to laminar hook

- Contraindications to open reduction internal fixation (instead, use posterior spine fusion)
  - >30 yo
  - Early disc degeneration
  - >2-mm slippage across fracture site
  - L5

SPONDYLOLISTHESIS

- Slippages <50% (grade I, II)
  - Xr every year until mature to rule out progression
  - Avoid heavy labor, contact sports
  - TLSO if still painful despite rest
  - OR if failed nonoperative treatment or progression
  - In situ L5-S1 PSF—90% fusion
- Slippages >50% (grade III, IV)
  - L4-S1 fusion ± instrumentation even if asymptomatic
  - ? reduce if >75%, angle >45 degrees
  - If >100% (spondyloptosis), ? L5 vertebrectomy (Gaines)
  - If neurologic deficit, Gill procedure to decompress and remove L5 loose lamina
- Decompression without fusion contraindicated in kids because will increase progression
- Reduction with instrumentation is controversial
  - 20% sensory, 30% motor deficits but mostly transient

Reference

Wiltse LL, Jackson DW. Treatment of spondylolisthesis and spondylolysis in children. Clin Orthop Relat Res 1976;(117): 92–100.

Recommended Reading

Meyerding HW. Spondylolisthesis; surgical fusion of lumbosacral portion of spinal column and interarticular facets; use of autogenous bone grafts for relief of disabling backache. J Int Coll Surg 1956;26(5 Part 1):566–591.

T-spine—Disc Disease

- 1% of all clinically relevant discs
- High false positive on MR
- Most common on T8-12
- Location
  - **Central very common**
- Etiology
  - Genetic, torsional activities
- P/w back pain, myelopathy, or thoracic radiculopathy (chest pain)
- TL junction HNP can cause low back pain
- Ca^{2+} in canal in disc space level is pathognomic for thoracic HNP

INDICATIONS FOR SURGERY

- Myelopathy (gait, bowel/bladder)
- Radiculopathy
- Axial pain alone is NOT indication because poor results

Approach

- **Transthoracic for central HNP**
- Costotransversectomy or transpedicular for lateral HNP
- Laminectomy alone is contraindicated

LS-spine Total Disc Replacement

- Must endure 1 billion cycles over 40 yr (Kostuik)
- Nucleus-only replacement requires normal annulus
- End plates oblique for L5-S1, parallel for all other levels

INDICATIONS

- Same indications as interbody fusion
- Symptom disc disease at one or more levels
- Disc resorption with loss of height
- Postdiscectomy pain
- Lateral recess stenosis due to decreased disc height

REQUIREMENTS

- Posterior elements must be intact to share load

CONTRAINDICATIONS

- Osteoporosis (subsidence)
- Infection, cancer
- Spondylolisthesis
- Central stenosis
- Instability from loss of post elements

ADVANTAGES

- Reproduces normal biomechanics
- Reduces adjacent segment load transmission
- Restores disc height and avoids foraminal root compression

RESULTS

- RCT Single level ProDisc vs. fusion
  - 77% success vs 65% for fusion at 24 mo
  - (Zigler et al. Spine 2007)
- RCT Two level ProDisc vs fusion
  - 73% success vs 60% for fusion at 24 mo
  - (Delamarter et al. JBJS 2011)

References

Delamarter R, et al. Prospective, randomized, multicenter Food and Drug Administration investigational device exemption study of the ProDisc-L total disc replacement compared with circumferential arthrodesis for treatment of two-level lumbar degenerative disc disease: results at 24 month. J Bone Joint Surg Am 2011;93(8):705–715.

Zigler J, et al. Results of the prospective, randomized, multicenter Food and Drug Administration investigational device exemption study of the ProDisc-L total disc replacement versus circumferential fusion for the treatment of 1- level degenerative disc disease. Spine (Phila PA 1976) 2007;32(11):1155–1162; discussion 1163.

Recommended Reading

Sieber AN, Kostuik JP. Concepts in nuclear replacement. Spine J 2004;4(6 Suppl):322S–324S.

Trauma—Atlanto-occipital Dissociation

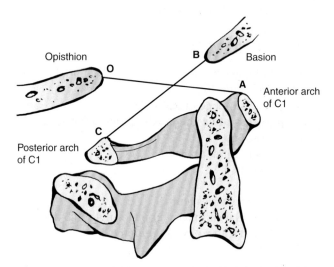

Power's ratio. The ratio of BC to AO normally equals 1. If the ratio is greater than 1, an anterior occipitoatlantal dislocation may exist. (From Bono C, Garfin SR, Orthopaedic Surgery Essentials: Spine Philadelphia: Lippincott Williams & Wilkins 2004 with permission.)

- Usually fatal
- Injury to cranial nerve VII to X, spino-medulla cord, vertebral/basilar artery, cervical roots
- Two times more common in children due to more horizontal atlanto-occipital junction in kids

TRAYNELIS CLASSIFICATION

- I—anterior displacement of occiput, 11%
- II—occiput displaced vertically, 3%
- III—occiput posterior, 2%
- IV—occiput displaced in oblique plane, 84%

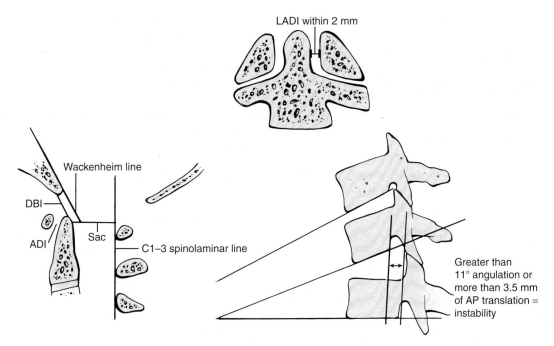

The spinolaminar junction and posterior vertebral body alignment lines. Note they are disrupted at the level of the injury (C5 dislocation). ADI, atlantodens interval; AP, anteroposterior; DBI, dens-basion interval; LADI, lateral atlantodens interval. (From Bono C, Garfin SR, Orthopaedic Surgery Essentials: Spine Philadelphia: Lippincott Williams & Wilkins 2004 with permission.)

DIAGNOSIS

- Odontoid tip avulsion fracture
- Wackenheim line
  - Posterior tip of clivus to posterior tip of dens, disrupted in atlanto-occipital dissociation
- Distance from tip of basion to tip of odontoid >10 mm in children and >5 mm in adults indicates vertical displacement
- Power's ratio—see figure at beginning of Trauma—Atlanto-occipital Dissociation section
  - Basion to anterior border of posterior arch of C1 divided by opisthion to posterior border of anterior arch of C1
  - Value >1 indicates anterior displacement
- Rule of 12s
  - Distance from basion tip to odontoid >12 mm
  - Line from basion to base of odontoid; atlanto-occipital displacement if posterior aspect of dens is >12 mm behind line
- Wallenberg syndrome
  - CN 7, 9, 10, 11 with ipsilateral Horner and contralateral pain/temperature loss, paralysis

TREATMENT

- All are unstable
- Avoid traction

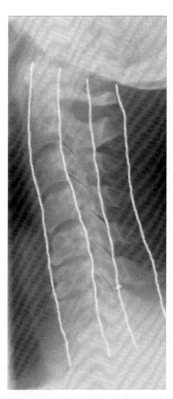

Diagram depicting cervical spine radiographic parameters of instability. (From Bono C, Garfin SR, Orthopaedic Surgery Essentials: Spine Philadelphia: Lippincott Williams & Wilkins 2004 with permission.)

– Reduce and immobilize with halo vest
– All need occipito-cervical operative stabilization because of severe ligamentous injury

Trauma—C-spine Radiographs

LATERAL VIEW

– 85% of significant injuries detected on lateral xr
– Anterior, posterior, and spinal laminar lines
– Basilar line of Wackenheim—line drawn along posterior clivus should be tangential to posterior dens
– Check each vertebral body to rule out loss of height or rotational deformity
– Inspect posterior structures to rule out facet dislocation or spinous process fracture
– Atlanto-dens interval should be <3 mm in the adult (5 mm in child)
– Torg/Pavlov ratio (canal/body) <0.8 suggests developmental stenosis
– Prevertebral soft tissues
  – C1 = 10 mm
  – C3 = 4–5 mm
  – C6 = 15–20 mm
  – In children
    – Crying can cause swelling
    – Base of C2—7 mm
    – Base of C6—14 mm
    – In children, swelling up to 1/2 of body higher and 1 body lower OK
    – Posterior spinolaminar line of Swischuk from C1-C3 to differentiate normal C2-C3 subluxation from pathologic
    – Pseudosubluxation seen in those <4–8 yo
      – Because facets more horizontal
      – No compensatory lordosis
      – Reverses on extension
    – For children <8 yo, 90% of injuries are at C3 or above

AP VIEW

– Interspinous distance
  – Vertical widening at a given level >1.5 times the level above or below suggests posterior instability
– Inspect the lateral masses for disruption
– Inspect the facet joints

OPEN-MOUTH VIEW

– Unable to do open mouth in intubated patients, thus do O-C2 CT
– Evaluate for odontoid fracture
– In open-mouth view, suspect fracture of C1 with transverse ligament disruption if sum of lateral mass "spread" >7 mm

– Odontoid should be centered—suspect C1 fracture if lateral atlas dens interval varies from left to right by >2 mm
– Evaluate C1-2 lateral mass junction spaces
– Rotation of C1 can give unilateral lateral mass overhang
– If CT for C7-T1 junction, must do sagittal recon
– MR if neurologic deficit without demonstrated instability on xr or CT

C-SPINE FLEXION/EXTENSION VIEWS

(Wang et al., 1999)
– 290 patients with h/o major trauma from 1990 to 1995 at UCLA, neurology intact, with neck pain, routinely had flexion/extension views acutely in ER
– One (0.34%) had positive finding of instability (>3.5-mm translation, sagittal plane angulation difference >11 degrees between two adjacent levels); this patient had prior C-spine disease, asymptomatic at 1 mo follow-up
– One third of patients could not flex/extend enough to get adequate study (<10-degree change from C2 to C7 from flexion to extension); thus, study was inconclusive
– Average motion in patients with adequate study was 40 degrees
– 2-yr follow-up on 40% of patients, all without C-spine problems
– Should wait 1–2 wk postinjury to do flexion/extension radiographs

MRI

(Klein et al., 1999)
– With CT as gold standard, 14% sensitivity and 97% specificity for posterior element fracture
– 37% sensitivity and 98% specificity for anterior element fracture
– Study of choice for occult vascular injury, HNP, hematomas, and ligament Injury, but need CT to detect and classify

References

Klein GR, et al. Efficacy of magnetic resonance imaging in the evaluation of posterior cervical spine fractures. Spine 1999; 24(8):771–774.
Wang JC, et al. Cervical flexion and extension radiographs in acutely injured patients. Clin Orthop Relat Res 1999; (365):111–116.

Trauma—C1 Fracture

– Easily missed
– Isolated injury <50% of time so check for other spine injuries especially in posterior arch fractures
– Neurologic injury rare due to large space available for the cord (SAC) and decompressive effect of fracture

- If neurologic deficit, look for other things
- Displaced lateral masses may impinge on CN 9, 11, or 12
- Cortical bone of posterior arch thinnest
- Look for disruption of spinolaminar line from C1 to C2
- Arch fracture hard to see on xr, need CT
- Levine & Edwards (1991)
  - I—posterior arch fracture
    - Most common, due to extension and axial load
    - Second fracture in 50% of cases
    - Second fracture most common is hangman's or dens
  - II—lateral mass fracture
  - III—Jefferson fracture
- **Stability depends on integrity of transverse ligament**

TREATMENT

- Most treated nonsurgically, halo
- Isolated anterior or posterior arch fracture stable; rule out C1-2 instability with flexion-extension xr's, then hard collar

JEFFERSON BURST FRACTURE

- Axial load
- Most common involves anterior and posterior arches
- Three to four fracture lines present
- Not associated with neurologic symptoms
- Unstable if lateral masses overhang by total >6.9 mm on open-mouth view because indicates transverse ligament injury—must be more aggressive with immobilization
- Transverse ligament intact likely if overhang sum <5.7 mm
- Usually treatment is halo for 3 mo first
- Flexion/extension xr's at end of treatment to detect C1-2 instability
- Surgery if odontoid fracture or transverse ligament midsubstance rupture with C1-2 instability, unable to tolerate halo
- Consider C2-1 Magerl screw to avoid postoperative halo
- ? transverse ligament rupture causing late instability
- ? need for reduction of lateral masses to prevent facet junction arthritis/pain

Reference
Levine AM, Edwards CC. Fractures of the atlas. J Bone Joint Surg Am 1991;73(5):680–691.

Trauma—C2—Odontoid Fracture

- One-fourth with neurologic deficit
- Anderson and d'Alonzo (1974)

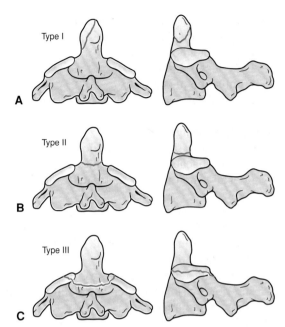

The odontoid fracture classification of Anderson and D'Alonzo. **(A)** Type I fractures of the odontoid tip represent alar ligament avulsions. **(B)** Type II fractures occur at the odontoid waist, above the C2 lateral masses. **(C)** Type III fractures extend below the odontoid waist to involve the body and lateral masses of C2. Hadley has added the type IIA fracture with segmental comminution at the base of the odontoid (not shown) (From Bucholz RW, Heckman JD, Court-Brown C, et al., eds. Rockwood and Green's Fractures in Adults, 6th ed. Philadelphia: Lippincott Williams & Wilkins, 2006.)

- Type I—rare
  - At tip from avulsion of alar ligament
  - Must rule out atlanto-occipital dissociation
  - Differential diagnosis—os odontoideum
  - Orthosis for 3 mo
- Type II
  - Most common
  - Junction of base and body, unstable
  - 30%–50% nonunion with reduction/halo
  - 100% nonunion if no treatment
- Initial closed reduction with traction, then collar or halo for 3 mo
- PSF or ORIF acute type II if
  - **Initial displacement >5 mm**
  - Angulation >10 degrees (irreducible)
  - Patient >50 yo
  - These are associated with nonunions
- Odontoid screw preserves rotation compared to C1-2 fusion and has 90% healing rate in acute fracture
- PSF if transverse ligament injury because healing not predictable and anterior screw alone will cause late instability

- Avoid ORIF with anterior screw fixation if
  - Anteriorly displaced fracture
  - Established nonunion
  - Imperfect reduction
  - Frontal oblique pattern
  - Barrel chest
  - Osteopenic
  - Transverse ligament injury
  - If nonunion, then C1-2 PSF; don't bother fixing fracture because only one-third go on to unite in established nonunions treated with anterior screw
- C1-2 PCF wiring techniques with >90% fusion rates but require halo
- Harms technique for C1-2 PCF if anterior screw contra-indicated
  - displaced irreducible fractures
  - anterior-inferior to posterior fracture pattern
  - comminuted fracture
- Type III
  - Within cancellous bone of body
  - Relatively stable
  - High union after reduction and immobilization
  - Anterior screw contraindicated
  - Treat in **halo**
  - Malunion in hard collar can lead to stenosis
- In children, surgery rarely needed
  - Postural reduction ± halo
  - Reduction easy due to anterior soft tissue hinge
  - Minerva cast or halo for 6 wk

ANTERIOR ODONTOID SCREW

- Preserves C1-2 rotation and may avoid halo
- Two K-wires to provisionally fix, remove one, tap, then place one to two screws
- Average length 40 mm
- Tip of screw through apical cortex of odontoid for additional stability
- Load to failure same for one or two screws
- Fails by screw bending in II and by cutout in III
- Stiffer in bending than wiring but no difference in rotation

Reference

Anderson LD, D'Alonzo RT. Fractures of the odontoid process of the axis. J Bone Joint Surg Am 1974;56(8):1663–1674.

Trauma—C2 Fracture (Hangman's)

- C2 traumatic spondylolisthesis due to bilateral fracture of C2 pars/pedicles
- Hyperextension force, then flexion
- 25%–40% immediate death
- Survivors usually no neurologic deficit
- 75% caused by motor vehicle accident
- Usually no neurologic injury in survivors
- Levine & Edwards (1985)
  - Type I
    - <3-mm displacement, no angulation
    - Hyperextension, axial load
    - C2-3 disc intact
    - Stable
    - Collar protection
    - 90% heal
  - Type II
    - >3-mm displacement, angulated
    - Associated C3 anterior wedge fracture
    - Hyperextension, axial load then flexion
    - Potentially unstable
    - Reduced by extension/distraction in halo, then halo vest
    - Alternatively, fuse C2-3 anteriorly, C1-3 with wiring or C2-3 with pedicle/lateral mass screws posteriorly
  - Type IIa
    - Minimal displacement, significant angulation without slippage
    - Different injury mechanism
    - Variant of C2-3 flexion distraction
    - Unstable due to posterior longitudinal ligament disruption
    - Tends to displace in traction
    - Reduction with gentle extension and **compression** in halo vest
    - Usually heals well and autofuses C2-3 anteriorly due to disc injury
  - Type III
    - Facet fracture-dislocation of C2-3, pars fracture
    - Flexion compression
    - Grossly unstable, anterior longitudinal ligament and PLL gone
    - Often irreducible—open reduction
    - Neurologic injury common, poor prognosis
    - Always surgery, C2-3 fusion
- Starr and Eismont
  - Variant in which fracture extends through posterior cortex of C2 body and 33% neurologic injury due to narrowing of canal

OVERALL

- Heals well despite displacement
- Generally reduce, then halo

Reference

Levine AM, Edwards CC. The management of traumatic spondylolisthesis of the axis. J Bone Joint Surg Am 1985;67(2):217–226.

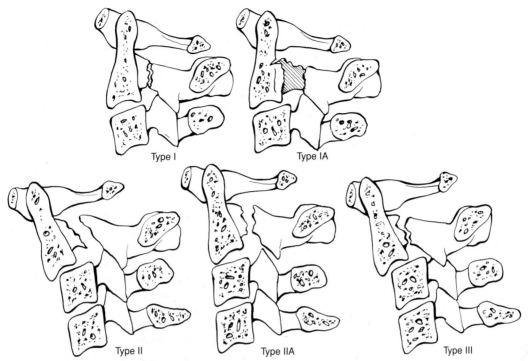

Classification of hangman's fractures. Type I—minimal separation of the fragments, without significant angulation or translation. Type IA—oblique fracture through posterior portion of vertebral body may be difficult to visualize on lateral radiograph. There may be apparent elongation of the vertebral body and pars. Type II—relatively vertical fracture with separation of the fragments, angulation, and translation of C2 on C3. Type IIA—oblique fracture line by failure of pars in tension, no translation, but significant angulation of C2 on C3. Type III—combined injury, with type I fracture of pars and C2-3 facet dislocation. (From Bono C, Garfin SR, Orthopaedic Surgery Essentials: Spine Philadelphia: Lippincott Williams & Wilkins 2004 with permission.)

Trauma—Cervical—Pediatric

- Rare in kids
- If child <8 yo, injury at C3 or higher in 87% and higher rate of fatality
- C-spine approaches adult size and shape by 8 yo
- Less slope in facet junctions—more mobile
- To accommodate big head, use spine board with occipital recess or elevate body

PSEUDOSUBLUXATION

- Most common at C2-3 (in 19% kids 1–7 yo)
- Also seen at C3-4
- Up to 4 mm or 40% normal in those <8 yo
- Posterior line of Swischuk

SPINAL CORD INJURY WITHOUT RADIOGRAPHIC ABNORMALITY

- Occurs because flexible neck in kids
- Spinal column can elongate 2 in. while cord ruptures after 0.25 in. of stretch

Trauma—Cervical Body Fracture

- Isolated vertical body fractures from axial load without flexion component are stable—immobilization alone if no neurologic deficit
- Teardrop component (flex, axial load injury with potential rupture of PLL)
  - High rate of neurologic injury
  - Unstable, needs surgery
  - Anterior corpectomy, strut, with plating
  - ASF/strut and PSF

Trauma—Cervical Facet Dislocation

- Mechanism is flexion distraction
- Most common at C5-6, C6-7
- 40% initially missed due to inadequate xr's
- Purely ligamentous injuries

UNILATERAL

- Rotated, ventral body dimensions changed
- Never >25% subluxation if unilateral

- "Bow-tie" laminae on lateral xr
- Spinous process deviation to side of dislocation on AP xr
- Can present with severe unilateral radiculopathy because dislocated side's foramen narrows
- Low risk of cord injury
- Can be harder to reduce, <50% success

BILATERAL

- Usually 50% subluxation
- 50% chance of cord injury, worse with more displacement

MRI

(Vaccaro et al., 2001)
- Unilateral and bilateral show damage to muscle, interspinous ligament, supraspinous ligament, ligamentum flavum, facet capsule
- Only bilateral consistently showed damage to PLL, anterior longitudinal ligament, and left capsule

TREATMENT

- Consider MRI to rule out HNP before reduction
  - Up to 54% HNP in these patients
  - Don't waste time with MR if spinal cord injury complete because quick reduction is best chance that patient has
  - Treatment of patients with incomplete injury is controversial
  - Intact patients should get MRI
  - Unconscious patients should get MR
  - MR after all successful reduction, failed closed reduction, or neurologic changes
- Closed reduction if alert
- Skeletal traction
  - Can go up to 140 lbs
  - Usually reduction with 40–70 lbs
  - Neurologic check with each weight
  - Too much if neurologic change or disc space >1 cm
  - Done early in trauma bay in cooperative patient
  - Early reduction associated with best neurologic recovery
- Usually all need fusion because of ligamentous nature of injury
- Usually PSF after reduction if no HNP
  - Shapiro (1993)—98% success in open reduction and posterior fusion
- Can try halo in unilateral but usually fails
  - Bucholz and Cheung (1989)—45% eventual surgery
- If HNP, ACDF first ± PSF
  - Anterior reduction often fails requiring posterior exposure after anterior decompression, followed by return anteriorly for fusion
- Irreducible—open reduction, PSF

References

Bucholz RD, Cheung KC. Halo vest versus spinal fusion for cervical injury: evidence from an outcome study. J Neurosurg 1989;70(6):884–892.

Shapiro SA. Management of unilateral locked facet of the cervical spine. Neurosurgery 1993;33(5):832–837; discussion 837.

Vaccaro AR, et al. Distraction extension injuries of the cervical spine. J Spinal Disord 2001;14(3):193–200.

Trauma—Cervical Stability List

- O-C1 instability
  - >8-degrees axial rotation to 1 side
  - >1 mm translation
- C1-2 instability
  - >6.9-mm combined overhang
  - >45-degree axial rotation to one side
  - >4-mm sagittal translation
  - <12-mm space available for the cord
  - Ruptured transverse ligament
- Panjabi and White
  - 5 or more—patient has unstable subaxial spine
  - 2—anterior elements shot
  - 2—posterior elements shot
  - 2—>3.5-mm relative sagittal translation
  - 2—>**11-degree relative sagittal angulation**
  - 2—positive stretch test
  - 2—cord damage
  - 1—root damage
  - 1—disc narrowing
  - 1—anticipated dangerous loading

Trauma—Cervical Subaxial Fractures

(Allen et al., 1982)
- 19% vertebral a. injury in C-spine trauma, most common with compression flexion and distraction flexion
- Bony disc resists compression and ligaments resist tension

COMPRESSION FLEXION (20%)

- Most common at C4, 5, 6
- MVA, diving
- Anterior compression, posterior distraction
- >25% body anterior height loss associated with posterior ligament injury
- CFs 1—anterior-superior body rounding and blunting
- CFs 2—beaking of anterior body due to greater compression
- CFs 1 and 2—mid- and post column OK
  - Neurologic loss rare
  - Orthosis/halo for 3 mo

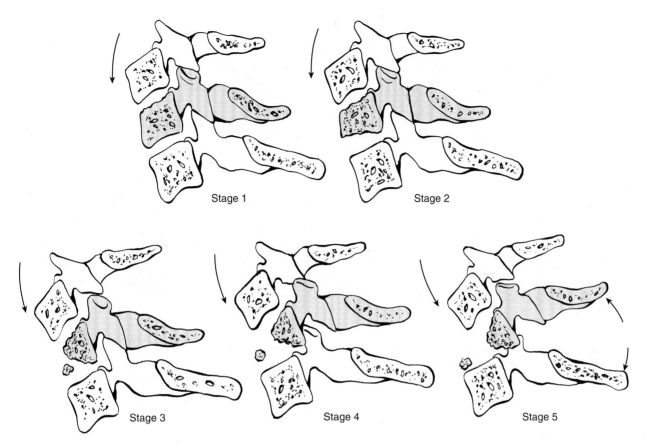

Compressive flexion injuries. Stage 1—blunting of anterosuperior vertebral margin. Stage 2—additional loss of height, involvement of inferior end plate. Stage 3—oblique fracture from anterosuperior surface to subchondral plate. Stage 4—posterior displacement (<3 mm) into neural canal. Stage 5—further disruption of posterior ligamentous complex and posterior displacement of vertebral body (>3 mm). (From Bono C, Garfin SR, Orthopaedic Surgery Essentials: Spine Philadelphia: Lippincott Williams & Wilkins 2004 with permission.)

- CFs 3—oblique fracture of anterior body beak into posterior-inferior end plate
  - 25% complete SCI
- CFs 4—<3-mm retrolisthesis of body into canal; "teardrop"
  - 38% complete SCI
- CFs 3–4
  - Get MRI to check post ligaments
  - Halo if stable (PLL OK)
  - Surgery if potential for late deformity
  - PSF or anterior corpx fusion
- CFs 5—three-column injury
  - >3-mm retrolisthesis
  - 91% complete SCI
  - Usually anterior/posterior corpx fusion

VERTICAL COMPRESSION (15%)

- Most common C6 and C7
- VCs 1—central cupping of end plate

- VCs 2—superior and inferior end plate fracture
- VCs 3—VCs 2 with displacement of body into canal
- All three usually stable and halo if neurologically intact
- Usually anterior corpx, fusion if neurologic deficit

DISTRACTIVE FLEXION (10%)

- These are facet dislocations
- DFs 1—spinous process divergence and <25% subluxation
- DFs 2—unilateral facet dislocation, 25%–50%
- DFs 3—bilateral facet dislocation, >50%
- DFs 4—full-width body displacement anteriorly
- Immediate closed reduction needed
- Then usually posterior fusion, stabilization
- If HNP, anterior discectomy and fusion with plating sufficient

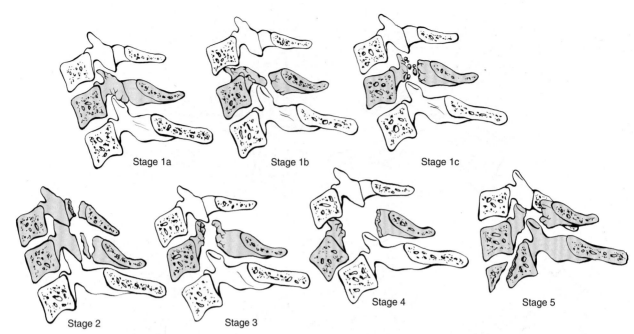

Compressive extension injuries. Stage 1 involves unilateral fracture through the articular process, pedicle, or lamina. Stage 2 involves bilaminar fracture, which often occurs at multiple contiguous levels. Stages 3 and 4 are hypothetical stages, not seen in Allen's initial observations. Stage 5 involves three contiguous levels, anterior displacement, and shear injury through the adjacent inferior centrum. (From Bono C, Garfin SR, Orthopaedic Surgery Essentials: Spine Philadelphia: Lippincott Williams & Wilkins 2004 with permission.)

COMPRESSION EXTENSION

- CEs 1—unilateral arch fracture
  - CEs 1a—articular process fracture
  - CEs 1b—pedicle fracture
  - CEs 1c—lamina fracture
- CEs 2—bilateral arch fracture
  - usually collar/halo for CEs 1 and 2
- CEs 3—progressive injury to posterior elements without body displacement
  - usually halo or PSF
- CEs 4—bilateral posterior element fracture with partial body displacement
- CEs 5—100% body displacement
  - Usually reduction/PSF for CEs 4 and 5

DISTRACTIVE EXTENSION (22%)

- In elderly with ankylosing spondylitis or diffuse idiopathic skeletal hyperostosis
- Xr appears benign
- DEs 1—anterior ligament failure or transverse fracture through vertebral body
  - Disc space wide on xr
  - If bony, usually halo

- If thru disc, ? ACDF with anterior tension band instrumentation
- DEs 2—with disruption of posterior ligaments
  - Always unstable, needs ACDF
- Vaccaro et al., 2001
  - 42% mortality in this elderly population
  - Anterior graft and tension plate ideal for acute jury (ALL and disc)
  - Type II may need posterior approach to realign, then anterior reconstruction
  - Avoid anterior overdistraction with graft because it leads to neurologic injury

LATERAL FLEXION (20%)

- Seen in football, missed on plain xr
- SCI rare but brachial plexus and root injury not uncommon
- LFs 1—nondisplacement arch fracture with asymmetric compression fracture
  - Stable, no displacement on AP xr
  - Hard collar
- LFs 2—contralateral ligament failure
  - Reduction with skeletal traction
  - PSF, anterior decompression if cord injury

References

Allen BL Jr, et al. A mechanistic classification of closed, indirect fractures and dislocations of the lower cervical spine. Spine 1982;7(1):1–27.

Vaccaro AR, et al. Distraction extension injuries of the cervical spine. J Spinal Disord 2001;14(3):193–200.

Trauma—Halo, Tongs

HALO

- Ideal orthosis of upper C-spine
- Fixes skull relative to torso
- Unreliable for lower C-spine because allows intercalated paradoxical subaxial motion
- 1 cm superior to orbital rim, cephalad to the lateral two-thirds of the orbit, below the greatest circumference of skull
- Watch out for supraorbital n. in medial one-third of brow; if you get even more medial, you get supratrochlear n, then frontal sinus
- Pins should be 1 cm above superior aspect of ear, never touch ear
- Stay out of temporalis fossa to avoid increasing pin loosening in weak bone, infection
- Pins placed with eyes SHUT
- Total four pins, 8 lb of torque each

Diagram of the safe zone for placement of anterior halo fixator pins. (From Bono C, Garfin SR, Orthopaedic Surgery Essentials: Spine Philadelphia: Lippincott Williams & Wilkins 2004 with permission.)

- In children six to eight pins, 4–5 lb
  - Minerva cast if child <2 yo

Complications

- Pin loosening—change pins
- Infection
- Dural puncture rare

GARDNER-WELLS TONGS

- Use stainless steel pins if expect >50 lb of traction because MRI-compatible carbon fiber ones will bend

Trauma—Occipital Condyle Fracture

- High energy
- Concomitant head injury
- Injury to CNs IX–XII
- Usually fatal
- Unable to diagnose on xr, need CT
- Anderson and Montesano
- Type I
  - Impaction of condyles with comminution
  - Due to axial load
  - Stable, hard collar for 3 mo

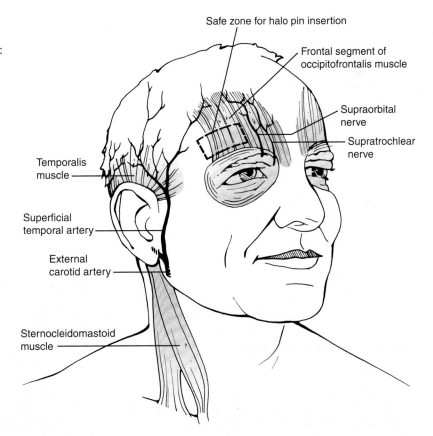

- Type II
  - Basilar skull fracture associated with fracture of condyles
  - Stable, halo vest for 3 mo
- Type III
  - Avulsion of alar ligament with tip of condyle
  - Tectorial membrane (PLL) may be torn
  - Often bilateral
  - With AOD in 30%–50%
  - Unstable, must rule out atlanto-occipital dissociation
  - Halo or occipital-C2 fusion

Reference

Anderson LD, D'Alonzo RT. Fractures of the odontoid process of the axis. J Bone Joint Surg Am 1974;56(8):1663–1674.

Trauma—Sacrum Fracture

- Osteoporotic insufficiency or high-energy fracture
- Bladder and urethral injury common
- Up to 50% neurologic injury in high-energy fracture
- Neurologic exam for sacral roots
  - Anal tone
  - Anal sensation
  - Bladder function
- AP, inlet, outlet, CT
- XR signs of pelvic instability
  - >1 cm posterior or vertical displacement
  - Lumbar L5 TP fracture
  - Ischial spine avulsion fracture
  - Asymmetric sacral foramina
  - Cephalad migration of hemipelvis
  - SI gap instead of compression

VERTICAL FRACTURE

- Zone 1—lateral extraforaminal (50%)
  - rare neurologic (6%), bladder injury
  - L5 is most common injured
- Zone 2—traverses foramen (35%)
  - 30% neurologic injury—L5, S1, S2
  - 97% of missed diagnoses are in zones 1 and 2
- Zone 3—medial extraforaminal with central canal involvement (15%)
  - 60% neurologic injury—bowel/bladder, sexual
- Vertical fracture treated nonoperatively, PWB if pelvis stable and no neurologic deficit

TRANSVERSE FRACTURE

- Usually at S1-3
- Associated with bladder dysfunction
- Transverse fracture needs posterior decompression and stabilization (lateral mass plates)

H-SHAPED FRACTURE

- Usually high energy
- Avoid partially threaded lag screws if fracture through neural foramen
- Presence of preoperative neurologic injury most important to predict outcome

Trauma—Spinal Cord Injury

- Males, age 19
- 50% from MVA, gun shot wound increasing
- 5%–10% of those with closed head injury and unconscious have C-spine injury
- Number one cause of death is pneumonia
- 25% vertical a. injury with blunt cervical trauma; thus, image if you plan to go back years later for surgery

ASIA SCALE MOTOR SOURCE

- C5—elbow flexors
- C6—wrist extensors
- C7—elbow extensors
- C8—middle finger flexors
- T1—small finger abductor
- L2—hip flexors
- L3—knee extensors
- L4—ankle dorsiflexors
- L5—hallux extensors
- S1—ankle plantarflexors

FRANKEL/ASIA CLASSIFICATION

- A—no motor, no sensory
- B—no motor, some sensory
- C—some motor below level, some sensory
- D—useful motor below level, some sensory
- E—normal motor and normal sensory
- Level is most caudal level with normal sensory and motor function on both sides
- Motor level is level that is 3/5
- Sensory graded as absent, 0; impaired, 1; or normal, 2

MOTOR INDEX SCORE

- 100-point maximum
- 0–5 points at each of 10 levels bilaterally
- Complete
  - C6 quadriplegia with wrist extension has better function
  - Can transfer out of wheelchair with C7
  - In lower C-spine, one can get one to two levels back from complete loss with decompression ("root

return" makes no functional difference in thoracic spine)
- Thus, relative indication to operate on complete loss in lower C-spine
- Incomplete
  - Sacral sparing with voluntary anal sphincter control and perineal sensation indicates INCOMPLETE injury with good prognosis for continued improvement
- Bulbocavernosus reflex
  - Anal contraction with squeezing of glans, clitoris, or pulling Foley
  - Return in 24–48 hr indicative of end of spinal shock
  - Can't judge whether injury is complete or not until this comes back (or deem that it's not coming back based on injury to conus)
  - First to return because it is lowest cord-mediated reflex (S3-4)
- Anal wink
  - Contraction of sphincter with scratching of perianal skin
  - Mediated by S2-4
- MRI poor prognosis factors for functional motor recovery
  - Edema more than two levels
  - Hematoma within cord

TREATMENT

- Initial
  - Avoid low blood pressure, hypoxia
  - Ulcer pphy is key
  - Deep venous thrombosis pphy—boots, inferior vena cava filter
  - Foley
  - Nasogastric tube except if face fracture
- Steroids
- Apply skeletal traction, reduce
- MRI
  - For suspected HNP
  - Incomplete injury, with normal alignment

Spinal cord injury syndromes. Incomplete spinal cord lesions are described according to the predominant area of injury. Each of the four types is associated with a different prognosis for neurologic recovery: central cord syndrome (A), Brown-Sequard syndrome (B), anterior cord syndrome (C), and posterior cord syndrome (D). (From Bucholz RW, MD and Heckman JD, MD. Rockwood & Green's Fractures in Adults, 5th ed. Phialdelphia:Lippincott, Williams & Wilkins, 2001.)

- Before open reduction (general anesthesia)
- If neurologic worsening
- For spinal cord injury without radiological abnormality
- Generally GSW nonoperative except if it involves conus or cauda equina or through colon
- Surgical indications—decompression
  - Persistent stenosis with incomplete injury
  - Worsening neurologic status
  - Complete SCI to facilitate rehab off brace or for lower cervical root return

COMPLICATIONS

- Neurogenic shock—decreased BP with relative bradycardia
  - Swan-Ganz, **pressors**
- Autonomic dysreflexia
  - Rare in level below T6
  - Headache, agitation, hypertension
  - Sweating, dilated pupils
  - Caused by noxious stimuli
  - Check Foley, disimpact, then treat hypertension
- Urosepsis
- Skin breakdown
- Posttraumatic syringomyelia
  - In 3% of spinal cord injuries
  - Onset months to years after injury
  - Progressive motor and sensory loss greater than initial injury
  - Charcot shoulder
  - Hand blisters from burns/temperature insensitivity

Trauma—Spinal Cord Syndromes

- Central cord syndrome—**most common**
  - Motor loss in upper extremities, worse in hands; LEs spared because lateral corticospinal tract has UE closer to center
  - Sacral sparing

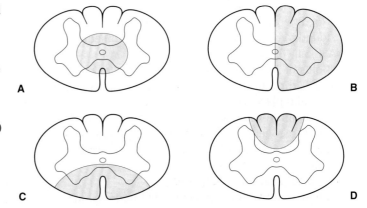

- Varying degree of sensory loss
- Late—LMN signs in UE, UMN signs in LE
- ? related to ischemia, seen in **elderly** after extension injury
- Recovery fair to poor
- Walks, some bladder control, clumsy hands
- Anterior cord syndrome
  - Usually flexion compression mechanism
  - Usually vascular insult, anterior two-thirds
  - Motor loss below level (pyramidal tract) with LE worse than UE
  - ± spinothalamus tract (pain, temperature, touch)
  - Posterior tract OK (vibration and position)
  - Worse prognosis when severe
- Brown-Sequard syndrome
  - Half cord injured, rare
  - Ipsilateral motor and proprioception loss (these fibers ascent ipsilaterally, then cross in midbrain)
  - Contra pain, temperature, touch loss (these fibers cross through ventral commissure, then ascend)
  - Excellent prognosis for ambulation
- Posterior cord syndrome—rare
  - Loss of vibration, position sense
  - Functional outcome fair

Trauma—Steroids

PROTOCOL

- Methylprednisolone 30 mg/kg over first hour, then 5.4 mg/kg/hr drip
  - 23 hr if before 3 hr from injury
  - 48 hr if between 3 and 8 hr from injury
  - Not useful after 8 hr from injury

CONTRAINDICATIONS

- GSW
- Pregnancy
- Patient <13 yo
- National Acute Spinal Cord Injury Study I (NASCIS), (Bracken JAMA 1984)
  - Natural acute spinal cord injury study
  - Low- vs. high-dose methylprednisolone
  - No difference in neurologic recovery but doses found to be too low in animal studies subsequently
- NASCIS II (Bracken NEJM 1990)
  - Bolus of 30 mg/kg of methylprednisolone, then 5.4 mg/kg/hr infusion for 23 hr compared with naloxone and placebo
  - Methylprednisolone within 8 hr after injury had more recovery regardless of whether injury was initially complete or incomplete (one to two levels gained)
- NASCIS III (Bracken JAMA 1997)
  - Compared two regimens of methylprednisolone

- 30 mg/kg bolus, then 5.4 mg/kg/hr for 24 hr vs. 48 hr
- Third group of patients got 30 mg/kg bolus, then boluses of 2.5 mg/kg of tirilazad mesylate q6h for 48 hr
- When given within 3 hr of injury, no difference between three groups
- When given 3–8 hr from injury, 48-hr infusion of methylprednisolone was best

Reference

Bracken MB, et al. Efficacy of methylprednisolone in acute spinal cord injury. JAMA 1984;251(1):45–52.

Bracken MB, et al. A randomized, controlled trial of methylprednisolone or naloxone in the treatment of acute spinal-cord injury. Results of the second national acute spinal cord injury study. N Engl J Med 1990;322(20):1405–1411.

Bracken MB, et al. Administration of methylprednisolone for 24 or 48 hours or tiriazad mesylate for 48 hours in treatment of acute spinal cord injury. Results of the Third National Acute Spinal Cord Injury Study Randomized Controlled Trial. JAMA 1997;277(20):1597–1604.

Trauma—Thoracolumbar Fracture

- Mid-T fracture is a common cause of widened mediastinum
- T2-10 fractures are usually stable because of fourth column, the rib cage, and sternum, but have high risk of neurologic injury because it takes lots of energy to disrupt four columns
- T11-L1 fracture—isolated conus injuries, mixed neurologic pattern
- L2 down—cauda equina, better prognosis
- Denis (1984): Three columns
  - Anterior—ALL, front half body
  - Middle—back half body, PLL
  - Posterior—posterior elements
  - Two of three columns disrupted = unstable
- Ferguson and Allen (1984): seven types
- 1—compressive flexion (three subtypes)
  - Most common, 48%
  - I—anterior compressed
  - II—ant compression, post tension, midcolumn is axis of rotation
  - III—midcolumn fails and is retropulsed, most common
- 2—distractive flexion
  - Tension failure of all three columns
  - Flexion-distraction seatbelt injuries
- 3—lateral flexion
- 4—translational—shear
- 5—torsional flexion—rotation
- 6—vertical compression
  - Two to three columns fail in compression
- 7—distractive extension
  - Tension anterior, compression posterior

STABILITY

- **Any translation in TL spine—unstable, needs to be fused/stabilized even if neurologic exam normal**
- Complete SCI with unstable injury needs to be stabilized for rehab
- Incomplete spinal cord injury with unstable injury needs first needs to be stabilized to protect recovery and then decompress at plateau early
- If posterior ligament injury, operate because it doesn't heal to restore stability

References

Denis F. Spinal instability as defined by the three-column spine concept in acute spinal trauma. Clin Orthop Relat Res 1984;(189):65–76.

Ferguson RL, Allen BL Jr. A mechanistic classification of thoracolumbar spine fractures. Clin Orthop Relat Res 1984;(189): 77–88.

Trauma—TL Burst Fracture

- Compression failure anterior and middle
- Centrifugal displacement of fracture fragments with retropulsed fragment into canal
- Possible compression or tensile failure of posterior column
- Most common in TL region due to transition from rigid to mobile segments; also, TL junction is straight, thus axial force > compression of all columns
- Biphasic age distribution in young and elderly
- Almost 50% neurologic injury
- Over 50% concomitant thoracic or abdominal injury
- Must document progression of neurologic changes since injury
- Neurologic deficit due to initial force vs. residual canal deformity and neural compression
- One-third of patients with local tenderness after trauma to TL spine with negative xr's will have occult injury
- 5%–10% incidence of concomitant multilevel spine injury
- 50% of concomitant multilevel spinal injury missed with average delay in diagnosis of 50 days and 25% of those have neurologic deterioration due to improper immobilization
- Xr entire spine after one injury seen
- Xr can only differentiate burst from simple compression 54% of the time
- MR can see cord compression by disc, epidural hematoma, flavum invagination, subtle ligament injuries
  - T2 sees post ligament injuries
  - "Black stripe sign" indicates injury to PLL or supraspinous ligament
  - High signal in interspinous area indicates injury
- Stable vs. unstable burst (McAfee et al., 1983)

- Anterior body compression >50%
- Segmental kyphosis >20–30 degrees
- (Facet subluxation or interspinous widening)
- (Progressive neurologic deterioration)
- Nonoperative
  - Bedrest until ileus resolves
  - Custom total contact thoraco-lumbo-sacral-orthosis for 3–6 mo
  - Serial xr's
  - Indicated in
    - <20-degree segmental kyphosis
    - <45% canal compromise
    - Neurologically intact
    - No posterior column disruption
  - Flexion/extension xr's to check for dynamic stability prior to mobilization
  - Instability does not always mean surgery
  - Residual canal compromise and mild kyphosis do not correlate with outcome
  - Lower lumbar burst with unilateral root deficit, especially if L5, has been shown to heal in brace with improved neurologic function
- Surgery
  - Decision for surgery depends on injury morphology, neurologic status, and presence of posterior ligamentous injury
  - OR if translational or distraction injury, usually posterior stabilization
  - OR if neurologic injury, usually anterior approach to decompress +/− posterior stabilization
  - OR if associated posterior ligamentous injury, usually posterior stabilization
- Burst fracture in lower lumbar spine
  - 4% of all spine fractures
  - Vertical lamina fracture may entrap dura and cause tear or entrap rootlet
  - Look for this in patient with no stenosis but with isolated single root deficit
  - Do lami first, then decompression and stabilization
  - Lower lumbar burst usually treated nonoperatively

Reference

McAfee PC, et al. The value of computed tomography in thoracolumbar fractures. an analysis of one hundred consecutive cases and a new classification. J Bone Joint Surg Am 1983;65(4):461–473.

Vaccaro, et al. Surgical decision making for unstable thoracolumbar spine injuries: results of a consensus panel review by the Spine Trauma Study Group. J Spinal Disord Tech 2006;19(1):1–10.

Trauma—TL Compression Fracture

- Anterior column failure, middle OK
- Usually in elderly
- Stable due to rib cage support

TREATMENT

– Analgesia, early ambulation
– Hyperextension orthosis if
  – Anterior body compression >50%
  – Segmental kyphosis >30 degrees
  – These are potentially unstable due to possible posterior ligament disruption
  – Multiple adjacent levels—late kyphosis
  – Soft corset in elderly
– Surgery if
  – Unstable
  – Documented deformity progression
  – Threatened neurologic status

– Posterior approach
– Compression construct

BENIGN VS. MALIGNANT FRACTURE

– Acute benign fracture
  – High on T1 in body (Fat replaced marrow)
  – Becomes normal in 1–3 mo (medium on T1, low on T2)
– Acute malignant fracture
  – Irregular marrow replacement (Low on T1, high on T2)
  – Pedicle, posterior involved

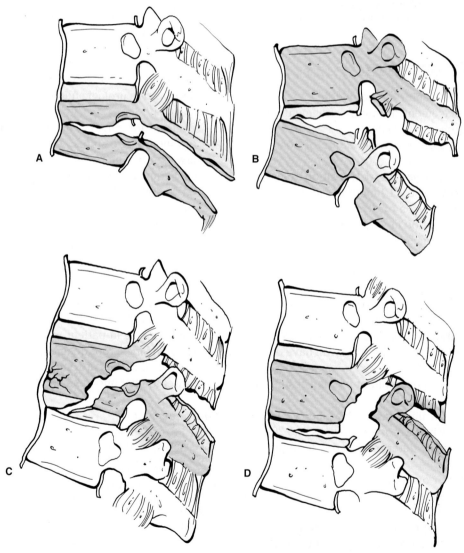

Denis's classification of flexion/distraction injuries. These may occur at one level through the bone **(A)**, at one level through the ligaments and disc **(B)**, at two levels with the middle column injured through the bone **(C)**, or at two levels with the middle column injured through the ligament and disc **(D)**. (From Bono C, Garfin SR, Orthopaedic Surgery Essentials: Spine Philadelphia: Lippincott Williams & Wilkins 2004 with permission.)

Trauma—TL Flexion Distraction (Seat Belt)

- Lap seat belt injury
- Axis of rotation anterior to spine generally
- The axis can shift into the body, causing secondary axial load, leading to an element of burst or compression to body
- Entire spine sees distraction force
- Through bone alone, bone and ligaments, or ligaments alone
- Bony flexion-distraction (Chance fracture, figure A above) most common at L1-3
- Osteoligamentous injury (ligamentous Chance fracture, figure B above) at T-L junction and has poorer healing
- Associated with retroperitoneal **visceral injuries**
- Consider nonoperative treatment for purely bony injury
    - Initially bedrest
    - TLSO with molded hyperextension when abd injury is cleared
    - 3 mo, serial xr's
    - Dynamic xr's before d/c cast
- If through soft tissue, operate
    - Posterior approach, compression construct
    - Neutralization construct if associated burst
    - If HNP, hemilaminotomy and discectomy before reduction and PSF

Recommended Reading
Bradford DS, McBride GG. Surgical management of thoracolumbar spine fractures with incomplete neurologic deficits. Clin Orthop Relat Res 1987;(218):201–216.

Trauma—TL Fracture-Dislocation

- High-energy, combination forces
- Goal to stabilize and mobilize
- Usually posterior approach with fracture reduction
- "Empty facet" sign on CT

Trauma—Gun Shot Wound

- GSW associated with perforation of colon is controversial—removal of bullet, débride, and antibiotics vs. antibiotics alone
- Bullet removal in complete cord injury in T-spine is of minimal benefit
- Bullet removal increases nerve root recovery in TL and L injuries with incomplete neurologic injury
- Usually only decompression is required unless iatrogenic instability

INDEX

Note: Page number followed by f indicates figure only.

A

Accessory navicular syndrome, 175–176
  classification, 176
  clinical manifestations, 175
  radiographs, 176
  treatment, 176
Accuracy, 443
Acetabular fracture, 279–288
  anatomy, 279, 279f, 280f
  anterior column fractures, 281
  anterior column, posterior
      hemitransverse, 281
  anterior wall fractures, 281
  approaches
    extended iliofemoral approach, 283
    fixation, 283
    ilioinguinal incision, 283
    Kocher-Langenbeck (K-L) approach,
        283
  both columns, 281–282, 282f
  classification, 281f
  complications, 283
  contraindications to surgery, 283
  CT scan, 282
  high energy, 280
  indications, 283
  left hemipelvis, 282f
  Letournel's associated fracture, 280
  Letournel's elementary fracture, 280
  low energy, 280
  nonoperative criteria, 282–283
  operative anatomy, 284f–288f
    anatomy of Kocher-Langenbeck,
        283
    gluteus maximus, 285
    sciatic and piriformis variations, 283,
        285, 285f
  OR tips and tricks
    ilioinguinal approach., 285–288,
        286f–288f
  polytrauma victim with, 287f
  posterior column fractures, 281
  posterior wall fractures, 281
  prognosis, poor, 283
  radiographs, 280, 280f
  six lines, 280
  transverse fractures, 281
  treatment, 282
  T-type, 281
Achilles tendon disorders, 570
  history, 570
  imaging, 570
  physical examination, 570
  treatment, 570
    paratenonitis, 570
    tendinosis, 570
    tendon rupture, 570–571, 571f
Achondroplasia, 113
  etiology, 113
  manifestations, 113–114
  treatment, 114
ACL. See Anterior cruciate ligament (ACL)

Acromioclavicular (AC) joint injury
  anatomy, 90
  classification, 90, 91f
  imaging, 90
  treatment, 92
Acromioplasty, arthroscopic
  contraindications, 92
  failures, categories of, 93
  indications, 92
  results, 93
Acute lymphocytic leukemia (ALL).
    See Leukemia
Acute respiratory distress syndrome,
    186f, 187–188, 187f
Adamantinoma, 462, 463f
  history and physical examination,
      463
  pathology, 463
  treatment, 463
  x-ray, 462
Adhesive capsulitis, 93f
  classification, 93
  clinical stages, 93–94
  differential diagnosis, 93
  evaluation, 93
  treatment, 94
Adriamycin (Doxorubicin), 463–464
Alkaptonuria, 423
Amniotic band syndrome, 113
Amputations
  Chopart (midtarsal) disarticulation, 582
  determination of level, 579
  indications, 579
  Lisfranc (tarsometatarsal)
      disarticulation, 582
  ray amputation, 581
  surgical considerations, 579
  Syme ankle disarticulation, 581f, 582
  toe disarticulations, 579, 581
  transmetatarsal amputation,
      580f, 581
Amyoplasia, 118
Amyotrophic lateral sclerosis (ALS),
    423
Aneurysmal bone cyst, 461, 461f, 462f
  differential diagnosis, 462
  history and physical examination,
      461
  imaging, 462
  pathology, 462
  treatment, 462
Anion gap (AG), 423–424
Ankle arthroplasty
  contraindications, 589–590
  indication, 589
  patient selection, 589
  preoperative considerations, 590
  surgical procedure, 590
  treatment options, 590
Ankle fracture, 345–354
  anatomy, 345
  classification, 345

Lauge Hansen classification, 347–348,
    350f, 351f
  syndesmosis, 345, 347
  Weber, 345, 349f
distal fibular plates, 353f
high fibula fracture, 352f
open, 354, 354f
OR tips and tricks, 355f, 356f
  lateral approach, 356–357
  medial approach, 357
  posterolateral approach, 355–356
pediatric, 418–421
postoperative course, 357–358
pronation-abduction ankle fracture,
    352f
special considerations
  posterior malleolus, 349
  posttraumatic arthritis, 349
treatment, 348–349
X-ray normal ankle, 352f
Ankle instability, 568
  Chrisman-Snook reconstruction, 569f
  history, 568
  modified Broström repair, 568f
  physical examination, 568
  treatment, 568
Ankle sprain, 568
Ankylosing spondylitis (AS), 424, 585
Anterior cruciate ligament (ACL)
  anterior drawer test, 78f
  arthroscopic procedure transtibial
      technique, 80
  grafts, 78f
  natural history, 78
  pathophysiology, 78
  pediatric, 80–81
  rehab, 80
  ruptures, 79f
  treatment, 78, 80
Antibiotics, 424
  antibacterial drug classes, 425f
  bone and joint infections, 426
  open fractures, 426
  surgical prophylaxis, 424
  total joint arthroplasty (TJA) patients,
      425
Anticoagulation
  aspirin, 427
  coagulation cascade, 426f
  heparin, 427
  heparinoids, 427
  prior to surgery, 426
  venous thromboembolism, 426–427
  Virchow triad, 427
  warfarin, 427
Apert syndrome, 117–118
Apophyseal ring fracture
  and back pain in children, 145
Arthritis episode, acute, 431
Arthrodesis
  of ankle and hindfoot, 586
    ankle arthrodesis, 586, 587f

Arthrodesis (Contd.)
  nonoperative treatment, 586
  pantalar arthrodesis, 587–588
  preoperative considerations, 586
  subtalar arthrodesis, 586–587, 587f
  surgical options, 586
  tibiocalcaneal arthrodesis, 587
  triple arthrodesis, 587, 588f
  of midfoot and forefoot
    first interphalangeal joint, 588–589
    first metatarsophalangeal joint
      arthrodesis, 588, 589f
    Lisfranc arthrodesis, 589
Arthrogryposis, 118, 118f
Arthroplasty
  complications, 44–61
    heterotopic ossification, 52–53
    hip dislocation, 54–56
    infection, 44–48
    patellar problems, 58–59
    periprosthetic femoral fractures,
      56–58
    periprosthetic knee fractures, 60–61
    soft tissue complications, 52
    venous thromboembolic disease,
      48–52
    wear and loosening, 53–54, 59–60
  hip, 4–30
  inflammatory arthritis and, 1–2
  knee, 30–44
  osteoarthritis and, 2–4
  revision, 61–65
    total hip replacement, 61–64
    total knee arthroplasty, 64–65
Arthroscopy, foor and ankle, 555–556,
  555f
Atlanto-occipital dissociation
  diagnosis, 641
  Traynelis classification, 640
  treatment, 641–642
Avascular necrosis, 9–10
  classification systems, 10
  core decompression, 10
  imaging
    MRI, 9–10
    plain film, 9
  presentation, 9
  treatment, 10

B

Back pain, in children, 145
  apophyseal ring fracture and, 146
  differential diagnosis, 145
  herniated nucleus pulposus and, 145
  history, 145
  idiopathic juvenile osteoporosis and,
    146
  leukemia and, 145
  physical exam, 145
  tumor versus infection on MRI, 146
  workup, 145
Back pain, low, 612
Basal joint osteoarthritis, 544–545
Becker muscular dystrophy, 128
Benign lytic bone lesions
  age older than 30 years, 452
  aneurysmal bone cyst, 452
  chondroblastoma, 452
  chondromyxoid fibroma, 452
  differential diagnosis, 452–453
  enchondroma, 451–452
  eosinophilic granuloma, 452

  epiphyseal, 452
  expansile, lytic, posterior spine, 452
  fibrous dysplasia, 451
  giant cell tumor, 452
  hyperparathyroidism, 452
  infection, 452
  mnemonic for, 451
  multiple, 452
  myeloma, metastases, 452
  nonossifying fibroma, 452
  osteoblastoma, 452
  pain or periostitis, 452
  sacral lesions, 453
  sequestrations, 452
  simple bone cyst/unicameral bone cyst,
    452
Biopsy
  excisional, indications for, 453
  high complication rate, 453
  no need for biopsy, 453
  practical tips, 453
  and shape of bone hole, 453
  and size of bone hole, 453–454
  types of, 453
Bisphosphonates, 427–428
Blount disease, 164–167
  adolescent/late-onset, 165
  differential diagnosis, 165
  infantile, 165
  lower-limb alignment, in infants, 165f
  physical exam, 165
  radiographic findings, 165, 166
  staging, 166
  treatment, 166–167
    bracing, 166
    late-onset, 167
    surgical, 166–167
Bone age, 112
Bone grafts, 428
  allografts, 428
  autografts, 428
  bone morphogenetic protein (BMP), 428
  demineralized bone matrix, 428
  synthetic, 428
Bone island, 463
Bone metastases, 455
  acrometastases, 455
  better survival outcomes, 455
  biopsy, 455
  blastic versus lytic, 455
  metastatic bladder, 455
  metastatic breast, 455
  metastatic colon, 455
  metastatic lung, 455
  presenting symptoms, 455
Bone, physiology of, 437–438
  osteoblasts, 437
  osteocalcin, 437
  osteoclasts, 437
  RANKL/OPG, 437–438
Boutonniere deformity, 535–536, 536f
Boutonniere thumb, 542
Brachial plexus, 86f, 522–523, 523f
Brachial plexus injury, 215–216, 216f
  background, 215
  pre- vs. postganglionic injury, 215
  reconstructive options, 215
  surgical management, 215
Brachial plexus obstetric palsy, 112–113
Brachytherapy, 460
Bunionette, 566
  causes, 566
  history and physical examination, 566

  imaging, 566
  radiographic staging, 566
  treatment
    distal osteotomy, 566
    lateral condylectomy and
      capsulorrhaphy, 566
    metatarsal head resection, 566
    midshaft osteotomy, 566
    nonoperative, 566
    proximal osteotomy, 566
Burch-Schneider ring, 58f

C

Caffey disease, 139
Calcaneovalgus foot, 176
Calcaneus fracture, 364–367
  anatomy, 364
  background, 364
  complications, 366–367
  imaging
    Bohler's angle, 364, 365f, 366f
    Broden's view, 364–365
    crucial angle of Gissane, 364, 366f
    Harris heel axial view, 365
  nonoperative treatment, 365
  OR tips and tricks, 365–366
  percutaneous pin technique of
    Tornetta, 366f
  Sanders classification of, 365, 365f
Calcitonin, 432
Calcium hydroxyapatite deposition, 2
Calcium pyrophosphate dihydrate
  (CPPD). See Pseudogout
Camptodactyly, 545–546
Capitellar fracture, 243–245
  background, 243–244
  classification, 244, 244f
  Hahn-Steinthal, 244f
  mechanism, 244
  related anatomy, 244, 244f
  treatment, 244–245
Carpal tunnel syndrome, 525, 525f
  carpal tunnel contents, 525
  carpal tunnel release technique,
    526–527
  diagnosis, 525–526
  endoscopic carpal tunnel release, 526
  predisposing factors, 525
  revision carpal tunnel release, 526
  standard carpal tunnel release, 526
  transverse carpal ligament
    attachments, 525
Cartilage, physiology of, 438
Case control, 430
Case series, 430
Cauda equina syndrome, 607
Cavus foot, 176–177
  clinical manifestations, 176
  evaluation, 176
  radiographs, 176–177
  treatment, 177
Cerebral palsy (CP), 130
  ambulation prognosis, 131
  anatomic patterns
    diplegia, 130
    hemiplegia, 130
    quadriplegia, 130
  hip, 132, 132f
    causative factors, 132
    clinical manifestations, 132
    dislocation, treatment of, 133
    natural history, 132

osteotomies for subluxation, 133
painful chronic hip dislocations salvage, 133
physical exam, 132
radiographs, 132
soft tissue releases for hip, 132–133
treatment, 132–133
lower extremity, 133
clinical manifestations, 133–134
treatment, 134–135
neuropathic patterns
ataxic, 130
athetoid, 130
spastic, 130
presentation, 130–131
reflexes
postural, 131
primitive, 131
spine
natural history, 136
neuromuscular scoliosis in, 136
treatment, 136
types, 136
treatment, 131
upper extremity, 135
clinical manifestations, 135
treatment, 135–136
Cervical facet dislocation, 645–646
bilateral, 646
MRI, 646
treatment, 646
unilateral, 645–646
Cervical myelopathy, 601–603
causes, 601
complications, 603
diagnosis, 602
natural history, 601
pathology, 601
presentation, 601–602
prognosis, 603
spondylotic myelopathy, 601
treatment, 602–603
Cervical radiculopathy, 605–607
anatomy, 605
causes, 605
differential diagnosis, 605–606
epidemiology, 605
natural history, 605
presentation, 605
treatment, 606–607
Cervical spine
ACDF
advantages of, 597
bone graft, 599
complications, 599–600
corpectomy, 599
landmarks, 597, 598f
plates, 600
surgical approach, 597
anatomy of, 593
cervical lateral masses, 593–594
vertebral artery, 594
disc disease, 600–601
myelopathy, 601–603
radiculopathy, 605–607
rheumatoid arthritis, 603–605
Cervical subaxial fractures, 646–648
compression extension, 648, 648f
compression flexion, 646–647, 647f
distractive extension, 648
distractive flexion, 647
lateral flexion, 648
vertical compression, 647

Charcot arthropathy, 576, 577f
etiology, 576
history and physical examination, 576
imaging, 576–577
staging, 577
treatment, 577
Charcot-Marie-Tooth disease, 137, 137f
Dejerine-Sottas disease, 138
hypertrophic, 137–138
neuronal, 138
Chemical burns, 537
Chemotherapy
adriamycin, 463–464
cisplatin, 464
ifosfamide, 464
vincristine, 464–465
Children. See Pediatrics
Chondral defects, 82
acute cartilage injury, 82
options, 82–83
treatment considerations, 83
Chondroblastoma, 465, 466f
differential diagnosis, 465
history and physical examination, 465
imaging, 465
natural history, 465
pathology, 465
treatment, 465
Chondrocalcinosis, 2
Chondromalacia, 76
Chondromyxoid fibroma, 467, 467f
history and physical examination, 467
imaging, 467
pathology, 467
treatment, 467
Chondrosarcoma, 467
chondrosarcoma in situ, 468
differential diagnosis, 469
vs. enchondroma, 468
histologic subtypes, 468
history and physical examination, 467
imaging, 467–468
low-grade, 468f
metastasis, 469
moderate-grade, 469f
vs. osteochondroma, 468
pathology, 468–469
treatment, 469
Chordoma, 470–471, 470f
differential diagnosis, 471
history and physical examination, 471
imaging, 471
pathology, 471
prognosis, 471
treatment, 471
Chronic recurrent osteomyelitis. See Kasser disease
Cisplatin, 464
Clavicle
anatomy, 209
functions, 210
radiographs, 209–210
Clavicle fracture, 207–211, 208f–211f
classification, 207–209, 208f
displacing forces on, 210f, 211f
evaluation, 210f
sternoclavicular dislocations, 210
treatment, 210–211
Claw toe, 565
Clear cell sarcoma, 471
pathology, 471
treatment, 471
Cleidocranial dysplasia, 114–115

Clinodactyly, 545
Closed reduction (CR), for developmental dysplasia of hip, 153–155
Club foot, 177–178
diagnosis, 177
etiology, 177
physical exam, 177
radiographs, 177
treatment, 177–178
Cobra plate technique, for hip arthrodesis, 12f, 13
Codman Tumor. See Chondroblastoma
Concussions, 109
Congenital constriction band syndrome. See Amniotic band syndrome
Congenital muscular torticollis, 149
Congenital pseudoarthrosis of clavicle, 113
Congenital talipes equinovarus. See Club foot
Congenital vertical talus, 178, 179f
clinical manifestations, 178
differential diagnosis, 178
radiographs, 178
treatment, 178
Congenital vertical talus (CVT), 118
Coxa vara, 150, 150f
acquired, 150
clinical presentation, 151
congenital, 150
developmental, 150–151
hilgenreiner-epiphyseal (H-E) angle, 151f
natural history, 152
neck-shaft angle, evolution of, 151f
pathology, 151
radiographs, 152
treatment, 152
valgus rotational osteotomies, 152
CP. See Cerebral palsy (CP)
C-reactive protein (CRP), 429
Crossed adduction test, 88
Crystal disease, 2
Cubital tunnel syndrome, 527
diagnosis, 527
subcutaneous transposition, 527
treatment, 527
Cuboid fracture, 374–375, 375f
background, 374
diagnosis, 374
mechanism, 374
treatment, 375
Curly toe, 178

D
Deep vein thrombosis (DVT), 48–51
Dejerine-Sottas disease, 138
Delta phalanx, 180
natural history, 180
radiographs, 180
treatment, 180
Desmoid (fibromatosis), 472, 472f
history and physical examination, 472
imaging, 472
pathology, 472
treatment, 472
Developmental dysplasia of hip, 10–11, 11f
in children
closed reduction (CR), 153–155
diagnosis, 152
open reduction, 155
Pavlik, 152–153, 154f
treatment, 152

Developmental dysplasia of hip (*Contd.*)
  epidemiology, 11
  imaging, 11
  presentation, 10–11
  treatment, 11
Diabetes mellitus (DM), 429
Diabetic foot ulcers, 577
  classification, 578
  etiology, 577–578
  and infection, 578
    diagnosis, 578
    nonoperative treatment, 578
    operative treatment, 579
  nonoperative treatment, 578
  surgical treatment, 578
Diastrophic dysplasia, 115, 115f
Diazepam (Valium), pediatric dosage, 375
Diffuse idiopathic skeletal hhyperostosis
    (DISH), 429
Disc calcification syndrome, 607
Discitis, 140
  clinical presentation, 140–141
  imaging, 141
  laboratory evaluation, 141
  treatment, 141
Discoid meniscus, 167, 168f
  clinical presentation, 167
  differential diagnosis, 167
  radiographic findings, 167
  treatment, 167
  Watanabe classification, 167, 168f
Distal arthrogryposis syndrome, 118, 118f
Distal biceps rupture, 106
  anatomy, 106
  natural history, 106
  operative techniques, 106
  results, 106
Distal femoral epiphyseal fractures,
    pediatric, 406–410
Distal humerus fractures, 237–243
  anatomy, 237
  background, 237
  classification
    AO/OTA Classification, 239f–242f
    Jupiter classification, 238
    Muller/AO classification, 237–238
    Posada's fracture, 237
  complications, 240, 243
  history and physical examination, 237
  radiographs, 237
  related anatomy, 237
  treatment/approach
    fixation, 238–239
    olecranon osteotomy, 238
    total elbow arthroplasty, 239–240
    triceps reflecting, 238
    triceps sparing approach, 238
    triceps splitting, 238
Distal radius fracture, 260, 262f–267f
  classification
    Fernandez, 260
    Frykman, 260
  complications
    median nerve dysfunction, 263
    posttraumatic arthritis, 263–264
  fracture patterns, 261–262
  imaging, 260–261
  OR tips and trick
    closed reduction percutaneous
        pinning, 266–267
    dorsal buttress plate, 265–266
    volar buttress plate, 264–265
  related anatomy, 260

treatment
  external fixation, 262–263
  open reduction internal fixation,
      263
  percutaneous pinning, 262, 263f
Dorsal intercalated segment instability
    (DISI), 548
Dorsal wrist ganglion, 529, 529f
Down syndrome, 126
  atlantoaxial instability in, 126, 128
  cervical spine abnormalities in, 127f
  foot deformity in, 128
  hip instability in, 126
  medical manifestations, 126
  orthopaedic delayed ambulation, 126
  patellar instability in, 128
Dual energy x-ray absorptiometry (DEXA),
    436
Duchenne muscular dystrophy, 128
  clinical manifestations, 129
  natural history, 129
  pathology, 129
  scoliosis in, 129
  treatment, 129
Dupuytren contracture, 530, 530f
  cords formed, 530
  Luck's stages, 530
  non-surgical management, 531
  operating room tips, 531
  structures affected, 530
  structures not affected, 530
  surgical management, 531
    and complications, 531
    indications, 531

E

Ehlers-Danlos syndrome
  clinical manifestations, 119
  treatment, 119
  types, 119
Elbow arthroscopy, 106
  lateral portals, 106–107
  medial portals, 107
  posterior portals, 107
Elbow dislocation, 245–248, 245f–248f
  anatomy, 245
  associated ligamentous injuries, 247
  classification, 247–248
  evaluation, 245–246
  natural history, 247
  posterolateral rotatory instability
      (PLRI) and, 247f
  reduction, 246
  treatment, 248
Elbow MCL injury, 107, 107f, 108f
  anatomy, 107
  anterior pain, 108
  arthroscopic test, 108–109
  lateral pain, 108
  medial pain, 108
  pathophysiology, 107–108
  physical examination, 108
  reconstruction, 109
  rehabilitation, 109
  repair, 109
  x-ray studies, 108
Electromyography (EMG), 435
Embolism, 48
Enchondroma, 473–475, 473f
  history and physical examination, 473
  imaging, 473
  natural history, 475

pathology, 473
treatment, 475
Engelmann-Camurati disease, 115–116
Enostosis. *See* Bone island
Eosinophilic granuloma, 475
Epidemiology/study types, 429–430
Exertional compartment syndrome,
    109
Extensor mechanism injuries, 321–325
  chronic quadriceps tendon rupture,
      324–325
  history and physical examination, 321
  imaging, 321
  patellar tendon ruptures, 321, 322f
  quadriceps tendon ruptures, 321,
      323–324, 323f
Extensor tendon injury, 534f
  anatomy, 534
  extension of individual joints, 534
  extensor zones, 534
  intrinsic tightness, 535
  outcomes of repair, 534
  principles of treatment, 534

F

Facioscapulohumeral dystrophy, 128
Fat embolism syndrome, 186
Femoral anteversion, 168
  derotational osteotomy, 168
  physical exam, 168
  treatment, 168
Femoral head fracture, 292–295, 292f–294f
  anterior and anterolateral approach,
      293f
  background, 292
  classification, 293
    Brumback, 292f
    Pipkin, 293f
  imaging, 292–293
  internal fixation of, 294f
  treatment, 294–295
    immediate, 293
    nonoperative approach, 294–295
    open reduction internal fixation, 295
Femoral neck fractures, 295–299
  algorithm for treatment of, 296f
  background, 295
  closed reduction and internal fixation,
      298f
  complications
    associated pathology, 297–298
    avascular necrosis, 298–299
    infection, 299
    mortality, 297
    nonunion, 298
    transfusion, 299
  Garden classification, 295, 297f
  hip joint area cross section, 298f
  Pauwels classification, 295, 298f
  physical examination
    high energy, 295
    low energy, 295
  treatment
    determinants of treatment modality,
        295
    displaced fractures, elderly, 296
    displaced fractures, young, 296
    nondisplaced/valgus impacted,
        elderly, 295
Femoral shaft fracture, 307–311
  background, 307
  deforming muscle forces on femur, 308f

OR tips and tricks
  femoral nail, 310–311
sites of vascular injury after, 308f
traction, 307
treatment, 307–308, 309f–311f
  concomitant shaft and neck fracture,
    309–310
  gunshot wound, 308
  intramedullary nails, 308
  plate, 308
  retrograde nail, indications for, 308
  temporary external fixation, 308, 309f
  union rates, 308–309
  Winquist-Hansen classification, 307,
    308f
Femoral subtrochanteric fracture,
    304–307, 304f–306f
  anatomy, 304
  background, 304
  implant selection variables, 304f
  OR tips and tricks
    trochanteric fixation nail, 306–307
  with proximal extension and
    comminution, 306f
  Russell-Taylor classification, 304–305,
    305f
  Seinsheimer classification, 305, 305f
Femur fractures, pediatric, 404–406
Femur, periprosthetic fracture of, 56, 57f
Femur, supracondylar fracture of,
    311–316
  associated injuries, 313
  background, 311–312
  classification, 312
  definition, 312
  deforming forces, 312
  direct open reduction and internal
    fixation, 313f, 314f, 315f
  distal femur fracture, 312f
  imaging, 312
  implants
    blade plate 95 degrees, 313
    condylar buttress plate, 313
    dynamic compression screw, 313
    IM nails, 314
    less invasive stabilization system
      (LISS) plate, 314
  muscle attachments and deforming
    forces, 313f
  OR tips and tricks
    retrograde femoral nail, 314–316, 314f
  treatment, 312–313
Fibrous dysplasia, 478, 479f
  imaging, 478
  pathology, 479
  treatment, 479
Fibrous lesions
  benign fibrous histiocytosis (BFH), 454
  desmoplastic fibroma, 454
  fibrosarcoma, 454
  fibrous cortical defect, 454
  malignant fibrous histiocytoma (MFH),
    454
  nonossifying fibroma, 454
Fibular hemimelia, 168–169
  classification, 169, 169f, 171f
  treatment, 169
Fifth metatarsal/jones fracture, 371–372
  anatomy, 371
  background, 371
  fracture of fifth metatarsal base, 372f
  treatment, 371
    dancer's fracture, 372

diaphyseal stress fracture, 372
Jones fracture, 371
zones of proximal fifth metatarsal
    fracture, 372f
Fight bite, 531–532
Flaps, 537–538
Flatfoot, in adults, 573
  anatomy, 573
  differential diagnosis, 574
  etiology, 573–574
  pathology, 573
  physical examination, 574
  posttibial tendon insufficiency clinical
    staging, 574
  radiographs, 574
  treatment, 574
Flexible flatfoot, 180–181, 181f
  clinical presentation, 180
  differential diagnosis, 180
  physical exam, 180
  radiographs, 180, 181f
  treatment, 180–181
Flexor digitorum longus tendon, 553
Flexor digitorum profundus avulsion, 535
Flexor hallucis longus tendon
  anatomy, 553
  differential diagnosis, 553
  disorders, 553
  findings, 553
  treatment, 553
Flexor tendon injury
  functional anatomy, 532–533
  fundamentals, 532
  postoperative protocols, 533
  tendon healing, phases of, 533
Flexor tendon zones, 533–534, 533f
Flexor tenosynovitis, 531, 532f
Floating knee, 318–321
  background, 318
  Fraser-Wadell classification, 318
  OR tips and tricks
    external fixation of knee, 320–321
  treatment, 318–320, 319f, 320f
    interlocking nails, 320f
    open knee wound, 319f
Flumazenil, pediatric dosage, 376
Foot and ankle. See also specific disorders
  arthritis, 584–590
  arthroscopy, 555–556
  diabetes and neurologic disorders,
    576–584
  forefoot disorders, 557–567
  gait and foot biomechanics, 551–552
    float phase, 551
    gait cycle, 552f
    joint motions, 552
    stance phase, 551
    swing phase, 551
  midfoot and hindfoot disorders,
    568–576
  Os peroneum, 556
  Os trigonum, 556
  plantar fasciitis, 554–555
  tendon disorders, 552–554
  tendons, 552
Foot drop, 582
  evaluation, 582
  nonoperative treatment, 582
  operative treatment, 582
    arthrodesis, 582–583
    tendon transfer, 582, 583f
    tenodesis, 582
Forearm fractures, 256

AO/OTA classification, 257f
background, 256
classification, 256
imaging, 256
physical examination, 256
treatment, 256
Freiberg infraction, 567, 567f
  history and physical examination, 567
  imaging, 567
  nonoperative treatment, 567
  operative treatment, 567
  staging, 567
Friedreich's ataxia, 138
  clinical manifestations, 138
  natural history, 138
  treatment
    cavovarus, 138
    scoliosis, 138
Frostbite, 430
Frozen shoulder. See Adhesive capsulitis

G
Galeazzi fracture, 255–256, 255f, 256f
  radiographic evaluation, 255
  treatment, 255–256
  Walsh classification, 256f
Gamekeeper's thumb, 536–537, 542
GAP cup, 58f
Gaucher disease, 139, 139f
Gentamicin, 430
  dosing, 430
  nephrotoxicity, 430
  ototoxicity, 430
Genu valgum, 169
  differential diagnosis, 169–170
  hemiepiphysiodesis, 170
  osteotomy, 170
  radiographs, 170
  treatment, 170
Giant cell tumor, 479
  differential diagnosis, 482
  distal radius, 480f
  histology, 481–482
  history and physical examination, 481
  imaging, 481
  metastases, 482
  prognosis, 482
  proximal lateral tibia, 481f
  tendon sheath, 504
  treatment, 482
Glasgow Coma Scale (GSC), 188–189
Glenohumeral joint, 85f. See also Shoulder
Glomus tumor, 482
  differential diagnosis, 482
  history and physical examination, 482
  treatment, 482
Gout, 2, 430, 586
  recurrent, 431
Growth plates, 112
Guillain-Barré syndrome, 431
Gun shot wound, 655
Guyon canal, 528

H
Haglund deformity, 571, 572f
  history and physical examination, 571
  imaging, 571
  nonoperative treatment, 571
  operative treatment, 571
    calcaneal osteotomy, 572
    ostectomy, 571

Hallux rigidus, 563–564
  history and physical examination, 564
  imaging, 564
  nonoperative treatment, 564
  operative treatment
    cheilectomy, 564
    metatarsophalangeal arthrodesis, 564
    Moberg osteotomy, 564
    modified Keller interpositional
      arthroplasty, 564
Hallux valgus, 181–182
  adolescent, 557–559
    Akin osteotomy, 558f
    Chevron osteotomy, 558f
    distal metatarsal articular angle, 558f
    double first metatarsal (MT)
      osteotomy, 559f
    general description, 557
    nonoperative treatment, 557
    operative treatment, 557
    radiographic measurements, 557f
  adult, 559–561
    anatomy, 559
    causes, 559
    Chevron osteotomy, 561f
    decision making, 559–560
    imaging, 559
    physical examination, 559
    special considerations, 560
    treatment algorithm, 560f
  children vs. adults, 181
  distal soft tissue procedure, 561f, 562
  etiology, 181
  radiographs, 181
  scarf osteotomy, 562
  treatment, 181–182, 562–563
    Akin procedure, 562
    Chevron osteotomy, 562
    distal soft tissue procedure and
      proximal MT osteotomy, 563
    Keller, 563
    metatarsal-cuneiform fusion, 563
    metatarsal-phalanx fusion, 563
    Mitchell distal metatarsal osteotomy,
      563
    modified McBride procedure, 563
Hammer toe, 565
Hand. See also specific syndromes
  anatomy
    abbreviation, 511–512
    median nerve, 515–516, 515f
    palm landmarks, 514–515
    radial nerve, 516–517
    surface, 515f
    ulnar nerve, 517–518, 517f
    Vascular, 514
  anteroposterior radiograph, 522f
  approaches
    dorsal approach, 519
    dorsal Thompson approach, 519
    Kocher "J" lateral elbow, 519
    Morrey posterior elbow approach,
      519
    volar Henry approach to radius, 519
  brachial plexus, 522–523, 523f
  carpal bones, ossification of, 512
    axillary artery, 512–514
    brachialis innervation, 514
    lateral antebrachial cutaneous nerve,
      512
    radial artery, 512
    triceps, 514
    ulnar artery, 512

dislocations, 540–541
dorsal wrist compartments, 518–519
fracture
  and angulation, 539
  commonly fractured bones, 539
  metacarpal, 538–539
  open, 531
  phalangeal, 539
  treatment, 539–540
Lateral view, 521f
muscles of forearm and wrist, 513f
nerve injury, 523–524
  differential diagnosis, 524
  injury patterns, 524
  natural history, 524
  nerve function failure, sequence of,
    524
  nerve function recovery, sequence of,
    524
  recovery, 524
  Seddon nerve injury classification,
    523–524
  signs and symptoms, 524
  sites of compression, 524
physical examination, 519–521
  intrinsic minus, 520
  intrinsic plus, 520
  lumbrical plus, 520
  quadrigia effect, 521
  retinacular test, 520
wrist block, 518
and wrist, bony structures of, 511f
wrist radiograph, 521, 522f
Hand-Schüller-Christian disease, 475
Hangman's fracture, 644, 645f
Hemangioma, 482–483, 483f
  imaging, 483
  intramuscular, 484
  pathology, 483
  treatment/prognosis, 484
Hemipelvectomy, 484
Hemophilia, 431–432
Herniated nucleus pulposus (HNP), in
    children, 145
Heterotopic ossification, 52–53
High tibial osteotomy (HTO), 83
  lateral closing technique, 83
  medial opening technique, 83
Hinge total knee replacement (TKR), 484
Hip, anatomy of
  bones
    acetabulum, 6
    femur, 7
  muscle/tendon, 4
    abductors, 4
    adductors, 4
    extensors, 4
    external rotators, 4–5
    flexors, 4
    insertions into greater trochanter, 5
  neurovascular, 5–6
    obturator nerve, 5
    sciatic nerve, 6
    superficial lateral femoral cutaneous
      nerve, 5
  surface, 4
  vascular, 6
Hip arthritis
  nonarthroplasty options for, 12–18
    arthrodesis, 12–13, 12f
    arthroscopy, 16–18
    intertrochanteric osteotomy, 13–15,
      14f

osteotomy, 13, 13f
  periacetabular osteotomy, 15–16
  nonsurgical management for, 11–12
    pharmacologic therapy, 12
    physical therapy, 11
Hip arthroplasty, 4–30
  anatomy of hip, 4–7, 5f–7f
  approaches
    anterior, 7
    anterolateral, 7
    lateral, 7, 9f
    medial, 8
    posterior, 7–8
    surgical dislocation, 8
  avascular necrosis and, 9–10
  bearing surfaces, 29–30
    alternate bearing surfaces, 29–30
    combinations, 29
    polyethylene, 29
  developmental dysplasia of hip and,
    10–11
  implant type
    acetabulum, 23–24
    femur, 26–29
  total hip arthroplasty, 19–23
Hip dislocation, 54–56, 288–292
  anterior, Allis maneuver for, 291f
  background, 288
  classification, 288–289, 290f
  CT scan for intraarticular fragments,
    291f
  with femoral head fractures, Brumback
    classification of, 292f
  femoral head vascular anatomy, 289–290
  fragments in joint prior to hip
    reduction, 292f
  imaging, 288
  management algorithm, 289f
  mechanism, 288
  pediatric, 399–403
  posterior, Allis reduction technique for,
    291f
  treatment, 290–292
Hip fracture
  femoral neck, 295–299
  intertrochanteric, 299–304
  pediatric, 399–403
Hip pain, in athlete
  differential diagnosis, 83
    labral tear, 84
    by physical exam, 84
    sports hernia, 84
  hip snapping, 84
Homocystinuria, 139
  clinical manifestations, 139–140
  treatment, 140
Humeral shaft fractures, 227–237,
    229f–236f
  anterolateral surgical approach to, 235f
  aseptic nonunion and reoperation,
    234f
  atrophic nonunion of, 233f
  background, 227
  OR tips and tricks
    anterolateral, 233
    lateral, 237
    posterior triceps splitting, 233, 237
  OTA classification, 228, 229f–232f
  physical examination, 227
  posterior surgical approach to, 235f
  radial nerve palsy, 227–228
  radiographs, 228
  surgical approaches, 233

treatment
bracing, 228
intramedullary nail, 228, 236f
open reduction with internal fixation, 228, 236f
plating, 228, 236f
upper arm, neurovascular anatomy of, 234f
Hunter syndrome, 140
Hurler syndrome, 140
Hyperparathyroidism, 432
Hypochondroplasia, 114
Hypophosphatemic rickets. See Rickets

I
Idiopathic juvenile osteoporosis and back pain in children, 146
Ifosfamide, 464
Iliac crest bone graft (ICBG), 607
Impingement sign, 87–88, 88f
Implants
acetabulum, 23–24, 24f–26f
cemented, 24
noncemented, 23–24
femur, 26–29, 27f–29f, 43
cemented, 27–29
noncemented, 26–27
surface finish, 26
tibia
cemented, 43
noncemented, 43
Incidence, defined, 429
Infantile tibia vara, 165, 166
Injury severity score, 185–186
Internal impingement, shoulder, 96
Internal tibial torsion, 170
Intertrochanteric hip fractures, 299–304
background, 299
characteristics
stable fractures, 299, 302f
unstable fractures, 299, 303f
classification, 301f
compression hip screw components, 300f
imaging, 299
intramedullary approach, 302f, 303f
lateral surgical approach, 301f
OR tips and tricks
dynamic hip screw, 300–301
gamma nail, 302–304, 302f
reverse obliquity right fracture, 303f
sliding hip screw, 302f, 303f
tip-apex distance (TAD), 301f
treatment
95-degree fixed-angle device, 300
dynamic hip screw, 299–300
intramedullary nail, 300
In-toeing, 170

J
Jansen type metaphyseal chondrodysplasia, 116
Jefferson burst fracture, 643
Jersey finger, 535
Jumper's knee. See Patellar tendonitis
Juvenile rheumatoid arthritis (JRA), 2
diagnostic criteria, 122
differential diagnosis, 122
pauciarticular, 122
polyarticular, 122
systemic still disease, 122
treatment, 122

K
Kasser disease, 141
Ketamine, pediatric dosage, 376
Kienböck's disease, 549–550
definition, 549
epidemiology, 550
etiology, 549–550
nonoperative treatment, 550
operative treatment, 550
presentation, 550
radiographic staging, 550
Kirner deformity, 545
Klippel-Feil syndrome, 609–610
Knee
anatomy
ACL, 68
LCL, 68
MCL, 68
medial knee, 69
menisci, 68
patella, 68–69
PCL, 68
posterolateral, 69–70
injuries, 79f
MRI, 74–75
basics, 75
cartilage, 75
collaterals, 75
cruciates, 75
grades, 75
menisci, 75
meniscofemoral ligaments, 75
physical exam
ACL, 70, 70f
menisci, 71–72
patella, 72
PCL, 71
PF joint, 70
PLc, 71
varus, valgus instability, 70
x-ray, 72
meniscal tears, 72–73, 72f–74f
Knee arthroplasty, 30–44, 35f
anatomy of knee, 30f, 31–33, 31f
approaches, 33
avascular necrosis and osteonecrosis, 33–34, 34f
nonarthroplasty options, 35–36
nonsurgical management, 34
bearing surfaces
alternate bearings, 44
PCL retaining, 43–44
posterior stabilized, 44
rotating platform, 44
tensioners, 44
biomechanics, 30
computer-assisted surgery, 42–43
diagnostic arthroscopy, 36
high tibial osteotomy, 37f
implant types
femur, 43
tibia, 43
knee deformities, 33f
partial knee replacement, 40–42
skin incision, approach for, 32f
total knee arthroplasty, 37–40
Knee dislocations, 316–318
ACL/PCL tears on MRI, 317f
arterial routes and knee joint, 318f
background, 316
classification, 316
imaging/radiographs, 316
medial exposure of knee, 317f
physical examination, 316
posterior cruciate ligament intact dislocation, 317f
reduction of, technique for, 317f
treatment
nonoperative, 317
operative, 317–318, 317f–318f
Kniest dysplasia, 117
Kugelberg-Welander disease, 130
Kyphoplasty, 610
Kyphosis
adult, 610–611
Scheuermann, 611

L
Lachman test, for anterior cruciate ligament insufficiency, 70f
Larsen syndrome, 120f, 123
Lateral condyle fracture, pediatric, 385–387
Lateral pivot shift test, 71f
Legg-Calvé-Perthes disease, 155, 156f–161f
Catterall classification, 156f–160f, 161
clinical presentation, 155
lateral pillar classification, 161, 161f
prognosis, 161–162
radiographs, 155, 160–161
Salter-Thompson classification, 161
treatment, 162
Leg length discrepancy (LLD), 170, 172–173
epiphysiodesis, 173
etiology, 172
Green/Anderson growth remaining method for, 172
leg lengthening for, 173
limb lengthening for, 173
multiplier method for, 172
radiographs, 172
treatment, 172–173
White/Menelaus arithmetic method for, 170
Lesser toe deformities, 565
anatomy, 565
claw toe, 565
hammer toe, 565
intractable plantar keratosis, 566
mallet toe, 565
Letterer-Siwe disease, 475
Leukemia, 485
and back pain in children, 145
history and physical examination, 485
laboratory values, 485
prognosis, 485
treatment, 485
Limping child, 173
Lipoblast, 486
Lipoma, 485
history and physical examination, 485
imaging, 485
intramuscular, 485
pathology, 485
treatment, 485
variants, 485
Lipomeningocoele, 146
Liposarcoma, 485–486, 486f, 487f
imaging, 486
metastases, 486
pathology, 486
subtypes, 486
treatment and prognosis, 486

Lisfranc injury
  anatomy, 369
  atypical, 370f, 371f
  background, 369
  classification, 369
  imaging, 369–370, 370f
  Lisfranc dislocation, 370f
  Myerson classification, 370f
  tarsometatarsal joints of foot, 369f
  treatment, 370–371
Lorazepam (Ativan), pediatric dosage, 375
The Lower Extremity Assessment Project
      (LEAP), 339
Lumbar spine
  anatomy of, 594
    axial plane levels, 594–595
    lumbar pedicles, 594
    sagittal plane levels, 595
  degenerative scoliosis, 612–613
  disc herniation/radiculopathy, 613–615
  low back pain, 612
  pedicle screws, 615–616
  spinal stenosis, 616–620
  total disc replacement, 640
Lyme disease, 432–433
Lymphoma of bone, 487
  history and physical examination, 487
  imaging, 487
  pathology, 487
  treatment, 488
Lytic bone lesions, benign. See Benign
      lytic bone lesions

M
Maffucci syndrome, 475
Malignant bone tumors, 455
  and age, 455
  with bone edema, 455
  mimics, 455
  x-ray signs, 455
Malignant fibrous histiocytoma, 488f, 489
  of bone, 489–490
  history and physical examination, 489
  metastases, 489
  pathology, 489
  prognosis, 489
  subtypes, 489
  treatment, 489
Malignant peripheral nerve sheath tumor
      (MPNST), 494
Mallet finger, 535
  with fracture, 535
Mallet toe, 565
Malnutrition, 433
Marfan syndrome, 119, 121f
  clinical manifestations, 120
  differential diagnosis, 119
  scoliosis and protrusio of hips in,
      121f
  treatment, 122
Material science, 433
  CoCr, 433
  stainless steel, 433–434
  titanium, 433
McKusick type metaphyseal
      chondrodysplasia, 116
McMurray test, 71, 71f
Medial epicondyle fractures, pediatric,
      387–389
Medial patellofemoral ligament (MPFL), 77
Medial tibial stress syndrome, 109
Meningocoele, 146

Menisci
  anatomy, 68
  McMurray test, 71, 71f
  physical exam, 71–72
  tears, 72
    classification by location, 72
    complications, 73
    Fairbanks changes, 73
    partial meniscectomy, 73
    popliteal cysts, 73
    posterior horn of lateral meniscus, 73f
    postrepair MRI, 73
    repair techniques, 73, 73f, 74f
    type, 72, 72f
Menkes kinky hair syndrome, 140
Meperidine (Demerol), pediatric dosage,
      375
Metabolic bone diseases, 434
Metacarpal fracture, 538–539
Metaphysial chondrodysplasia, 116
Metastatic carcinoma. See Bone
      metastases
Metatarsophalangeal joint dislocation, 565
Metatarsus adductus, 182, 182f
  natural history, 182
  physical exam, 182
  radiographs, 182
  treatment, 182
Midazolam (Versed), 376
Midfoot sprain, 569
MNEMONIC, benign lytic bone lesions, 451
Monteggia fracture, 248–250
  background, 248
  classification
    bado, 248, 249f
    Jupiter, 248, 250
  late diagnosis, 250
  radiographs, 248
Morphine, 376
Morquio disease, 140
Morton interdigital neuroma, 583
Mucopolysaccharidoses, 140
Mucous cyst, 530
Multiple epiphyseal dysplasia (MED), 116
Multiple hereditary osteochondromas
      (MHO)
  differential diagnosis, 491
  natural history, 491
  presentation, 491
  surgery, 491
Multiple myeloma, 491
  clinical variants, 491
  diagnosis, 492
  imaging, 492
  laboratory values, 492
  pathology, 492
  presentation, 492
  prognosis, 492
  staging, 492
  treatment, 492
Muscle, physiology of, 438
Musculoskeletal tumors
  benign bone, 456
  benign cartilage, 456
  benign soft tissue, 456
  bone dysplasia, 456
  malignant bone, 456
  malignant soft tissue, 456
  nerve sheath tumors, 456
  nontumors, 456
  synovial tumors, 456
Myelomeningocele (MMC), 146
  ambulation, 147

  etiology, 146
  foot and, 148
  hip and, 147
  knee and, 148
  level of defect, 146–147
  mental status, change in, 147
  natural history, 146
  prevention, 146
  spectrum of defects, 146
  spine and, 148–149
Myositis ossificans, 492
  imaging, 493
  pathology, 493
  treatment, 493

N
Naloxone (Narcan), 376
National acute spinal cord injury studies
      (NASCIS), 445
Navicular fracture, 372–374
  background, 372
  classification, 372–373, 373f
  fixation methods, 374f
  imaging, 372
  treatment, 373, 374f
Negative predictive value (NPV), 443
Neonates, osteomyelitis in, 141. See also
      Osteomyelitis, in children
Nerve conduction velocity, 434–435
Nerve endings
  Meissner corpuscle, 438
  Merkel cells, 438
  neuromuscular junction, 439f
  Pacinian corpuscle, 438
  Ruffini end organs, 439
Nerve sheath tumors, 494
Neurilemoma (Schwannoma), 494
Neurofibroma, 494
Neurofibromatosis (NF), 123
  radiographic findings, 123–124
  treatment, 124
  type 1, 123
    clinical manifestations, 123
    congenital tibial dysplasia, 123
    orthopedic manifestations, 123
  type 2, 124
Niemann-pick disease, 140
Nonossifying fibroma, 494f, 495f
  differential diagnosis, 494
  histology, 494
  history and physical examination,
      494
  imaging, 494
  natural history, 495
  treatment, 495
Noonan syndrome, 124

O
Obrien active compression test, 88
Obturator nerve, 5
Occipital condyle fracture, 649–650
Olecranon fracture, 250–253
  background, 250
  classification
    Mayo, 250, 250f
    Schatzker, 250
  comminuted, 253f
  complications, 253
  imaging, 250
  physical examination, 250
  tension band wiring, 251f–252f

treatment, 251
  cancellous screw tension band, 253
  excision of fragment and triceps
    advancement, 253
  figure-of-8 tension band, 251, 253
  nonoperative, 251
  operative, 251
  plate fixation, 253
Ollier disease, 475
Open hand fractures, 531
Open reduction (CR), for developmental
    dysplasia of hip, 155
Os acromiale, 95
Os odontoideum, 626
Os peroneum, 556
Ossiculum terminale, 626
Ossifying fibroma, 495
Osteoarthritis (OA), 2–3, 3f, 4f
  diagnosis, 3
  imaging, 3
  knee, 435
  pathophysiology, 3–4
  posttraumatic, 3
  risk factors, 435
  types, 3
Osteoblastoma, 495–496
  differential diagnosis, 496
  imaging, 496
  pathology, 496
  treatment, 496
Osteochondritis dessicans (OCD), 75–76,
    76f
Osteochondroma, 496, 496f
  differential diagnosis, 496
  imaging, 496
  natural history, 496
  pathology, 496
  treatment, 496
Osteofibrous dysplasia, 462
Osteogenesis imperfecta (OI), 124, 125f
  clinical manifestations, 124
  radiographic findings, 125
  Silence classification, 124–125
  treatment, 125–126
Osteogenic sarcoma
  classic high grade, 497, 498f–499f
    differential diagnosis, 497
    history and physical examination, 497
    imaging, 497
    metastases, 497
    molecular staging, 500
    pathology, 497
    prognosis, 500
    treatment, 497, 500
  primary osteosarcoma, 500
  secondary osteosarcoma, 500
Osteoid osteoma, 501, 501f, 502f
  differential diagnosis, 501
  history and physical examination, 501
  imaging, 501
  pathology, 501
  prostaglandin, 501
  treatment, 501
Osteomalacia, 432. See also Rickets
Osteomyelitis, in children, 141, 142f
  causative organisms, 143
  differential diagnosis, 141
  laboratory findings, 141, 143
  radiographic findings
    bone scan, 143
    MRI, 143
  treatment, 143
Osteopetrosis, 435

Osteoporosis, 435
  bisphosphonates, 437
  calcium, 437
  DEXA, 436
  estrogen, 437
  exercise, 437
  hip protectors, 436
  PTH, 437
  WHO criteria, 436
  workup, 436
Osteoprotegerin (OPG), 438
Os trigonum, 556
Overlapping fifth toe, 182–183

P
Paget disease, 502
  differential diagnosis, 502
  history and physical examination, 502
  imaging, 502
  laboratory values, 502
  medical treatment, 503
  oncologic problems, 503
  pathology, 502–503
  surgical treatment, 503
Paratenonitis, 552, 553
Parathyroid hormone (PTH), 432
Partial knee replacement, 40
  indication, 40
  limitations, 40
  patellofemoral arthroplasty, 42
  tibial hemiarthroplasty, 40
Patellar dislocation, 76–77, 76f
  anatomy, 77
  natural history, 77
Patellar fracture, 325–327
  background, 325
  classification, 325f
  complications, 327
  history and physical examination, 325
  patterns and examples of internal
    fixation, 326f
  radiographs, 325
  treatment
    nonoperative, 325
    operative, 325
    surgical approach, 325–327
Patellar tendonitis, 77
Patellar tendon ruptures, 321, 322f
Patellofemoral pain
  merchant view, 77
  nonoperative treatment, 77
  operative treatment, 77
  patellar subluxation, 77
  patellar tilt, 77
  rehab, 77–78
Pathological fracture, 456
  after soft tissue sarcoma resection, 457
  mortality and prognosis, 456–457
Pavlik harness treatment, for
    developmental dysplasia of hip,
    152–153, 154f
PCL. See Posterior cruciate ligament (PCL)
Pediatrics. See also specific disorder
  ankle fractures, 418–421
  anterior cruciate ligament, 80–81
  congenital disorders, 112–113
  conscious sedation, 375–376
  development, 112
  distal femoral epiphyseal fractures,
    406–410
  femur fractures, 404–406
  foot/ankle, 175–184

general pediatric medicine, 112
  genetics/syndromes, 117–128
  hip, 150–164, 399–403
  infection, 140–145
  lateral condyle fracture, 385–387
  lower extremity injuries, 393–421
  medial epicondyle fractures, 387–389
  metabolic disorders, 139–140
  muscular dystrophies, 128–130
  neuromuscular disorders, 130–138
  pediatric elbow, 379
  pelvic/acetabular fractures, 393–397
  physeal injuries, 421
  proximal humerus fractures, 376–378
  radial head and neck fractures, 389–391
  radius and ulnar shaft fractures,
    391–392
  septic hip, 397–398
  skeletal dysplasias, 113–117
  spine, 145–149
  spondylolisthesis, 638–639
  supracondylar humerus fractures,
    379–385
  thigh/knee/leg, 164–175
  tibial eminence fracture, 410–413
  tibial shaft fractures, 415–418
  tibial tubercle fractures, 413–415
  transphyseal humerus fracture, 379
  upper extremity, 149
Pelvic fractures, 267–279
  anatomy/biomechanics, pelvis, 270
    external rotation force, 270
    internal rotation force, 270
  bladder rupture and urethral
    disruption, 277f
  bony architecture of pelvic ring, 268f
  classifications, 270–275
    anterior posterior compression I,
      271f, 275
    anterior posterior compression II,
      271f, 275
    anterior posterior compression III,
      272f, 275
    combined mechanism, 275, 275f
    lateral compression I, 273f, 275
    lateral compression II, 273f, 275
    lateral compression III, 274f, 275
    tile classification, 270
    vertical shear, 274f, 275
    young and burgess classification, 275
  evaluation, 267
    genitourinary, 269
    neurologic, 269
    open fractures, 269
    radiographic signs of instability, 267,
      269
    shock and mortality, 269
    stability, 267, 269
    venous thromboembolism, 269
  imaging
    CT scan, 270
    radiographs, pelvis views, 269–270,
      270f
  ligamentous structures of pelvic ring,
    269f
  OR tips and tricks
    SI screw, 278–279, 278f, 279f
  treatment
    external fixation, 276, 277f
    iliac wing external fixation, 276
    lateral compression fractures,
      surgery for, 278
    nonoperative, 278

Pelvic fractures (*Contd.*)
    operative fixation, indications for, 278
    supracetabular pins, 276–277, 277f
    vascular and ligamentous structures relationship, 276f
Periosteal chondroma, 503
    imaging, 503
    natural history, 503
    pathology, 503
    treatment, 503
Peripheral neuroectodermal tumor, 475–476
    chemotherapy, 476
    Ewing sarcoma, 476f–478f
    histologic response to chemotherapy, 478
    history and physical examination, 476
    imaging, 476
    metastases, 476
    pathology, 476
    prognosis, 478
    radiation therapy, 476, 478
    small round cell tumors and age, 476
    treatment, 476
Peroneal tendons, 553
    anatomy, 553
    differential diagnosis, 554
    dislocation, 572
    disorders, 554
    findings, 554
    treatment, 554
Pes planus
    clinical history, 573
    etiology, 573
    incidence/natural history, 572
    pathoanatomy, 572
    physical examination, 573
    radiography, 573
    treatment, 573
Phalangeal fracture, 539
Phalen test, 526f
Physeal injuries, pediatric, 421
Physiology
    bone, 437–438
    cartilage, 438
    muscle, 438
    nerve endings, 438–439
Pigmented villonodular synovitis, 503, 504f
    imaging, 503
    pathology, 504
    treatment, 504
Pilon fractures, 342–345
    classification
        AO/OTA, 342–343
        ruedi-algower, 342, 343f
    complications, 344–345
    fixation considerations, 343
    history and physical examination, 342
    imaging, 342
    mechanism of energy, 342
    OR tips and tricks
        anterolateral approach, 344
        external fixation, 345
        posterolateral approach to fibula/tibia, 344
        treatment, 343–344, 344f
    outcomes, 344
Plantar fasciitis
    anatomy, 554
    conservative treatment, 554–555

differential diagnosis, 554
    heel pain, differential diagnosis, 554
Polio, 439
Polio-associated scoliosis, 439
Popliteal artery entrapment syndrome, 110
Positive predictive value (PPV), 443
Posterior cruciate ligament (PCL), 81, 81f
    indications, 81
    MRI, 81
    primary repair, 81
    reconstruction, 81
    ruptures, 79f
Posterior interosseous nerve syndrome, 528
Posterior tibial tendon dysfunction (PTTD), 575
    anatomy, 575
    diagnosis, 575
    radiography, 575
    staging, 575
Posterolateral corner (PLc), 70
    anatomy, 82
    imaging, 82
    physical examination, 82
    treatment, 82
Postradiation sarcoma of bone, 503
Prader-Willi syndrome, 126
Precision, 443
Prevalence, defined, 429
Pronator syndrome, 528
Prospective cohort, 430
Proximal femoral focal deficiency (PFFD), 174
    aitken classification, 174
    clinical presentation, 174
    treatment, 174
Proximal humerus fractures
    background, 216
    classification, 218–220
    fracture fragments, displacement of, 218f
    incision from coracoid to deltoid insertion, 223f
    Neer classification, 217f
    nonreconstructable fractures, 225f
    OR tips and tricks
        anterolateral, 221–223
        deltopectoral, 221
        hemiarthroplasty, 223, 225
    pediatric, 376–378
    related anatomy, 216
        blood supply, 217
        nerve supply, 217
        radiographs, 218
    reverse shoulder arthroplasty joint, 225f
    soft-tissue anatomy of shoulder, 222f
    three-part fracture dislocation of, 226f
    traction injury to axillary nerve, 227f
    trauma series, 219f
    treatment, 220–221, 222f–227f
        blade plate, 221, 226f
        closed reduction and percutaneous pinning, 221, 226f
        hemiarthroplasty, 220f, 221, 226f
        locked intramedullary nail, 221
        proximal humeral locking plate, 221
Proximal interphalangeal joint, 536
    dislocations, 541f
        dorsal dislocation, 540
        volar dislocation, 540–541
Prune belly syndrome, 113
Pseudoachondroplasia, 114

Pseudogout, 439–440. *See also* Gout
Psoriatic arthritis, 585

Q

Quadriceps tendon ruptures, 321, 323–324, 323f

R

Rachischisis, 146
Radial head fractures, 253–255
    background, 253–254
    classification, 254
    history and physical examination, 254
    imaging, 254
    OR tips and tricks, 255
    outcomes/results, 255
    radial head arthroplasty, 255
    treatment, 254
Radial tunnel syndrome, 527
    etiology, 527
    radial tunnel, 527
        and posterior interosseous nerve, 527
    treatment, 527
Radiation therapy
    complications, 460
    high sensitivity, 460
    intraoperative, 460
    low sensitivity, 460
    moderate sensitivity, 460
    for soft tissue sarcoma, 460
Radiocarpal ligaments
    dorsal radiocarpal ligaments, 548
    intrinsic ligaments of wrist, 548
    volar radiocarpal ligaments, 547–548
Radioulnar synostosis, 549
Radius, dorsal Thompson approach to, 258
RANK ligand (RANKL), 438
Reiter syndrome, 585
Relocation test, 87f
Renal cell carcinoma (RCC), metastatic, 490
    prognosis, 490
    treatment, 490
Renal osteodystrophy, 440
Replants, 537
Rett syndrome, 126
Revision total hip replacement
    revision cup
        acetabular deficiencies, 61, 62f
        DeLee-Charnley zones for cup, 61
        epidemiology, 61
        treatment, 61–62
    revision stem
        caveats, 63–64
        epidemiology, 62
        femoral bone defects, 63, 63f
        modes of loosening, 62
        treatment, 63
    surgical approaches, 64
Revision total knee arthroplasty, 64–65, 65f
    bone defects, 64–65
    laxity, 64
    stages, 64
    stems, 64
Rhabdomyolysis (RML), 440
Rhabdomyosarcoma, 504
    differential diagnosis, 505
    history and physical examination, 504

pathology, 505
subtypes, 504–505
treatment, 505
Rheumatoid arthritis (RA), 440–441, 584. *See also* Arthroplasty; Systemic lupus erythematosus (SLE)
boutonniere deformity, 542–543
of cervical spine, 603–605
atlantoaxial impaction, 604
atlantoaxial subluxation, 603
combinations, 604
complications, 605
natural history, 605
radiographic parameters, 604, 604f
Ranawat's clinical grades, 604
subaxial subluxation, 604
in hand, 441
imaging, 2
knee joint, 2f
pathology, 1–2
presentation, 1
radiographs, 584
thumb deformity types, 542
treatment
medical, 2
nonoperative, 584–585
operative, 2, 585
Rickets, 441–442
Ring avulsion injuries, 537
Roos test, 87
Rotator cuff disease, 94–95, 94f
imaging, 95
pathophysiology, 94–95
treatment, 95
Runner, leg pain, 109–110

S

Sacral agenesis, 146
Sacroiliitis, 149
Sacrum fracture, 650
Sagittal band rupture, 537
Sandifer syndrome, 126
Sanfilippo syndrome, 140
Sarcoidosis, 442
Scapholunate advanced collapse, 549
Scapholunate dissociation, 548
Scapholunate instability, 548
Scapular fractures, 212–215, 213f, 214f
associated injuries, 212
classification, 212
history and physical exam, 212
imaging, 212
OTA classification of, 213f
outcomes/complications, 215
scapulothoracic dissociation, 215
treatment, 212–215
open reduction internal fixation, 214–215
surgical indications, 214
Scheuermann kyphosis, 611
differential diagnosis, 611
natural history, 611
treatment, 611
Schmid type metaphyseal chondrodysplasia, 116
Sciatic nerve, 6
Scoliosis. *See also* Spine
adolescent, 626–630
adult, 630–631
congenital, 631–633
in Friedreich's ataxia, 138
history and physical examination, 633

infantile, 636
juvenile, 634
King-Moe classification, 635
Lenke classification, 635–636
in myelomeningocele, 148–149
neuromuscular, 636–637
selection of fusion levels, 637
selective fusion, 637–638
Scurvy, 442
Sensitivity, 443
Septic arthritis, 143
causative organisms, 144
differential diagnosis, 143
laboratory workup, 143–144
in neonate, 144
radiographic findings, 144
bone scan, 144
MRI, 144
SI joint and, 144
Septic hip, pediatric, 397–398
Seronegative arthropathies, 443. *See also* Ankylosing spondylitis (AS)
Seronegative spondyloarthropathies. *See* Seronegative arthropathies
Seronegative spondyloarthropathy, 585
Serpentine foot, 182
Serratus anterior, paralysis of, 96f
Sesamoids, 567
Shoulder
anatomy, 84–86, 85f
nerves, 86–87, 86f
MRI
biceps tendon, 90
labrum, 90
RTC tear, 90
systematic approach, 89
physical exam, 87–88, 87f, 88f
x-ray studies
AP, 88
axillary lateral, 89
bicipital groove view, 89
30-degree caudal tilt view, 89
Garth, 89
Hobbs, 89
serendipity, 89
stryker notch, 89
supraspinatus outlet, 89
west point, 89
Zanca, 89
Shoulder arthroscopy, 101–102, 102f
Bankart, 101
capsular shift, 102
SAD/RTC repair, 101–102
SLAP (superior labral tears anterior to posterior), 101
Shoulder dislocation, 96–97
complications, 97–98
recurrence, 97
Shoulder instability
anterior, 98
arthroscopic repairs, 100
biomechanics, 98
open repairs, 101
pathologic lesions, 98
static restraints, 98
chronic locked posterior dislocation, 100
multidirectional, 98–99
history and physical examination, 98
pathophysiology, 98
treatment, 98–99
posterior, 99–100
imaging, 99

pathophysiology, 99
treatment, 99–100
Sickle cell disease, 443–444
Sinus tarsi syndrome, 569
Skeletal metastases, of unknown origin, 457
Skewfoot. *See* Serpentine foot
SLAP lesions, 102–103, 103f
classification, 102–103
differential diagnosis, 103
treatment, 103
Slipped capital femoral epiphysis (SCFE), 162, 163f, 164f
classification, 163
clinical presentation, 163
etiology, 162
pathoanatomy, 163f
radiographic findings, 163
radiographic grading, 163
treatment, 163–164
Soft tissue complications, 52
Soft tissue sarcomas, 457
chemotherapy, 458
grading, 458
of hand, 457
metastases workup, 458
prognosis, 458
spread through lymph nodes, 457
treatment, 458
types, 457
Somatosensory-evoked potential (SSEP), EMG
acetabulum, 444
neuromuscular scoliosis, 444
spine, 444
Specificity, 443
Speed test, 88
Spina bifida occulta, 146
Spinal cord injury, 650–651
Asia scale motor source, 650
complications, 651
Frankel/Asia classification, 650
motor index score, 650–651
treatment, 651
Spinal muscular atrophy, 129
treatment, 130
types, 129–130
Spinal stenosis, 616
classification, 616
diagnosis, 618
differential diagnosis, 617–618
MRI findings, 618
pathophysiology, 616
stenosis locations, 617
treatment, 618–620
Spinal trauma
atlanto-occipital dissociation, 640–642
cervical body fracture, 645
cervical facet dislocation, 645–646
cervical, pediatric, 645
cervical stability list, 646
cervical subaxial fractures, 646–648
C1 fracture, 642–643
C2 Hangman's fracture, 644, 645f
C2 odontoid fracture, 643–644, 643f
C-spine radiographs
AP view, 642
flexion/extension views, 642
lateral view, 642
MRI, 642
open-mouth view, 642
gun shot wound, 655

Spinal trauma (*Contd.*)
    halo, 649, 649f
    occipital condyle fracture, 649–650
    sacrum fracture, 650
        H-shaped fracture, 650
        transverse fracture, 650
        vertical fracture, 650
    spinal cord injury, 650–651
    spinal cord syndromes, 651–652
    steroids, 652
    thoracolumbar fracture, 652–653
    TL burst fracture, 653
    TL compression fracture, 653–564
    TL flexion distraction, 655
    TL fracture-dislocation, 655
    tongs, 649
Spine
    atlantoaxial rotatory displacement,
        596–597
        Grisel syndrome, 596
        transverse ligament injury, 597
        traumatic, 596–597
    cervical (*see* Cervical spine)
    infections
        postoperative, 607–608
        spondylodiscitis/osteomyelitis,
            608–609
        tuberculosis, 609
    lumbar (*see* Lumbar spine)
    MRI
        abnormal annulus, 620
        abnormal nucleus, 620
        arachnoiditis, 621
        axial cuts, 620
        contrast, 620
        disc morphology, 620–621
        facets, 621
        intraosseous herniated nucleus
            pulposis, 621
        normal disc, 620
        postoperative, 621
        sagittal cuts, 620
        scar *vs.* disc, 621
        spinous processes, 621
    neurologic exam, 621
        anterior and posterior sensory
            dermatomes, 623f
        cervical and peripheral nerves,
            622
        clinical testing of C5-T1 nerve roots,
            624f
        clinical testing of L4-S1 nerve roots,
            625f
        lower extremity, 622
        lower motor neuron signs, 622
        quick, 622–625
        upper motor neuron signs, 621–622
    neurologic injury, 625–626
    thoracic spine, anatomy of, 595
        and disc disease, 639–640
        radicular artery of Adamkiewicz, 596
        thoracic pedicles, 595–596
    trauma (*see* Spinal trauma)
Spine metastatic tumors, 459
    imaging, 459
    posterolateral transpedicle approach
        (PTA), 459
    surgery principles, 459
    treatment, 459
Spine tumors, 458–459
Spondyloepiphyseal dysplasia
    congenita, 116
    tarda, 116–117

Spondylolisthesis
    adult, 638
    pediatric, 638–639
Spondylolysis, pediatric, 638–639
Sports, 68–110. *See also specific topics*
Spurling test, 88
Staging, tumors
    benign Enneking system, 459–460
    malignant bone (AJCC-6), 460
    malignant Enneking system, 460
    musculoskeletal tumor staging, 459
    soft tissue (AJCC-6), 460
    soft tissue tumor staging (AJCC-5), 460
    types of excisions, 460
Statistics, 444–445
Stenosing tenosynovitis, 553
Steroids, 445
Streeter constriction band syndrome. *See*
    Amniotic band syndrome
Stress fractures, 109–110
Subscapularis tear, 96
Subtalar dislocation
    background, 367
    classifications/treatment
        lateral, 368f, 369
        medial, 367, 367f, 368f
    imaging, 367
    physical exam, 367
Subtalar sprain, 569
Subungual exostosis, 183
Sulcus sign, 87
Superficial lateral femoral cutaneous
    nerve, 5
Superficial peroneal nerve (SPN),
    583–584
Supracondylar humerus fractures,
    pediatric, 379–385
Suprascapular neuropathy, 103
Swan neck deformity, 541–542, 541f
Syndactyly, 546
Syndesmosis injury, 569
Synovial chondromatosis, 507
Synovial cyst, of wrist, 529f
Synovial sarcoma, 507
    imaging, 507
    metastases, 507
    pathology, 507
    prognosis, 508
    treatment, 507
Systemic lupus erythematosus (SLE), 2,
    445–446

T

Talus fractures, 358–364
    background, 358
    Canale and Kelly view of foot, 360f
    classification
        AO/OTA classification, 361,
            362f–363f
        talar body classification, 361
        talar neck classification, 360f, 361
    history and physical exam, 358
    imaging, 358–359
    open reduction and internal fixation,
        359f
    osteonecrosis of talar body, 361f
    outcomes/complications, 364
    talar blood supply, 359–361, 360f
    treatment, 361
        body fractures, 362, 364
        head fractures, 364
        neck fractures, 361–362

Talus osteochondritis dissecans, 576
    Berndt and Harty classification system,
        576
    CT-based classification system, 576
    imaging, 576
Tarsal coalition, 183–184
    clinical presentation, 183
    differential diagnosis, 183
    evaluation, 183
    radiographs, 183–184
    treatment, 184
Tarsal tunnel syndrome, 584
Temporal arteritis, 446
Tendinosis, 552, 553
Tenosynovitis, 553
Thoracic outlet syndrome, 103–104,
    104f
Thoracolumbar fracture, 652–653
Thumb hypoplasia, 546–547
Thyroid cancer, metastatic, 491
Tibial bowing
    anterolateral, 174–175
    anteromedial, 175
    posteromedial, 175
Tibial dysplasia, in neurofibromatosis
    type 1, 123, 124
Tibial eminence fracture, pediatric,
    410–413
Tibial hemimelia, 175
    classification, 175
    clinical presentation, 175
    treatment, 175
Tibialis anterior tendon
    anatomy, 552
    differential diagnosis, 553
    disorders, 552–553
    findings, 553
    treatment, 553
Tibial plateau fractures, 327–332
    background, 327
    history and physical exam, 327
    imaging, 327
    local compression fracture, 329f
    nonoperative treatment, 328
    operative treatment
        depressed, 328
        external fixation, 328
        internal fixation, 328
        Schatzker VI, 328
        split/depressed, 328
        splits, 328
    OR tips and tricks
        anterolateral approach, 328, 330
    outcomes/complications, 330–332
    posteromedial approach to medial tibial
        plateau, 330f
    Schatzker classification, 327, 329f
Tibial shaft fracture, 332–342
    AO/OTA classification, 332, 333f–335f
    background, 332
    blocking screw technique, 339f
    exchange nailing, indications for, 339
    healing complications, 339
    high-energy injuries, 332
    history and physical examination, 332
    imaging, 332
    low-energy injuries, 332
    open tibia fractures, 337
    OR tips and tricks, 340–342, 340f–341f
    outcomes/complications, 337, 339
    treatment, 337f–339f
        distal metaphyseal fractures, 336
        external fixation, 337

intramedullary nailing, 332, 336
nonoperative, 332
operative, 332
plating, 337
proximal third fracture and
intramedullary nail, 336
Tscherne classification of closed
fractures, 336f
Tibial shaft fractures, pediatric, 415–418
Tibial tubercle fractures, pediatric,
413–415
Tinel sign, 526f
Torticollis, congenital muscular, 149
clinical presentation, 149
differential diagnosis, 149
evaluation, 149
treatment, 149
Total hip arthroplasty, 19–23
brief operative note, 20
and hip dislocation, 54–56
infection in, 44–45
aspiration, 44–45
classification, 45
epidemiology, 44
histology, 45
presentation, 44
prevention, 45
radiographic evaluation, 44
risk factors, 44
treatment options, 45, 47f
operative technique for posterior
approach, 22–23
pulmonary embolism in, 48
resurfacing arthroplasty, 21–22
templating
acetabulum, 19
femur, 19–20
wear and loosening in, 53–54
Total knee arthroplasty (TKA), 37–40
deep vein thrombosis in, 49–51
infection in, 45–46, 48
in juvenile rheumatoid arthritis, 122
knee balancing techniques, 38–40
asymmetric gaps, 39–40
component rotational positioning, 39
coronal balancing, 38
order of release in valgus deformity,
38–39
order of release in varus deformity, 38
patellar tracking, 39
sagittal balance, 39
symmetric gaps, 39
measured resection *vs.* gap balancing,
40
mini-TKA, 40
and patellar problems, 58–59
patellar resurfacing, 40
and periprosthetic knee fractures,
60–61
procedure, 37–38, 38f
wear and loosening in, 59–60
Total shoulder arthroplasty
contraindications, 104
indications, 105–106
operative pearls, 105
rehabilitation, 105
results, 105
technique, 104–105
Transfusion, 446–447
Transient synovitis, 144
differential diagnosis, 144–145
laboratory findings, 145
natural history, 144

presentation, 145
radiographic findings, 145
treatment, 145
ultrasound, 145
Transphyseal humerus fracture, pediatric,
379
Trauma
general principles
acute compartment syndrome,
194–199
acute respiratory distress syndrome,
186f, 187–188, 187f
arthrocentesis/injections, 204–205
brain injury, 188, 188f
fat embolism syndrome, 186, 187f
fracture blisters, 199, 199f
fracture healing stages, 199–201
Glasgow Coma Scale, 188–189
gunshot wounds, 192, 193f
hemorrhagic shock, 189
hypotension, causes of, 189
injury severity score, 185–186
mangled extremity severity score
(MESS), 192, 194
metabolic response to, 186
open fractures, 190–192
osteomyelitis, 201–204
ring fixator/Ilizarov method, 206–207
shock, 189, 189f
lower extremity
acetabular fracture, 279–288
ankle fracture, 345–354
calcaneus fracture, 364–367
cuboid fracture, 374–375
extensor mechanism injuries,
321–325
femoral head fracture, 292–295
femoral neck fractures, 295–299
femoral shaft fracture, 307–311
femoral subtrochanteric fracture,
304–307
fifth metatarsal/jones fracture,
371–372
floating knee, 318–321
hip dislocation, 288–292
intertrochanteric hip fractures,
299–304
knee dislocations, 316–318
Lisfranc injury, 369–371
navicular fracture, 372–374
open ankle fracture, 354–358
patellar fracture, 325–327
pelvic fractures, 267–279
pilon fractures, 342–345
subtalar dislocation, 367–369
supracondylar femoral fracture,
311–316
talus fractures, 358–364
tibial plateau fractures, 327–332
tibial shaft fracture, 332–342
pediatric
ankle fractures, 418–421
conscious sedation, 375–376
distal femoral epiphyseal fractures,
406–410
femur fractures, 404–406
hip fractures and dislocations,
399–403
lateral condyle fracture, 385–387
lower extremity injuries, 393–421
medial epicondyle fractures, 387–389
pediatric elbow, 379
pelvic/acetabular fractures, 393–397

physeal injuries, 421
proximal humerus fractures, 376–378
radial head and neck fractures,
389–391
radius and ulnar shaft fractures,
391–392
septic hip, 397–398
supracondylar humerus fractures,
379–385
tibial eminence fracture, 410–413
tibial shaft fractures, 415–418
tibial tubercle fractures, 413–415
transphyseal humerus fracture, 379
upper extremity
approaches to ulna and radius,
257–260
brachial plexus injury, 215–216
capitellar fracture, 243–245
clavicle fracture, 207–211
distal humerus fractures, 237–243
distal radius fracture, 260–267
elbow dislocation, 245–248
forearm fractures, 256, 257f
Galeazzi fracture, 255–256
humeral shaft fractures., 227–237
Monteggia fracture, 248–250
olecranon fracture, 250–253
proximal humerus fractures,
216–227
radial head fractures, 253–255
scapular fractures, 212–215
ulnar shaft fractures, 260
Trevor disease, 117
Triangular fibrocartilage complex, 549
Trigger finger, 53f, 543–544, 544f
background, 543
finger pulleys, 543
history and physical examination, 543
mechanics, 543
operative treatment, 543–544
steroid injection, 543
Trigger thumb, in children, 149
Trisomy 21. *See* Down syndrome
Tuberculosis, spinal, 609
differential diagnosis, 609
pathology, 609
surgery, 609
Tumoral calcinosis, 508
history and physical examination, 508
imaging, 508
pathology, 508
treatment, 508
Turf toe, 567
Turner syndrome, 128

U
Ulna and radius, surgical approaches to,
258f–259f
complications
malunion, 259
nonunion, 259
refracture, 60
synostosis, 259
direct approach to ulna, 258
dorsal Thompson approach, 258
open fractures, 258
volar approach to radius, 257
Ulnar impaction, 547
Ulnar (medial) collateral ligament, 108f.
See also Elbow MCL injury
injury of, 536–537
associated injuries, 536

Ulnar (medial) collateral ligament, 108f.
See also Elbow MCL injury (Contd.)
diagnosis and treatment, 537
Stener lesion, 536
surgical treatment, 537
Ulnar shaft fractures, 260
background, 260
classification, 260
imaging, 260
treatment, 260
Ulnar tunnel syndrome, 528
Ulnar variance, 547, 547f
Unicameral bone cyst, 505, 505f, 506f
differential diagnosis, 505
imaging, 505
pathology, 505
prognosis, 505
treatment, 506

V
Vancomycin, 447
Vincristine, 464–465
Vitamin D, 441–442
photobiosynthesis and activation, 436
Volar intercalated segment instability (VISI), 548–549
Von Recklinghausen disease. See Neurofibromatosis (NF)
Von Willebrand disease, 432

W
Wartenberg syndrome, 528
diagnosis, 528
etiology, 528
treatment, 529

Werdnig-Hoffman disease, 129
Winged scapula, 96f
World health organization (WHO) criteria, of osteoporosis, 436

X
X-rays and radiation doses, 447

Y
Yergason test, 88

Z
Z-foot. See Serpentine foot